Advances in
VIRUS RESEARCH

VOLUME **79**

Research Advances in Rabies

Advances in
VIRUS RESEARCH

VOLUME **79**

Research Advances in Rabies

Edited by

ALAN C. JACKSON

Departments of Internal Medicine
(Neurology) and of Medical Microbiology
University of Manitoba
Winnipeg, Manitoba, Canada

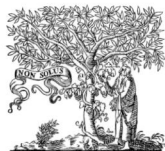

ELSEVIER

AMSTERDAM • BOSTON • HEIDELBERG • LONDON
NEW YORK • OXFORD • PARIS • SAN DIEGO
SAN FRANCISCO • SINGAPORE • SYDNEY • TOKYO
Academic Press is an imprint of Elsevier

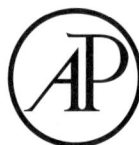

Academic Press is an imprint of Elsevier

32 Jamestown Road, London, NW1 7BY, UK
Radarweg 29, PO Box 211, 1000 AE Amsterdam, The Netherlands
225 Wyman Street, Waltham, MA 02451, USA
525 B Street, Suite 1900, San Diego, CA 92101-4495, USA

First edition 2011

Library of Congress Cataloging-in-Publication Data

A catalog record for this book is available from the Library of Congress

British Library Cataloguing-in-Publication Data

A catalogue record for this book is available from the British Library

ISBN: 978-0-12-387040-7
ISSN: 0065-3527

For information on all Academic Press publications
visit our website at elsevierdirect.com

Printed and bound in USA
11 12 13 14   10 9 8 7 6 5 4 3 2 1

Working together to grow
libraries in developing countries

www.elsevier.com | www.bookaid.org | www.sabre.org

ELSEVIER   BOOK AID International   Sabre Foundation

CONTENTS

Aurélie A. V. Albertini
UPR 3296 CNRS, Virologie Moléculaire et Structurale, Gif sur Yvette, France

Ashley C. Banyard
Rabies and Wildlife Zoonoses Group, Department of Virology, Veterinary Laboratories Agency, Weybridge, New Haw, Addlestone, Surrey, United Kingdom

Darryll A. Barkhouse
Center for Neurovirology, Department of Cancer Biology, Thomas Jefferson University, Philadelphia, Pennsylvania, USA

Denise Bélanger
Faculté de médecine vétérinaire, Département de pathologie et microbiologie, GREZOSP Université de Montréal, Saint-Hyacinthe, Quebec, Canada

Danielle Blondel
UPR 3296 CNRS, Virologie Moléculaire et Structurale, Gif sur Yvette, France

Karl-Klaus Conzelmann
Max von Pettenkofer Institute and Gene Center, Ludwig-Maximilians-University Munich, Munich, Germany

Bernhard Dietzschold
Center for Neurovirology, Department of Microbiology and Immunology, Thomas Jefferson University, Philadelphia, Pennsylvania, USA

Milosz Faber
Center for Neurovirology, Department of Microbiology and Immunology, Thomas Jefferson University, Philadelphia, Pennsylvania, USA

Paul Fernyhough
Division of Neurodegenerative Disorders, St. Boniface Hospital Research Centre, and Department of Pharmacology and Therapeutics, University of Manitoba, Winnipeg, Manitoba, Canada

Anthony R. Fooks
Rabies and Wildlife Zoonoses Group, Department of Virology, Veterinary Laboratories Agency, Weybridge, New Haw, Addlestone, Surrey, and National Centre for Zoonosis Research, University of Liverpool, Leahurst, Neston, Wirral, United Kingdom

Richard Franka
Poxvirus and Rabies Branch, Centers for Disease Control and Prevention, Atlanta, Georgia, USA

Zhen F. Fu
Departments of Pathology, University of Georgia, Athens, Georgia, USA

Emily A. Gomme
Department of Microbiology and Immunology, Jefferson Medical College, Thomas Jefferson University, Philadelphia, Pennsylvania, USA

Ronald N. Harty
Department of Pathobiology, School of Veterinary Medicine, University of Pennsylvania, Philadelphia, Pennsylvania, USA

David Hayman
Rabies and Wildlife Zoonoses Group, Department of Virology, Veterinary Laboratories Agency, Weybridge, New Haw, Addlestone, Surrey, and Cambridge Infectious Diseases Consortium, Department of Veterinary Medicine, Cambridge; Institute of Zoology, Regent's Park, London, United Kingdom

Thiravat Hemachudha
Department of Medicine (Neurology) and WHO Collaborating Center in Research and Training on Viral Zoonoses, Faculty of Medicine, Chulalongkorn University, Bangkok, Thailand

D. Craig Hooper
Center for Neurovirology, Department of Cancer Biology, and Department of Neurological Surgery, Thomas Jefferson University, Philadelphia, Pennsylvania, USA

Nipan Israsena
Department of Pharmacology, Faculty of Medicine, Chulalongkorn University, Bangkok, Thailand

Alan C. Jackson
Department of Internal Medicine (Neurology), and Department of Medical Microbiology, University of Manitoba, Winnipeg, Manitoba, Canada

Nicholas Johnson
Rabies and Wildlife Zoonoses Group, Department of Virology, Veterinary Laboratories Agency, Weybridge, New Haw, Addlestone, Surrey, United Kingdom

Wafa Kammouni
Department of Internal Medicine (Neurology), University of Manitoba, Winnipeg, Manitoba, Canada

Rhonda B. Kean
Center for Neurovirology, Department of Cancer Biology, Thomas Jefferson University, Philadelphia, Pennsylvania, USA

Monique Lafon
Unité de Neuroimmunologie Virale, Département de Virologie, Institut Pasteur, Paris, France

Jiraporn Laothamatas
Advanced Diagnostic Imaging and Image-Guided Minimal Invasive Therapy Center (AIMC) and Department of Radiology, Ramathibodi Hospital, Faculty of Medicine, Mahidol University, Bangkok, Thailand

Jianwei Li
Center for Neurovirology, Department of Cancer Biology, Thomas Jefferson University, Philadelphia, Pennsylvania, USA

Boonlert Lumlertdacha
Queen Saovabha Memorial Institute, Thai Red Cross Society, Bangkok, Thailand

Aekkapol Mahavihakanont
Department of Medicine (Neurology) and WHO Collaborating Center in Research and Training on Viral Zoonoses, Faculty of Medicine, Chulalongkorn University, Bangkok, Thailand

Lorraine McElhinney
Rabies and Wildlife Zoonoses Group, Department of Virology, Veterinary Laboratories Agency, Weybridge, New Haw, Addlestone, Surrey,

and National Centre for Zoonosis Research, University of Liverpool, Leahurst, Neston, Wirral, United Kingdom

Susan A. Nadin-Davis
Centre of Expertise for Rabies, Ottawa Laboratory Fallowfield, Canadian Food Inspection Agency, Ottawa, Ontario, Canada

Xuefeng Niu
Departments of Pathology, University of Georgia, Athens, Georgia, USA

Atsushi Okumura
Department of Pathobiology, School of Veterinary Medicine, University of Pennsylvania, Philadelphia, Pennsylvania, USA

Vijay G. Panjeti
Department of Biology and Center for Disease Ecology, Emory University, Atlanta, Georgia, USA

Bruce A. Pond
Wildlife Research and Development Section, Ontario Ministry of Natural Resources, Peterborough, Ontario, Canada

Leslie A. Real
Department of Biology and Center for Disease Ecology, Emory University, Atlanta, Georgia, USA

Erin E. Rees
Faculté de médecine vétérinaire, Département de pathologie et microbiologie, GREZOSP Université de Montréal, Saint-Hyacinthe, Quebec, Canada

Martina Rieder
Max von Pettenkofer Institute and Gene Center, Ludwig-Maximilians-University Munich, Munich, Germany

Rick Rosatte
Ontario Ministry of Natural Resources, Wildlife Research and Development Section, Trent University, Peterborough, Ontario, Canada

Anirban Roy
Center for Neurovirology, Department of Cancer Biology, Thomas Jefferson University, Philadelphia, Pennsylvania, USA

Rob W. H. Ruigrok
UMI 3265 UJF-EMBL-CNRS, Unit of Virus Host Cell Interactions, Grenoble, France

Charles E. Rupprecht
Poxvirus and Rabies Branch, Centers for Disease Control and Prevention, Atlanta, Georgia, USA

Matthias J. Schnell
Department of Microbiology and Immunology, and Jefferson Vaccine Center, Jefferson Medical College, Thomas Jefferson University, Philadelphia, Pennsylvania, USA

Prapimporn Shantavasinkul
Queen Saovabha Memorial Institute, The Thai Red Cross Society (World Health Organization Collaborating Center for Research on Rabies Pathogenesis and Prevention), Bangkok, Thailand

Todd G. Smith
Poxvirus and Rabies Branch, Centers for Disease Control and Prevention, Atlanta, Georgia, USA

Witaya Sungkarat
Advanced Diagnostic Imaging and Image-Guided Minimal Invasive Therapy Center (AIMC) and Department of Radiology, Ramathibodi Hospital, Faculty of Medicine, Mahidol University, Bangkok, Thailand

Rowland R. Tinline
Department of Geography, Queen's University, Kingston, Ontario, Canada

Gabriella Ugolini
Neurobiologie et Développement, UPR3294 CNRS, Institut de Neurobiologie Alfred Fessard (INAF), 1 Avenue de la Terrasse, Bât. 32, 91198 Gif-sur-Yvette, France

Hualei Wang
Departments of Pathology, University of Georgia, Athens, Georgia, USA

Celestine N. Wanjalla
Department of Microbiology and Immunology, Jefferson Medical College, Thomas Jefferson University, Philadelphia, Pennsylvania, USA

Henry Wilde
WHO-CC for Research and Training on Viral Zoonoses, Faculty of Medicine, Chulalongkorn University, Bangkok, Thailand

Christoph Wirblich
Department of Microbiology and Immunology, Jefferson Medical College, Thomas Jefferson University, Philadelphia, Pennsylvania, USA

Xianfu Wu
Poxvirus and Rabies Branch, Centers for Disease Control and Prevention, Atlanta, Georgia, USA

Rabies is an ancient disease that unfortunately remains an important public health problem in humans. There have been many important research advances extending from our understanding of how rabies virus replicates and assembles to how the disease can be prevented and treated in humans and how rabies can be controlled in wildlife hosts. The vaccination of Joseph Meister by Louis Pasteur and colleagues in 1885 was just one of many important landmarks of our advances against a truly diabolical virus that infects the brain of its vectors and alters behavior, resulting in transmission by biting at a time when the deadly virus is secreted in the saliva. There has been much progress in many different areas, but many challenges remain involving our understanding of rabies virus infection. Only further basic research will give us a better understanding of mechanisms involved in all aspects of the infection, including at the level of the cell and of the host and also in human and animal populations. This knowledge is needed to develop strategies to better combat all aspects of the disease. In addition, rabies virus is now recognized as the best available tool for the study of neuronal circuits in the nervous system and neuroscientists will certainly use it much more in the future.

I would like to express my appreciation to the series editors, Karl Maramorosch and Frederick Murphy, and to Lisa Tickner at Elsevier for giving me the opportunity of putting together a research volume on rabies and to our many contributors, who are all experts in their fields, for their hard work in preparing insightful and up-to-date chapters that summarize our current state of knowledge in diverse aspects of this very interesting and important viral disease.

ALAN C. JACKSON
Winnipeg, Manitoba, Canada
December 2010

CHAPTER 1

Rabies Virus Transcription and Replication

Aurélie A. V. Albertini,* Rob W. H. Ruigrok,† and Danielle Blondel*

Contents

Abstract

Rabies virus (RABV) is a negative-stranded RNA virus. Its genome is tightly encapsidated by the viral nucleoprotein (N) and this RNA–N complex is the template for transcription and replication by the

* UPR 3296 CNRS, Virologie Moléculaire et Structurale, Gif sur Yvette, France
† UMI 3265 UJF-EMBL-CNRS, Unit of Virus Host Cell Interactions, Grenoble, France

Advances in Virus Research, Volume 79
ISSN 0065-3527, DOI: 10.1016/B978-0-12-387040-7.00001-9

viral RNA-dependent RNA polymerase (L) and its cofactor, the phosphoprotein (P). We present molecular, structural, and cellular aspects of RABV transcription and replication. We first summarize the characteristics and molecular biology of both RNA synthesis processes. We then discuss biochemical and structural data on the viral proteins (N, P, and L) and their interactions with regard to their role in viral transcription and replication. Finally, we review evidence that rabies viral transcription and replication take place in cytoplasmic inclusion bodies formed in RABV-infected cells and discuss the role of this cellular compartmentalization.

I. INTRODUCTION

Rabies virus (RABV) and rabies-related viruses belong to the *Lyssavirus* genus of the *Rhabdoviridae* family, which also includes the *Vesiculovirus* genus with the prototype vesicular stomatitis virus (VSV). However, the natural histories of RABV and VSV are very different. RABV is a prototype neurotropic virus that causes fatal disease in humans and animals, whereas VSV is an arthropod-borne virus that primarily affects rodents, cattle, swine, and horses and can cause mild symptoms upon infection of humans and other species. *Rhabdoviridae* are part of the *Mononegavirales* order, which includes other virus families such as the *Paramyxoviridae*, the *Filoviridae*, and the *Bornaviridae*.

RNA transcription and replication of rhabdoviruses require an intricate interplay of the nucleoprotein N, the RNA-dependent RNA polymerase (RdRp) L, a nonenzymatic polymerase cofactor P, and the RNA genome enwrapped by N, also called the nucleocapsid. During RNA synthesis, P binds L to the N–RNA template through an N–P interaction that involves two adjacent N proteins in the nucleocapsid. L–P binding to the N–RNA probably triggers conformational changes that allow access of the polymerase to the RNA.

II. MOLECULAR ASPECTS OF VIRAL TRANSCRIPTION AND REPLICATION

A. Virion structure

Rabies virions have a bullet-like shape, with a diameter of 75 nm and a length of 100–300 nm depending on the strain (Matsumoto, 1962; Tordo and Poch, 1988b). One end is conical, and the other end is flat (Fig. 1). The viral RNA is encapsidated by the nucleoprotein N (450 amino acids (aa)) to form a helical nucleocapsid in which each N protomer binds to nine nucleotides like for VSV (Iseni *et al.*, 1998; Thomas *et al.*, 1985). The nucleocapsid is associated with a significant amount of phosphoprotein P (297 aa),

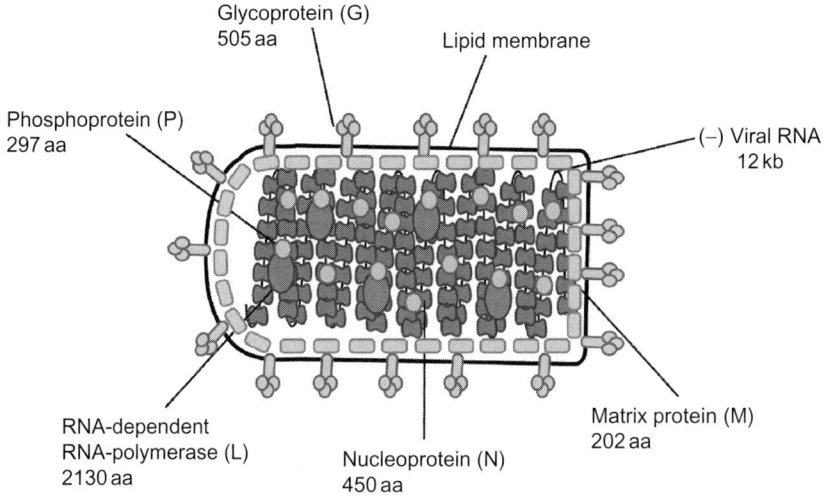

FIGURE 1 *Schematic representation of the rabies virus particle.* Viral proteins (N for nucleoprotein, P for phosphoprotein, M for matrix protein, G for glycoprotein, and L for large protein) and their length in amino acids are indicated. The viral membrane is covered by the glycoprotein G, and M is located beneath the membrane. N is bound to the genomic RNA and together with P and L forms the ribonucleoprotein that constitutes the active viral replication unit. (See Page 1 in Color Section at the back of the book.)

some of which carry copies of the RdRp (L for large protein 2130 aa). The RNA plus N, P, and L form the ribonucleoprotein (RNP), which is the component that is active in transcription and replication. The RNP is enwrapped by a lipid bilayer derived from the host cell plasma membrane during the budding process. The matrix protein M (202 aa) and the glycoprotein G (505 aa) are membrane-associated proteins. M protein is located beneath the viral membrane and bridges the nucleocapsid and the lipid bilayer. G protein is an integral transmembrane protein that is involved in viral entry. In the case of VSV, the organization of the compacted nucleocapsid and its mode of interaction with M in the bullet-shaped virion have recently been determined by cryo-electron microscopy (Ge *et al.*, 2010).

B. Genome organization

The *Lyssavirus* genome consists of a single negative-stranded RNA molecule of about 12 kb that encodes the five viral proteins in the order of 3'-N-P-M-G-L-5' (Fig. 2). The N, M, and L proteins are similar in structure and length among all lyssavirus species and strains, whereas the length of P and cytoplasmic domain of G are variable (Le Mercier *et al.*, 1997; Marston *et al.*, 2007).

1424 nt   991 nt   805 nt   1675 nt   ψ   6475 nt   TIS

3′ Leader [N] [P] [M] [G] [L] Trailer 5′ vRNA (−)   TTP

Variable
IGR

Intergenomic   A/UCUUUUU   G(N)   UUGURR$_n$GA   Signals at the   3′ UGCGAAUUGUU
signals: Transcription   Transcription   genomic termini : 5′ ACGCUUAACAA
    termination polyadenylation   initiation
        signal

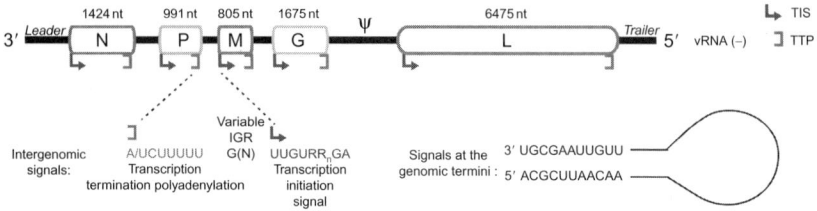

FIGURE 2 *Rabies virus genome organization.* Transcription initiation signals (TIS) and transcription termination and polyadenylation signals (TTP) are indicated on the genome. Genes are separated by variable intergenic regions (IGRs). Noncoding sequences at the genome termini constitute the 3′ leader and 5′ trailer. The first and last nine nucleotides (nt) of the viral RNA are inversely complementary and conserved.

1. Genome signals and intergenic sequences

Each gene is composed of an internal coding region flanked by noncoding regions (NCRs) that are bordered by transcription initiation signals (TISs) and transcription termination polyadenylation (TTP) signals (Fig. 2). These signals are composed of about 10 nucleotides that are closely related to those of VSV (Tordo *et al.*, 1986). The TIS consensus sequence (3′-U-U-G-U-R-R-n-GA-5′) is strictly conserved in all *Lyssavirus* genomes. The TTP consensus sequence (3′-A/U-C-U-U-U-U-U-U-U-G-5′) contains a sequence of seven uridine residues, which are reiteratively copied by the RNA polymerase to produce the polyadenylated tail of each mRNA before reinitiating at the next start signal. In some RABV strains, there are two consecutive TTPs for the M and G cistrons (Tordo and Poch, 1988a). These sequences modulate the activity of the polymerase during transcription but are ignored or inactive during the replication process.

The genes are usually separated by conserved nontranscribed intergenic regions (IGRs; Fig. 2). The IGRs are short (2–6 nucleotides) except for the M-G IGR in Mokola virus and Lagos bat (16 nucleotides) and for G/L IGRs in all lyssaviruses (19–28 nucleotides) (Tordo *et al.*, 1986). In the case of VSV, the four IGRs consist of the same GA dinucleotide (Rose, 1980).

2. Signals at the genome termini

The five genes are flanked by two short NCRs at the 3′- and 5′–ends: the 3′ leader (le) and 5′ trailer (tr) (Fig. 2). These sequences, respectively, initiate and terminate genome transcription and replication. The leader and trailer are very rich in U and A nucleotides. The leader region is strictly conserved in length (58 nucleotides) and the first nine nucleotides are identical in all lyssaviruses. The length and sequence of the trailer region are more variable (around 70 nucleotides). The sequences of the 3′- and 5′-ends of the genome are inversely complementary (Bourhy *et al.*, 1989; Conzelmann and Schnell, 1994; Tordo *et al.*, 1988). This complementarity is another classical feature of the *Mononegavirales*. Reverse genetic experiments have shown that the termini contain essential promoter sequences for transcription and replication and also signals for encapsidation of newly made viral RNAs (Conzelmann and Schnell, 1994).

C. Viral cycle

The viral cycle is cytoplasmic (Fig. 3A). After receptor binding, the virus enters the cell via the endocytic pathway. The acidic environment of the endosome induces a change in the conformation of the glycoprotein G that mediates fusion of the viral envelope with the cellular membrane. The negative-sense RNP is then released in the cytoplasm and constitutes the template for viral gene expression and replication by the viral RNA polymerase (the L–P polymerase complex). It has been recently shown that RABV transcription and replication take place within Negri bodies (NBs) that are inclusion bodies (IBs) formed during viral infection (see Section IV). During transcription, a positive-stranded leader RNA and five capped and polyadenylated mRNAs are synthesized (Fig. 3B). The replication process yields nucleocapsids containing full-length antigenome-sense RNA, which in turn serve as templates for the synthesis of genome-sense RNA. During their synthesis, both the nascent antigenome and the genome are encapsidated by N protein. The neo-synthesized genomic RNP either serves as a template for secondary transcription or is transported to the cell membrane and assembles with the M and G proteins for the budding of neo-synthesized virions (Fig. 3A).

D. Viral transcription and replication

In many aspects, transcription and replication of the single-stranded, negative-sense RNA viruses are similar and much of the understanding of RABV transcription and replication comes from studies on VSV (Banerjee, 1987; Emerson, 1987; Wagner, 1991). The template for viral transcription and replication is a helical complex consisting of the viral RNA and the nucleoprotein (N) (Arnheiter *et al.*, 1985). Figure 4A shows a negative stain electron micrograph of the helical N–RNA structure in which the individual N-protomers can easily be distinguished. The RNA is protected and hidden inside this helical structure.

A

B

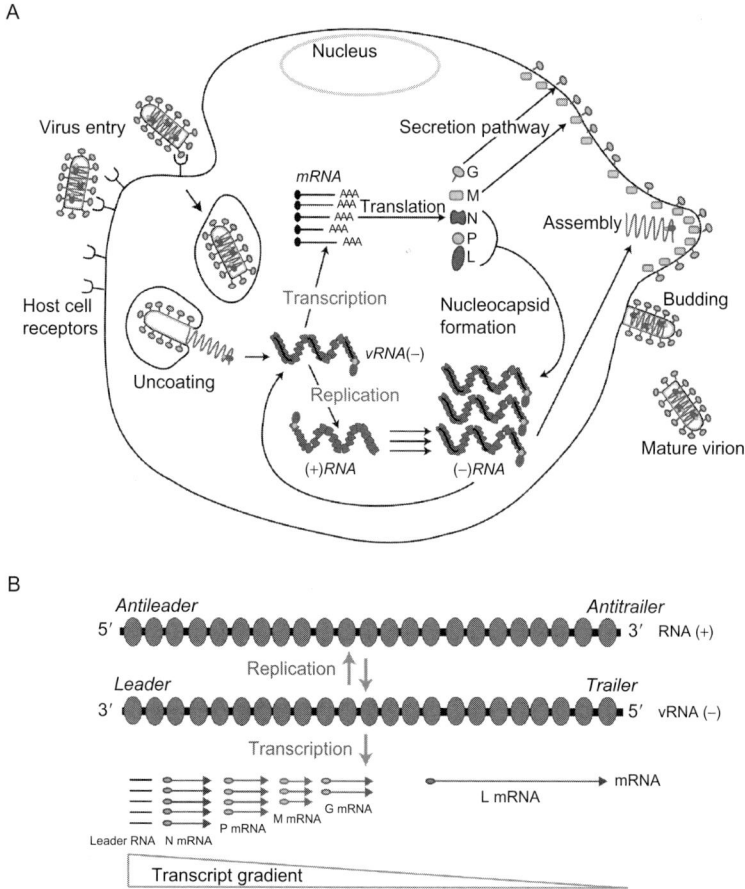

FIGURE 3 *Viral cycle.* (A) Rabies virus replicates in the cytoplasm of the host cell. Several phases can be observed: receptor binding, endocytosis followed by membrane fusion and nucleocapsid release, then transcription, replication, and finally virus assembly and progeny virion budding. (B) Overview of RNA synthesis events during the rabies virus infectious cycle. Viral mRNAs produced during transcription are naked (free of N), the leader RNA is neither polyadenylated nor capped, whereas viral mRNAs are polyadenylated at the 3′-end and capped at the 5′-extremity by the L subunit. Reinitiation of the transcription at each TIS does not always occur, generating a gradient of amounts of transcript (leader RNA > mRNA G > mRNA N > mRNA P > mRNA M > mRNA G > mRNA L). Viral RNA (−) and RNA (+) produced during replication are always associated with N, P, and L.

1. Transcription

The polymerase complex gains access to the vRNA in a, as yet, poorly understood manner (Fig. 4B). It is thought to recognize a specific promoter at the 3′-end of the genome and progress toward the 5′-end by a stop–start

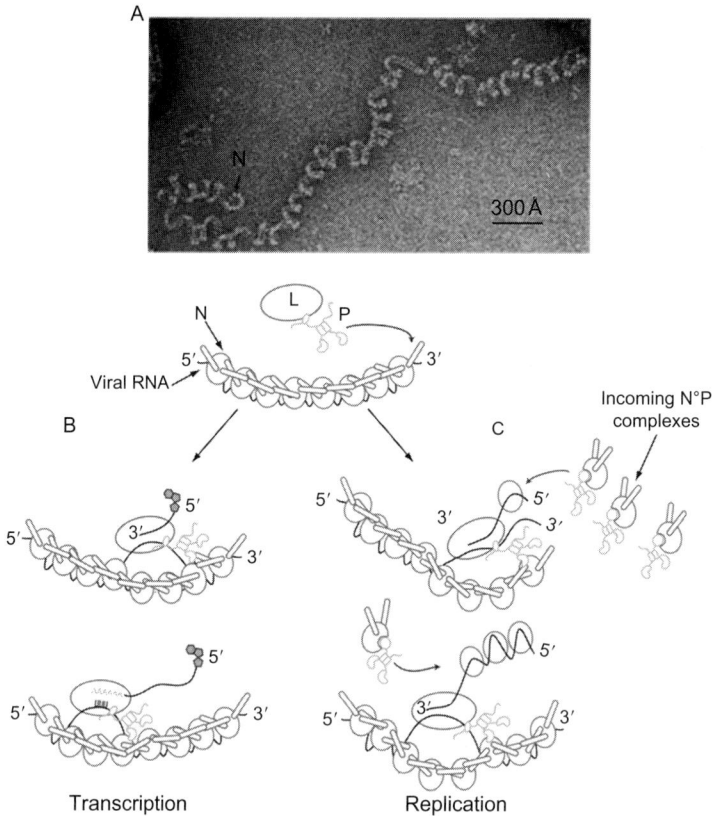

FIGURE 4 *Transcription and replication by rabies virus.* (A) Electron micrograph of negatively stained rabies virus nucleocapsid purified from infected cells by CsCl gradient density centrifugation. Individual nucleoprotein subunits on the viral RNA can be easily distinguished. The scale bar indicates 30 nm. (B and C) Schematic models of rabies virus transcription (B) and replication (C). During transcription and replication, the catalytic subunit of the polymerase (L) is associated with a phosphoprotein dimer; L–P binding to N subunits in the nucleocapsid probably triggers a local RNA release allowing access of the polymerase to the viral RNA. During transcription (B), the mRNA is capped and methylated on its nascent 5′ extremity at the end of the gene. During replication (C), the newly synthesized RNA is instantly encapsidated by incoming N°–P complexes. Extension of the replication process leads to the production of a new full-length encapsidated genomic or antigenomic N–RNA complex. (See Page 1 in Color Section at the back of the book.)

mechanism, producing six consecutive transcripts: first, the leader RNA and then the five successive mRNAs coding for the N, P, M, G, and L proteins (Fig. 3B). The leader RNA is uncapped and nonpolyadenylated, while all mRNAs are capped and polyadenylated by the polymerase complex. The 3′-poly-A tail is synthesized by the polymerase through slippage on the short poly-U stretch in the TTP (Barr *et al.*, 1997). To control the sequential progression of the synthesis of the mRNAs, the polymerase complex recognizes transcription initiation, transcription termination, and polyadenylation signals flanking the cistrons (described in the Section II. B.1). The complex is thought to dissociate from the template at each stop signal and to reinitiate poorly at the next start signal. The process continues until the enzyme reaches the end of the L gene and results in a concentration gradient of the amount of each mRNA depending on its order and its distance from the 3'-end: leader > N > P > M > G > L (Fig. 3B).

Results obtained during the past 10 years indicate that (i) the VSV RNA polymerase can initiate transcription directly at the N gene start and not exclusively at the 3'-end of the genome (Whelan and Wertz, 2002); (ii) two RNA polymerase complexes isolated from VSV-infected cells are separately responsible for transcription and replication in infected cells: a transcriptase containing P–L and the EF1 host factor initiating at the N gene start and a replicase containing N–P–L initiating at the 3'-end of the genome (Qanungo *et al.*, 2004). Although the stop–start model of viral transcription and replication is admitted, these results raise discussions about the detailed mechanisms of RNA synthesis (Curran and Kolakofsky, 2008; Whelan, 2008). New approaches are required to understand the precise mechanisms of these processes.

2. Replication

Unlike transcription, replication requires ongoing protein synthesis to provide a source of soluble N protein (N^0) necessary to encapsidate the nascent RNA; the activity of the polymerase P–L complex switches from transcription to replication to produce a full-length positive RNA strand complementary to the complete genome (Figs. 3B and 4C). Replication is asymmetric, producing an up to 50-fold excess of genomes over antigenomes for RABV (Finke and Conzelmann, 1997). These positive-stranded RNAs are also encapsidated by the N protein, bind the L–P complex, and are used as template to amplify negative-stranded genomes for the progeny virions. It is thought that a promoter for encapsidation exists near their 5'-end to initiate the concomitant encapsidation of the nascent RNA. Newly synthesized N^0 protein binds to nascent leader RNA and prevents recognition of termination signals (Fig. 4C). This association of N protein to the viral genome or antigenome is regulated by the P protein, which plays the role of chaperone in the form of an N^0–P complex, preventing the N protein from binding to cellular RNA and from aggregating (Fig. 4C; Peluso and Moyer, 1988).

3. Regulation of viral RNA synthesis and gene expression

Accurate regulation of viral gene expression is required for successful RABV infection. Indeed, RABV gene expression and genome replication differ in some respects from those of VSV. Whereas the highly cytopathic VSV should replicate very fast, RABV regulates viral gene expression to produce viral components in sufficient amounts for viral spread, but low enough to maintain host cell survival and to escape from antiviral host cell responses. RABV has evolved different mechanisms to regulate viral gene expression.

a. Alternative termination of M and G cistrons   A typical feature of transcription of the RABV genome is the phenomenon of alternative termination due to the presence of two consecutive TTPs for the M and G cistrons separated from each other by around 400 nucleotides (Conzelmann *et al.*, 1990; Tordo and Poch, 1988a). This alternative synthesis of mRNAs with longer or shorter 3'-NCRs may influence the efficiency of transcription of the distal gene by modifying the size of the IGRs. The fact that the ratio between the large and the small messengers varies during the course of infection and is different in fibroblast and neuronal cells suggests that alternative termination is a mechanism for regulating the expression of the rabies genome. Interestingly, alternative termination is only observed with some laboratory strains (SAD, PV, ERA) and not in most of the other strains for which only the distal TTP is used (Bourhy *et al.*, 1993; Kuzmin *et al.*, 2008; Marston *et al.*, 2007; Sacramento *et al.*, 1992).

b. Role of IGRs in differential gene expression   Sequential synthesis of mRNA according to the stop–start model is a common feature of all negative-stranded RNA viruses and provides means to differentially express individual genes. The major determinant is the relative distance of a gene from the 3'-promoter. The other determinant is the attenuation at gene borders. In the case of VSV, the genes are usually separated by a conserved IGR consisting of the GA dinucleotide (Rose, 1980). At each gene border of VSV, around one-third of the polymerases that terminate an upstream mRNA fail to initiate transcription of the downstream gene, resulting in a transcription gradient. The IGRs of the RABV genome (described in Section II.B.1) that increase in length along the genome result in a severe attenuation at the G/L border and, consequently, to a drastic downregulation of L synthesis (Finke *et al.*, 2000). Interestingly, the switch of the IGRs in a recombinant rabies genome alters the mRNA and protein levels of the downstream genes indicating that the length of the IGRs plays an important role in regulating gene expression (Finke *et al.*, 2000).

c. Role of the matrix protein in the regulation of the balance between transcription and replication   The RABV matrix protein is a multifunctional protein that plays an essential role in viral assembly and budding, M is responsible for recruiting RNPs to the cell membrane, their condensation into tight helical structures and for the budding of virus (Mebatsion *et al.*, 1999). The M proteins of *Rhabdoviridae* have also been shown to play a regulatory role in the balance of virus transcription and replication (Finke and Conzelmann, 2003; Finke *et al.*, 2003); M protein inhibits viral transcription and stimulates viral replication.

III. STRUCTURAL ASPECT OF RABV TRANSCRIPTION AND REPLICATION; PROTEINS INVOLVED IN TRANSCRIPTION AND REPLICATION

A. Nucleoprotein

Viral nucleocapsids are very flexible structures, and in order to determine the structure of N, a regular form or complex had to be found. When N is expressed by itself in bacterial or eukaryotic cells, it binds to cellular RNA and forms long helical N–RNA complexes or closed N–RNA rings, depending on the length of the encapsidated RNA (Iseni *et al.*, 1998). After separation of these rings in distinct size classes, they could be crystallized and their atomic structure determined (Albertini *et al.*, 2006, 2007). This artificial way of obtaining regular N–RNA structures was also successful for the structure determination of the N–RNAs of VSV and RSV (Green *et al.*, 2006; Tawar *et al.*, 2009). The structure of the N–RNA ring is shown in Fig. 5A.

N is a two-domain protein with a positively charged cleft between the two domains (Fig. 5C–E). Both domains have extensions that reach over to the backs of the neighboring N-protomers to strengthen and rigidify the N–RNA structure. Part of the C-terminal extension is flexible and not visible in the structure (dots in Fig. 5D). The very C-terminus of the protein comes back to its own protomer to complete the C-terminal domain. The RNA follows a wavy path, indicated in black, at the inside of the ring. In Fig. 5B, the ring is cut open to show the RNA. Each N-protomer binds exactly nine ribonucleotides that are completely enclosed by the protein (Fig. 5C and D). The RNA is recognized through its sugar-phosphate backbone through electrostatic interactions between positively charged amino acid side chains with the phosphates and the 2′ oxygen of the ribose, without any nucleotide base specificity. The manner in which the RNA is bound to N suggests that this structure represents an RNA storage state in which the RNA is hidden from cellular RNAses and factors that recognize foreign nucleic acids in order to start interferon production. The L protein cannot have access to the RNA in this state and a conformational change in N will be necessary in order to make the RNA available for transcription or replication.

B. Phosphoprotein

The phosphoproteins of RABV and VSV form elongated dimers (Gerard *et al.*, 2007) that contain three ordered and functional domains separated by two intrinsically disordered regions (Gerard *et al.*, 2009; Fig. 6A and B).

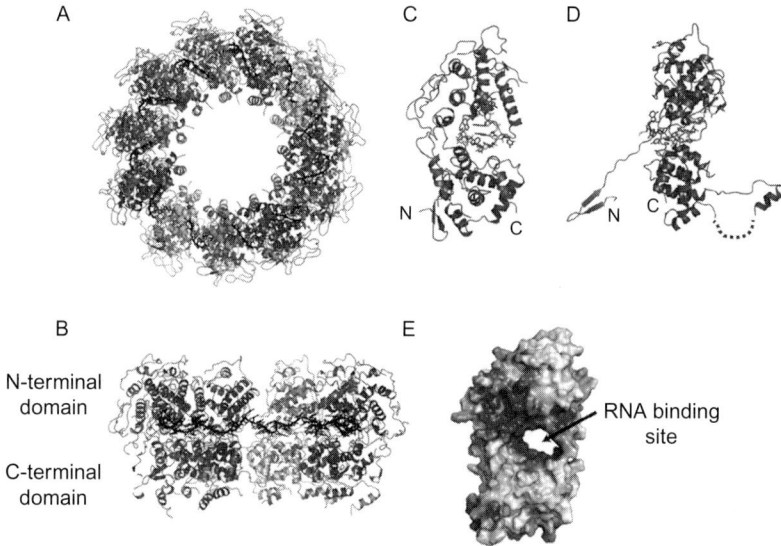

FIGURE 5 *Crystal structure of the rabies virus N–RNA complex.* (A) Ribbon diagram of the rabies N_{11}–RNA ring structure as viewed from the top (PDB code: 2GTT). The 99 nt RNA molecule is shown as black sticks. (B) View of the inside of the ring with the N-terminal domain (NTD) of N at the top and the C-terminal domain (CTD) of N at the bottom. The RNA molecule is shown as a ribbon and black sticks in a clockwise 5′–3′ orientation. (C) Ribbon diagram of the N protomer viewed from the side showing the enclosure of the RNA (represented as sticks) by the N protomer. (D) Ribbon diagram of the N protomer viewed from the inside of the ring displaying the two main domains (top NTD and bottom CTD) and two subdomains NTD arm and CTD arm. (E) Electrostatic potential surface of an N protomer revealing the basic cavity (blue) located between the NTD and the CTD which constitutes the RNA binding site. (See Page 2 in Color Section at the back of the book.)

Such unfolded regions are often involved in transient interactions with partner proteins and may fold upon binding to these partners (Dyson and Wright, 2002). In the case of rabies P, part of the N-terminal unfolded region interacts with L (Castel *et al.*, 2009; Chenik *et al.*, 1998) and a domain in the C-terminal unfolded region interacts with the cytoplasmic dynein light chain, LC8 (Jacob *et al.*, 2000; Raux *et al.*, 2000). Folding upon binding may allow high specificity without very tight binding, which may be important for dynamic processes.

The N-terminal functional domain is predicted to be folded into a pair of α-helices but is not very structured when expressed on its own (Gerard *et al.*, 2009). The first 40 amino acids are involved in forming the N^0–P complex (Castel *et al.*, 2009; Mavrakis *et al.*, 2006). In this complex, in which one molecule of N^0 binds a dimer of P (Mavrakis *et al.*, 2003), P has a chaperone function and binds to N that is not yet bound to viral

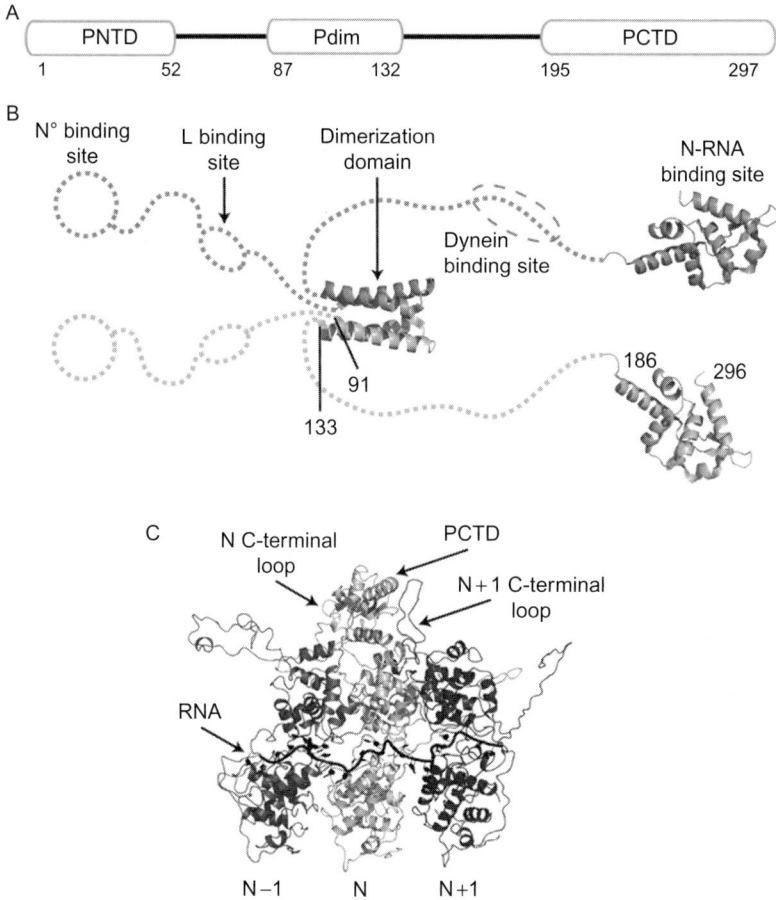

FIGURE 6 *Structural data on the rabies virus phosphoprotein.* (A) Schematic drawing of the rabies virus phosphoprotein. Folded domains are depicted as boxes (PNTD stands for phosphoprotein N-terminal domain, Pdim for phosphoprotein dimerization domain, and PCTD for phosphoprotein C-terminal domain). (B) Structural model of the P dimer showing the known X-ray structures (dimerization domain (PDB code: 3L32) and C-terminal domain (PDB code: 1VYI). Disordered regions are represented by dotted lines. Regions of the protein that are susceptible of being folded upon binding to a partner are shown as dotted circles. (C) Ribbon diagram of the rabies N–RNA–P complex showing the positioning of the PCTD on the surface of the N–RNA complex. Three adjacent N protomers are represented in blue and PCTD is colored in orange. Note that the orientation of N in this figure is upside down compared to its orientation in Fig. 5. (See Page 3 in Color Section at the back of the book.)

RNA in order to keep it from binding nonspecifically to cellular RNA (Masters and Banerjee, 1988a,b) and to prevent it from oligomerizing with other molecules of N^0 (Fig. 4C). Although no structural information has yet been published on the N^0–P complex, the highly acidic nature of this domain of P suggests that it may bind in the RNA binding groove on N and perhaps also interfere with the two extensions on N that are involved in interprotomer contacts in the N–RNA structure. A mutant of the nucleoprotein of VSV that is incapable of binding RNA is, however, still capable to oligomerize (Zhang *et al.*, 2008), suggesting that these two activities are independent and that both will have to be inhibited in the N^0–P complex. Expression or transfection of a peptide containing the first 57 residues of P leads to significant inhibition of virus infection, probably by out-competing the viral phosphoprotein in binding to N^0 (Castel *et al.*, 2009).

The middle domain of P is the dimerization domain (Gerard *et al.*, 2009). Both P proteins from VSV and RABV form dimers, but the structures of the dimerization domains are quite different. For VSV, the domain consists of two parallel helices flanked by β-sheets on both sides but with the N- and C-terminal unfolded regions coming out of this domain at opposite sides (Ding *et al.*, 2006). For RABV, the domain consists of two helical hairpins that stick together and are stabilized by extensive hydrophobic contacts (Ivanov *et al.*, 2010). In this case, the N- and C-terminal unfolded regions come out at the same side of the domain (Fig. 6B), which may be necessary for the close opposition of the two unfolded regions or for the interaction of binding partners on both regions. The biological role for dimerization is not known since a mutant of Mokola virus P that lacks this domain is still active in transcription (Jacob *et al.*, 2001).

The C-terminal domain of P binds to the viral N–RNA and, as such, attaches the polymerase complex to its template (Gerard *et al.*, 2009; Mavrakis *et al.*, 2004). This highly structured domain has the shape of a lengthwise cut pear with a large number of charged amino acid residues on both the round and the flat sides that are involved in binding to the N–RNA (Jacob *et al.*, 2001; Mavrakis *et al.*, 2004). The corresponding domain of the VSV phosphoprotein is clearly homologous in structure but misses a number of helices making it considerably smaller (Ribeiro *et al.*, 2008). Early proteolysis experiments on N–RNA showed that removal of the C-terminal domain of N (residue 377 up to the C-terminal residue 450) prevented binding of P to N–RNA, suggesting that the C-terminal extension of N and, in particular, its unfolded part (dots in Fig. 5D) is involved in binding to P (Schoehn *et al.*, 2001). It was not possible to crystallize the recombinant RABV N–RNA rings with bound phosphoprotein or with a bound C-terminal domain of P. However, probably due to the smaller size of the N–RNA binding domain of VSV P, it was possible to do so for VSV and it was observed that the C-terminal domain of VSV P binds to the tip of the C-terminal domain of N and is enclosed by two C-terminal loops of the same N-protomer and that of the neighboring protomer that have now become ordered in this complex (Green and Luo, 2009). In parallel, performing small angle X-ray scattering experiments on the RABV N–RNA–P complex, combined with biochemical characterization and model building, the equivalent position for RABV P on the N–RNA complex was identified (Ribeiro *et al.*, 2009; Fig. 6C). The contacts between the C-terminal domain of P and the C-terminal loops of N and N − 1 (Fig. 4C) are more extensive than for VSV, and due to the larger size of the P-domain, the loops are significantly distorted and will not allow the binding of P onto the neighboring N. At most, one monomer of P can bind per two protomers of N or one dimer of P per four protomers of N, which is very close to the estimated N–P ratio of 1.9 in the virus particle (Flamand *et al.*, 1993). The charged residues in P that were identified to be involved in binding to N (Jacob *et al.*, 2001) are involved in salt bridges with residues on the N loops. In the infected cell, binding of P to N–RNA is accompanied by phosphorylation of N at Ser389, which enhances the affinity of P for N (Toriumi and Kawai, 2004). In the structure, the phosphates on two subsequent N loops were modeled and these made new interactions with positively charged residues on both faces of the P domain (Ribeiro *et al.*, 2009). Finally, the manner in which this domain of P becomes enveloped by the C-terminal loops of two consecutive N-protomers in an N–RNA structure also excludes that this domain can bind to soluble N^0. Although the effect of P binding to long, noncircular N–RNA complexes, similar to N–RNA complexes isolated from virus, has not yet been tested, the specific binding of P to two subsequent N-protomers is likely to impose a particular curvature to the N–RNA, which may be necessary for the accessibility of the RNA to L. The P protein is phosphorylated at multiple serine residues by protein kinase-C and another cellular kinase (Gupta *et al.*, 2000). Phosphorylation of P is not required for its oligomerization (Gigant *et al.*, 2000), and no effects of the phosphorylation of P on viral transcription and replication are known to date.

C. Large protein

The large protein (L) is the enzymatic component of the L–P polymerase complex and is responsible for nucleotide addition to the neosynthesized RNA chain (RdRp activity) and for the synthesis of the cap-structure for the viral mRNAs. Apart from sequence analyses, very little is known about the large protein of RABV because no easy system exists for reconstituting *in vitro* transcription or replication. Hence, mutational analyses, such as have been done for the polymerases of VSV and the paramyxovirus Sendai virus, have not been possible for rabies L. Sequence analysis of L showed that it contains the same six conserved regions as other nonsegmented negative-stranded RNA virus polymerases (Poch *et al.*, 1990; Fig. 7A). For VSV, regions I–IV are supposed to fold into the RdRp, domain V is involved in placing a GDP onto the 5′-end of monophosphorylated mRNA (Li *et al.*, 2008; Ogino *et al.*, 2010), and domain VI is active in methylating the N7G and the 2′O of the cap (Li *et al.*, 2005). As has been described for the capping enzyme of bluetongue virus, a rotavirus (Sutton *et al.*, 2007), it is likely that the domains involved in the capping reactions are arranged in a sequential manner so that the newly made mRNA first receives the G(5′)PPP(5′)N on domain V and is subsequently methylated on domain VI. Such a process would most likely slow down the early steps in the transcription process. Studies on L–P interaction have shown that domain VI located in the C-terminus part of L is involved in the binding to P (Chenik *et al.*, 1998). Although it is likely that the transcription active L–P complex has other posttranslational modifications or binds to other host factors than the replication active complex, for RABV nothing is known yet. Recently, Whelan and coworkers produced new insights into the structure of VSV L (Rahmeh *et al.*, 2010). They expressed and purified a full-length active VSV L protein from insect cells and visualized it by electron microscopy. Their results show that L is organized in several structural domains: a ring-shaped domain that harbors the RNA polymerase activity and a set of three globular domains

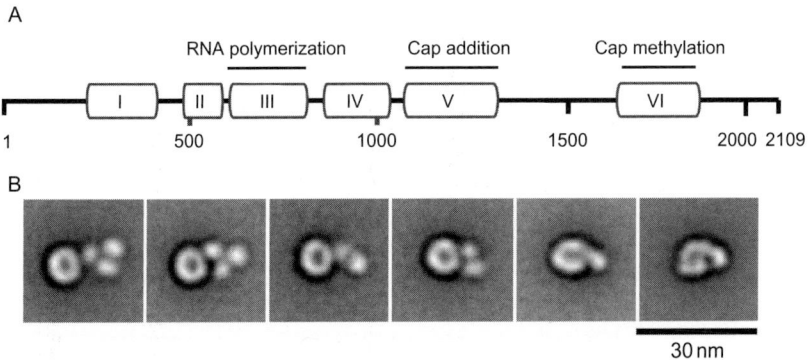

FIGURE 7   *Domain organization of L protein and electron micrographs of VSV L.* (A) Schematic drawing of the VSV large protein. Conserved regions among negative-stranded RNA virus are depicted as boxes (I–VI). Location of RNA polymerization, cap addition, and cap methylation is indicated. (B) Electron microscopic characterization of VSV L: six class averages of negatively stained L show its overall appearance consisting of a ring-shaped domain ($\sim$100 Å in diameter) and a variable appendage that comprises three globular domains ($\sim$50 Å in diameter for each). In several averages, only two globular domains are visible, suggesting the presence of flexible linkers between the ring domain and the smaller domains (scale bar = 30 nm). Images courtesy of Dr. Sean Whelan (Rahmeh *et al.*, 2010).

carrying the capping machinery (Fig. 7B). Electron microscopy images of purified L–P complexes indicate that, upon binding of P, VSV L undergoes an important structural rearrangement. L needs to be associated with the phosphoprotein to be active for RNA synthesis; thus, these conformational changes may reflect an optimal positioning of the domains of L for RNA synthesis.

IV. CELLULAR ASPECT OF RABIES TRANSCRIPTION AND REPLICATION: IBS FORMED IN INFECTED CELLS ARE THE SITES OF VIRAL RNA SYNTHESIS

RABV infection induces the formation of cytoplasmic IBs termed NBs (Negri, 1903). As these structures are typical of RABV infection of the brain, they have a diagnostic value and have been used as definite histological proof of such infection. These spherical structures having a diameter of a few micrometers (2–10 μm) are found in the cytoplasm of infected nerve cells. IBs are also present in nonneuronal cells (Lahaye *et al.*, 2009; Menager *et al.*, 2009). Consistent with the known properties of NBs, these inclusions could be stained with the Seller's solution containing the dye, basic fushin (Lahaye *et al.*, 2009). Thus, the staining characteristics, the size, and the shape of the IBs formed in infected cells indicate that these structures can be considered as Negri body-like structures (NBLs). NBLs are full of N (Fig. 8A) and P (Fig. 8D) and contain also the polymerase L (Finke *et al.*, 2004), but M and G are excluded. Electron microscopic observations indicate that NBLs progressively associate with a double membrane that could be derived from the RER (16-h postinfection, Fig. 8B). NBLs have been considered for a long time as side products of the infectious process due to the passive accumulation of large quantities of proteins produced in excess during infection. It has now been demonstrated that NBLs are functional structures where viral transcription and replication take place (Lahaye *et al.*, 2009). Specifically, *in situ* fluorescent hybridization (FISH) techniques reveal that all viral mRNAs plus genome and antigenome are located inside the IBs (Fig. 8C). Interestingly, viral RNAs synthesized inside the NBLs appear to be surrounded by a cage formed by N that may protect them from degradation. Although the FISH method does not allow a precise quantification, it clearly indicated that N mRNA is more abundant than L mRNA, in agreement with the gradient of decreasing mRNAs concentration that reflects the gene order (data not shown). In addition, short-term RNA labeling in the presence of Bromo UTP (BrUTP) indicates that the RABV polymerase incorporates BrUTP into RNA that is actively synthesized within the NBLs (Fig. 8D). This provides evidence that the NBs are not RNA storage compartments, but active sites of viral transcription and replication. Similar results have

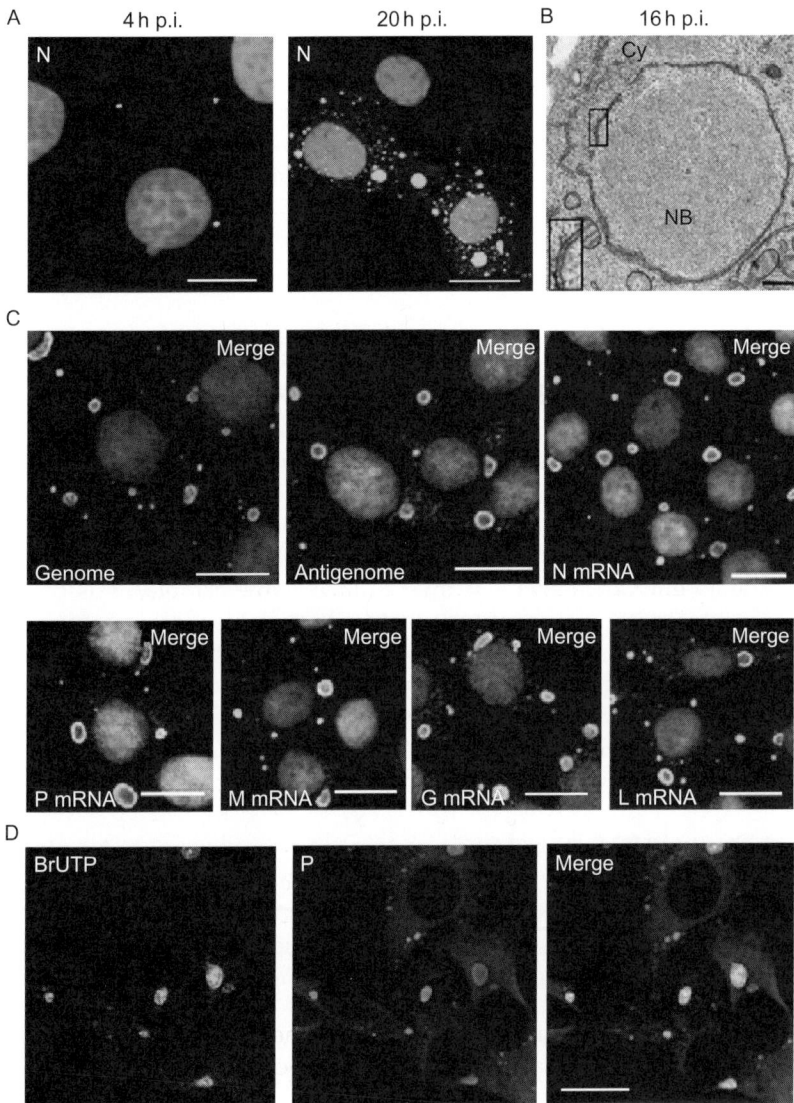

FIGURE 8 *Negri body-like structures are the sites of viral transcription and replication.*
(A) Evolution of NBLs during the viral cycle. BSR cells were infected with rabies virus
and analyzed at different times postinfection (p.i.) by confocal microscopy and by using
an antibody directed against the viral N protein that is the major component of
NBLs. At an early stage of infection (4-h p.i.), infected cells present one or two viral
inclusions that grow in size at a later stage of infection with the appearance of smaller
structures (20-h p.i.). (B) Ultrastructural aspect of one NBL present in BSR infected
cells. NBLs display a granular dense structure that is surrounded by a double membrane.
(C) All viral RNAs are detected in the NBLs (16-h p.i.) as shown by FISH experiments
with biotinylated oligonucleotides followed by incubation with streptavidin conjugated
to Cy3. The N protein (green) forms a cage around the viral RNAs (red). (D) Viral RNAs
are synthesized inside the NBLs. Short-term RNA labeling was performed in the presence
of BrUTP and actinomycin D (inhibitor of cellular transcription). (See Page 4 in Color
Section at the back of the book.)

recently been reported for VSV for which the viral replication machinery is also localized in cytoplasmic inclusions (Heinrich *et al.*, 2010). However, the confinement of VSV RNA to inclusions appears to be dependent on the time of the viral cycle. Primary RNA synthesis seems to occur throughout the cytoplasm and then protein expression induces the formation of inclusions to which RNA synthesis is redirected. This could also be the case for RABV, but such early events have not been analyzed. Compartmentalization of the viral replication machinery, a common property of many positive-stranded RNA viruses, might also be generalized among viruses of the *Mononegavirales* order. Until now the functional significance of such compartments has not been elucidated; it is not known whether they serve to concentrate host and viral components in one place to facilitate viral replication and/or to immobilize and inactivate proteins that would otherwise inhibit infection, or whether they reflect a cellular response to infection. Further studies on the characterization of NBLs, such as the identification of cellular factors associated with these structures, should provide a better knowledge of their function. Interestingly, this cellular confinement with the recruitment of cellular factors may explain the failure to perform *in vitro* transcription with RNPs purified from RABV or from infected cells. Electron microscopy and tomography will help to obtain structural information on the organization of these macromolecular complexes and their communication with organelles.

V. CONCLUDING REMARKS

Important progress has been made in understanding viral transcription and replication of the *Mononegavirales*. Molecular biology and reverse genetics approaches have allowed a more detailed analysis of the regulatory mechanisms of these RNA synthesis processes. Structural studies have increased the knowledge of the structural dynamics of the transcription/replication machinery. The atomic structure of the intact L protein of the *Mononegavirales* or of functional domains of L that are missing today should reveal new mechanistic insights into polymerase function. Advances in the identification of host factors recruited for the polymerase activity will provide a complete structure–function analysis of the polymerase complex.

ACKNOWLEDGMENTS

We thank our colleagues in Gif-sur-Yvette and Grenoble for extensive discussions. We thank Dr. Sean Whelan, Harvard Medical School, Boston, for discussions and for the pictures shown in Fig. 7B. The work of R. W. H. R. was supported by grants from the French ANR (ANR-07-001-01; ANRAGE) and from the FINOVI foundation. We acknowledge support from the CNRS.

REFERENCES

Albertini, A. A., Wernimont, A. K., Muziol, T., Ravelli, R. B., Clapier, C. R., Schoehn, G., Weissenhorn, W., and Ruigrok, R. W. (2006). Crystal structure of the rabies virus nucleo-protein-RNA complex. *Science* **313**:360–363.
Albertini, A. A., Clapier, C. R., Wernimont, A. K., Schoehn, G., Weissenhorn, W., and Ruigrok, R. W. (2007). Isolation and crystallization of a unique size category of recombinant rabies virus nucleoprotein-RNA rings. *J. Struct. Biol.* **158**:129–133.
Arnheiter, H., Davis, N. L., Wertz, G., Schubert, M., and Lazzarini, R. A. (1985). Role of the nucleocapsid protein in regulating vesicular stomatitis virus RNA synthesis. *Cell* **41**:259–267.
Banerjee, A. K. (1987). Transcription and replication of rhabdoviruses. *Microbiol. Rev.* **51**:66–87.
Barr, J. N., Whelan, S. P., and Wertz, G. W. (1997). Role of the intergenic dinucleotide in vesicular stomatitis virus RNA transcription. *J. Virol.* **71**:1794–1801.
Bourhy, H., Tordo, N., Lafon, M., and Sureau, P. (1989). Complete cloning and molecular organization of a rabies-related virus, Mokola virus. *J. Gen. Virol.* **70**:2063–2074.
Bourhy, H., Kissi, B., and Tordo, N. (1993). Molecular diversity of the Lyssavirus genus. *Virology* **194**:70–81.
Castel, G., Chteoui, M., Caignard, G., Prehaud, C., Mehouas, S., Real, E., Jallet, C., Jacob, Y., Ruigrok, R. W., and Tordo, N. (2009). Peptides that mimic the amino-terminal end of the rabies virus phosphoprotein have antiviral activity. *J. Virol.* **83**:10808–10820.
Chenik, M., Schnell, M., Conzelmann, K. K., and Blondel, D. (1998). Mapping the interacting domains between the rabies virus polymerase and phosphoprotein. *J. Virol.* **72**:1925–1930.
Conzelmann, K. K., and Schnell, M. (1994). Rescue of synthetic genomic RNA analogs of rabies virus by plasmid-encoded proteins. *J. Virol.* **68**:713–719.
Conzelmann, K. K., Cox, J. H., Schneider, L. G., and Thiel, H. J. (1990). Molecular cloning and complete nucleotide sequence of the attenuated rabies virus SAD B19. *Virology* **175**:485–499.
Curran, J., and Kolakofsky, D. (2008). Nonsegmented negative-strand RNA virus RNA synthesis in vivo. *Virology* **371**:227–230.
Ding, H., Green, T. J., Lu, S., and Luo, M. (2006). Crystal structure of the oligomerization domain of the phosphoprotein of vesicular stomatitis virus. *J. Virol.* **80**:2808–2814.
Dyson, H. J., and Wright, P. E. (2002). Coupling of folding and binding for unstructured proteins. *Curr. Opin. Struct. Biol.* **12**:54–60.
Emerson, S. U. (1987). Transcription of vesicular stomatitis virus. *In* "The Rhabdoviruses" (R. R. Wagner, ed.), pp. 245–269. The Rhabdoviruses. Plenum Press, New York.
Finke, S., and Conzelmann, K. K. (1997). Ambisense gene expression from recombinant rabies virus: Random packaging of positive- and negative-strand ribonucleoprotein complexes into rabies virions. *J. Virol.* **71**:7281–7288.
Finke, S., and Conzelmann, K. K. (2003). Dissociation of rabies virus matrix protein functions in regulation of viral RNA synthesis and virus assembly. *J. Virol.* **77**:12074–12082.
Finke, S., Cox, J. H., and Conzelmann, K. K. (2000). Differential transcription attenuation of rabies virus genes by intergenic regions: Generation of recombinant viruses overexpressing the polymerase gene. *J. Virol.* **74**:7261–7269.
Finke, S., Mueller-Waldeck, R., and Conzelmann, K. K. (2003). Rabies virus matrix protein regulates the balance of virus transcription and replication. *J. Gen. Virol.* **84**:1613–1621.
Finke, S., Brzozka, K., and Conzelmann, K. K. (2004). Tracking fluorescence-labeled rabies virus: Enhanced green fluorescent protein-tagged phosphoprotein P supports virus gene expression and formation of infectious particles. *J. Virol.* **78**:12333–12343.
Flamand, A., Raux, H., Gaudin, Y., and Ruigrok, R. W. (1993). Mechanisms of rabies virus neutralization. *Virology* **194**:302–313.

Ge, P., Tsao, J., Schein, S., Green, T. J., Luo, M., and Zhou, Z. H. (2010). Cryo-EM model of the bullet-shaped vesicular stomatitis virus. *Science* **327:**689–693.

Gerard, F. C., Ribeiro Ede, A., Jr., Albertini, A. A., Gutsche, I., Zaccai, G., Ruigrok, R. W., and Jamin, M. (2007). Unphosphorylated rhabdoviridae phosphoproteins form elongated dimers in solution. *Biochemistry* **46:**10328–10338.

Gerard, F. C., Ribeiro, E. D., Jr., Leyrat, C., Ivanov, I., Blondel, D., Longhi, S., Ruigrok, R. W., and Jamin, M. (2009). Modular organization of rabies virus phosphoprotein. *J. Mol. Biol.* **338:**978–996.

Gigant, B., Iseni, F., Gaudin, Y., Knossow, M., and Blondel, D. (2000). Neither phosphorylation nor the amino-terminal part of rabies virus phosphoprotein is required for its oligomerization. *J. Gen. Virol.* **81:**1757–1761.

Green, T. J., and Luo, M. (2009). Structure of the vesicular stomatitis virus nucleocapsid in complex with the nucleocapsid-binding domain of the small polymerase cofactor, P. *Proc. Natl. Acad. Sci. USA* **106:**11713–11718.

Green, T. J., Zhang, X., Wertz, G. W., and Luo, M. (2006). Structure of the vesicular stomatitis virus nucleoprotein-RNA complex. *Science* **313:**357–360.

Gupta, A. K., Blondel, D., Choudhary, S., and Banerjee, A. K. (2000). The phosphoprotein of rabies virus is phosphorylated by a unique cellular protein kinase and specific isomers of protein kinase C. *J. Virol.* **74:**91–98.

Heinrich, B. S., Cureton, D. K., Rahmeh, A. A., and Whelan, S. P. (2010). Protein expression redirects vesicular stomatitis virus RNA synthesis to cytoplasmic inclusions. *PLoS Pathog.* **6:**e1000958.

Iseni, F., Barge, A., Baudin, F., Blondel, D., and Ruigrok, R. W. (1998). Characterization of rabies virus nucleocapsids and recombinant nucleocapsid-like structures. *J. Gen. Virol.* **79** (Pt. 12):2909–2919.

Ivanov, I., Crepin, T., Jamin, M., and Ruigrok, R. W. (2010). Structure of the dimerization domain of the rabies virus phosphoprotein. *J. Virol.* **84:**3707–3710.

Jacob, Y., Badrane, H., Ceccaldi, P. E., and Tordo, N. (2000). Cytoplasmic dynein LC8 interacts with lyssavirus phosphoprotein. *J. Virol.* **74:**10217–10222.

Jacob, Y., Real, E., and Tordo, N. (2001). Functional interaction map of lyssavirus phosphoprotein: Identification of the minimal transcription domains. *J. Virol.* **75:**9613–9622.

Kuzmin, I. V., Wu, X., Tordo, N., and Rupprecht, C. E. (2008). Complete genomes of Aravan, Khujand, Irkut and West Caucasian bat viruses, with special attention to the polymerase gene and non-coding regions. *Virus Res.* **136:**81–90.

Lahaye, X., Vidy, A., Pomier, C., Obiang, L., Harper, F., Gaudin, Y., and Blondel, D. (2009). Functional characterization of Negri bodies (NBs) in rabies virus-infected cells: Evidence that NBs are sites of viral transcription and replication. *J. Virol.* **83:**7948–7958.

Le Mercier, P., Jacob, Y., and Tordo, N. (1997). The complete Mokola virus genome sequence: Structure of the RNA-dependent RNA polymerase. *J. Gen. Virol.* **78**(Pt. 7):1571–1576.

Li, J., Fontaine-Rodriguez, E. C., and Whelan, S. P. (2005). Amino acid residues within conserved domain VI of the vesicular stomatitis virus large polymerase protein essential for mRNA cap methyltransferase activity. *J. Virol.* **79:**13373–13384.

Li, J., Rahmeh, A., Morelli, M., and Whelan, S. P. (2008). A conserved motif in region v of the large polymerase proteins of nonsegmented negative-sense RNA viruses that is essential for mRNA capping. *J. Virol.* **82:**775–784.

Marston, D. A., McElhinney, L. M., Johnson, N., Muller, T., Conzelmann, K. K., Tordo, N., and Fooks, A. R. (2007). Comparative analysis of the full genome sequence of European bat lyssavirus type 1 and type 2 with other lyssaviruses and evidence for a conserved transcription termination and polyadenylation motif in the G-L 3′ non-translated region. *J. Gen. Virol.* **88:**1302–1314.

Masters, P. S., and Banerjee, A. K. (1988a). Complex formation with vesicular stomatitis virus phosphoprotein NS prevents binding of nucleocapsid protein N to nonspecific RNA. *J. Virol.* **62:**2658–2664.

Masters, P. S., and Banerjee, A. K. (1988b). Resolution of multiple complexes of phosphoprotein NS with nucleocapsid protein N of vesicular stomatitis virus. *J. Virol.* **62:**2651–2657.

Matsumoto, S. (1962). Electron microscopy of nerve cells infected with street rabies virus. *Virology* **17:**198–202.

Mavrakis, M., Iseni, F., Mazza, C., Schoehn, G., Ebel, C., Gentzel, M., Franz, T., and Ruigrok, R. W. (2003). Isolation and characterisation of the rabies virus N degrees-P complex produced in insect cells. *Virology* **305:**406–414.

Mavrakis, M., McCarthy, A. A., Roche, S., Blondel, D., and Ruigrok, R. W. (2004). Structure and function of the C-terminal domain of the polymerase cofactor of rabies virus. *J. Mol. Biol.* **343:**819–831.

Mavrakis, M., Mehouas, S., Real, E., Iseni, F., Blondel, D., Tordo, N., and Ruigrok, R. W. (2006). Rabies virus chaperone: Identification of the phosphoprotein peptide that keeps nucleoprotein soluble and free from non-specific RNA. *Virology* **439:**422–429.

Mebatsion, T., Weiland, F., and Conzelmann, K. K. (1999). Matrix protein of rabies virus is responsible for the assembly and budding of bullet-shaped particles and interacts with the transmembrane spike glycoprotein G. *J. Virol.* **73:**242–250.

Menager, P., Roux, P., Megret, F., Bourgeois, J. P., Le Sourd, A. M., Danckaert, A., Lafage, M., Prehaud, C., and Lafon, M. (2009). Toll-like receptor 3 (TLR3) plays a major role in the formation of rabies virus Negri bodies. *PLoS Pathog.* **5:**e1000315.

Negri, A. (1903). Contributo allo studio dell eziologia della rabia. *Bol. Soc. Med. Chir.* **2:**88–114.

Ogino, T., Yadav, S. P., and Banerjee, A. K. (2010). Histidine-mediated RNA transfer to GDP for unique mRNA capping by vesicular stomatitis virus RNA polymerase. *Proc. Natl. Acad. Sci. USA* **107:**3463–3468.

Peluso, R. W., and Moyer, S. A. (1988). Viral proteins required for the in vitro replication of vesicular stomatitis virus defective interfering particle genome RNA. *Virology* **162:**369–376.

Poch, O., Blumberg, B. M., Bougueleret, L., and Tordo, N. (1990). Sequence comparison of five polymerases (L proteins) of unsegmented negative-strand RNA viruses: Theoretical assignment of functional domains. *J. Gen. Virol.* **71**(Pt 5):1153–1162.

Qanungo, K. R., Shaji, D., Mathur, M., and Banerjee, A. K. (2004). Two RNA polymerase complexes from vesicular stomatitis virus-infected cells that carry out transcription and replication of genome RNA. *Proc. Natl. Acad. Sci. USA* **101:**5952–5957.

Rahmeh, A. A., Schenk, A. D., Danek, E. I., Kranzusch, P. J., Liang, B., Walz, T., and Whelan, S. P. (2010). Molecular architecture of the vesicular stomatitis virus RNA polymerase. *Proc. Natl. Acad. Sci. USA* **107:**20075–20080.

Raux, H., Flamand, A., and Blondel, D. (2000). Interaction of the rabies virus P protein with the LC8 dynein light chain. *J. Virol.* **74:**10212–10216.

Ribeiro, E. A., Jr., Favier, A., Gerard, F. C., Leyrat, C., Brutscher, B., Blondel, D., Ruigrok, R. W., Blackledge, M., and Jamin, M. (2008). Solution structure of the C-terminal nucleoprotein-RNA binding domain of the vesicular stomatitis virus phosphoprotein. *J. Mol. Biol.* **382:**525–538.

Ribeiro, A., Jr., Leyrat, C., Gerard, F. C., Albertini, A. A., Falk, C., Ruigrok, R. W., and Jamin, M. (2009). Binding of rabies virus polymerase cofactor to recombinant circular nucleoprotein-RNA complexes. *J. Mol. Biol.* **394:**558–575.

Rose, J. K. (1980). Complete intergenic and flanking gene sequences from the genome of vesicular stomatitis virus. *Cell* **19:**415–421.

Sacramento, D., Badrane, H., Bourhy, H., and Tordo, N. (1992). Molecular epidemiology of rabies virus in France: Comparison with vaccine strains. *J. Gen. Virol.* **73**(Pt. 5):1149–1158.

Schoehn, G., Iseni, F., Mavrakis, M., Blondel, D., and Ruigrok, R. W. (2001). Structure of recombinant rabies virus nucleoprotein-RNA complex and identification of the phosphoprotein binding site. *J. Virol.* **75:**490–498.

Sutton, G., Grimes, J. M., Stuart, D. I., and Roy, P. (2007). Bluetongue virus VP4 is an RNA-capping assembly line. *Nat. Struct. Mol. Biol.* **14:**449–451.

Tawar, R. G., Duquerroy, S., Vonrhein, C., Varela, P. F., Damier-Piolle, L., Castagne, N., MacLellan, K., Bedouelle, H., Bricogne, G., Bhella, D., Eleouet, J. F., and Rey, F. A. (2009). Crystal structure of a nucleocapsid-like nucleoprotein-RNA complex of respiratory syncytial virus. *Science* **326:**1279–1283.

Thomas, D., Newcomb, W. W., Brown, J. C., Wall, J. S., Hainfeld, J. F., Trus, B. L., and Steven, A. C. (1985). Mass and molecular composition of vesicular stomatitis virus: A scanning transmission electron microscopy analysis. *J. Virol.* **54:**598–607.

Tordo, N., and Poch, O. (1988a). Strong and weak transcription signals within the rabies genome. *Virus Res.* **11:**30–32.

Tordo, N., and Poch, O. (1988b). Structure of rabies virus. *In* "Rabies" (J. B. Campbell and K. M. Charlton, eds.), pp. 25–45. Rabies. Kluwer Academic Publishers, Boston.

Tordo, N., Poch, O., Ermine, A., Keith, G., and Rougeon, F. (1986). Walking along the rabies genome: Is the large G-L intergenic region a remnant gene? *Proc. Natl. Acad. Sci. USA* **83:**3914–3918.

Tordo, N., Poch, O., Ermine, A., Keith, G., and Rougeon, F. (1988). Completion of the rabies virus genome sequence determination: Highly conserved domains among the L (polymerase) proteins of unsegmented negative-strand RNA viruses. *Virology* **165:**565–576.

Toriumi, H., and Kawai, A. (2004). Association of rabies virus nominal phosphoprotein (P) with viral nucleocapsid (NC) is enhanced by phosphorylation of the viral nucleoprotein (N). *Microbiol. Immunol.* **48:**399–409.

Wagner, R. R. (1991). *Rhabdoviridae* and their replication. *In* "Fundamental Virology" (B. N. Fields and D. M. Knipe, eds.), pp. 489–503. Raven Press, New York.

Whelan, S. P. (2008). Response to "Non-segmented negative-strand RNA virus RNA synthesis in vivo" *Virology* **371:**234–237.

Whelan, S. P., and Wertz, G. W. (2002). Transcription and replication initiate at separate sites on the vesicular stomatitis virus genome. *Proc. Natl. Acad. Sci. USA* **99:**9178–9183.

Zhang, X., Green, T. J., Tsao, J., Qiu, S., and Luo, M. (2008). Role of intermolecular interactions of vesicular stomatitis virus nucleoprotein in RNA encapsidation. *J. Virol.* **82:**674–682.

CHAPTER 2

Rabies Virus Assembly and Budding

Atsushi Okumura and Ronald N. Harty

Abstract

Rabies virus (RABV) and other negative-strand RNA viruses are the causes of serious diseases in humans and animals worldwide. Assembly and budding are important late events in the replication cycles of these negative-strand RNA viruses that have received much attention in the past decade. Indeed, important insights into the molecular mechanisms by which rhabdoviral proteins usurp and/or interact with host proteins to promote efficient virion assembly and egress has greatly enhanced our understanding of the budding process. Assembly/budding of rhabdoviruses is driven largely by the matrix (M) protein. RABV M protein contains a late budding domain that mediates the recruitment of host proteins linked to the vacuolar protein sorting pathway of the cell to facilitate virus–cell separation. This chapter summarizes our current knowledge of the roles that both RABV M protein and interacting host proteins play during the budding process.

Department of Pathobiology, School of Veterinary Medicine, University of Pennsylvania, Philadelphia, Pennsylvania, USA

Advances in Virus Research, Volume 79
ISSN 0065-3527, DOI: 10.1016/B978-0-12-387040-7.00002-0

I. INTRODUCTION

Rabies virus (RABV) is a nonsegmented, negative-stranded RNA virus within the *Rhabdoviridae* family. The prototypic member of the *Lyssavirus* genus is RABV, whereas the prototypic member of the *Vesiculovirus* genus is vesicular stomatitis virus (VSV). Both RABV and VSV are enveloped, bullet-shaped virions averaging approximately 180 nm in length and 80 nm in width. RABV encodes five subgenomic mRNAs that are translated to yield five proteins, all of which are components of the mature virion. The viral proteins include (i) the nucleoprotein (N), which encapsidates the genomic and antigenomic RNA to form the ribonucleoprotein (RNP) complex; (ii) the phosphoprotein (P), which is the noncatalytic subunit of the RNA polymerase complex; (iii) the viral polymerase protein (L), which transcribes and replicates the RNA genome; (iv) the transmembrane glycoprotein (G), which is the surface spike protein involved in attachment to host cells; and (v) the matrix protein (M), which is the major structural protein involved in virion assembly and egress. As with many other negative-stranded RNA viruses, the viral matrix protein plays a key role in virus budding and is thought to recruit host proteins to facilitate efficient virion egress. Compared to our in-depth understanding of VSV M protein structure and function, our knowledge of RABV M protein structure and function is less complete. Nevertheless, recent findings on the role of both viral and interacting host proteins in the process of RABV budding have been reported and will be the focus of this chapter.

II. RABIES VIRUS M PROTEIN

The RABV M protein is small (20–25 kDa; 202 amino acids), yet plays a number of roles during the replication cycle of RABV. For example, RABV M is an important structural component of rabies virions and plays a role in RNP condensation. RABV M is thought to form a layer between the glycoprotein (G) within the virion envelope and the helical nucleocapsid core composed of the RNA genome and the N, L, and P proteins (Lenard and Vanderoef, 1990; Mebatsion *et al.*, 1999; Zakowski and Wagner, 1980). In addition, RABV M modulates genome replication and transcription (Finke and Conzelmann, 2003; Finke *et al.*, 2003), and has been shown recently to activate host cell caspases and induce apoptosis (Larrous *et al.*, 2010). Lastly, RABV M is known to be a determinant of pathogenicity and may also contribute to host tropism (Faber *et al.*, 2004; Finke *et al.*, 2010; Pulmanausahakul *et al.*, 2008).

III. THE CENTRAL ROLE OF M AND SUPPORTING ROLE OF G IN RABV BUDDING

One of the first studies to provide direct evidence that RABV M protein is important for virus assembly and budding was reported by Mebatsion *et al.*, who used reverse genetics (Schnell *et al.*, 1994) to recover an M-deficient mutant of RABV (Mebatsion *et al.*, 1999). Strikingly, removal of RABV M from the RABV genome reduced budding of this mutant by 500,000-fold compared to that of wild-type virus (Mebatsion *et al.*, 1999). Studies to evaluate virion production and budding efficiency of this M-deficient mutant as well as those of a G-deficient mutant revealed that the M protein was the main contributor to virus budding and virion morphogenesis, whereas the G protein plays more of a supportive role in these processes (Mebatsion *et al.*, 1996, 1999). Indeed, a model for rhabdovirus assembly was proposed in which M protein is the major determinant for budding and G protein supports this process by contributing to the formation of an M protein lattice, which promotes membrane curvature to form the bud site (Garoff *et al.*, 1998; Schnell *et al.*, 1998). Expression of the RABV G protein was shown to enhance the efficiency of virion budding by approximately 10- to 30-fold for both RABV and VSV (Mebatsion *et al.*, 1996; Robison and Whitt, 2000), suggesting that G also possesses an autonomous exocytic activity. These findings were supported by data from a study using Semliki Forest Virus (SFV) replicons encoding VSV G protein in which high-level expression of G protein from the SFV vector resulted in the release of G-containing vesicles (Rolls *et al.*, 1994). Therefore it appears that the exocytic activity of G protein creates a "pull" effect from the outside of the membrane to aid the "push" function of M protein from the inside of the membrane (Cadd *et al.*, 1997; Mebatsion *et al.*, 1996). In sum, these models emphasize the concerted contributions of both M and G proteins in RABV assembly and egress.

IV. FEATURES OF M PROTEIN IMPORTANT FOR BUDDING

As the rhabdoviral M protein plays a central role in virion assembly and egress, it is of interest to determine the mechanism of M-mediated budding. Early studies on the VSV M protein revealed that M was able to bud from mammalian cells in the form of virus-like particles (VLPs) in the absence of any other viral protein (Justice *et al.*, 1995; Li *et al.*, 1993). These studies indicated that essentially all of the information necessary for virus budding was contained within the M protein alone. Results from more recent studies (Harty *et al.*, 2001; Irie *et al.*, 2004a; Wirblich *et al.*, 2008) demonstrate that RABV M protein shares this autonomous budding property with VSV M and with a growing number of functionally homologous proteins from other RNA viruses, including the Gag protein of retroviruses and the VP40 protein of filoviruses (for review, see Chen and Lamb, 2008). At least three features shared by all of these viral matrix proteins are important for efficient budding including (i) the ability to interact with lipid bilayers at the site of budding (e.g., plasma membrane), (ii) the ability to self-assemble into homo-oligomers, and (iii) the presence of one or more domains referred to as "late" budding domains (L-domains) to mediate efficient virus–cell separation (Chen and Lamb, 2008).

The functional significance of the viral L-domains in mediating budding has received much attention since the L-domains were shown to promote virus budding by interacting with host proteins, most of which are components of the vacuolar protein sorting (vps) or endosomal sorting complex required for transport (ESCRT) pathways (Chen and Lamb, 2008; Jayakar et al., 2004). As the name implies, the L-domain functions at a late step in virus–cell separation. Indeed, mutations that disrupt the L-domain sequences result in budding defective virions or VLPs, many of which remain tethered to the plasma membrane and are unable to "pinch-off" from the host cell. Intriguingly, the viral L-domains are believed to function in budding by hijacking host cell proteins that help to facilitate the budding process (described below). Four L-domain core motifs have been identified thus far (PPxY, PT/SAP, YxxL, and FPIV, where x can be any amino acid), and each of these L-domains interacts with a specific host protein (Chen and Lamb, 2008). For RABV M protein, the L-domain motif is composed of a PPEY core and is located at the N-terminus of the protein at amino acids 35–38 (Harty et al., 1999; Wirblich et al., 2008). The RABV L-domain motif is similar in location and sequence to that present in the M protein of VSV (PPPY motif at amino acids 24–27). Interestingly, a second potential L-domain motif (YxxL) is also present in the RABV M protein and is organized in an overlapping fashion (PPxYxxL), similar to that described for the VP40 matrix protein of Ebola virus (Harty et al., 2000; Licata et al., 2004). However, the ability of the YxxL motif within RABV M protein to function as a bona fide L-domain remains to be determined.

V. VIRAL L-DOMAIN/HOST INTERACTIONS

Two of the best-characterized L-domain core motifs include the PPxY and PT/SAP motifs. For example, the viral PPxY motif has been shown to serve as a ligand for binding to WW-domains present within the HECT family of E3 ubiquitin ligases, such as Nedd4 (Blot et al., 2004; Harty et al.,

1999, 2000; Irie and Harty, 2005; Longnecker *et al.*, 2000; Martin-Serrano *et al.*, 2005; Sakurai *et al.*, 2004; Strack *et al.*, 2000; Timmins *et al.*, 2003; Yasuda *et al.*, 2003). The PT/SAP motif is known to interact directly with host protein Tsg101, a component of the ESCRT-I complex and the MVB sorting pathway within mammalian cells (Bouamr *et al.*, 2003; Garrus *et al.*, 2001; Irie and Harty, 2005; Irie *et al.*, 2005; Licata *et al.*, 2003; Martin-Serrano *et al.*, 2001; Myers and Allen, 2002; Pornillos *et al.*, 2002a,b; VerPlank *et al.*, 2001). Both Nedd4 and Tsg101 contribute to the function of the ESCRT pathway in sorting ubiquitinated target proteins into inwardly budding vesicles that form the multivesicular body (MVB) in mammalian cells. The inward invagination of these vesicles away from the cytoplasm is topologically identical to that of a virus particle budding from the plasma membrane (Fig. 1). Results from early studies suggested that host protein Vps4 and the ESCRT pathway may not be important for budding of rhabdoviruses (Chen and Lamb, 2008; Irie *et al.*, 2004b);

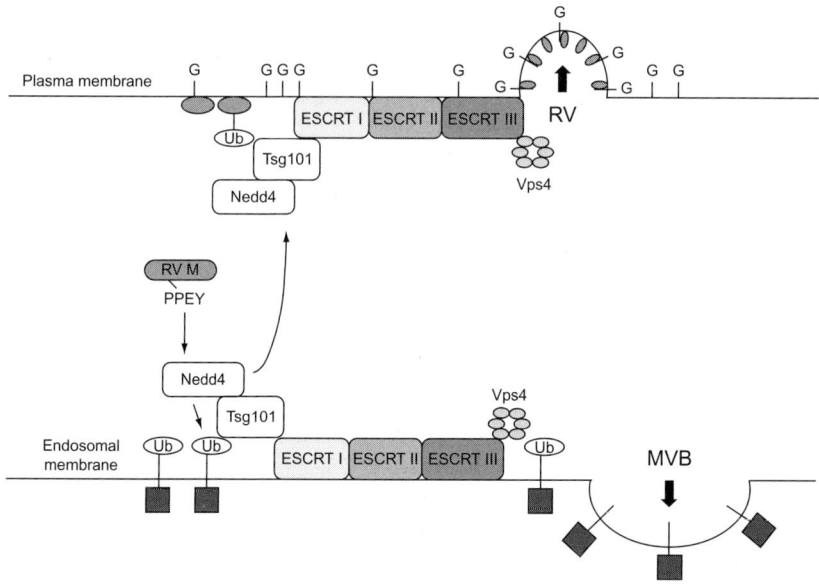

FIGURE 1 *Working model depicting the potential recruitment of the host VPS machinery by RABV M protein to facilitate virion budding.* The PPEY motif of RABV M protein interacts with host Nedd4 E3 ubiquitin ligase leading to the relocalization of the ESCRT machinery (Tsg101, ESCRTI–III complexes, and Vps4) from the endosomal membrane to the site of virus budding at the plasma membrane. The ubiquitination of RABV M by host Nedd4 remains to be determined. The topology of the outwardly budding virion and the inwardly budding vesicle is identical. Black square, host cargo protein; gray oval, RABV M protein; Ub, ubiquitination; MVB, multivesicular body; G, RABV glycoprotein.

however, subsequent studies using stable cell lines expressing Vps4 suggest that there is a role for the ESCRT machinery in rhabdoviral egress (Taylor *et al.*, 2007). Thus, by interacting with components of the host ESCRT pathway, the viral L-domains are thought to recruit and relocalize the ESCRT pathway to the site of virus budding where this machinery can then facilitate virion egress (Fig. 1).

VI. UBIQUITINATION AND RABV BUDDING

Specifically for RABV, the PPEY L-domain motif within the M protein was first shown to interact with WW-domains of host proteins, including Nedd4, by using GST fusion proteins and far-Western blotting (Harty *et al.*, 1999). A single point mutation that changed the PPEY motif to PPEA abolished the ability of RABV M protein to interact with host WW-domains (Harty *et al.*, 1999). In subsequent studies, host protein-mediated ubiquitination of rhabdoviral M proteins was postulated to play a role in the efficient egress of both RABV and VSV (Harty *et al.*, 2001). For example, the VSV M protein was shown to interact both physically and functionally with E3 ubiquitin ligase Rsp5 (the yeast homolog of Nedd4) in an *in vitro* ubiquitination assay (Harty *et al.*, 2001). Indeed, wild-type VSV M protein was ubiquitinated *in vitro* in the presence of Rsp5; however, a PPxY mutant of VSV M was not ubiquitinated (Harty *et al.*, 2001). To further prove that host-mediated ubiquitination is important for rhabdovirus budding, RABV- or VSV-infected cells were treated with the proteasome inhibitor, MG132, to decrease the cellular levels of free ubiquitin. Viral titers from MG132-treated cells were found to be 10- to 20-fold lower than those measured from untreated control cells (Harty *et al.*, 2001). These findings were confirmed in a later study (Taylor *et al.*, 2007) and together provide strong evidence that cellular ubiquitination and rhabdoviral L-domain-mediated interactions with host ubiquitin ligases are important for efficient budding of RABV and VSV. In addition to rhabdoviral budding, ubiquitination and the Nedd4 family of E3 ubiquitin ligases have been implicated in facilitating egress of retroviruses and filoviruses as well (for review, see Chen and Lamb, 2008).

Despite the findings described earlier, the biological relevance of the PPEY L-domain motif of RABV M protein during the virus life cycle remained to be determined. In order to address this gap in our understanding of M-mediated budding of RABV, Wirblich *et al.* generated a series of recombinant RABVs by reverse genetics that contained mutations within the PPEY motif and analyzed their effects on viral replication and RABV pathogenicity (Wirblich *et al.*, 2008). Results from these experiments indicated that P35 was critical for viral replication, whereas mutations of P36 and/or Y38 had less of an impact (Wirblich *et al.*, 2008).

Since there was no major impact on viral RNA synthesis, the defect in viral replication was likely due to an inhibitory effect on virion egress. In addition, several of the PPEY mutant viruses exhibited a cell-associated phenotype and a reduced focus size, suggesting that the PPEY motif played a role in RABV release (Wirblich *et al.*, 2008). Last, the PPEY L-domain mutants were found to be highly attenuated in mice compared to wild-type RABV (Wirblich *et al.*, 2008). Taken together, these findings strongly suggested that the RABV PPEY motif possesses L-domain activity in the context of a virus infection and may be important for the pathogenic potential of the virus in an animal model.

VII. SUMMARY

In summary, the working model for assembly and budding of RABV is thought to occur in the following stepwise manner: (i) The nucleocapsid core forms as the N protein interacts with newly synthesized genomic RNA. The polymerization of the N protein onto the RNA backbone is facilitated by the release of N protein from N–P dimers in the cytoplasm. The RABV M protein is also able to recognize and interact with the newly forming RNP structures in the cytoplasm. (ii) Simultaneously with RNP formation, the RABV G protein localizes to the plasma membrane, the site of virion formation and budding. (iii) RABV M protein accumulates on the cytoplasmic side of G-enriched microdomains on the plasma membrane as the RNPs condense into tightly coiled structures by interacting with M protein. (iv) The microdomains containing high levels of G protein along with the continued condensation of M-RNP structures are thought to facilitate outward membrane curvature and eventual virion egress. (v) Last, the PPEY motif of RABV M engages host Nedd4 E3 ligase and likely recruits the cellular vps machinery to the site of RABV budding to facilitate the final step of virus–cell separation (Jayakar *et al.*, 2004).

ACKNOWLEDGMENTS

We wish to acknowledge the generosity and contributions of Dr. Matthias Schnell and his laboratory to some of the work described in this chapter. This work was supported in part by NIH Grant AI46499 to R. N. H.

REFERENCES

Blot, V., Perugi, F., Gay, B., Prevost, M. C., Briant, L., Tangy, F., Abriel, H., Staub, O., Dokhelar, M. C., and Pique, C. (2004). Nedd4.1-mediated ubiquitination and subsequent recruitment of Tsg101 ensure HTLV-1 Gag trafficking towards the multivesicular body pathway prior to virus budding. *J. Cell Sci.* **117:**2357–2367.

Bouamr, F., Melillo, J. A., Wang, M. Q., Nagashima, K., de Los Santos, M., Rein, A., and Goff, S. P. (2003). PPPYVEPTAP motif is the late domain of human T-cell leukemia virus type 1 Gag and mediates its functional interaction with cellular proteins Nedd4 and Tsg101 [corrected]. *J. Virol.* **77:**11882–11895.

Cadd, T. L., Skoging, U., and Liljestrom, P. (1997). Budding of enveloped viruses from the plasma membrane. *Bioessays* **19:**993–1000.

Chen, B. J., and Lamb, R. A. (2008). Mechanisms for enveloped virus budding: Can some viruses do without an ESCRT? *Virology* **372:**221–232.

Faber, M., Pulmanausahakul, R., Nagao, K., Prosniak, M., Rice, A. B., Koprowski, H., Schnell, M. J., and Dietzschold, B. (2004). Identification of viral genomic elements responsible for rabies virus neuroinvasiveness. *Proc. Natl. Acad. Sci. USA* **101:**16328–16332.

Finke, S., and Conzelmann, K. K. (2003). Dissociation of rabies virus matrix protein functions in regulation of viral RNA synthesis and virus assembly. *J. Virol.* **77:**12074–12082.

Finke, S., Mueller-Waldeck, R., and Conzelmann, K. K. (2003). Rabies virus matrix protein regulates the balance of virus transcription and replication. *J. Gen. Virol.* **84:**1613–1621.

Finke, S., Granzow, H., Hurst, J., Pollin, R., and Mettenleiter, T. C. (2010). Intergenotypic replacement of lyssavirus matrix proteins demonstrates the role of lyssavirus M proteins in intracellular virus accumulation. *J. Virol.* **84:**1816–1827.

Garoff, H., Hewson, R., and Opstelten, D. J. (1998). Virus maturation by budding. *Microbiol. Mol. Biol. Rev.* **62:**1171–1190.

Garrus, J. E., von Schwedler, U. K., Pornillos, O. W., Morham, S. G., Zavitz, K. H., Wang, H. E., Wettstein, D. A., Stray, K. M., Cote, M., Rich, R. L., Myszka, D. G., and Sundquist, W. I. (2001). Tsg101 and the vacuolar protein sorting pathway are essential for HIV-1 budding. *Cell* **107:**55–65.

Harty, R. N., Paragas, J., Sudol, M., and Palese, P. (1999). A proline-rich motif within the matrix protein of vesicular stomatitis virus and rabies virus interacts with WW domains of cellular proteins: Implications for viral budding. *J. Virol.* **73:**2921–2929.

Harty, R. N., Brown, M. E., Wang, G., Huibregtse, J., and Hayes, F. P. (2000). A PPxY motif within the VP40 protein of Ebola virus interacts physically and functionally with a ubiquitin ligase: Implications for filovirus budding. *Proc. Natl. Acad. Sci. USA* **97:**13871–13876.

Harty, R. N., Brown, M. E., McGettigan, J. P., Wang, G., Jayakar, H. R., Huibregtse, J. M., Whitt, M. A., and Schnell, M. J. (2001). Rhabdoviruses and the cellular ubiquitin-proteasome system: A budding interaction. *J. Virol.* **75:**10623–10629.

Irie, T., and Harty, R. N. (2005). L-domain flanking sequences are important for host interactions and efficient budding of vesicular stomatitis virus recombinants. *J. Virol.* **79:**12617–12622.

Irie, T., Licata, J. M., Jayakar, H. R., Whitt, M. A., Bell, P., and Harty, R. N. (2004a). Functional analysis of late-budding domain activity associated with the PSAP motif within the vesicular stomatitis virus M protein. *J. Virol.* **78:**7823–7827.

Irie, T., Licata, J. M., McGettigan, J. P., Schnell, M. J., and Harty, R. N. (2004b). Budding of PPxY-containing rhabdoviruses is not dependent on host proteins TGS101 and VPS4A. *J. Virol.* **78:**2657–2665.

Irie, T., Licata, J. M., and Harty, R. N. (2005). Functional characterization of Ebola virus L-domains using VSV recombinants. *Virology* **336:**291–298.

Jayakar, H. R., Jeetendra, E., and Whitt, M. A. (2004). Rhabdovirus assembly and budding. *Virus Res.* **106:**117–132.

Justice, P. A., Sun, W., Li, Y., Ye, Z., Grigera, P. R., and Wagner, R. R. (1995). Membrane vesiculation function and exocytosis of wild-type and mutant matrix proteins of vesicular stomatitis virus. *J. Virol.* **69:**3156–3160.

Larrous, F., Gholami, A., Mouhamad, S., Estaquier, J., and Bourhy, H. (2010). Two overlapping domains of a lyssavirus matrix protein that acts on different cell death pathways. *J. Virol.* **84:**9897–9906.

Lenard, J., and Vanderoef, R. (1990). Localization of the membrane-associated region of vesicular stomatitis virus M protein at the N terminus, using the hydrophobic, photoreactive probe 125I-TID. *J. Virol.* **64:**3486–3491.

Li, Y., Luo, L., Schubert, M., Wagner, R. R., and Kang, C. Y. (1993). Viral liposomes released from insect cells infected with recombinant baculovirus expressing the matrix protein of vesicular stomatitis virus. *J. Virol.* **67:**4415–4420.

Licata, J. M., Simpson-Holley, M., Wright, N. T., Han, Z., Paragas, J., and Harty, R. N. (2003). Overlapping motifs (PTAP and PPEY) within the Ebola virus VP40 protein function independently as late budding domains: Involvement of host proteins TSG101 and VPS-4. *J. Virol.* **77:**1812–1819.

Licata, J. M., Johnson, R. F., Han, Z., and Harty, R. N. (2004). Contribution of ebola virus glycoprotein, nucleoprotein, and VP24 to budding of VP40 virus-like particles. *J. Virol.* **78:**7344–7351.

Longnecker, R., Merchant, M., Brown, M. E., Fruehling, S., Bickford, J. O., Ikeda, M., and Harty, R. N. (2000). WW- and SH3-domain interactions with Epstein-Barr virus LMP2A. *Exp. Cell Res.* **257:**332–340.

Martin-Serrano, J., Zang, T., and Bieniasz, P. D. (2001). HIV-1 and Ebola virus encode small peptide motifs that recruit Tsg101 to sites of particle assembly to facilitate egress. *Nat. Med.* **7:**1313–1319.

Martin-Serrano, J., Eastman, S. W., Chung, W., and Bieniasz, P. D. (2005). HECT ubiquitin ligases link viral and cellular PPXY motifs to the vacuolar protein-sorting pathway. *J. Cell Biol.* **168:**89–101.

Mebatsion, T., Konig, M., and Conzelmann, K. K. (1996). Budding of rabies virus particles in the absence of the spike glycoprotein. *Cell* **84:**941–951.

Mebatsion, T., Weiland, F., and Conzelmann, K. K. (1999). Matrix protein of rabies virus is responsible for the assembly and budding of bullet-shaped particles and interacts with the transmembrane spike glycoprotein G. *J. Virol.* **73:**242–250.

Myers, E. L., and Allen, J. F. (2002). Tsg101, an inactive homologue of ubiquitin ligase e2, interacts specifically with human immunodeficiency virus type 2 gag polyprotein and results in increased levels of ubiquitinated gag. *J. Virol.* **76:**11226–11235.

Pornillos, O., Alam, S. L., Davis, D. R., and Sundquist, W. I. (2002a). Structure of the Tsg101 UEV domain in complex with the PTAP motif of the HIV-1 p6 protein. *Nat. Struct. Biol.* **9:**812–817.

Pornillos, O., Alam, S. L., Rich, R. L., Myszka, D. G., Davis, D. R., and Sundquist, W. I. (2002b). Structure and functional interactions of the Tsg101 UEV domain. *EMBO J.* **21:**2397–2406.

Pulmanausahakul, R., Li, J., Schnell, M. J., and Dietzschold, B. (2008). The glycoprotein and the matrix protein of rabies virus affect pathogenicity by regulating viral replication and facilitating cell-to-cell spread. *J. Virol.* **82:**2330–2338.

Robison, C. S., and Whitt, M. A. (2000). The membrane-proximal stem region of vesicular stomatitis virus G protein confers efficient virus assembly. *J. Virol.* **74:**2239–2246.

Rolls, M. M., Webster, P., Balba, N. H., and Rose, J. K. (1994). Novel infectious particles generated by expression of the vesicular stomatitis virus glycoprotein from a self-replicating RNA. *Cell* **79:**497–506.

Sakurai, A., Yasuda, J., Takano, H., Tanaka, Y., Hatakeyama, M., and Shida, H. (2004). Regulation of human T-cell leukemia virus type 1 (HTLV-1) budding by ubiquitin ligase Nedd4. *Microbes Infect.* **6:**150–156.

Schnell, M. J., Mebatsion, T., and Conzelmann, K. K. (1994). Infectious rabies viruses from cloned cDNA. *EMBO J.* **13:**4195–4203.

Schnell, M. J., Buonocore, L., Boritz, E., Ghosh, H. P., Chernish, R., and Rose, J. K. (1998). Requirement for a non-specific glycoprotein cytoplasmic domain sequence to drive efficient budding of vesicular stomatitis virus. *EMBO J.* **17:**1289–1296.

Strack, B., Calistri, A., Accola, M. A., Palu, G., and Gottlinger, H. G. (2000). A role for ubiquitin ligase recruitment in retrovirus release. *Proc. Natl. Acad. Sci. USA* **97:**13063–13068.

Taylor, G. M., Hanson, P. I., and Kielian, M. (2007). Ubiquitin depletion and dominant-negative VPS4 inhibit rhabdovirus budding without affecting alphavirus budding. *J. Virol.* **81:**13631–13639.

Timmins, J., Schoehn, G., Ricard-Blum, S., Scianimanico, S., Vernet, T., Ruigrok, R. W., and Weissenhorn, W. (2003). Ebola virus matrix protein VP40 interaction with human cellular factors Tsg101 and Nedd4. *J. Mol. Biol.* **326:**493–502.

VerPlank, L., Bouamr, F., LaGrassa, T. J., Agresta, B., Kikonyogo, A., Leis, J., and Carter, C. A. (2001). Tsg101, a homologue of ubiquitin-conjugating (E2) enzymes, binds the L domain in HIV type 1 Pr55(Gag). *Proc. Natl. Acad. Sci. USA* **98:**7724–7729.

Wirblich, C., Tan, G. S., Papaneri, A., Godlewski, P. J., Orenstein, J. M., Harty, R. N., and Schnell, M. J. (2008). PPEY motif within the rabies virus (RV) matrix protein is essential for efficient virion release and RV pathogenicity. *J. Virol.* **82:**9730–9738.

Yasuda, J., Nakao, M., Kawaoka, Y., and Shida, H. (2003). Nedd4 regulates egress of Ebola virus-like particles from host cells. *J. Virol.* **77:**9987–9992.

Zakowski, J. J., and Wagner, R. R. (1980). Localization of membrane-associated proteins in vesicular stomatitis virus by use of hydrophobic membrane probes and cross-linking reagents. *J. Virol.* **36:**93–102.

CHAPTER 3

Evasive Strategies in Rabies Virus Infection

Monique Lafon

Contents

Abstract

Rabies virus (RABV) is a strictly neurotropic virus that slowly propagates in the nervous system (NS) of the infected host from the site of entry (usually due to a bite) up to the site of exit (salivary glands). Successful achievement of the virus cycle relies on the preservation of the neuronal network. Once RABV has entered the NS, its progression is not interrupted either by destruction of

Unité de Neuroimmunologie Virale, Département de Virologie, Institut Pasteur, Paris, France

Advances in Virus Research, Volume 79
ISSN 0065-3527, DOI: 10.1016/B978-0-12-387040-7.00003-2

the infected neurons or by the immune response, which are major host mechanisms for combating viral infection. RABV has developed two main mechanisms to escape the host defenses: (1) its ability to kill protective migrating T cells and (2) its ability to sneak into the NS without triggering apoptosis of the infected neurons and preserving the integrity of neurites.

I. INTRODUCTION

Viruses are obligatory parasites. Successful completion of virus cycle and subsequent transmission to a new host relies upon the evolution of strategies that exploit the cellular machinery and modulate host cell signaling pathways, in particular, that governing premature cell death and promoting cell survival. Rabies virus (RABV), a neurotropic virus causing fatal encephalitis, is transmitted by saliva of an infected animal (mainly dogs but also bats) after bites or scratches. RABV enters the nervous system (NS) through the neuromuscular junction via a motor neuron or through nerve spindles via a sensory nerve. Infecting neurons almost exclusively, it travels from one neuron to the next in the spinal cord to the brainstem, from where it reaches the salivary glands via cranial nerves (facial and glossopharyngeal nerves). Once RABV has reached the salivary glands, it is excreted in saliva and can be transmitted to a new host. After the successful completion of the virus cycle, death of the host occurs because of exhaustion of infected neurons accompanied with structural damage involving neuronal processes and associated severe neuronal dysfunction (Jackson *et al.*, 2010; Scott *et al.*, 2008).

Intriguingly, once the RABV has entered the NS, its progression is not interrupted either by destruction of the infected neuron or by the immune response, the two major host mechanisms for combating viral infection. RABV has two complementary characteristics particularly relevant to successful invasion of the NS: (1) RABV escapes the host immune response and (2) protects the infected neurons against apoptosis or premature destruction of neurites.

II. EVASION FROM HOST IMMUNE RESPONSES

Most pathogenesis studies have been performed in mice using laboratory-adapted RABV strains injected by intramuscular or intraplantar (footpad) route to mimic natural transmission by bite. Fatal rabies encephalitis can be reproduced in this animal model using the challenge virus standard, CVS. This virus invades the spinal cord and brain regions and causes fatal encephalitis (Camelo *et al.*, 2000; Park *et al.*, 2006; Xiang *et al.*, 1995). Some mutant strains of RABV with attenuated pathogenicity cause only transient infection of the NS. This is the case, among others, of Pasteur virus (PV) resulting in a nonfatal abortive disease characterized by a transient and restricted infection of the NS followed by irreversible paralysis of the limbs (Galelli *et al.*, 2000; Hooper *et al.*, 1998; Irwin *et al.*, 1999; Weiland *et al.*, 1992; Xiang *et al.*, 1995).

A. The killing of migratory T cells

Most of infections of the NS are controlled by infiltrating T cells. This is, for example, observed during the course of West Nile virus brain infection, where $CD8^+$ T cells attracted by the chemokines produced by inflammatory cells in the infected NS are a critical factor for controlling the infection (Klein *et al.*, 2005; Zhang *et al.*, 2008). In rabies, sterilization of the infection by T cells is inefficient and is specifically inactivated by the virus (Lafon, 2008). Immunohistochemical studies performed on rabies autopsy cases revealed that the cells undergoing death were leukocytes and not neurons (Hemachudha *et al.*, 2005; Tobiume *et al.*, 2009). This observation was reproduced in mice infected with the encephalitic RABV strain CVS. Immunocytochemistry of brain and spinal cord slices revealed that despite a heavy loading with viral antigens, infected neurons do not undergo death. In contrast, the migrating T cells ($CD3^+$) were apoptotic (Baloul and Lafon, 2003; Baloul *et al.*, 2004; Kojima *et al.*, 2009; Lafon, 2005; Rossiter *et al.*, 2009). Moreover, pathogenicity of the CVS strain was similar in immunocompetent mice Balb/c mice and in Nu/Nu Balb/c mice, indicating that T cells do not control the outcome of encephalitic rabies (Lafon, 2005). In striking contrast, deprivation of T cells transformed an abortive infection into a encephalitic rabies similar to those caused by the encephalitic strain CVS infection, showing that T cells is a critical factor in the restriction of the NS infection caused by an abortive RABV strain. Indeed, when apoptosis was analyzed in the spinal cord of immunocompetent mice infected with the abortive RABV strain PV, killing of T cells was not observed; instead, infected neurons died (Galelli *et al.*, 2000). Altogether, these observations indicated that T cells have a protective potential to control RABV infection in the NS nevertheless, their capacity to control RABV infection is impeded with the encephalitic RABV strain. The mechanisms by which the encephalitic RABV strain evades the host T-cell response was further studied as described below.

B. Impeded capacity controlling the infection in the NS is not the result of an abortive T-cell response in the periphery

The reason why T cells are protective in the case of an abortive strain of RABV infection and not after an infection by the encephalitic strain might simply result from differences in the level of T-cell activation in the periphery: strong activation of T cells after abortive RABV infection and low activation after encephalitic RABV infection. This is an unlikely hypothesis because, after a virus injection in the periphery, the immune response (neutralizing antibodies, CD4$^+$, CD8$^+$ T-cells response) was not different after injection of an encephalitic RABV bat strain (silver-haired bat rabies virus, SHBRV) or after a less pathogenic virus (CVS-F3, mutant of CVS encoding a mutation in the G protein Roy and Hooper, 2007).

Mononuclear leukocytes, monocytes, and macrophages are able to be recruited to the NS in pathological conditions, including infections by neurotropic viruses (Davoust *et al.*, 2008). Once activated, the T and B cells and macrophages from the periphery expressing surface adhesion molecules have the capacity to enter the NS (Engelhardt, 2008). This entry is independent of blood–brain barrier (BBB) integrity that modulates entry of solutes and not cells (Bechmann *et al.*, 2007). The absence of T-cell protection against an infection by the encephalitic RABV strain might be related to a low entry of T cells into the NS. This is likely not the case because after infection with an encephalitic RABV strain, blood T-cells expressed markers of activation (CD69) and were highly positive for collapsing response mediator protein 2 (CRMP2), a marker of T-cell polarization and migration. The brain was enriched with this type of cells, indicating they have migratory properties (Vuaillat *et al.*, 2008). Thus, activation and entry into the NS are not limiting factors for T-cell protective function. The presence of T cells in the infected NS of mice was observed in mice infected either with an abortive or an encephalitic RABV strain (Baloul *et al.*, 2004). As the infection of the NS progresses, the parenchyma became invaded by infiltrating T cells. However, this phenomenon was interrupted after a few days of infection by an encephalitic strain, whereas CD3$^+$ T-cell accumulation in PV-infected NS was continuous. Disappearance of T cells in the CVS-infected brain and an increase in number of apoptotic cells in the NS were concomitant events. These observations strongly suggest that CVS strain, but not PV strain, triggers unfavorable conditions for T-cell survival in the infected NS.

C. T-cell death is caused by the upregulation of FasL and B7-H1 in the infected NS

After their entry into the NS, migratory immune cells face unfavorable conditions for survival. This general feature of the NS, which results of a series of parameters controlled by neurons, seriously dampens T-cell activity. For example, secretion of several neuropeptides and neurotransmitters by neurons such as vasointestinal peptide, calcitonin-gene-related peptide, norepinephrine, and alpha-melanocyte-stimulating hormone downregulate the activity of T cells (Niederkorn, 2006).

It can be surmised that RABV exploits these intrinsic features of the NS to reduce the activity of the migratory T cells. Indeed, it has been observed that RABV-infected brain (mainly noninfected neurons) upregulates the expression of calcitonin-related gene peptide, somatostatin, and vasointestinal peptides, three molecules known to contribute to limit T-cell activity in the NS (Weihe *et al.*, 2008). Nevertheless, these observations have been obtained using an attenuated RABV strain, and whether encephalitic RABV exacerbates the expression of these molecules to enhance the restriction of T cells is currently unknown.

Tumors evade immune surveillance by multiple mechanisms, including the inhibition of tumor-specific T-cell immunity. In order to escape attack from protective T cells, tumor cells upregulate expression of certain surface molecules such as B7-H1, FasL, and HLA-G, which triggers death signaling in activated T cells expressing the corresponding ligands PD-1 for B7-H1, Fas for FasL, and CD8 among others for HLA-G (Dong *et al.*, 2002; Gratas *et al.*, 1998; Rouas-Freiss *et al.*, 2003). Studies evaluating whether RABV-infected neurons upregulate immunosubversive molecules to kill activated T cells following an evasive strategy similar to that selected by tumors cells have been undertaken both *in vivo* and *in vitro*. *In vitro*, RABV infection was found to upregulate the expression of HLA-G at the surface of human neurons (Lafon *et al.*, 2005; Megret *et al.*, 2007). *In vivo*, comparison of experimental rabies in mice caused by CVS, which kills T cells, or by PV, which does not kill T cells, leads to the finding that the CVS-infected NS, but not the PV-infected NS, upregulates the expression of FasL. In mice lacking a functional FasL, there was less T-cell apoptosis in the NS than in control mice. Remarkably, RABV morbidity and mortality were reduced in these mice. In addition, RABV-infected brain upregulates the expression of another immunosubversive molecule, B7-H1 (Lafon *et al.*, 2008). Whereas noninfected NS was almost devoid of B7-H1 expression, RABV infection triggers neural B7-H1 expression that increases as the infection progresses. Infected neurons and also noninfected neural cells, including astrocyte-like cells, were found positive for B7-H1. RABV infection of B7-H1 deficient mice resulted in a drastic reduction in clinical signs and mortality. Reduction of RABV virulence in B7H1$^{-/-}$ mice was concomitant of a reduction of CD8$^+$ T-cell apoptosis among the migratory T cells.

RABV drives T cells into an apoptosis pathway by upregulating the expression of molecules such as FasL and B7-H1 in the NS (especially in neurons); these molecules trigger the death pathway in T cells expressing the corresponding ligands, Fas and PD-1, similar to what is observed in tumor cells. In mice lacking functional FasL or B7-H1, virulence was drastically attenuated indicating the critical role of this mechanism for virus neuroinvasiveness. Thus, RABV uses immunosubversive molecules as a protection to evade host T-cell defenses.

D. How does RABV upregulate B7-H1 expression?

B7-H1 (also known as PD-L1 or CD274) is a B7 family member that inhibits T-cell activation and cell-mediated toxic function of T cells. Interferons (IFNs), tumor necrosis factor alpha (TNF-alpha), and Toll-like receptor (TLR) stimulation are potent activators of B7-H1 expression (Lafon *et al.*, 2008; Liu *et al.*, 2007; Pulko *et al.*, 2009; Schreiner *et al.*, 2004). Treatment of human neurons with recombinant human IFN-beta triggers expression of B7-H1. IFN-gamma and TNF-alpha are less potent activators (Lafon *et al.*, 2008). Therefore, in order to express neural B7-H1 in the infected NS, the RABV-infected NS, and neurons in particular, should require IFN to be produced during the course of RABV infection. This may be seen as an unexpected situation, as IFN is supposed to fight infection instead of promoting infection.

The innate immune response is the first line of defense against infectious agents. The innate immune system can sense the presence of microorganisms through "pattern recognition receptors" molecules that recognize the conserved danger pattern expressed by microbes. TLRs or RIG-like receptors (RLRs) are important molecules for the recognition of viral dsRNAs and ssRNAs. Resulting signal transduction cascades trigger production of antiviral molecules such as type I IFN.

The NS parenchyma, similar to most tissues, has the capacity to sense viral infection. The innate immune response triggered *in situ* by the entry of pathogens into the brain is characterized by the production of type I IFN (predominantly IFN-beta in the brain, no IFN-alpha, and no type III IFN-lambda; Delhaye *et al.*, 2006; Prehaud *et al.*, 2005; Sommereyns *et al.*, 2008). Microglia, astrocytes, and recently neurons have been identified as main innate keepers of the brain (Delhaye *et al.*, 2006; Lafon *et al.*, 2006; Olson and Miller, 2004; Yang *et al.*, 2000; Zhou *et al.*, 2009). Cells of the NS, mainly glial cells, express receptors such as TLR or RLR that allow them to recognize and respond to the presence of danger signals and pathogen-associated molecular patterns encoded by pathogens (Furr *et al.*, 2008; Olson and Miller, 2004). Neurons were also found to express TLRs and RLRs (Lafon *et al.*, 2006; Peltier *et al.*, 2010; Tang *et al.*, 2007, 2008) and to mount type I IFN response after RABV infection (Prehaud *et al.*, 2005).

RIG-I is described as the RABV innate immune sensor (Faul *et al.*, 2010; Hornung *et al.*, 2006). RABV, like most viruses (Randall and Goodbourn, 2008), has developed a strategy to counteract the host IFN response and escape this first line of host defense (Masatani *et al.*, 2010; Rieder and Conzelmann, 2009). Dampening the IFN response favors RABV infection as demonstrated with the death of mice intracerebrally infected with P protein RABV mutants lacking the capacity to reduce the host type I IFN response (Ito *et al.*, 2010). Nevertheless, IFN induction in the RABV-infected NS is far from being abrogated (Lafon *et al.*, 2008). Indeed, after injection of RABV into the hindlimbs, a progressive infection within the spinal cord and the brain is accompanied by a robust innate immune response characterized by a type I IFN response as well as chemoattractive and inflammatory responses. Downregulation of the IFN response is indeed noticed *in vitro*. For example, in RABV-infected human postmitotic neurons (NT2-N), transcription of *IFN-beta* gene is seen as early as 6 h postinfection, and IFN-beta protein is produced during the first 24-h postinfection even if it declines thereafter (Prehaud *et al.*, 2005). This transient type I IFN response might be sufficient to upregulate type I IFN-dependent gene transcription such as B7-H1 transcription, not only in neurons but also in the neighboring noninfected cells, provided these cells express receptor for type I IFN. This should be the case as demonstrated for human neurons and astrocytes which are fully susceptible to an IFN-beta treatment in absence of infection (Lafon *et al.*, 2005).

Viral proteins control mechanisms by which RABV escapes the IFN response. Therefore, they are functional in infected neurons only, because these neurons express viral proteins, but they are not functional in noninfected neighboring glial cells that do not express viral proteins. This heterocellular production of IFN was found in other viral models to be essential for host defense (Chen *et al.*, 2010). In RABV, the virus to enhance the expression of molecules promoting its infection could hijack this function. Indeed, in RABV-infected mixed cultures of human neurons and astrocytes (NT2-N/A) and also in the infected mouse brain, B7-H1 expression could be detected not only in neurons but also in nonneuronal cells (Lafon *et al.*, 2008). It is likely that RABV infection can take advantage of minute amounts of IFN produced by neurons early in the infection to establish an immunoevasive tissue environment.

In conclusion, IFN might be required to promote B7-H1-mediated immune evasion because *B7-H1* is an IFN-dependent gene. As B7-H1 is critical for the successful immunoevasive strategy of RABV, it can be surmised that RABV pathogenicity relies paradoxically on the protective mechanism of IFN production, which is triggered by the host to fight the infection.

E. Other functions that may contribute to RABV-mediated immunoevasive strategies

Another intrinsic property of the NS is the limitation of inflammation in the NS following NS injury or toxic insults. This results from the capacity of neurons to reduce inflammation and regulate microglial phenotype during infection or injury (Meuth *et al.*, 2008). Control of local glial inflammation occurs via the expression by neurons of receptors such as CD47, CD22, CD200, and by their ligands on glial cells (Griffiths *et al.*, 2007; Hoek *et al.*, 2000; Wright *et al.*, 2000).

Despite the existence of mechanisms limiting neuroinflammation, inflammation is still triggered in the NS by most virus infections. For example, inflammation favors West Nile virus access to the NS (Brehin et al., 2008; Wang et al., 2004). In contrast, encephalitic RABV strains, compared with other encephalitic virus infection such as Borna virus, trigger only limited inflammation (Fu et al., 1993; Shankar et al., 1992).

RABV seems to minimize the inflammation in the nervous tissues it infects. The more pathogenic the virus strain is, the less acute is the inflammatory response (Baloul and Lafon, 2003; Hicks et al., 2009; Laothamatas et al., 2008; Wang et al., 2005). Dogs infected with RABV causing paralytic rabies showed longer period of illness and more intense nuclear magnetic resonance (NMR) signals than dogs infected with strains causing furious rabies, and the pattern of cytokines and chemokines mRNAs expression was greater in paralytic than in furious rabies (Laothamatas et al., 2008). Mice immunization with proinflammatory myelin basic protein (MBP) prior to RABV infection improved the survival to a challenge with SHBRV and, conversely, treatment with a steroid hormone decreasing brain inflammation and with minocycline, a tetracycline derivate with anti-inflammatory properties, increased the mortality rate (Jackson et al., 2007; Roy and Hooper, 2007). Also, overexpression of TNF-alpha (a proinflammatory cytokine) by a recombinant RABV attenuates replication by inducing strong T-cell infiltration and microglial activation (Faber et al., 2005). These two last examples illustrate that increasing the inflammatory response may be negative factors for RABV neuroinvasiveness. How RABV limits neuroinflammation is not yet well understood.

It has also been proposed that RABV pathogenicity is related to the impermeability of the BBB, with nonpathogenic RABV strains triggering a transient opening of the BBB, but not pathogenic strains (Phares et al., 2006; Roy et al., 2007). Mechanisms by which pathogenic RABV strains control the BBB impermeability, which may be linked to the low inflammation triggered by pathogenic RABV strains, deserve further investigation.

Neutralizing antibodies have been described as a critical factor for protection against RABV (Hooper et al., 1998; Montano-Hirose et al., 1993; Wiktor et al., 1984; Wunner et al., 1983). The entry of B cells into the RABV-infected NS and the local secretion of antibody contribute to the clearance of attenuated RABV from NS (Hooper et al., 2009). It is striking to note that during the course of encephalitic RABV infection, B cells are almost undetectable in brain (Camelo et al., 2000; Kojima et al., 2010), suggesting that restricted entry or specific destruction of migratory B cells could also contribute to RABV virulence.

III. PRESERVATION OF NEURON AND NEURONAL NETWORK INTEGRITY

Protection of axon, dendrites, and synapses is a critical factor for success-ful infection of neurotropic viruses that spread in the NS using axonal transport and virus transmission at synapses. Demonstration of this state-ment was obtained in a model of NS infection with Theiler's virus. By using a mouse strain in which axonal degeneration is impeded (the Wallerian degeneration slow mouse mutant, C57Bl Wld[s]), Ikwo Tsunoda demonstrated that pathogenicity of Theiler's virus was increased when axonal degeneration was impeded (Tsunoda *et al.*, 2007). In the same line, axonal degeneration might be a self-defense mechanism set up by the host limiting the infection for neurotropic viruses using axonal transport and synapses transmission. It can be expected that these viruses have specific mechanisms to counteract such a host defense mechanism.

RABV propagates in the host NS by transneural transfer exclusively in a retrograde direction. After entry at the neuromuscular junction or passage through the synapse, RABV particles propagate in axonal vesi-cles (Klingen *et al.*, 2008). Virus replication occurs in the cell bodies. Viral proteins are detected in the dendrites, but not in axons (Ugolini, 1995; Ugolini, 2010). Dendrites are described as active sites of protein synthesis with their rough endoplasmic reticulum and "Golgi outposts" in corre-spondence to spines or within the spines, whereas axons, with smooth reticulum endoplasm and rare polysomes, are poorly active sites for protein synthesis (Meldolesi, 2010). According to the distinct features of axons and dendrites, it is likely that RABV protein synthesis and viral particle assembly occur not only in cell bodies but also in dendrites, whereas axons are devoted to transport viral particles to the next order neuron. Successful RABV propagation should require that neurites and axons from the infected neuron are protected in the period necessary for transport of virus particles up to the cell body, protein synthesis in cell bodies and dendrites, virus particle assembly, and transmission through synapses. Indeed, in a model of RABV infection of nonhuman primates 4 days after infection, infected motor neurons show no signs of degenera-tion with normal size, morphology, and Nissl staining (Ugolini, 2010). *In vitro*, rat spinal motoneurons never encounter death (Guigoni and Coulon, 2002). Neuronal apoptosis is a rare event in natural rabies (Jackson *et al.*, 2008). Later in the infection, when the brain is already infected, dendrites showed beading, degenerative changes are seen in dendrites and axons, and peripheral nerve dysfunction occurs (Jackson *et al.*, 2010; Juntrakul *et al.*, 2005; Kojima *et al.*, 2009; Rossiter *et al.*, 2009; Scott *et al.*, 2008). Nerve cell destruction is characterized by accumulation of Nissl bodies, shrunken nuclei, cytoplasm vacuolization, and swollen mitochondria, which is a pattern distinct from apoptosis (Baloul and Lafon, 2003; Iwasaki et al., 1977; Jackson et al., 2008; Kojima et al., 2009; Ugolini, 2010).

Altogether, these data lead to the conclusion that successful RABV propagation in the NS requires that neuronal cell bodies are not damaged by premature apoptosis and that the integrity of axons and dendrites is preserved, at least during the period of time required for the virus to reach the salivary glands.

A. Death or survival of RABV-infected neurons is controlled by the RABV G protein

Suicide of viral-infected cells can be considered an early defense against viral infection. It has been proposed that mature neurons, because they are poorly renewable cells, would not be prone to follow this mechanism of defense (Allsopp et al., 1998), but this is not a general feature since poliovirus or West Nile virus kill motor neurons efficiently (Girard et al., 1999; Schafernak and Bigio, 2006). Resistance to neuronal death and promotion of neuronal survival during RABV infection are likely actively controlled by RABV.

In order to analyze how RABV actively controls the fate of infected neurons, comparison of two different types of laboratory RABV strains, CVS-NIV and ERA-NIV, was undertaken in human neuroblastoma cell lines (Prehaud et al., 2010). CVS-NIV causes fatal encephalitic rabies when inoculated intramuscularly in the hindlimbs of adult mice (Camelo et al., 2000) and engages the human neuron toward a survival-signaling program. This survival is characterized by the stimulation of neurite elongation, acquisition of resistance against oxidative stress, and growth cone collapsing drug (lysophosphatidic acid), and the activation of the AKT signaling pathway (Phosphorylation of AKT, P-AKT). In contrast, ERA-NIV is an attenuated laboratory strain identified in the search for candidate live vaccines (Megret et al., 2005), which has lost neurotropism after intramuscular injection and causes apoptosis of the infected cells triggering both caspase-dependent and caspase-independent pathways (Prehaud et al., 2003; Thoulouze et al., 1997, 2003).

Treatment of cells with UV-inactivated ERA-NIV is not sufficient to trigger death or proliferation. Induction of apoptosis and survival requires virus replication. This suggests that infected neurons could engage into one of the two competing pathways, the choice being controlled by newly synthesized viral components. Transfection experiments and analysis of recombinant gene expression of the various viral proteins showed that apoptosis/survival decisions are largely determined by the nature of the G protein (Prehaud et al., 2010). Another group suggested that protection against apoptosis might be determined by the level of expression of the RABV G protein: the weaker the G protein expression, the less apoptosis (Faber *et al.*, 2002; Morimoto *et al.*, 1999). However, in a system of maximal expression of viral proteins, the replacement of a proapoptotic *G* gene by a nonapoptotic *G* gene CVS-NIV was sufficient to prevent destruction of the infected cells by apoptosis, increase the pool of P-AKT, and trigger protection of neurites. Therefore, it is likely that commitment to apoptosis or survival depends mainly on determinants in the sequence of the G protein and is largely independent of the level of transcription or replication (Prehaud *et al.*, 2010). The molecular basis of RABV-induced survival/apoptosis of neurons was largely unknown. Breakthroughs in this field have been recently obtained (Prehaud *et al.*, 2010). At first, the cytoplasmic domain of G protein (Cyto-G) has been identified as a critical element for the survival and apoptotic phenotypes. Moreover, the G of CVS-NIV and ERA-NIV strains are different by only six aa, two of which are located in the 44 aa long Cyto-G. Chimeric and endswap G recombinant RABV mutants isolated by reverse genetics showed without ambiguity that the control by the Cyto-G for death or survival relies on the nature of the last COOH terminal four aa. These last four aa form a consensus-binding site for a PDZ domain (PDZ-BS). PDZ domains are globular structures, 80–100 amino acids long, that contain a groove into which the C-terminal segment of a partner protein, PDZ-BS, inserts. PDZ domains play a central role in cell signaling by favoring spatial contacts between enzymes and their substrates, or more generally by assembling and/or regulating protein networks (Harris and Lim, 2001; Lee and Zheng, 2010; Sheng and Sala, 2001). Remarkably, one single mutation (Q to E) in the PDZ-BS was sufficient to switch the fate of the infected cell from survival to apoptosis. The nature of the PDZ-BS governs the interaction of the viral protein with the PDZ domains of different cell partners. High-scale two-hybrid experiments were undertaken with a human brain bank and cellular interactors were identified. The fished cell proteins all harbor PDZ domains. Cyto-G of both CVS-NIV and ERA-NIV strains targeted the PDZ of the microtubule serine-threonine kinase 2, MAST2. The Q to E change increases the number of cellular partners for PDZ-BS in the infected cells, with attenuated RABV strain G protein interacting with the PDZ domain of the human nonreceptor tyrosine phosphatase PTPN4. Since interaction of Cyto-G with the PDZ of MAST2 triggers neurosurvival and not apoptosis, it is likely that interaction of Cyto-G of ERA-NIV with the PDZ of PTPN4 triggering apoptosis is a dominant trait supplanting the survival-signaling pathway governed by the Cyto-G interaction with MAST2-PDZ.

Silencing of *MAST2* and silencing of *PTPN4* showed that MAST2 is an inhibitor of neurite outgrowth, whereas PTPN4 guards cells against apoptosis (Loh *et al.*, 2008; Prehaud *et al.*, 2010). Disruption of the complexes formed by PDZ domains and their ligands can trigger profound altera-tions in the relevant signaling pathways (Aarts *et al.*, 2002; Hou *et al.*, 2010; Nourry *et al.*, 2003; Yanagisawa *et al.*, 1997). Comparisons with other models of signals controlled by PDZ domains (Hou *et al.*, 2010; Yanagisawa *et al.*, 1997) suggest that a peptide could trigger apoptosis or survival by simply disrupting a crucial cellular interaction. In RABV-infected cells, Cyto-G of ERA-NIV would interrupt crucial interaction between the PTPN4-PDZ and the PDZ-BS of a yet unidentified endoge-nous PTPN4 ligand. In RABV-infected neurons, Cyto-G of CVS-NIV would interrupt crucial interactions between MAST2-PDZ and the PDZ-BS of endogenous MAST2 ligand. In both cases, Cyto-G functions as an inhibitor of MAST2 and PTPN4 functions. By doing so, G protein of ERA-NIV could annihilate the antiapoptotic function of PTPN4 and trigger cell death. In the same line, G protein of CVS-NIV could inhibit the antisurvival function of MAST2.

In conclusion, RABV neuroinvasiveness may be favored by the capac-ity of its G protein to promote survival-signaling in the infected neuron. The study of the molecular basis of RABV pathogenesis illustrates how viruses divert host cell signaling for their benefit. The additional finding that intracellularly delivered short peptides encoding the viral PDZ-BS mimic the virus phenotypes, triggering cell death or survival properties according to their sequences (Prehaud *et al.*, 2010), might open new therapeutic applications in neurodegenerative and cancer diseases.

B. Sequestration of TLR3 into Negri bodies

Neuronal expression of TLR3 seems to play a major role in the control of neurotropic viral infection, either decreasing viral replication in the case of West Nile virus infections or, more surprisingly, by promoting virus neuronal infection as shown in the case of RABV (Daffis *et al.*, 2008; Menager *et al.*, 2009). TLR3 is produced by neurons, human NT2N in culture, human neurons in autopsy cases and in motor neurons and sensory neurons, and human neuroblastoma cell lines as well as in peripheral nerves (Barajon *et al.*, 2009; Goethals *et al.*, 2010; Jackson *et al.*, 2006; Menager *et al.*, 2009; Prehaud *et al.*, 2005). The sequence of the *TLR3* gene of human neurons was determined (Genbank DQ445682). It was strictly identical to human dendritic cells TLR3 counterpart, suggesting that TLR3 expressed by neurons is fully functional. It was observed that in cultures of infected human neurons, RABV infection redistributed cyto-plasmic TLR-3 localization. In the absence of infection, TLR3 molecules are located in endosomes (late and early). Following RABV infection, TLR3 is present not only in endosomes and multivesicular bodies but also in detergent-resistant inclusion bodies located near the nucleus. Besides TLR3, these inclusion bodies contain RABV proteins (N and P, but no G) and viral genome. The size of the inclusion bodies (3–5 μm), their composition, and the absence of surrounded membrane as shown by electronic microscopy suggest that they correspond to the previously described Negri bodies, which appear in neurons in the course of RABV infection (Kristensson *et al.*, 1996) and have been described as viral factories (Lahaye *et al.*, 2009). Confocal microscopic analysis and three-dimensional models indicate that the structure of Negri bodies is strictly organized with a nuclear core containing TLR3 surrounded by a shell composed of viral N and P proteins. TLR3 expression is required for Negri body formation to occur, since in absence of TLR3, Negri bodies do not form, suggesting that Negri bodies and TLR3 entrapping have essential functions in RABV multiplication.

Negri bodies exhibit most of the characteristics of aggresomes. Aggresomes are perinuclear structures where proteins produced in excess or misfolded proteins are stored before elimination (Johnston *et al.*, 1998; Kopito, 2000). Aggresomes may also function as storage structures regulating the pool of active proteins (Kolodziejska *et al.*, 2005). Since sequestration of cellular protein in aggresomes could be a mechanism of posttranscriptional regulation of proteins, it can thus be proposed that TLR3 sequestration in Negri bodies dampens TLR3 properties.

Besides its role in triggering innate immune response against RNA virus nucleic acids, additional functions have been described for TLR3 (Cameron *et al.*, 2007; Chiron *et al.*, 2009; Lathia *et al.*, 2008). TLR3 accumulates in the growth cones at the tip end of dorsal root ganglia (DRG) neurites and treatment of DRG with Poly:IC (an agonist of TLR3) resulted in the inhibition of the axonal growth (Cameron *et al.*, 2007). This effect was not observed in TLR3$^{-/-}$ mice. Moreover, in the presence of IFN, TLR3 activation triggers cell death (Chiron *et al.*, 2009). Since protection against apoptosis and protection of neurite integrity are main features of the pathogenic RABV strain (see above), the hijacking of TLR3 into Negri bodies could be an attempt of the virus to protect the infected neuron against apoptosis and to favor the integrity of axons. Thus, besides their role in virus multiplication, Negri bodies can also contribute to the survival strategy of RABV.

IV. CONCLUSIONS ON RABV EVASIVE STRATEGIES

RABV has selected multiple sophisticated strategies to achieve its virus cycle into the host NS from the site of entry (bite) up to the salivary glands, where it will be excreted to infect a new host. From the experiments listed above, we suggest the following scheme of events (Fig. 1). After entry into the NS, RABV promotes neuronal survival and avoids premature cell death of the neurons it infects by triggering survival pathways.

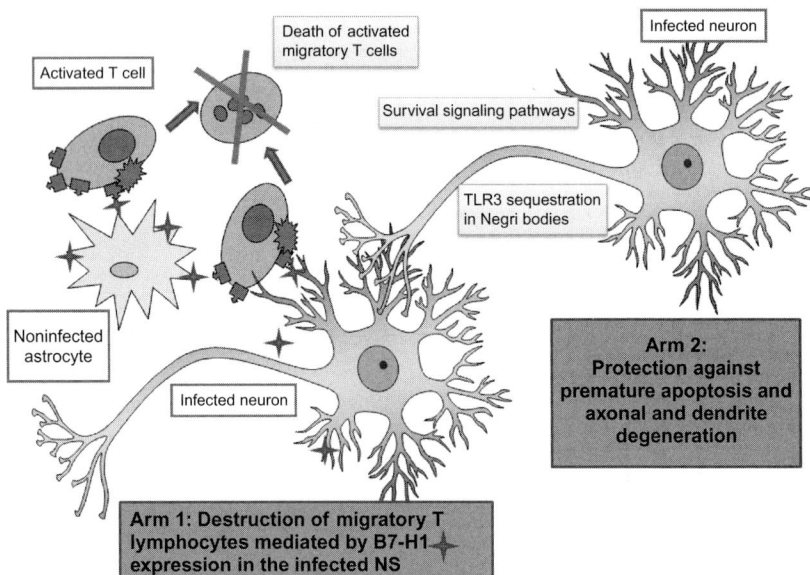

FIGURE 1 *RABV preserves the integrity of the neuronal network.* RABV evasion of the host response is a two-armed strategy: Arm 1: Infected neurons express not only immunosubversive molecules such as B7-H1 (red stars) but also HLA-G and FasL. Surface expression of these molecules triggers death into migratory T cells expressing the corresponding ligands. *B7-H1* and *HLA-G* are IFN-dependent genes. Heterocellular IFN production by noninfected astrocytes could be an additional source of IFN-mediated B7-H1 (and HLA-G) expression. Arm 2: Infected neurons are protected against premature apoptosis and axon or dendrite degeneration. RABV infection activates survival-signaling pathway in the infected neuron and confers a G protein-mediated protection. In addition, TLR3, a molecule described as an inhibitor of axonal elongation with proapoptotic function, is sequestered into Negri bodies. (For interpretation of the references to color in this figure legend, the reader is referred to the Web version of this chapter.)

The cytoplasmic portion of the G protein and the COOH terminal PDZ-BS control this function. Sequestration in Negri bodies of molecules such as TLR3, which may function as a proapoptotic protein and as an inhibitor of axonal growth, could also contribute to the survival of infected neurons. Early after NS infection by RABV, neuronal cells mount an innate immune response, including RIG-I, TLR signaling, and IFN-beta production leading to B7-H1, HLA-G, and FasL expression. These immunosubversive molecules proteins subsequently reach the cell surface of infected neurons or the surrounding noninfected astrocytes, where they can interact with their corresponding receptors (Fas for FasL, PD-1 for B7-H1, and CD8 for HLA-G) expressed by the migratory T cells attracted by the local modest inflammation in the NS. Interaction of these immunosubversive molecules with their respective ligands then triggers the exhaustion of $CD3^+/CD8^+$ T cells (e.g., by reducing cell expansion or by promoting active elimination) and thus favors viral invasion of the NS. This pathway appears to be crucial for the progression of disease in the NS because mice eliminate the invading virus much more efficiently when the immunosubversive molecules are not expressed (mice deficient for B7-H1 or FasL). As a result, there is a global subversion of the host immune defenses by RABV. This can be seen as a successful well-tailored adaptation of RABV to the host. One would expect that the host's natural capacity to fight such a well-adapted virus is severely restricted. For these reasons, post exposure treatment has to be applied without delay. Because of the difficulty of access to prompt post exposure treatment once the contamination has occured, antirabies vaccination campaigns in children could be an efficient stealth to limit the risk of post exposure treatment protection failure.

REFERENCES

Aarts, M., Liu, Y., Liu, L., Besshoh, S., Arundine, M., Gurd, J. W., Wang, Y. T., Salter, M. W., and Tymianski, M. (2002). Treatment of ischemic brain damage by perturbing NMDA receptor- PSD-95 protein interactions. *Science* 298(5594):846–850.

Allsopp, T. E., Scallan, M. F., Williams, A., and Fazakerley, J. K. (1998). Virus infection induces neuronal apoptosis: A comparison with trophic factor withdrawal. *Cell Death Differ.* 5(1):50–59.

Baloul, L., and Lafon, M. (2003). Apoptosis and rabies virus neuroinvasion. *Biochimie* 85(8):777–788.

Baloul, L., Camelo, S., and Lafon, M. (2004). Up-regulation of Fas ligand (FasL) in the central nervous system: A mechanism of immune evasion by rabies virus. *J. Neurovirol.* 10(6):372–382.

Barajon, I., Serrao, G., Arnaboldi, F., Opizzi, E., Ripamonti, G., Balsari, A., and Rumio, C. (2009). Toll-like receptors 3, 4, and 7 are expressed in the enteric nervous system and dorsal root ganglia. *J. Histochem. Cytochem.* 57(11):1013–1023.

Bechmann, I., Galea, I., and Perry, V. H. (2007). What is the blood-brain barrier (not)? *Trends Immunol.* 28(1):5–11.

Brehin, A.-C., Mouries, J., Frenkiel, M.-P., Dadaglio, G., Despres, P., Lafon, M., and Couderc, T. (2008). Dynamics of immune cell recruitment during West Nile encephalitis and identification of a new CD19+ B220- BST-2+ leukocyte population. *J. Immunol.* 180 (10):6760–6767.

Camelo, S., Lafage, M., and Lafon, M. (2000). Absence of the p55 Kd TNF-alpha receptor promotes survival in rabies virus acute encephalitis. *J. Neurovirol.* 6(6):507–518.

Cameron, J. S., Alexopoulou, L., Sloane, J. A., DiBernardo, A. B., Ma, Y., Kosaras, B., Flavell, R., Strittmatter, S. M., Volpe, J., Sidman, R., and Vartanian, T. (2007). Toll-like receptor 3 is a potent negative regulator of axonal growth in mammals. *J. Neurosci.* 27(47):13033–13041.

Chen, S., Short, J. A., Young, D. F., Killip, M. J., Schneider, M., Goodbourn, S., and Randall, R. E. (2010). Heterocellular induction of interferon by negative-sense RNA viruses. *Virology* 407(2):247–255.

Chiron, D., Pellat-Deceunynck, C., Amiot, M., Bataille, R., and Jego, G. (2009). TLR3 ligand induces NF-{kappa}B activation and various fates of multiple myeloma cells depending on IFN-{alpha} production. *J. Immunol.* **182**(7):4471–4478.

Daffis, S., Samuel, M. A., Suthar, M. S., Gale, M., Jr., and Diamond, M. S. (2008). Toll-like receptor 3 has a protective role against West Nile virus infection. *J. Virol.* **82**(21): 10349–10358.

Davoust, N., Vuaillat, C., Androdias, G., and Nataf, S. (2008). From bone marrow to microglia: Barriers and avenues. *Trends Immunol.* **29**(5):227–234.

Delhaye, S., Paul, S., Blakqori, G., Minet, M., Weber, F., Staeheli, P., and Michiels, T. (2006). Neurons produce type I interferon during viral encephalitis. *Proc. Natl. Acad. Sci. USA* **103** (20):7835–7840.

Dong, H., Strome, S. E., Salomao, D. R., Tamura, H., Hirano, F., Flies, D. B., Roche, P. C., Lu, J., Zhu, G., Tamada, K., Lennon, V. A., Celis, E., *et al.* (2002). Tumor-associated B7-H1 promotes T-cell apoptosis: A potential mechanism of immune evasion. *Nat. Med.* **8**(8): 793–800.

Engelhardt, B. (2008). The blood-central nervous system barriers actively control immune cell entry into the central nervous system. *Curr. Pharm. Des.* **14**(16):1555–1565.

Faber, M., Pulmanausahakul, R., Hodawadekar, S. S., Spitsin, S., McGettigan, J. P., Schnell, M. J., and Dietzschold, B. (2002). Overexpression of the rabies virus glycoprotein results in enhancement of apoptosis and antiviral immune response. *J. Virol.* **76**(7):3374–3381.

Faber, M., Bette, M., Preuss, M. A., Pulmanausahakul, R., Rehnelt, J., Schnell, M. J., Dietzschold, B., and Weihe, E. (2005). Overexpression of tumor necrosis factor alpha by a recombinant rabies virus attenuates replication in neurons and prevents lethal infection in mice. *J. Virol.* **79**(24):15405–15416.

Faul, E. J., Wanjalla, C. N., Suthar, M. S., Gale, M., Wirblich, C., and Schnell, M. J. (2010). Rabies virus infection induces type I interferon production in an IPS-1 dependent manner while dendritic cell activation relies on IFNAR signaling. *PLoS Pathog.* **6**(7):e1001016.

Fu, Z. F., Weihe, E., Zheng, Y. M., Schafer, M. K., Sheng, H., Corisdeo, S., Rauscher, F. J., 3rd, Koprowski, H., and Dietzschold, B. (1993). Differential effects of rabies and borna disease viruses on immediate-early- and late-response gene expression in brain tissues. *J. Virol.* **67**(11):6674–6681.

Furr, S. R., Chauhan, V. S., Sterka, D., Jr., Grdzelishvili, V., and Marriott, I. (2008). Characterization of retinoic acid-inducible gene-I expression in primary murine glia following exposure to vesicular stomatitis virus. *J. Neurovirol.* **14**(6):503–513.

Galelli, A., Baloul, L., and Lafon, M. (2000). Abortive rabies virus central nervous infection is controlled by T lymphocyte local recruitment and induction of apoptosis. *J. Neurovirol.* **6**(5):359–372.

Girard, S., Couderc, T., Destombes, J., Thiesson, D., Delpeyroux, F., and Blondel, B. (1999). Poliovirus induces apoptosis in the mouse central nervous system. *J. Virol.* **73** (7):6066–6072.

Goethals, S., Ydens, E., Timmerman, V., and Janssens, S. (2010). Toll-like receptor expression in the peripheral nerve. *Glia* **58**(14):1701–1709.

Gratas, C., Tohma, Y., Barnas, C., Taniere, P., Hainaut, P., and Ohgaki, H. (1998). Upregulation of Fas (APO-1/CD95) ligand and down-regulation of Fas expression in human esophageal cancer. *Cancer Res.* **58**(10):2057–2062.

Griffiths, M., Neal, J. W., and Gasque, P. (2007). Innate immunity and protective neuroinflammation: New emphasis on the role of neuroimmune regulatory proteins. *Int. Rev. Neurobiol.* **82**:29–55.

Guigoni, C., and Coulon, P. (2002). Rabies virus is not cytolytic for rat spinal motoneurons in vitro. *J. Neurovirol.* **8**(4):306–317.

Harris, B. Z., and Lim, W. A. (2001). Mechanism and role of PDZ domains in signaling complex assembly. *J. Cell Sci.* **114**(Pt 18):3219–3231.

Hemachudha, T., Wacharapluesadee, S., Mitrabhakdi, E., Wilde, H., Morimoto, K., and Lewis, R. A. (2005). Pathophysiology of human paralytic rabies. *J. Neurovirol.* **11**(1):93–100.

Hicks, D. J., Nunez, A., Healy, D. M., Brookes, S. M., Johnson, N., and Fooks, A. R. (2009). Comparative pathological study of the murine brain after experimental infection with classical rabies virus and European bat lyssaviruses. *J. Comp. Pathol.* **140**(2–3):113–126.

Hoek, R. M., Ruuls, S. R., Murphy, C. A., Wright, G. J., Goddard, R., Zurawski, S. M., Blom, B., Homola, M. E., Streit, W. J., Brown, M. H., Barclay, A. N., and Sedgwick, J. D. (2000). Down-regulation of the macrophage lineage through interaction with OX2 (CD200). *Science* **290**(5497):1768–1771.

Hooper, D. C., Morimoto, K., Bette, M., Weihe, E., Koprowski, H., and Dietzschold, B. (1998). Collaboration of antibody and inflammation in clearance of rabies virus from the central nervous system. *J. Virol.* **72**(5):3711–3719.

Hooper, D. C., Phares, T. W., Fabis, M. J., and Roy, A. (2009). The production of antibody by invading B cells is required for the clearance of rabies virus from the central nervous system. *PLoS Negl. Trop. Dis.* **3**(10):e535.

Hornung, V., Ellegast, J., Kim, S., Brzozka, K., Jung, A., Kato, H., Poeck, H., Akira, S., Conzelmann, K. K., Schlee, M., Endres, S., and Hartmann, G. (2006). 5′-Triphosphate RNA is the ligand for RIG-I. *Science* **314**(5801):994–997.

Hou, S. W., Zhi, H. Y., Pohl, N., Loesch, M., Qi, X. M., Li, R. S., Basir, Z., and Chen, G. (2010). PTPH1 dephosphorylates and cooperates with p38gamma MAPK to increase ras oncogenesis through PDZ-mediated interaction. *Cancer Res.* **70**(7):2901–2910.

Irwin, D. J., Wunner, W. H., Ertl, H. C., and Jackson, A. C. (1999). Basis of rabies virus neurovirulence in mice: Expression of major histocompatibility complex class I and class II mRNAs. *J. Neurovirol.* **5**(5):485–494.

Ito, N., Moseley, G. W., Blondel, D., Shimizu, K., Rowe, C. L., Ito, Y., Masatani, T., Nakagawa, K., Jans, D. A., and Sugiyama, M. (2010). Role of interferon antagonist activity of rabies virus phosphoprotein in viral pathogenicity. *J. Virol.* **84**(13):6699–6710.

Iwasaki, Y., Gerhard, W., and Clark, H. F. (1977). Role of host immune response in the development of either encephalitic or paralytic disease after experimental rabies infection in mice. *Infect. Immun.* **18**(1):220–225.

Jackson, A. C., Rossiter, J. P., and Lafon, M. (2006). Expression of Toll-like receptor 3 in the human cerebellar cortex in rabies, herpes simplex encephalitis, and other neurological diseases. *J. Neurovirol.* **12**(3):229–234.

Jackson, A. C., Scott, C. A., Owen, J., Weli, S. C., and Rossiter, J. P. (2007). Therapy with minocycline aggravates experimental rabies in mice. *J. Virol.* **81**(12):6248–6253.

Jackson, A. C., Randle, E., Lawrance, G., and Rossiter, J. P. (2008). Neuronal apoptosis does not play an important role in human rabies encephalitis. *J. Neurovirol.* **14**(5):368–375.

Jackson, A. C., Kammouni, W., Zherebitskaya, E., and Fernyhough, P. (2010). Role of oxidative stress in rabies virus infection of adult mouse dorsal root ganglion neurons. *J. Virol.* **84**(9):4697–4705.

Johnston, J. A., Ward, C. L., and Kopito, R. R. (1998). Aggresomes: A cellular response to misfolded proteins. *J. Cell Biol.* **143**(7):1883–1898.

Juntrakul, S., Ruangvejvorachai, P., Shuangshoti, S., Wacharapluesadee, S., and Hemachudha, T. (2005). Mechanisms of escape phenomenon of spinal cord and brainstem in human rabies. *BMC Infect. Dis.* **5**:104.

Klein, R. S., Lin, E., Zhang, B., Luster, A. D., Tollett, J., Samuel, M. A., Engle, M., and Diamond, M. S. (2005). Neuronal CXCL10 directs CD8+ T-cell recruitment and control of West Nile virus encephalitis. *J. Virol.* **79**(17):11457–11466.

Klingen, Y., Conzelmann, K. K., and Finke, S. (2008). Double-labeled rabies virus: Live tracking of enveloped virus transport. *J. Virol.* **82**(1):237–245.

Kojima, D., Park, C. H., Satoh, Y., Inoue, S., Noguchi, A., and Oyamada, T. (2009). Pathology of the spinal cord of C57BL/6J mice infected with rabies virus (CVS-11 strain). *J. Vet. Med. Sci.* **71**(3):319–324.

Kojima, D., Park, C. H., Tsujikawa, S., Kohara, K., Hatai, H., Oyamada, T., Noguchi, A., and Inoue, S. (2010). Lesions of the central nervous system induced by intracerebral inoculation of BALB/c mice with rabies virus (CVS-11). *J. Vet. Med. Sci.* **72**(8):1011–1016.

Kolodziejska, K. E., Burns, A. R., Moore, R. H., Stenoien, D. L., and Eissa, N. T. (2005). Regulation of inducible nitric oxide synthase by aggresome formation. *Proc. Natl. Acad. Sci. USA* **102**(13):4854–4859.

Kopito, R. R. (2000). Aggresomes, inclusion bodies and protein aggregation. *Trends Cell Biol.* **10**(12):524–530.

Kristensson, K., Dastur, D. K., Manghani, D. K., Tsiang, H., and Bentivoglio, M. (1996). Rabies: Interactions between neurons and viruses. A review of the history of Negri inclusion bodies. *Neuropathol. Appl. Neurobiol.* **22**(3):179–187.

Lafon, M. (2005). Modulation of the immune response in the nervous system by rabies virus. *Curr. Top. Microbiol. Immunol.* **289**:239–258.

Lafon, M. (2008). Immune evasion, a critical strategy for rabies virus. *Dev. Biol. (Basel)* **131**:413–419.

Lafon, M., Prehaud, C., Megret, F., Lafage, M., Mouillot, G., Roa, M., Moreau, P., Rouas-Freiss, N., and Carosella, E. D. (2005). Modulation of HLA-G expression in human neural cells after neurotropic viral infections. *J. Virol.* **79**(24):15226–15237.

Lafon, M., Megret, F., Lafage, M., and Prehaud, C. (2006). The innate immune facet of brain: Human neurons express TLR-3 and sense viral dsRNA. *J. Mol. Neurosci.* **29**(3):185–194.

Lafon, M., Megret, F., Meuth, S. G., Simon, O., Velandia Romero, M. L., Lafage, M., Chen, L., Alexopoulou, L., Flavell, R. A., Prehaud, C., and Wiendl, H. (2008). Detrimental contribution of the immuno-inhibitor b7-h1 to rabies virus encephalitis. *J. Immunol.* **180**(11): 7506–7515.

Lahaye, X., Vidy, A., Pomier, C., Obiang, L., Harper, F., Gaudin, Y., and Blondel, D. (2009). Functional characterization of Negri bodies (NBs) in rabies virus infected cells: Evidence that NBs are sites of viral transcription and replication. *J. Virol.* **83**(16):7948–7958.

Laothamatas, J., Wacharapluesadee, S., Lumlertdacha, B., Ampawong, S., Tepsumethanon, V., Shuangshoti, S., Phumesin, P., Asavaphatiboon, S., Worapruekjaru, L., Avihingsanon, Y., Israsena, N., Lafon, M., *et al.* (2008). Furious and paralytic rabies of canine origin: Neuroimaging with virological and cytokine studies. *J. Neurovirol.* **14**(2):119–129.

Lathia, J. D., Okun, E., Tang, S. C., Griffioen, K., Cheng, A., Mughal, M. R., Laryea, G., Selvaraj, P. K., ffrench-Constant, C., Magnus, T., Arumugam, T. V., and Mattson, M. P. (2008). Toll-like receptor 3 is a negative regulator of embryonic neural progenitor cell proliferation. *J. Neurosci.* **28**(51):13978–13984.

Lee, H. J., and Zheng, J. J. (2010). PDZ domains and their binding partners: Structure, specificity, and modification. *Cell. Commun. Signal.* **8**:8.

Liu, J., Hamrouni, A., Wolowiec, D., Coiteux, V., Kuliczkowski, K., Hetuin, D., Saudemont, A., and Quesnel, B. (2007). Plasma cells from multiple myeloma patients express B7-H1 (PD-L1) and increase expression after stimulation with IFN-{gamma} and TLR ligands via a MyD88-, TRAF6-, and MEK-dependent pathway. *Blood* **110**(1):296–304.

Loh, S. H., Francescut, L., Lingor, P., Bahr, M., and Nicotera, P. (2008). Identification of new kinase clusters required for neurite outgrowth and retraction by a loss-of-function RNA interference screen. *Cell Death Differ.* **15**(2):283–298.

Masatani, T., Ito, N., Shimizu, K., Ito, Y., Nakagawa, K., Sawaki, Y., Koyama, H., and Sugiyama, M. (2010). Rabies virus nucleoprotein functions to evade activation of the RIG-I-mediated antiviral response. *J. Virol.* **84**(8):4002–4012.

Megret, F., Prehaud, C., Lafage, M., Batejat, C., Escriou, N., Lay, S., Thoulouze, M. I., and Lafon, M. (2005). Immunopotentiation of the antibody response against influenza HA with apoptotic bodies generated by rabies virus G-ERA protein-driven apoptosis. *Vaccine* **23**:5342–5350.

Megret, F., Prehaud, C., Lafage, M., Moreau, P., Rouas-Freiss, N., Carosella, E. D., and Lafon, M. (2007). Modulation of HLA-G and HLA-E expression in human neuronal cells after rabies virus or herpes virus simplex type 1 infections. *Hum. Immunol.* **68**(4):294–302.

Meldolesi, J. (2010). Neurite outgrowth: This process, first discovered by Santiago Ramon y Cajal, is sustained by the exocytosis of two distinct types of vesicles. *Brain. Res. Rev.* **66**(1-2):246–255.

Menager, P., Roux, P., Megret, F., Bourgeois, J. P., Le Sourd, A. M., Danckaert, A., Lafage, M., Prehaud, C., and Lafon, M. (2009). Toll-like receptor 3 (TLR3) plays a major role in the formation of rabies virus Negri Bodies. *PLoS Pathog.* **5**(2):e1000315.

Meuth, S. G., Simon, O. J., Grimm, A., Melzer, N., Herrmann, A. M., Spitzer, P., Landgraf, P., and Wiendl, H. (2008). CNS inflammation and neuronal degeneration is aggravated by impaired CD200-CD200R-mediated macrophage silencing. *J. Neuroimmunol.* **194**(1–2):62–69.

Montano-Hirose, J. A., Lafage, M., Weber, P., Badrane, H., Tordo, N., and Lafon, M. (1993). Protective activity of a murine monoclonal antibody against European bat lyssavirus 1 (EBL1) infection in mice. *Vaccine* **11**(12):1259–1266.

Morimoto, K., Hooper, D. C., Spitsin, S., Koprowski, H., and Dietzschold, B. (1999). Pathogenicity of different rabies virus variants inversely correlates with apoptosis and rabies virus glycoprotein expression in infected primary neuron cultures. *J. Virol.* **73**(1):510–518.

Niederkorn, J. Y. (2006). See no evil, hear no evil, do no evil: The lessons of immune privilege. *Nat. Immunol.* **7**(4):354–359.

Nourry, C., Grant, S. G., and Borg, J. P. (2003). PDZ domain proteins: Plug and play. *Sci. STKE* **2003**(179):RE7.

Olson, J. K., and Miller, S. D. (2004). Microglia initiate central nervous system innate and adaptive immune responses through multiple TLRs. *J. Immunol.* **173**(6):3916–3924.

Park, C. H., Kondo, M., Inoue, S., Noguchi, A., Oyamada, T., Yoshikawa, H., and Yamada, A. (2006). The histopathogenesis of paralytic rabies in six-week-old C57BL/6J mice following inoculation of the CVS-11 strain into the right triceps surae muscle. *J. Vet. Med. Sci.* **68**(6):589–595.

Peltier, D. C., Simms, A., Farmer, J. R., and Miller, D. J. (2010). Human neuronal cells possess functional cytoplasmic and TLR-mediated innate immune pathways influenced by phosphatidylinositol-3 kinase signaling. *J. Immunol.* **184**(12):7010–7021.

Phares, T. W., Kean, R. B., Mikheeva, T., and Hooper, D. C. (2006). Regional differences in blood-brain barrier permeability changes and inflammation in the apathogenic clearance of virus from the central nervous system. *J. Immunol.* **176**(12):7666–7675.

Prehaud, C., Lay, S., Dietzschold, B., and Lafon, M. (2003). Glycoprotein of nonpathogenic rabies viruses is a key determinant of human cell apoptosis. *J. Virol.* **77**(19):10537–10547.

Prehaud, C., Megret, F., Lafage, M., and Lafon, M. (2005). Virus infection switches TLR-3-positive human neurons to become strong producers of beta interferon. *J. Virol.* **79**(20):12893–12904.

Prehaud, C., Wolff, N., Terrien, E., Lafage, M., Megret, F., Babault, N., Cordier, F., Tan, G. S., Maitrepierre, E., Menager, P., Chopy, D., Hoos, S., *et al.* (2010). Attenuation of rabies virulence: Takeover by the cytoplasmic domain of its envelope protein. *Sci. Signal.* **3**(105):ra5.

Pulko, V., Liu, X., Krco, C. J., Harris, K. J., Frigola, X., Kwon, E. D., and Dong, H. (2009). TLR3-stimulated dendritic cells up-regulate B7-H1 expression and influence the magnitude of CD8 T cell responses to tumor vaccination. *J. Immunol.* **183**(6):3634–3641.

Randall, R. E., and Goodbourn, S. (2008). Interferons and viruses: An interplay between induction, signalling, antiviral responses and virus countermeasures. *J. Gen. Virol.* **89**(Pt 1):1–47.

Rieder, M., and Conzelmann, K. K. (2009). Rhabdovirus evasion of the interferon system. *J. Interferon Cytokine Res.* **29**(9):499–509.

Rossiter, J. P., Hsu, L., and Jackson, A. C. (2009). Selective vulnerability of dorsal root ganglia neurons in experimental rabies after peripheral inoculation of CVS-11 in adult mice. *Acta Neuropathol.* **118**(2):249–259.

Rouas-Freiss, N., Moreau, P., Menier, C., and Carosella, E. D. (2003). HLA-G in cancer: A way to turn off the immune system. *Semin. Cancer Biol.* **13**(5):325–336.

Roy, A., and Hooper, D. C. (2007). Lethal silver-haired bat rabies virus infection can be prevented by opening the blood-brain barrier. *J. Virol.* **81**(15):7993–7998.

Roy, A., Phares, T. W., Koprowski, H., and Hooper, D. C. (2007). Failure to open the blood-brain barrier and deliver immune effectors to central nervous system tissues leads to the lethal outcome of silver-haired bat rabies virus infection. *J. Virol.* **81**(3):1110–1118.

Schafernak, K. T., and Bigio, E. H. (2006). West Nile virus encephalomyelitis with polio-like paralysis & nigral degeneration. *Can. J. Neurol. Sci.* **33**(4):407–410.

Schreiner, B., Mitsdoerffer, M., Kieseier, B. C., Chen, L., Hartung, H. P., Weller, M., and Wiendl, H. (2004). Interferon-beta enhances monocyte and dendritic cell expression of B7-H1 (PD-L1), a strong inhibitor of autologous T-cell activation: Relevance for the immune modulatory effect in multiple sclerosis. *J. Neuroimmunol.* **155**(1–2):172–182.

Scott, C. A., Rossiter, J. P., Andrew, R. D., and Jackson, A. C. (2008). Structural abnormalities in neurons are sufficient to explain the clinical disease and fatal outcome of experimental rabies in yellow fluorescent protein-expressing transgenic mice. *J. Virol.* **82**(1):513–521.

Shankar, V., Kao, M., Hamir, A. N., Sheng, H., Koprowski, H., and Dietzschold, B. (1992). Kinetics of virus spread and changes in levels of several cytokine mRNAs in the brain after intranasal infection of rats with Borna disease virus. *J. Virol.* **66**(2):992–998.

Sheng, M., and Sala, C. (2001). PDZ domains and the organization of supramolecular complexes. *Annu. Rev. Neurosci.* **24**:1–29.

Sommereyns, C., Paul, S., Staeheli, P., and Michiels, T. (2008). IFN-lambda (IFN-lambda) is expressed in a tissue-dependent fashion and primarily acts on epithelial cells in vivo. *PLoS Pathog.* **4**(3):e1000017.

Tang, S. C., Arumugam, T. V., Xu, X., Cheng, A., Mughal, M. R., Jo, D. G., Lathia, J. D., Siler, D. A., Chigurupati, S., Ouyang, X., Magnus, T., Camandola, S., *et al.* (2007). Pivotal role for neuronal Toll-like receptors in ischemic brain injury and functional deficits. *Proc. Natl. Acad. Sci. USA* **104**(34):13798–13803.

Tang, S. C., Lathia, J. D., Selvaraj, P. K., Jo, D. G., Mughal, M. R., Cheng, A., Siler, D. A., Markesbery, W. R., Arumugam, T. V., and Mattson, M. P. (2008). Toll-like receptor-4 mediates neuronal apoptosis induced by amyloid beta-peptide and the membrane lipid peroxidation product 4-hydroxynonenal. *Exp. Neurol.* **213**(1):114–121.

Thoulouze, M. I., Lafage, M., Montano-Hirose, J. A., and Lafon, M. (1997). Rabies virus infects mouse and human lymphocytes and induces apoptosis. *J. Virol.* **71**(10):7372–7380.

Thoulouze, M. I., Lafage, M., Yuste, V. J., Baloul, L., Edelman, L., Kroemer, G., Israel, N., Susin, S. A., and Lafon, M. (2003). High level of Bcl-2 counteracts apoptosis mediated by a live rabies virus vaccine strain and induces long-term infection. *Virology* **314**(2):549–561.

Tobiume, M., Sato, Y., Katano, H., Nakajima, N., Tanaka, K., Noguchi, A., Inoue, S., Hasegawa, H., Iwasa, Y., Tanaka, J., Hayashi, H., Yoshida, S., *et al.* (2009). Rabies virus dissemination in neural tissues of autopsy cases due to rabies imported into Japan from the Philippines: Immunohistochemistry. *Pathol. Int.* **59**(8):555–566.

Tsunoda, I., Tanaka, T., Saijoh, Y., and Fujinami, R. S. (2007). Targeting inflammatory demyelinating lesions to sites of Wallerian degeneration. *Am. J. Pathol.* **171**(5):1563–1575.

Ugolini, G. (1995). Specificity of rabies virus as a transneuronal tracer of motor networks: Transfer from hypoglossal motoneurons to connected second-order and higher order central nervous system cell groups. *J. Comp. Neurol.* **356**(3):457–480.

Ugolini, G. (2010). Advances in viral transneuronal tracing. *J. Neurosci. Methods* **194**(1):2–20.

Vuaillat, C., Varrin-Doyer, M., Bernard, A., Sagardoy, I., Cavagna, S., Chounlamountri, I., Lafon, M., and Giraudon, P. (2008). High CRMP2 expression in peripheral T lymphocytes is associated with recruitment to the brain during virus-induced neuroinflammation. *J. Neuroimmunol.* **193**(1–2):38–51.

Wang, T., Town, T., Alexopoulou, L., Anderson, J. F., Fikrig, E., and Flavell, R. A. (2004). Toll-like receptor 3 mediates West Nile virus entry into the brain causing lethal encephalitis. *Nat. Med.* **10**(12):1366–1373.

Wang, Z. W., Sarmento, L., Wang, Y., Li, X. Q., Dhingra, V., Tseggai, T., Jiang, B., and Fu, Z. F. (2005). Attenuated rabies virus activates, while pathogenic rabies virus evades, the host innate immune responses in the central nervous system. *J. Virol.* **79**(19):12554–12565.

Weihe, E., Bette, M., Preuss, M. A., Faber, M., Schafer, M. K., Rehnelt, J., Schnell, M. J., and Dietzschold, B. (2008). Role of virus-induced neuropeptides in the brain in the pathogenesis of rabies. *Dev. Biol. (Basel)* **131**:73–81.

Weiland, F., Cox, J. H., Meyer, S., Dahme, E., and Reddehase, M. J. (1992). Rabies virus neuritic paralysis: Immunopathogenesis of nonfatal paralytic rabies. *J. Virol.* **66**(8): 5096–5099.

Wiktor, T. J., Macfarlan, R. I., Reagan, K. J., Dietzschold, B., Curtis, P. J., Wunner, W. H., Kieny, M. P., Lathe, R., Lecocq, J. P., Mackett, M., *et al.* (1984). Protection from rabies by a vaccinia virus recombinant containing the rabies virus glycoprotein gene. *Proc. Natl. Acad. Sci. USA* **81**(22):7194–7198.

Wright, G. J., Puklavec, M. J., Willis, A. C., Hoek, R. M., Sedgwick, J. D., Brown, M. H., and Barclay, A. N. (2000). Lymphoid/neuronal cell surface OX2 glycoprotein recognizes a novel receptor on macrophages implicated in the control of their function. *Immunity* **13**(2):233–242.

Wunner, W. H., Dietzschold, B., Curtis, P. J., and Wiktor, T. J. (1983). Rabies subunit vaccines. *J. Gen. Virol.* **64**(Pt 8):1649–1656.

Xiang, Z. Q., Knowles, B. B., McCarrick, J. W., and Ertl, H. C. (1995). Immune effector mechanisms required for protection to rabies virus. *Virology* **214**(2):398–404.

Yanagisawa, J., Takahashi, M., Kanki, H., Yano-Yanagisawa, H., Tazunoki, T., Sawa, E., Nishitoba, T., Kamishohara, M., Kobayashi, E., Kataoka, S., and Sato, T. (1997). The molecular interaction of Fas and FAP-1. A tripeptide blocker of human Fas interaction with FAP-1 promotes Fas-induced apoptosis. *J. Biol. Chem.* **272**(13):8539–8545.

Yang, L., Voytek, C. C., and Margolis, T. P. (2000). Immunohistochemical analysis of primary sensory neurons latently infected with herpes simplex virus type 1. *J. Virol.* **74**(1):209–217.

Zhang, B., Chan, Y. K., Lu, B., Diamond, M. S., and Klein, R. S. (2008). CXCR3 mediates region-specific antiviral T cell trafficking within the central nervous system during West Nile virus encephalitis. *J. Immunol.* **180**(4):2641–2649.

Zhou, L., Wang, X., Wang, Y. J., Zhou, Y., Hu, S., Ye, L., Hou, W., Li, H., and Ho, W. Z. (2009). Activation of toll-like receptor-3 induces interferon-lambda expression in human neuronal cells. *Neuroscience* **159**(2):629–637.

CHAPTER 4

Rabies Virus Clearance from the Central Nervous System

**D. Craig Hooper,*,† Anirban Roy,*,1 Darryll
A. Barkhouse,* Jianwei Li,* and Rhonda B. Kean***

Contents

* Center for Neurovirology, Department of Cancer Biology, Thomas Jefferson University, Philadelphia, Pennsylvania, USA
† Center for Neurovirology, Department of Neurological Surgery, Thomas Jefferson University, Philadelphia, Pennsylvania, USA
1 Current address: Department of Environmental Medicine, University of Rochester, Rochester, New York, USA

Advances in Virus Research, Volume 79
ISSN 0065-3527, DOI: 10.1016/B978-0-12-387040-7.00004-4

Abstract   Rabies, a neurological disease associated with replication in central nervous system (CNS) tissues of any of a number of rabies viruses endemic in nature, is generally fatal. Prophylactic medical intervention is immune mediated and directed at preventing the spread of the virus from a peripheral site of exposure to the CNS. While individuals rarely develop immune responses capable of clearing the virus from CNS tissues, a variety of laboratory-attenuated rabies viruses are readily cleared from the CNS tissues in animal models. By comparing immune responses to wild-type and attenuated rabies viruses in these models, we have discovered that the latter induce processes required for immune effector infiltration into CNS tissues that are absent from lethal infections. Predominant among these are activities of cells of the neurovascular unit (NVU) that promote an interaction with circulating immune cells. In the absence of this interaction, the specialized barrier function of the NVU remains intact and circulating virus-specific immune effectors are largely excluded from infected CNS tissues. Studies of mixed infections with wild-type and attenuated rabies viruses reveal that wild-type rabies viruses fail to trigger, rather than inhibit, the interactions between immune cells and the NVU required for virus clearance from the CNS. These studies provide insights into how immune effectors with the capacity to clear the virus may be delivered into CNS tissues to contain a wild-type rabies virus infection. However, to apply immunotherapeutic strategies beyond the initial stages of CNS infection, further insights into the fate of the infected cells during virus clearance are needed.

I. INTRODUCTION

Phenotypic and functional characteristics of rabies virus are detailed elsewhere in this volume; therefore, we will only briefly summarize features pertinent to viral clearance from the central nervous system (CNS) before reviewing the mechanisms that make this possible. It should be noted that rabies virus infection of the CNS, whether by wild-type or attenuated variants, is unique in avoiding the pathological CNS inflammation associated with most neurotropic viral infections (Roy *et al.*, 2007;

Wang *et al.*, 2006). Thus rabies virus clearance from the CNS represents an ideal model of therapeutic CNS immunity.

II. RABIES VIRUS

Rabies is caused by CNS infection with one of a variety of rabies viruses that are endemic in different animal species. Each animal that serves as a natural reservoir of the virus carries a variant of rabies virus that is genetically, if not antigenically, distinguishable from the strains carried by other reservoir species (Baer *et al.*, 1990). Thus, the origin of a variant of the virus that causes rabies in humans, who are not natural reservoirs of rabies virus, can be accurately established if virus is recovered. A lyssavirus, rabies virus, has an unsegmented, linear, negative sense RNA genome that encodes five genes. The rabies virus glycoprotein (G) is the target of virus-neutralizing antibodies (VNA) and is generally expressed at relatively low levels in cells infected with wild-type rabies viruses (Cox *et al.*, 1977). The low level of G expression likely enables the virus to at least partly escape immune recognition during an infection. Laboratory-attenuated strains of rabies viruses express high levels of glycoprotein and, somewhat paradoxically, are more cytotoxic. Both features likely contribute to the generation of more effective antiviral immunity (Morimoto *et al.*, 1999). However, the rabies virus particle is inherently immunogenic as the administration of several doses of inactivated virus induces strong immune responses capable of protecting against subsequent infection with all rabies virus variants and antigenically cross-reactive lyssaviruses. Inactivated rabies virus is the basis of all current human rabies vaccination.

III. ANIMAL RESERVOIRS OF THE RABIES VIRUS AND THE THREAT OF HUMAN RABIES

A. Domestic animals

Dogs have been associated with human rabies throughout recorded history, and elimination of the virus from this natural reservoir by vaccination represents the single most important advance in controlling human exposure in many countries (Hampson *et al.*, 2009). Nevertheless, there are still large areas where dogs are not vaccinated against rabies, and dog rabies continues to be the major cause of human rabies worldwide. The reasons for not vaccinating dogs against rabies can be complex, and it seems unlikely that dog rabies will be controlled globally in the foreseeable future despite the availability of relatively inexpensive vaccines.

Consequently, human exposure to dog rabies is expected to continue at relatively high rates in certain geographical areas. For example, there are annually upward of 50,000 human rabies cases of dog origin in India, where the limited availability or expense of effective reagents mitigates against postexposure prophylaxis (PEP). In this case, the unknown risk of developing rabies after a possible exposure may be considered to be acceptable and PEP not sought after. Immunotherapy that could clear the virus from the CNS when the earliest signs of rabies appear may have potential utility in these circumstances.

While other domestic animals are not natural carriers of rabies virus, all mammals can be infected with the virus. Thus, other animals that are in contact with both humans and wildlife, such as cats, can transmit the virus from a reservoir species to humans and should be considered as potential vectors with exposures. As is the case for dog exposures, aberrant behavior during contact with an animal and, particularly, aggression culminating in a bite or a scratch should emphasize the need for laboratory evaluation of the animal for rabies and PEP if warranted. However, the lack of a clear exposure from a rabies reservoir species may result in the failure to obtain PEP, necessitating rabies immunotherapy capable of clearing the virus from CNS tissues.

B. Terrestrial wildlife

Natural reservoirs of rabies virus differ in different geographic regions. Foxes were an important reservoir of rabies in Europe that has largely been controlled by vaccination. In different areas of North America, rabies is endemic in raccoons and skunks, and it was previously endemic in coyotes. These animals usually avoid humans, and the absence of fear of humans should raise the possibility of rabies. There is a requirement for further investigation and PEP if transdermal or mucosal exposure to the animal's saliva is probable. A treatment paradigm effective after the disease manifests would only be necessary if PEP is not administered promptly, or if there is evidence that it failed in preventing viral spread to the CNS.

C. Bats

Rabies viruses are borne by a number of bat species in the Americas, whereas bats in Europe and Australia can carry rabies-related lyssaviruses. Bat rabies represents the greatest risk of transmission to humans without an identifiable exposure incident. Moreover, individuals who come into contact with a bat carrying the virus are often unaware of the risk. The event that transfers the virus is certainly less obvious than that associated with the bite of a large carnivore.

The result is that a number of individuals die each year of rabies due to bat rabies virus variants because they had no idea that they were exposed and they did not seek PEP.

IV. HUMAN RABIES

A. Pathogenesis

Despite the long history of human rabies, the pathogenesis of the disease remains poorly understood. We know that in the first days after infection, while the virus is traveling through peripheral nerve axons to the CNS, there is no clinical evidence of the infection. Definitive signs of disease do not appear until the virus reaches the CNS, when a wide range of nonspecific physiological, as well as more pathognomonic signs begin to develop. As more aggressive therapies for human rabies are attempted, we are beginning to learn more about the physiological changes that occur as the disease progresses (Willoughby *et al.*, 2005). However, much of our understanding of rabies pathogenesis in humans has been obtained from end-stage disease and, while much information has been gained from studies in animal models of the disease, little is known about the extent of neuronal involvement at earlier stages in humans.

B. Immunity

Historical data tell us that the incidence of clinical rabies in untreated individuals bitten by rabid animals is approximately 50–60% (Baltazard and Ghodssi, 1954). A small number of exposed individuals may have infection without clinical disease and develop protective immunity. Naturally infected humans who do not receive PEP and develop rabies generally do not mount a strong immune response to rabies virus until relatively late in the disease (Centers for Disease Control and Prevention, 2006, 2008a). VNA can appear in the sera and CSF, but the titers are usually relatively low (Centers for Disease Control and Prevention, 2008a). This contrasts with animal models where strong peripheral immune responses to wild-type rabies viruses often develop prior to a lethal outcome (Roy and Hooper, 2007, 2008; Roy *et al.*, 2007). Wild-type rabies virus infection in animal models also triggers innate immune mechanisms in the infected CNS tissues (Roy and Hooper, 2007, 2008; Roy *et al.*, 2007). Whether this is the case for the early stages of virus replication in the CNS of humans is unknown. However, it is likely that both innate and adaptive immune mechanisms were responsible for virus clearance in the rare individuals who have survived clinical rabies (Willoughby *et al.*, 2005).

V. THE CURRENT RABIES POSTEXPOSURE TREATMENT PARADIGM

A. History

The origin of rabies PEP in the successful treatment of Joseph Meister in 1885 by Louis Pasteur based on studies with Emile Roux is well known (Pasteur, 1885). The initial vaccination consisted of a series of inoculations prepared from dried spinal cord tissues from rabbits that had died from rabies, the 13th dose consisting of the most virulent preparation (Pasteur, 1885). Consequently, the vaccine series progressed from a killed or highly attenuated preparation to live rabies virus. Inactivated nerve tissue vaccines became the basis of rabies PEP until Hilary Koprowski showed in 1954 that a combination of vaccine and rabies antiserum was more effective (Koprowski and Black, 1954). Modern PEP consists of proper wound management, the administration of inactivated rabies virus vaccine and rabies immune globulin (Centers for Disease Control and Prevention, 2008b).

B. Efficacy

Over 20,000 individuals receive rabies PEP each year in the United States, where there has been no reported PEP failure with approved reagents properly administered promptly after a possible exposure (Krebs *et al.*, 1998). However, PEP failures have been reported elsewhere that cannot be attributed to poor reagents or errors in administration (Wilde, 2007). Most have been associated with bites on the face or upper extremities and many with the relatively rapid onset of clinical rabies (Wilde, 2007). These observations are consistent with the concept that PEP acts by preventing rabies virus spread to the CNS and that neither passively administered VNA nor the adaptive immune mechanisms induced by inactivated rabies vaccine are effective if the virus reaches CNS tissues.

VI. OBSTACLES IN CLEARING WILD-TYPE RABIES VIRUS FROM THE CNS

A. Induction of rabies virus-specific immunity

A wide variety of natural and laboratory-generated rabies virus variants are available for comparative studies of antiviral immunity. Attenuated strains have been derived by antibody escape mutation (Dietzschold *et al.*, 1983), cloned from laboratory-passaged virus (Morimoto *et al.*, 1998), and reverse-engineered to express attenuating products including cytochrome *c* (Pulmanausahakul *et al.*, 2001), TNFα (Faber *et al.*, 2005), chemokines (Zhao *et al.*, 2009), and elevated amounts of glycoprotein (Faber *et al.*, 2002). All induce strong rabies virus-specific VNA responses, which are considered to be the principal antiviral immune effector (Hooper *et al.*, 1998). However, mouse model infections with wild-type rabies viruses also induce substantial VNA titers that are often indistinguishable from attenuated rabies viruses such as glycoprotein 333 mutant CVS-F3 (Roy and Hooper, 2007; Roy *et al.*, 2007). In normal mice, both attenuated and wild-type rabies viruses induce a Th1-type immune response characterized by a predominantly IgG2a and IgG2b antibody response (Roy *et al.*, 2007). While there may be subtle differences between peripheral immunity induced by infection with attenuated in comparison with wild-type rabies viruses, adoptive transfer experiments in mice demonstrate that immune effectors from the lymphoid organs of mice lethally infected with a silver-haired bat rabies virus (SHBRV) can clear attenuated CVS-F3 from T and B cell-deficient recipients (Roy *et al.*, 2007). Thus, wild-type rabies virus lethality in mice is unlikely to be the consequence of a defect in the development of rabies virus-specific immunity.

B. Delivery of rabies virus-specific immune effectors to the CNS

1. Blood–brain barrier integrity

With the exception of HEP-Flury in 129/SvEv mice, all of the rabies viruses that we have tested spread to the mouse CNS following intradermal inoculation (Roy and Hooper, 2008). Serum antibody and VNA titers are comparable at day 8 of infection regardless of the outcome (Roy and Hooper, 2008). In addition, the expression of proinflammatory cytokine and chemokine genes in the infected CNS tissues does not substantially differ (Roy and Hooper, 2008). Nevertheless, immune effectors, including T and B cells, appear in the CNS tissues of mice where attenuated rabies virus has spread to the CNS, but not in animals with wild-type virus in the CNS (Roy and Hooper, 2008). Moreover, the fluid-phase permeability associated with immune cell infiltration into the CNS tissues of mice infected with attenuated rabies virus is undetectable in mice infected with wild-type rabies virus (Roy and Hooper, 2008). This suggested to us that there may be a defect in the immune–blood–brain barrier (BBB) interaction that is required for immune cell entry into CNS tissues (Roy and Hooper, 2008). Under normal circumstances, the BBB limits contact between cells and factors in the circulation and those in the CNS. During the course of the clearance of attenuated rabies virus from CNS tissues, the BBB becomes permeable to fluid-phase markers, but not to larger molecules (Fabis *et al.*, 2008). This presumably allows immune cells adherent in the neurovasculature to detect chemoattractants produced in the CNS and move up the gradient across the BBB toward the infected tissues.

These and other findings led us to conclude that wild-type rabies viruses evade immune clearance from CNS tissues through the maintenance of BBB integrity (Fabis *et al.*, 2008; Roy and Hooper, 2007; Roy *et al.*, 2007).

2. Mechanisms of BBB permeability

In studies with CVS-F3 in mouse adoptive transfer models, we identified CD4 T cells as the principal effectors of the fluid-phase BBB permeability associated with immune effector entry into the CNS and virus clearance (Phares *et al.*, 2007). Elevated BBB permeability correlated with IFN-γ, but not with TNFα, mRNA levels in the surrounding CNS tissues (Phares *et al.*, 2007). IFN-γ treatment was found to induce permeability in an *in vitro* BBB model through a process dependent upon the activity of the peroxynitrite-dependent radical NO_2 (Phares *et al.*, 2007). We had long been aware of an association not only between the enhanced expression of NOS-2 in CNS tissues infected with attenuated rabies virus (Akaike *et al.*, 1995) but also with the role of NOS-2 and its oxidative products NO, peroxynitrite, and NO_2, in pathological CNS inflammation (Hooper *et al.*, 2000, 2001; Spitsin *et al.*, 2000). We therefore compared CNS tissues from CVS-F3-infected mice and mice with the autoimmune disease experimental allergic encephalomyelitis (EAE) and found that NOS-2 and an end-product of the peroxynitrite-dependent pathway, nitrated tyrosine residues, are restricted to the neurovasculature during CVS-F3 clearance as opposed to their association with more destructive invasive cells in EAE (Fabis *et al.*, 2008). This results in the production of radicals that can influence BBB function being focused in the neurovasculature and not elaborated deeper in the CNS parenchyma where their cytotoxicity would be problematic.

3. The immune–BBB interface

If functional changes in the BBB leading to immune cell infiltration of CNS tissues are induced by CD4[+] Th1 cells elaborating IFN-γ, it would be expected that there must be a close interaction between these cells and cells of the neurovascular unit (NVU). During the course of rabies virus infection with either attenuated or wild-type rabies viruses, neurovascular endothelial cells express the important adhesion molecule ICAM-1 in response to TNFα produced by CNS resident cells (Phares *et al.*, 2006; Roy *et al.*, 2007). This would allow activated, LFA-1[+] CD4 T cells to adhere in the neurovasculature, but induction of IFN-γ production would normally involve MHC class II-dependent antigen recognition. We therefore examined microvessels in CNS tissues from mice clearing CVS-F3 and found that they are indeed MHC class II-positive (Hooper *et al.*, submitted). This suggests the possibility that an interaction between the CD4 T cell receptor and MHC class II, possibly containing rabies virus peptide, which leads to IFN-γ production may be required for the entry of these cells into the CNS. While formal proof of this hypothesis in an intact animal will be a

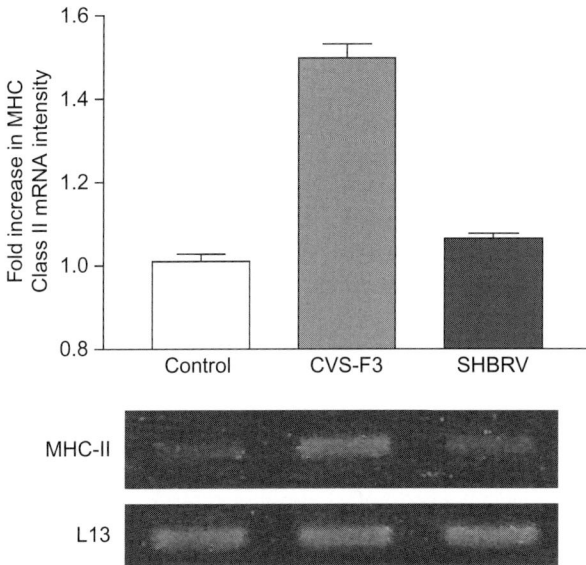

FIGURE 1 The expression of MHC class II in CNS tissues is deficient in mice infected with wild-type rabies virus. Microvessels were isolated from the CNS tissues of 129/SvEv mice infected intradermally in both ears with either 10^5 focus-forming units of the attenuated rabies virus strain CVS-F3 or 10^4 focus-forming units of the pathogenic strain SHBRV in 10 μL of PBS as previously described (Roy et al., 2007). RNA was extracted and subjected to RT-PCR using probes specific for I-A^b and the housekeeping gene L13 and the images of the gels assessed by ImageJ. MHC class II intensity was normalized to that of L13 and is expressed as a fold increase by comparison with the band in samples from normal mice.

challenge, it should be noted that infection with wild-type SHBRV does not induce MHC class II expression in the neurovasculature (Fig. 1) or immune cell invasion into the CNS (Roy et al., 2007). In addition, mice lacking Th1 cells (Tbet$^{-/-}$) have a deficit in the development of the capacity to clear rabies virus from the CNS. Administration of the GAS–GAS rabies vaccine raises a VNA response that is comparable in Tbet$^{-/-}$ and congenic controls, yet only the latter are fully protected against intracranial challenge with wild-type virus at 10 days after vaccination (Fig. 2). These observations support the concept that an interaction between IFN-γ-producing T cells and MHC class II-expressing cells associated with the NVU makes an important contribution to rabies virus clearance from the CNS.

4. CNS innate immunity

Chemoattractants produced by rabies virus-infected CNS tissues are necessary to induce immune cells adherent in the neurovasculature to cross the BBB and infiltrate the tissues. A wide variety of such cytokines and

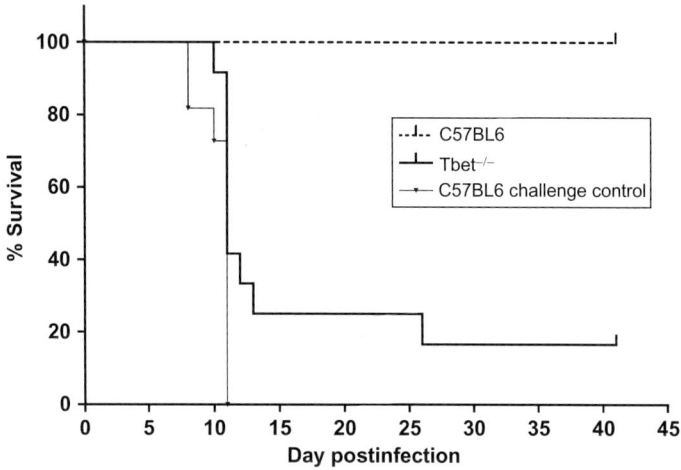

FIGURE 2 Tbet$^{-/-}$ mice are not protected against intracranial challenge with wild-type rabies virus after short-term immunization with live-attenuated rabies virus. Tbet$^{-/-}$ and C57BL/6 mice ($n = 10$) were infected with 10^5 FFU of recombinant SPBNGAS-GAS virus in the gastrocnemius muscle. Ten days later, the mice were intracranially infected with 10^3 FFU of virulent Dog4 rabies virus. Survival was monitored for 7 weeks.

chemokines are induced in the CNS by rabies virus infection (Phares *et al.*, 2006; Roy *et al.*, 2007). While we have not detected any clear difference between the levels and types of factors triggered by infection with attenuated versus wild-type rabies virus infection (Roy *et al.*, 2007), subtle differences have been detected by others (Wang *et al.*, 2005). We expect that MHC class II may be expressed in the neurovasculature of CVS-F3-infected mice, but not in animals infected with SHBRV as a consequence of differences in the innate responses to these viruses as the discrepancy is apparent in T and B cell-deficient rag-2$^{-/-}$ mice (data not shown). This raises the issue as to whether or not certain aspects of the innate response culminating in the maintenance of BBB integrity are inhibited by wild-type rabies virus infection. We do not consider this to be the case because mixed infections with attenuated and wild-type viruses are cleared (Hooper *et al.*, submitted). We speculate that, for some as yet unknown reason, infection with wild-type rabies viruses fails to trigger this element of the innate response.

C. Antiviral immunity in the CNS

The clearance of attenuated rabies virus from the CNS is temporally associated with the appearance of T and B cells as well as antibody production in CNS tissues (Phares *et al.*, 2006). Early containment of rabies virus replication and spread may not be entirely dependent on antibody. However, as CVS-F3 replication in the CNS of B cell-deficient JHD$^{-/-}$

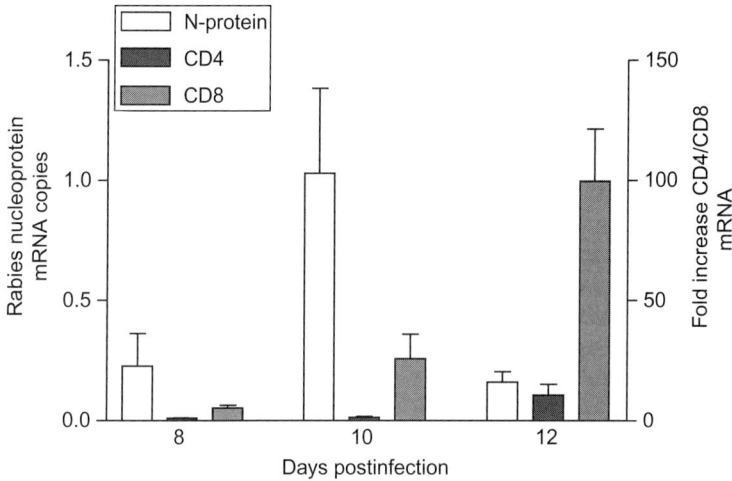

FIGURE 3   Rabies nucleoprotein mRNA levels decrease concomitantly with an increase in T cell mRNA accumulation in the CNS tissues of B cell-deficient mice. JhD$^{-/-}$ mice ($n = 5$–11) were infected intranasally with 10^5 FFU of CVS-F3 rabies virus. At the time points indicated, cerebellar tissues were collected and levels of mRNAs specific for rabies virus nucleoprotein (N-Protein), *CD4* and *CD8* genes were measured using QRT-PCR as previously described (Spitsin *et al.*, 2000). Nucleoprotein mRNA levels are expressed as the mean $\pm$ SEM copy number per copy of mRNA for the housekeeping gene L13. CD4 and CD8 levels are expressed as the mean fold increase $\pm$ SEM in samples over the copy number in samples from uninfected mouse tissues, normalized to L13 mRNA content.

mice is curtailed as T cells accumulate in the infected tissues (Fig. 3). We speculate that IFN-γ production by infiltrating T cells activates innate antiviral mechanisms, including, for example, the production of type 1 interferons. CD8 T cells may also participate in this mechanism as CD8-deficient mice can clear CVS-F3 from CNS tissues, but over a prolonged time period (Hooper *et al.*, 1998). It is unknown whether or not CD8 T cells contribute to rabies virus immunity in the CNS through cytotoxic mechanisms. In fact, the fate of the infected neuron during rabies virus clearance is unknown. Rabies virus infection is not cytolytic but causes functional changes in neurons (Fu and Jackson, 2005). While we may conclude that antibody and T cell functions collaborate to clear the virus from CNS tissues, it remains unclear whether or not the virus can be cleared without neuronal loss. This is an important question with respect to the extent of infection that is amenable to immunotherapy.

An aspect of immunity that likely contributes to whether or not a rabies virus can be cleared from the CNS is immune regulation. Certain rabies viruses induce processes that interfere with their clearance. For example, the T cells that infiltrate CNS tissues infected with a pathogenic CVS variant undergo apoptosis rather than contribute to protective immunity (Baloul *et al.*, 2004).

D. CNS immunopathology

In both humans and mice that have died of wild-type rabies virus infection, there is often little evidence of immunopathology as may be expected if immune cell infiltration across the BBB does not occur. Nevertheless, there are circumstances where the immune response to a rabies virus may be expected to cause pathology. Clearly, there would be a greater risk of immunopathology, whether mediated by antibody or cellular mechanisms, when the immune response develops relatively late in the infection and the virus has spread more extensively through the CNS. Virus strains that spread rapidly and trigger the processes that facilitate immune cell infiltration into CNS tissues would likely present a greater risk of immunopathology. Rabies viruses that rapidly spread to the CNS but induce immune cell infiltration across the BBB may be expected to cause some immunopathology. For example, the spontaneous development of rabies virus immunity was associated with the survival, with neurological sequelae, of one-third of mice infected in the hindlimb footpad with a fox street rabies virus (Jackson *et al.*, 1989). The likelihood that immunopathology contributed to the neurological impairments seen in the survivors is supported by evidence of acute inflammation in the brainstem and spinal cord and neuronal degeneration in the spinal cord and dorsal roots of the animals (Jackson *et al.*, 1989). We theorize that the absence of inflammatory CNS pathology during the clearance of certain attenuated rabies viruses is a consequence of limited virus spread in the CNS tissues together with the nature of the immune response. In comparative studies, we identified the infiltration of mononuclear cells expressing NOS-2 as a key difference between autoimmune CNS inflammation and CVS-F3 clearance from the CNS (Fabis *et al.*, 2008). Evidently, the activation of these highly pathogenic, CNS-infiltrating cells is avoided during CVS-F3 clearance, which is unexpected for a Th1-centered immune response and appears to be unique to protective rabies virus immunity.

VII. PROSPECTS FOR HUMAN RABIES IMMUNOTHERAPY THROUGH VIRUS CLEARANCE FROM THE CNS

A. Rabies virus-specific immunity

Unlike the experimental situation in mice, humans do not usually mount a strong peripheral immune response to natural wild-type rabies virus infection until late in the infection (Baltazard and Ghodssi, 1954; Centers

TABLE I Comparison of antibody response in C57BL/6 mice after immunization with live or inactivated rabies virus vaccine[a]

	IgG1	IgG2a	IgG2b
Live virus	−	++	+++
UV-inactivated virus	+++	+	+++

Serum samples with an absorbance over half the maximum are denoted by +++, between one-third to half of the maximum by ++, and significantly higher than background (normal sera) but less than one-third of the maximum by +. A level that is not significantly higher than background is denoted by −.
[a] Isotype of rabies virus-specific antibody in sera was determined by ELISA using isotype-specific secondary antibodies as previously described (Wang *et al.*, 2005).

for Disease Control and Prevention, 2006). The rapid induction of rabies virus-specific immune effectors is the primary objective of PEP, with the initial aim of preventing spread of the virus to the CNS. For this purpose, a Th2 response may be adequate, as vaccinated Tbet$^{-/-}$ mice are protected against a peripheral challenge (Li and Hooper, unpublished observations). To clear virus from the CNS, however, a Th1 response is more appropriate (Hooper *et al.*, 1998; Phares *et al.*, 2007). Thus a vaccine that rapidly induces a Th1 response to rabies viral antigens is a first requirement. However, in mice, inactivated rabies vaccines primarily induce IgG1 and IgG2b antibodies (Table I) suggesting that a Th2 response has been induced. The Th bias of the immune response to current human rabies vaccines has not been extensively studied.

B. Targeting effectors to the CNS

Introduction of wild-type virus into a highly innervated site or a delay in seeking treatment increases the chance that the virus might reach the CNS where it is inaccessible to the response generated by conventional PEP. Accumulated experience with PEP failures in individuals with facial and upper extremity dog bites in dog rabies endemic areas attests to this possibility (Wilde, 2007). Whether or not inactivated vaccines can be modified to generate a strong Th1 response with a single dose may be a moot point, as it is unlikely that the effectors would cross the BBB and enter CNS tissues in the absence of an innate response due to CNS infection. Ideally, wild-type virus replication would be limited in the CNS tissues when virus-specific immune effectors arrive, which would necessitate some means of triggering functional changes in the BBB and proinflammatory cytokine and chemokine production by CNS tissues. In the mouse model, postexposure administration of inactivated vaccine is ineffective, but modern, live-attenuated vaccines can protect up to several days after administration of a lethal dose of wild-type rabies virus (Faber *et al.*, 2009). Based on what we know about rabies virus clearance from the CNS, this is not unexpected. Regardless of whether or not the killed vaccine is as immunogenic as its attenuated counterpart, the peripheral immune response to wild-type rabies virus infection is strong in mice (Roy and Hooper, 2008) and unlikely to be substantially altered by the delayed administration of vaccine. However, wild-type rabies virus infection fails to induce the functional changes in the neurovasculature necessary to promote immune cell extravasation into the CNS tissues (Roy and Hooper, 2008; Roy *et al.*, 2007). Inactivated virus applied to the periphery is very unlikely to induce such changes, which appear to be a consequence of the innate response of CNS resident cells to attenuated rabies virus infection. In fact, direct intracranial inoculation of the live-attenuated Triple-GAS virus into the CNS is effective in promoting postexposure survival from wild-type rabies virus infection for several days longer than with administration of this vaccine strain in the gastrocnemius (Faber *et al.*, 2009). This provides additional support for the hypothesis that rapid targeting of innate CNS immunity is an important element of wild-type rabies virus clearance from the CNS. At present, the only means of accomplishing this is through the spread of attenuated rabies virus to the CNS.

Currently, passive administration of rabies virus VNA is an integral part of PEP. VNA probably limit spread of the virus from the periphery to the CNS but are unlikely to be effective after the virus has reached CNS tissues. This is well illustrated by the fact that mice immunized with inactivated rabies vaccine have high levels of circulating VNA but are poorly protected against an intracranial challenge with a virus that has little effect when given intramuscularly (Fig. 4). If attenuated rabies virus

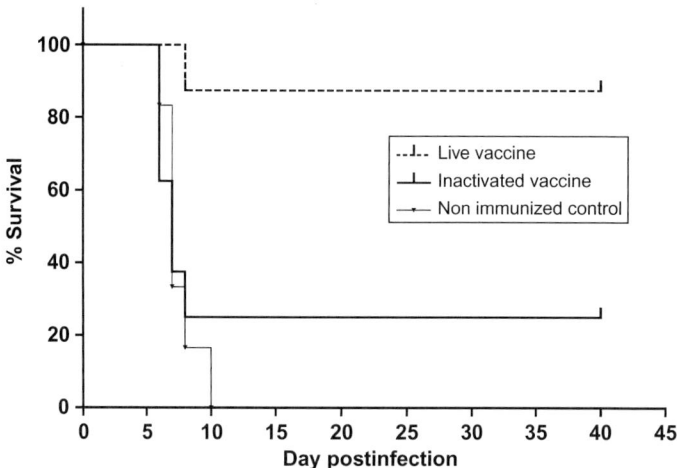

FIGURE 4 Live-attenuated, but not inactivated rabies virus vaccine, protects mice against intracranial challenge. Groups of Swiss Webster mice ($n = 10$) were immunized with 10^5 FFU of live or 10^8 FFU of UV-inactivated CVS-F3 in the gastrocnemius with 10 mice being left untreated. Twenty-one days later, the mice were challenged i.c. with 10^3 FFU of SHBRV-17 and survival was monitored.

is used to target the CNS mechanisms that promote immune effector delivery to the CNS, passive antibody administration would be contraindicated. We speculate that the best approach to clearing rabies virus from the human CNS may be to administer live-attenuated and inactivated vaccine simultaneously. This may raise a strong immune response as well as target it to the CNS. The outcome would then depend on the extent of wild-type rabies virus infection in the CNS tissues and whether or not immune clearance causes substantial neuronal loss.

ACKNOWLEDGMENTS

This work was supported by the National Institutes of Health Grants AI 077033, AI 060005 and AI083046. We thank Drs. Faber and Dietzschold for provision of SPBNGAS-GAS live-attenuated rabies vaccine virus and the Dog4 challenge strain.

REFERENCES

Akaike, T., Weihe, E., Schaefer, M., Fu, Z. F., Zheng, Y. M., Vogel, W., Schmidt, H., Koprowski, H., and Dietzschold, B. (1995). Effect of neurotropic virus infection on neuronal and inducible nitric oxide synthase activity in rat brain. *J. Neurovirol.* **1** (1):118–125.

Baer, G. M., Bellini, W. J., and Fishbein, D. B. (1990). Rhabdoviruses. *In* "Virology" (B. N. Fields, ed.), 2nd edn. pp. 883–930. Raven press, New York.

Baloul, L., Camelo, S., and Lafon, M. (2004). Up-regulation of Fas ligand (FasL) in the central nervous system: A mechanism of immune evasion by rabies virus. *J. Neurovirol.* **10** (6):372–382.

Baltazard, M., and Ghodssi, M. (1954). Prevention of human rabies: Treatment of persons bitten by rapid wolves in Iran. *Bull. World Health Organ.* **10**:799–803.

Centers for Disease Control and Prevention (2006). Human rabies—Mississippi, 2005. *MMWR Morb. Mortal. Wkly. Rep.* **55**:207–208.

Centers for Disease Control and Prevention (2008a). Human rabies—Minnesota, 2007. *MMWR Morb. Mortal. Wkly. Rep.* **57**:460–462.

Centers for Disease Control and Prevention (2008b). Human rabies prevention—United States, 2008. Recommendations of the Advisory Committee on immunization practices. *MMWR Morb. Mortal. Wkly. Report.* **57**(RR-3):1–28.

Cox, J. H., Dietzschold, B., and Schneider, L. G. (1977). Rabies virus glycoprotein. II. Biological and serological characterization. *Infect. Immun.* **16**(3):754–759.

Dietzschold, B., Wunner, W. H., Wiktor, T. J., Lopes, A. D., Lafon, M., Smith, C., and Koprowski, H. (1983). Characterization of an antigenic determinant of the glycoprotein which correlates with pathogenicity of rabies virus. *Proc. Natl. Acad. Sci. USA* **80**:70–74.

Faber, M., Pulmanausahakul, R., Hodawadekar, S. S., Spitsin, S., McGettigan, J. P., Schnell, M. J., and Dietzschold, B. (2002). Overexpression of the rabies virus glycoprotein results in enhancement of apoptosis and antiviral immune response. *J. Virol.* **76**:3374–3381.

Faber, M., Bette, M., Preuss, M. A., Pulmanausahakul, R., Rehnelt, J., Schnell, M. J., Dietzschold, B., and Weihe, E. (2005). Overexpression of tumor necrosis factor alpha by a recombinant rabies virus attenuates replication in neurons and prevents lethal infection in mice. *J. Virol.* **79**:15405–15416.

Faber, M., Li, J., Kean, R. B., Hooper, D. C., Alugupalli, K. R., and Dietzschold, B. (2009). Effective preexposure and postexposure prophylaxis of rabies with a highly attenuated recombinant rabies virus. *Proc. Natl. Acad. Sci. USA* **106**(27):11300–11305.

Fabis, M. J., Phares, T. W., Kean, R. B., Koprowski, H., and Hooper, D. C. (2008). Blood-brain barrier changes and cell invasion differ between therapeutic immune clearance of neurotrophic virus and CNS autoimmunity. *Proc. Natl. Acad. Sci. USA* **105**(40):15511–15516.

Fu, Z. F., and Jackson, A. C. (2005). Neuronal dysfunction and death in rabies virus infection. *J. Neurovirol.* **11**(1):101–106.

Hampson, K., Dushoff, J., Cleaveland, S., Haydon, D. T., Kaare, M., Packer, C., and Dobson, A. (2009). Transmission dynamics and prospects for the elimination of canine rabies. *PLoS Biol.* **7**(3):e53.

Hooper, D. C., Morimoto, K., Bette, M., Weihe, E., Koprowski, H., and Dietzschold, B. (1998). Collaboration of antibody and inflammation in clearance of rabies virus from the central nervous system. *J. Virol.* **72**(5):3711–3719.

Hooper, D. C., Scott, G. S., Zborek, A., Mikheeva, T., Kean, R. B., Koprowski, H., and Spitsin, S. V. (2000). Uric acid, a peroxynitrite scavenger, inhibits CNS inflammation, blood-CNS barrier permeability changes, and tissue damage in a mouse model of multiple sclerosis. *FASEB J.* **14**(5):691–698.

Hooper, D. C., Kean, R. B., Scott, G. S., Spitsin, S. V., Mikheeva, T., Morimoto, K., Bette, M., Röhrenbeck, A. M., Dietzschold, B., and Weihe, E. (2001). The central nervous system inflammatory response to neurotropic virus infection is peroxynitrite dependent. *J. Immunol.* **167**(6):3470–3477, 15.

Jackson, A. C., Reimer, D. L., and Ludwin, S. K. (1989). Spontaneous recovery from the encephalomyelitis in mice caused by street rabies virus. *Neuropathol. Appl. Neurobiol.* **15**:459–475.

Koprowski, H., and Black, J. (1954). Studies on chick-embryo-adapted rabies virus. V. Protection of animals with antiserum and living attenuated virus after exposure to street strain of rabies virus. *J. Immunol.* **72**(1):85–93.

Krebs, J. W., Long-Marin, S. C., and Childs, J. E. (1998). Causes, costs, and estimates of rabies postexposure prophylaxis treatments in the United States. *J. Public Health Manag. Pract.* **4**:56–62.

Morimoto, K., Hooper, D. C., Carbaugh, H., Fu, Z. F., Koprowski, H., and Dietzschold, B. (1998). Rabies virus quasispecies: Implications for pathogenesis. *Proc. Natl. Acad. Sci. USA* **95**(6):3152–3156.

Morimoto, K., Hooper, D. C., Spitsin, S., Koprowski, H., and Dietzschold, B. (1999). Pathogenicity of different rabies virus variants inversely correlates with apoptosis and rabies virus glycoprotein expression in infected primary neuron cultures. *J. Virol.* **73**(1):510–518.

Pasteur, L. (1885). Bulletin de l'Académie de médecine, séance du 27 octobre 1885, 2e sér., XIV, pp. 1431–1439.

Phares, T. W., Kean, R. B., Mikheeva, T., and Hooper, D. C. (2006). Regional differences in blood-brain barrier permeability changes and inflammation in the apathogenic clearance of virus from the central nervous system. *J. Immunol.* **176**(12):7666–7675.

Phares, T. W., Fabis, M. J., Brimer, C. M., Kean, R. B., and Hooper, D. C. (2007). A peroxynitrite-dependent pathway is responsible for blood-brain barrier permeability changes during a central nervous system inflammatory response: TNF-α is neither necessary nor sufficient. *J. Immunol.* **178**(11):7334–7343.

Pulmanausahakul, R., Faber, M., Morimoto, K., Spitsin, S., Weihe, E., Hooper, D. C., Schnell, M. J., and Dietzschold, B. (2001). Overexpression of cytochrome C by a recombinant rabies virus attenuates pathogenicity and enhances antiviral immunity. *J. Virol.* **75**:10800–10807.

Roy, A., and Hooper, D. C. (2007). Lethal silver-haired bat rabies virus infection can be prevented by opening the blood-brain barrier. *J. Virol.* **81**:7993–7998.

Roy, A., and Hooper, D. C. (2008). Immune evasion by rabies viruses through the mainte-nance of blood-brain barrier integrity. *J. Neurovirol.* **14**(5):401–411.

Roy, A., Phares, T. W., Koprowski, H., and Hooper, D. C. (2007). Failure to open the blood-brain barrier and deliver immune effectors to the CNS tissues leads to the lethal outcome of Silver-haired bat rabies virus infection. *J. Virol.* **81**(3):1110–1118.

Spitsin, S. V., Scott, G. S., Kean, R. B., Mikheeva, T., and Hooper, D. C. (2000). Protection of myelin basic protein immunized mice from free-radical mediated inflammatory cell invasion of the central nervous system by the natural peroxynitrite scavenger uric acid. *Neurosci. Lett.* **292**(2):137–141.

Wang, Z. W., Sarmento, L., Wang, Y., Li, X. Q., Dhingra, V., Tseggai, T., Jiang, B., and Fu, Z. F. (2005). Attenuated rabies virus activates, while pathogenic rabies virus evades, the host innate immune responses in the central nervous system. *J. Virol.* **79**(19):12554–12565.

Wang, T., Rumbaugh, J. A., and Nath, A. (2006). Viruses and the brain: From inflammation to dementia. *Clin. Sci.* **110**(4):393–407.

Wilde, H. (2007). Failures of post exposure prophylaxis. *Vaccine* **25**:7605–7609.

Willoughby, R. E., Jr., Tieves, K. S., Hoffman, G. M., Ghanayem, N. S., Amlie-Lefond, C. M., Schwabe, M. J., Chusid, M. J., and Rupprecht, C. E. (2005). Brief Report: Survival after treatment of rabies with induction of coma. *N. Engl. J. Med.* **352**:2508–2514.

Zhao, L., Toriumi, H., Kuang, Y., Chen, H., and Fu, Z. F. (2009). The roles of chemokines in rabies virus infection: Overexpression may not always be beneficial. *J. Virol.* **83**(22):11808–11818.

Role of Chemokines in Rabies Pathogenesis and Protection

Xuefeng Niu, Hualei Wang, and **Zhen F. Fu**

Contents

Abstract

Chemokines are a family of structurally related proteins that are expressed by almost all types of nucleated cells and mediate leukocyte activation and/or chemotactic activities. The role of chemokines in rabies pathogenesis and protection has only recently been investigated. Expression of chemokines is induced

Departments of Pathology, University of Georgia, Athens, Georgia, USA

Advances in Virus Research, Volume 79
ISSN 0065-3527, DOI: 10.1016/B978-0-12-387040-7.00005-6

by infection with laboratory-adapted, but not street, rabies viruses (RABVs), and it has been hypothesized that expression of chemokines is one of the mechanisms by which RABV is attenuated. To further define the role of chemokines in rabies pathogenesis and protection, chemokine genes such as MIP-1α, RANTES, IP-10, and macrophage-derived chemokine (MDC) have been cloned into RABV genome. It has been found that recombinant RABVs expressing RANTES or IP-10 induce high and persistent expression of these chemokines, resulting in massive infiltration of inflammatory cells into the central nervous system (CNS) and development of diseases and death in the mouse model. However, recombinant RABVs expressing MIP-1α, MDC, as well as GM-CSF further attenuate RABV by inducing a transient expression of chemokines, infiltration of inflammatory cells, enhancement of blood–brain barrier (BBB) permeability. Yet, these recombinant RABVs show increased adaptive immune responses by recruiting/activating dendritic cells, T and B cells in the periphery as well as in the CNS. Further, direct administration of these recombinant RABVs into the CNS can prevent mice from developing rabies days after infection with street RABV. All these studies together suggest that chemokines are both protective and pathogenic in RABV infections. Those with protective roles could be exploited for development of future RABV vaccines or therapeutic agents.

I. INTRODUCTION

Rabies continues to present a serious burden for both public health and the global economy. It causes more than 55,000 human deaths, and more than 10 million people undergo postexposure prophylaxis (PEP) every year around the globe (Martinez, 2000; Meslin *et al.*, 1994). Most human cases occur in the developing countries of Asia and Africa, where canine rabies is endemic and resources are limited (Fu, 1997). In more developed countries, human rabies has dramatically declined during the past 60 years as a direct consequence of routine vaccination of pet animals (Lackay *et al.*, 2008). However, wildlife rabies has emerged as a major threat (Morimoto *et al.*, 1996). Despite extensive investigation over more than 100 years, the pathogenetic mechanisms by which infection of street rabies virus (RABV) results in neurological diseases and death in humans are not well understood. Neuronal pathology or damage in the central nervous system (CNS) is limited in rabies patients with only mild inflammation (Miyamoto and Matsumoto, 1967; Murphy, 1977). However, laboratory-attenuated RABV induces extensive inflammation and neuronal degeneration in experimental animals (Miyamoto and Matsumoto, 1967;

Yan *et al.*, 2001). It is only recently that the roles of chemokines in rabies pathogenesis and protection have been investigated. This chapter will summarize recent research activities in this area.

II. CHEMOKINES

Chemokines are a family of structurally related proteins that are expressed by almost all types of nucleated cells and mediate leukocyte activation and/or chemotactic activities (Zlotnik and Yoshie, 2000). The majority of chemokines have molecular masses of 8–14 kDa and share approximately 20–50% sequence homology among each other at the protein level (Gale and McColl, 1999; Zlotnik and Yoshie, 2000). Chemokine proteins also share common gene sequences and tertiary structures, and all chemokines possess a number of conserved cysteine residues involved in intramolecular disulfide bond formation. Chemokines can be divided into four major subfamilies based on cysteine signature motifs: the C, CC, CXC, and CX3C families (Table I) (Gale and McColl, 1999; Zlotnik and Yoshie, 2000). Chemokines in which the C1 and C2 cysteine residues are adjacent are called CC chemokines and include RANTES, MCP-1, TARC, and eotaxin. Many CC chemokines exert their effects on monocytes and macrophages, but CC chemokines have been shown to be important for dendritic cell (DC) chemotaxis and some CC chemokines appear to act preferentially on Th2-type T cells (Gale and McColl, 1999; Zlotnik and Yoshie, 2000). Chemokines in which the C1 and C2 cysteine residues are separated by a single amino acid are called CXC chemokines and include IL-8, IP-10, I-TAC, and SDF-1. CXC chemokines act as chemoattractants for neutrophils and have been shown to be important mediators of T- and B-lymphocyte chemotaxis (Gale and McColl, 1999; Zlotnik and Yoshie, 2000). The C subfamily chemokine, lymphotactin, is a potent T-lymphocyte chemoattractant, and fractalkine is the only member of CX3C chemokine subfamily, which may chemoattract mononuclear leukocytes (Glabinski and Ransohoff, 1999). Chemokines are highly basic proteins and contain at least four cysteine residues that form two disulfide bonds (Ubogu *et al.*, 2006). This property may help mediate stable gradient formation by promoting interactions of chemokines with sulfated proteins and proteoglycans (Cyster, 1999). Chemokines may also be divided into inflammatory chemokines and homeostatic chemokines in terms of biological features and cellular distribution of chemokine receptors (Moser and Loetscher, 2001). The former are secreted by resident and infiltrated cells on inflammatory stimuli or contacting with pathogenic agents. These chemokines are responsible for recruiting cells related to inflammatory reactions

TABLE I   Chemokines and chemokine receptors

	Systematic name	Human/mouse ligand	Chemokine receptor
C family		Lymphotactin	XCR1
CC family	CCL1	I-309	CCR8
	CCL2	MCP-1	CCR2, CCR4
	CCL3	MIP-1α	CCR1, CCR5
	CCL4	MIP-1β	CCR5
	CCL5	RANTES	CCR1, CCR3, CCR5
	CCL6	C10, MRP-1	CCR1
	CCL7	MCP-3	CCR1, CCR2, CCR3
	CCL8	MCP-2	CCR1, CCR2B, CCR5
	CCL9	MRP-2, MIP-1γ	CCR1
	CCL11	eotaxin-1	CCR2, CCR3, CCR5
	CCL12	MCP-5	CCR2
	CCL13	MCP-4	CCR2, CCR3, CCR5
	CCL14	HCC-1	CCR1
	CCL15	HCC-2	CCR1, CCR3
	CCL16	HCC-4	CCR1, CCR2, CCR5, CCR8
	CCL17	TARC	CCR4
	CCL18	PARC	Unknown
	CCL19	MIP-3β	CCR7
	CCL20	LARC, MIP-3α	CCR6
	CCL21	6Ckine, SLC, exodus-2	CCR7
	CCL22	MDC	CCR4
	CCL23	MPIF-1	CCR1
	CCL24	MPIF-2, eotaxin-2	CCR3
	CCL25	TECK	CCR9
	CCL26	Eotaxin-3	CCR3
	CCL27	ILC, CTACK	CCR10
	CCL28	MEC	CCR3, CCR10
CXC family	CXCL1	GROα, MSGA-α	CXCR2
	CXCL2	GROβ, MSGA-β	CXCR2
	CXCL3	GROγ, MSGA-γ	CXCR2
	CXCL4	PF4	CXCR3
	CXCL5	ENA-78	CXCR2
	CXCL6	GCP-2	CXCR1, CXCR2
	CXCL7	NAP-2	CXCR2
	CXCL8	IL-8	CXCR1, CXCR2
	CXCL9	Mig	CXCR3

TABLE I   (*continued*)

	Systematic name	Human/mouse ligand	Chemokine receptor
	CXCL10	IP-10	CXCR3
	CXCL11	I-TAC, IP-9	CXCR3
	CXCL12	SDF-2	CXCR4
	CXCL13	BLC	CXCR5
	CXCL14	BRAK	Unknown
	CXCL15	Lungkine	Unknown
CX3C	CX3CL1	Fractalkine	CX3CR1

(Holman *et al.*, 2010). However, homeostatic chemokines are involved in maintaining trafficking and positioning of immune cells involved in adaptive immunity and antigen presentation in secondary lymphoid organs (Moser and Loetscher, 2001; Sallusto *et al.*, 1999).

Chemokines mediate their effects by binding to the seven transmembrane G-protein-coupled cell-surface receptors (Table I) (Rossi and Zlotnik, 2000; Zlotnik and Yoshie, 2000). Upon binding, the chemokine receptors initiate cellular signaling through changes in intracellular concentrations of calcium and cAMP. Many cellular chemokine receptors can bind more than one chemokine with similar affinities. For example, the chemokine receptors CCR1 and CCR5 may bind RANTES, MIP-1α, and MIP-1β, whereas the chemokine receptors CXCR1 and CXCR2 may bind IL-8 (Gale and McColl, 1999; Zlotnik and Yoshie, 2000). Based on the chemokine subfamilies, chemokine receptors have been named CCR1-9, CXCR1-5, XCR1, and CX3R1 (Zlotnik and Yoshie, 2000). Several chemokines can bind to one receptor, and one ligand can bind to more than one receptor (Ubogu *et al.*, 2006). These intricate complex interactions can provide adequate host defenses against infection with pathogens. However, viruses may mimic chemokine receptors to evade host defense mechanisms (Glabinski and Ransohoff, 1999).

III. THE ROLE OF CHEMOKINES IN THE CNS WHEN INFECTED BY VIRUSES

A recent review has provided an elegant illustration of the roles of chemokines in the CNS after viral infections (Hosking and Lane, 2010). Viral infections of the CNS can result in a temporal expression of several chemokines and chemokine receptors by CNS resident cells (astrocytes, microglia, as well as neurons) and by inflammatory cells infiltrated into the CNS (Hosking and Lane, 2010; Nakamichi *et al.*, 2005; Prehaud *et al.*, 2005). Astrocytes and microglia are the dominant source of chemokines following infection with neurotropic viruses (Hosking and Lane, 2010). Robust expression of numerous CC chemokines such as CCL2, CCL3, CCL4, and CCL5 (Zlotnik and Yoshie, 2000) was observed following infection with measles virus (Patterson *et al.*, 2003), mouse hepatitis virus (MHV) (Kim and Perlman, 2005), and human coronavirus (Chen *et al.*, 2010). Infection of rat astrocytes and microglia with paramyxoviruses resulted in rapid expression of mRNA transcripts for CCL5 and CXCL10 (Fisher *et al.*, 1995; Vanguri and Farber, 1994). In some virus infections, chemokine expression was found in a particular cell type. For example, CXCL10 was exclusively secreted by astrocytes in the neural parenchyma, but not by microglia in the brain or recruited bone marrow-derived cell types after infection with lymphocytic choriomeningitis virus (LCMV) (Christensen *et al.*, 2009). Induction of chemokine gene expression is promoted by toll-like receptors (TLRs) when recognizing viral DNA or RNA (Gibson *et al.*, 2002; So and Kim, 2009). For example, TLR2 and TLR3 cooperation leads to the expression of macrophage chemoattractants CCL2 and CCL5 during infection with Theiler's murine encephalitis virus (TMEV) (So and Kim, 2009). However, TLR2 and TLR9 mediate chemokine expression during HSV-1 infection (Aravalli *et al.*, 2008; Lima *et al.*, 2010).

The major activity of chemokines is modulating leukocyte trafficking into the CNS (Hosking and Lane, 2010). Both neuroprotective and neuropathologic effects of chemokine expression in the CNS have been reported, and these are largely due to attracting T lymphocytes and macrophages (Dorries, 2001; Lin *et al.*, 2009). On one hand, infiltration and antiviral activity of T lymphocytes are requisite for viral clearance and survival. For example, CXCL10 expressed in the CNS after infection with neurotropic viruses attracts activated T lymphocytes bearing the receptor CXCR3 (Zhang *et al.*, 2008). It has been reported that in many virus infections such as herpes simplex virus (HSV), MHV, and West Nile virus (WNV), ablation of CXCL10 expression by either depletion with neutralization antibodies or genetic knockout dramatically reduces infiltration of T cell into the CNS, which results in inefficient viral control and severe disease (Stiles *et al.*, 2009; Thapa and Carr, 2008; Zhang *et al.*, 2008). Another chemokine CCL5 and its receptors, CCR5, have also been found to promote leukocyte trafficking into the CNS and control of HSV and WNV infections (Glass *et al.*, 2005; Thapa *et al.*, 2007). CCR5 knockout showed an increased risk for symptomatic WNV infection (Glass *et al.*, 2006). On the other hand, excessive chemokine secretion and accumulation of leukocytes within the CNS lead to the development of neuropathology. It is well known that fatal meningoencephalitis induced by LCMV infection is mediated by infiltration of virus-specific cytotoxic T lymphocytes (CTLs) (Fung-Leung et al., 1991; Kim et al., 2009). Genetic silencing of CXCL10 or its receptor CXCR3 reduces the infiltration of CD8+ T cells, conferring either partial or near complete protection from immunopathology and death (Christensen et al., 2006; Hofer et al., 2008). Demyelinating disease during MHV infection is largely due to sustained CXCL10 and CCL5 expression, and abrogation of expression of either these chemokine reduces infiltration of immune cells, disease severity, and demyelination (Glass et al., 2004; Liu et al., 2001). There are numerous examples of neuroprotective and neuropathologic activities associated with the expression of chemokines during viral infections (Hosking and Lane, 2010).

IV. INDUCTION OF CHEMOKINE EXPRESSION IN RABV INFECTIONS

RABV induces a fatal neurological disease in humans and animals, and the roles of chemokines in rabies are just beginning to emerge. Using oligonucleotide microarray, we reported that chemokines were upregulated in the mouse brain after infection with laboratory-attenuated, but not with street virus (Wang et al., 2005). This includes both the CC and CXC subfamilies of proinflammatory chemokines. Among these chemokines, MIP-1α, RANTES, and IP-10 were increased more than 50- to 100-fold in infected versus sham-infected mice (Kuang et al., 2009; Wang et al., 2005). Further, the protein level of chemokines CXCL10 and CCL5 was dramatically upregulated in neuroblastoma cells after infection with laboratory-attenuated RABV (Masatani et al., 2010). It has also been reported that chemokine CXCL-10 and cytokines (IL-6, IFN-γ) were upregulated at the time of clinical disease in the CNS of mice infected with European bat lyssaviruses (EBLV) types 1 and 2 (Mansfield et al., 2008). Interestingly, a lower but significant increase of CXCL10 was also observed in the salivary glands (Mansfield et al., 2008). CXCL10 has also been reported to be activated by macrophages and microglia infected with RABV (Nakamichi et al., 2004, 2005).

The increased expression of chemokines in RABV infection in the CNS resulted in infiltration of inflammatory cells, induction of apoptosis, and enhancement of blood–brain barrier (BBB) permeability in mice infected with fixed (or laboratory-attenuated) RABV (Fabis et al., 2008; Kuang et al., 2009; Sarmento et al., 2005; Wang et al., 2005; Zhao et al., 2009). As a consequence, fixed RABV could be cleared from the CNS of mice when infected with low doses (Hooper et al., 2009; Sarmento et al., 2005). It is, therefore, hypothesized that induction of innate immunity, particularly with chemokines and IFN, is one of the mechanisms for RABV attenuation. However, mice infected with high dose of fixed RABV die with excessive inflammation in the CNS (Sarmento *et al.*, 2005; Wang *et al.*, 2005). Therefore, the pathogenetic mechanisms by which street and fixed RABV induce disease are different. In animals infected with a high dose of fixed RABV, it is the expression of chemokines and other innate immune molecules that results in the enhancement of BBB permeability and infiltration of inflammatory cells into the CNS, which is ultimately responsible for the demise of the infected animals (Kuang *et al.*, 2009; Wang *et al.*, 2005). On the contrary, street RABV invades the CNS without stimulating the innate immune responses. Although the exact mechanisms by which street RABV causes rabies are not known, it has been hypothesized that RABV induces CNS dysfunction (Dietzschold *et al.*, 2001). Recently, we have observed that infection of street RABV inhibits the expression of proteins involved in the fusion between neurotransmitter vesicle membrane and the presynaptic membrane, resulting in massive accumulation of neurotransmitter vesicles in presynapses (Dhingra *et al.*, 2007). These observations may also explain why very little neuronal pathology or damage is observed in the CNS of rabies patients (Miyamoto and Matsumoto, 1967; Murphy, 1977), whereas laboratory-attenuated RABV induces extensive inflammation and neuronal degeneration in experimentally infected animals (Miyamoto and Matsumoto, 1967; Yan *et al.*, 2001).

V. OVEREXPRESSION OF CHEMOKINES CAN BENEFIT THE HOST IF THE EXPRESSION IS TRANSIENT WHILE IT HARMS THE HOST IF THE EXPRESSION IS PERSISTENT DURING RABV INFECTIONS

To further explore the role of chemokines in RABV infections, chemokines MIP-1α, RANTES, or IP-10 were individually expressed in the genome of RABV HEP-Flurry strain (Zhao *et al.*, 2009, 2010). It was found that although the expression of MIP-1α further reduced RABV pathogenicity, expression of RANTES or IP-10 enhanced RABV pathogenicity in the mouse model. The differences in pathogenicity induced by these recombinant RABVs are not due to the rate of virus replication, but rather due to the level and the duration of the expression of chemokines (Zhao *et al.*, 2009). HEP-MIP1α induced the expression of MIP-1α in the mouse model but subsided quickly. In addition, only low to moderate levels of other chemokines were induced. Likewise, only low and transient infiltration of inflammatory cells (macrophages, neutrophils, and T cells) was observed in the infected mice. In contrast, HEP-RANTES and particularly HEP-IP10 induced not only high and persistent expression of the intended chemokines but also high expression of other chemokines. High and persistent infiltration of inflammatory cells was also observed in the CNS, which could produce neurotoxins, free radicals, and proinflammatory cytokines, causing CNS destruction (Hooper *et al.*, 2009; Zhao *et al.*, 2009). HEP-MIP1α enhanced the BBB permeability temporarily, while HEP-RANTES and HEP-IP10 induced more extensive and prolonged enhancement of BBB permeability. Further, HEP-IP10 induced BBB permeability to the extent that allowed large molecules (10 kDa) to enter the CNS. Although the consequence is not entirely clear, this may have allowed more inflammatory cells or other toxic substances enter into the CNS. Thus, these studies indicate that transient expression of chemokines may help attenuate RABV, whereas high and persistent expression of these chemokines, particularly IP-10, may be harmful to the host during RABV infections.

VI. CHEMOKINES EXPRESSION CORRELATES WITH THE ACTIVATION OF DENDRITIC CELLS AND ENHANCEMENT OF ADAPTIVE IMMUNITY

As chemokines play roles as attractants of naïve and effector T cells (Moser and Loetscher, 2001), these recombinant RABV expressing chemokines were tested for their ability to enhance adaptive immunity (Zhao *et al.*, 2009, 2010). Although overexpression of MIP-1α further attenuated RABV (Zhao *et al.*, 2010), it enhanced the adaptive immune responses by stimulating the production of high levels of virus-neutralizing antibodies (VNA). As MIP-1α is one of the major chemoattractants for monocytes, especially immature DCs and macrophages (Barouch *et al.*, 2003; Maurer and von Stebut, 2004; McKay *et al.*, 2004), it is possible that expression of MIP-1α recruits/activates DCs. Indeed, it was found that overexpression of MIP-1α resulted in the induction of a strong innate immune response at the local site and recruitment/activation of DCs as well as B cells in the draining lymph nodes and the peripheral blood, leading to the production of high levels of VNA (Zhao *et al.*, 2010). DCs are the most potent antigen presenting cells (APCs) (Clark, 1997), which process antigen, migrate to the T cell zone and stimulate the activation of antigen-specific naïve T cells. Activated T cells stimulate the proliferation and differentiation of antigen-specific naïve B cells into antibody-producing plasma cells (Dubois *et al.*, 1999).

To confirm that recruitment/activation of DCs is the major step in the induction of VNA in RABV immunization, DC-recruitment/activation molecules such as macrophage-derived chemokine (MDC) and granulocyte-macrophage colony-stimulating factor (GM-CSF), in addition to MIP-1α, were individually expressed in the RABV LBNSE strain (Wen *et al.*, 2011). MDC is known to preferentially attract Th2 cells and regulatory T cells via CCR4 (Iellem *et al.*, 2001; Imai *et al.*, 1999; Yoshie *et al.*, 2001). It is also a potent chemoattractant for additional cell types including DCs (Chantry *et al.*, 1999; Godiska *et al.*, 1997). MDC produced by DCs attracts CCR4-bearing activated (or memory) T cells to enhance immune responses and increase effector functions (Wu *et al.*, 2001), and it may allow for T–B cell interaction with subsequent formation of germinal centers (Schaniel *et al.*, 1998). GM-CSF regulates the production and functional activation of hemopoietic cells such as monocyte/macrophages and all granulocytes (Metcalf, 2008) and is a cytokine responsible for the recruitment, activation, and maturation of APC (Hamilton and Anderson, 2004). Each of these recombinant viruses stimulated more maturation/activation of murine bone marrow-derived DCs *in vitro* and more recruitment and/or activation of DCs, mature B cells as well as T cells in the periphery than the parent virus, which leads to higher levels of VNA and better protection (Wen *et al.*, 2011). Thus, our data suggest that the expression of chemokines can result in recruitment/activation of DCs, thus enhancing RABV immunogenicity and protection. Chemokines have been used as an adjuvant by incorporating into vaccine preparations to stimulate innate and adaptive immune responses (Han *et al.*, 2009; Kutzler *et al.*, 2010). Coadministration of chemokine and DNA encoding viral protective antigens increases trafficking of mature DCs into the secondary lymphoid tissues, presenting processed viral antigen to naïve T cells and provides protective immunity against virus challenge. RANTES, MCP-1, MIP-1β, and TRANCE have been used together with a truncated secreted version of the RABV glycoprotein in plasmid expression DNA vaccine to enhance immune responses (Pinto *et al.*, 2003). Together, these observations suggest that recombinant RABV expressing chemokines could be developed as potential vaccine candidates.

VII. RECOMBINANT RABV EXPRESSING CHEMOKINES/CYTOKINES CAN BE USED EFFECTIVELY TO PREVENT THE DEVELOPMENT OF RABIES

These recombinant RABV expressing chemokines/cytokines were also tested to determine whether they have the ability to prevent animals from developing rabies. Adult mice were infected with a lethal dose of street RABV and then treated with recombinant RABV at different time points after infection (Wang and Fu, unpublished data). As shown in Fig. 1, 60–70% of the mice intracerebrally treated with recombinant RABV expressing MDC, IP-10, MIP-1α, or GM-CSF at day 4 after infection with street RABV (a Mexican dog virus, DRV) were protected from developing rabies. The protection rate in mice treated with live recombinant RABV was significantly higher than that in sham-treated mice (20%). In contrast, treatment with UV-inactivated RABV did not provide significantly better protection than sham-treated mice despite the fact that VNAs

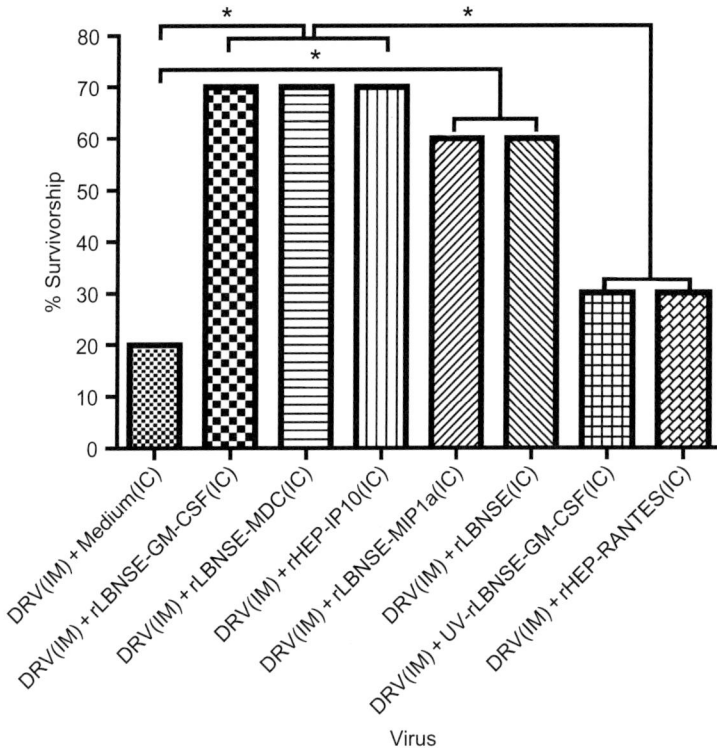

FIGURE 1 Recombinant RABVs expressing chemokines/cytokines prevent the development of rabies in the mouse model. ICR mice (4–6 weeks of age) were infected intramuscularly with street DRV and treated intracranially 4 days later with various recombinant RABVs or medium. Mice were observed daily for 2 weeks, and the survivorship was calculated and analyzed statistically.

were induced in these mice. Surprisingly, recombinant RABV expressing RANTES did not protect mice from developing rabies in these mice. Treatment with recombinant RABV by other routes (intramuscular, intradermal, or intranasal) was less effective (Wang and Fu, unpublished data). It was found that intracerebral treatment of mice with these recombinant RABVs induced significantly higher levels of chemokine/cytokine expression in the CNS and in the periphery, infiltration of inflammatory and immune cells into the CNS, and enhancement of BBB permeability than sham-treated mice or mice treated with UV-inactivated RABV. These studies indicate that there are two important factors for protection: VNA in the periphery and enhanced BBB permeability. To demonstrate this is the case, mice were treated with a chemokine (chemoattractant protein-1, MCP-1) with a dose known to enhance BBB permeability. Indeed, this treatment increased the protective efficacy of UV-inactivated RABV, but not in sham-treated mice. These data confirm that chemokines can induce infiltration of inflammatory cells in the CNS and thus enhance the BBB permeability, which allows immune effectors (VNA) enter into the CNS to clear the virus and prevent the development of rabies.

BBB is a separation of circulating blood and CSF in the CNS and protects the CNS tissues from circulating cells and factors (Pachter *et al.*, 2003). The enhancement of BBB permeability and inflammatory cells infiltration is often associated with pathological changes in the CNS. However, transiently increased BBB permeability has been found to be helpful in clearance of the attenuated RABV from the CNS (Phares *et al.*, 2006). Highly pathogenic RABV is correlated with the inability of infected animals to enhance BBB permeability and deliver immune effectors into the CNS (Roy *et al.*, 2007). Further studies have shown that lethal infection with pathogenic RABV could be prevented by increasing BBB permeability in infected animals through the induction of an autoimmune CNS inflammatory response that facilitates immune effectors entry into the CNS tissue and promotes virus clearance (Roy and Hooper, 2007). Chemokines can help enhance the BBB permeability by inducing inflammatory responses in the CNS, thus aiding immune effectors enter into and clear the virus from the CNS. One of the questions that remains unanswered in these studies is whether the immune effectors (in this case, VNA) need to be produced in the CNS as has been proposed (Hooper *et al.*, 1998, 2009) or whether VNA produced in the periphery and transported to the CNS is just as effective. Future studies should be directed to address this issue.

VIII. SUMMARY

This chapter summarizes recent studies on the role of chemokines in rabies pathogenesis and protection. It has been found that laboratory-adapted RABV is capable of inducing chemokine expression as part of innate immune responses, which is beneficial to the host by initiating infiltration of inflammatory cells into the CNS, enhancing the BBB permeability, and clearing the virus from the CNS (Kuang *et al.*, 2009; Sarmento *et al.*, 2005; Wang *et al.*, 2005). This is especially important when animals are infected with low doses of laboratory-adapted RABV. However, street RABV fails to induce the expression of chemokines and other innate immune molecules, leading to unblocked invasion of the virus into the CNS (Kuang *et al.*, 2009; Sarmento *et al.*, 2005; Wang *et al.*, 2005). However, excessive expression of chemokines and other innate immune molecules could induce neurological diseases by inducing extensive inflammation in the CNS when animals are infected with high doses of fixed RABV (Kuang *et al.*, 2009; Sarmento *et al.*, 2005; Wang *et al.*, 2005). Thus, expression of chemokines has both protective and pathogenetic roles in RABV infections. This contention has been further confirmed by over-expression of some of the chemokines (Zhao *et al.*, 2009). Overexpression of MIP-1α further attenuates RABV, while overexpression of RANTES and IP-10 increases RABV pathogenicity (Zhao *et al.*, 2009). However, overexpression of MIP-1α enhances the immunogenicity of RABV, and the recruitment/activation of DCs is the possible mechanism for the enhanced immunogenicity (Zhao *et al.*, 2010). Indeed, overexpression of chemokines or cytokines with the ability to activate DCs increased RABV immunogenicity and provided better protection (Wen *et al.*, 2011; Zhao *et al.*, 2010). Further, recombinant RABV expressing chemokines/cyto-kines can be used to prevent the development of rabies in the mouse model (Wang and Fu, unpublished data). Therefore, recombinant RBAVs expressing chemokines/cytokines could have the potential to be used not only for pre- and postexposure immunization but also for therapy in clinical rabies.

ACKNOWLEDGMENTS

This work is supported partially by Public Health Service Grant AI-051560 from the National Institute of Allergy and Infectious Diseases.

REFERENCES

Aravalli, R. N., Hu, S., and Lokensgard, J. R. (2008). Inhibition of toll-like receptor signaling in primary murine microglia. *J. Neuroimmune Pharmacol.* 3(1):5–11.
Barouch, D. H., McKay, P. F., Sumida, S. M., Santra, S., Jackson, S. S., Gorgone, D. A., Lifton, M. A., Chakrabarti, B. K., Xu, L., Nabel, G. J., and Letvin, N. L. (2003). Plasmid chemokines and colony-stimulating factors enhance the immunogenicity of DNA priming-viral vector boosting human immunodeficiency virus type 1 vaccines. *J. Virol.* 77(16):8729–8735.
Chantry, D., Romagnani, P., Raport, C. J., Wood, C. L., Epp, A., Romagnani, S., and Gray, P. W. (1999). Macrophage-derived chemokine is localized to thymic medullary epithelial cells and is a chemoattractant for CD3(+), CD4(+), CD8(low) thymocytes. *Blood* 94(6):1890–1898.
Chen, I. Y., Chang, S. C., Wu, H. Y., Yu, T. C., Wei, W. C., Lin, S., Chien, C. L., and Chang, M. F. (2010). Upregulation of the chemokine (C-C motif) ligand 2 via a severe acute respiratory syndrome coronavirus spike-ACE2 signaling pathway. *J. Virol.* 84 (15):7703–7712.
Christensen, J. E., de Lemos, C., Moos, T., Christensen, J. P., and Thomsen, A. R. (2006). CXCL10 is the key ligand for CXCR3 on CD8+ effector T cells involved in immune surveillance of the lymphocytic choriomeningitis virus-infected central nervous system. *J. Immunol.* 176(7):4235–4243.
Christensen, J. E., Simonsen, S., Fenger, C., Sorensen, M. R., Moos, T., Christensen, J. P., Finsen, B., and Thomsen, A. R. (2009). Fulminant lymphocytic choriomeningitis virus-induced inflammation of the CNS involves a cytokine-chemokine-cytokine-chemokine cascade. *J. Immunol.* 182(2):1079–1087.

Clark, E. A. (1997). Regulation of B lymphocytes by dendritic cells. *J. Exp. Med.* **185** (5):801–803.

Cyster, J. G. (1999). Chemokines and cell migration in secondary lymphoid organs. *Science* **286**(5447):2098–2102.

Dhingra, V., Li, X., Liu, Y., and Fu, Z. F. (2007). Proteomic profiling reveals that rabies virus infection results in differential expression of host proteins involved in ion homeostasis and synaptic physiology in the central nervous system. *J. Neurovirol.* **13**(2):107–117.

Dietzschold, B., Morimoto, K., and Hooper, D. C. (2001). Mechanisms of virus-induced neuronal damage and the clearance of viruses from the CNS. *Curr. Top. Microbiol. Immunol.* **253**:145–155.

Dorries, R. (2001). The role of T-cell-mediated mechanisms in virus infections of the nervous system. *Curr. Top. Microbiol. Immunol.* **253**:219–245.

Dubois, B., Bridon, J. M., Fayette, J., Barthelemy, C., Banchereau, J., Caux, C., and Briere, F. (1999). Dendritic cells directly modulate B cell growth and differentiation. *J. Leukoc. Biol.* **66**(2):224–230.

Fabis, M. J., Phares, T. W., Kean, R. B., Koprowski, H., and Hooper, D. C. (2008). Blood-brain barrier changes and cell invasion differ between therapeutic immune clearance of neurotrophic virus and CNS autoimmunity. *Proc. Natl. Acad. Sci. USA* **105**(40):15511–15516.

Fisher, S. N., Vanguri, P., Shin, H. S., and Shin, M. L. (1995). Regulatory mechanisms of MuRantes and CRG-2 chemokine gene induction in central nervous system glial cells by virus. *Brain Behav. Immun.* **9**(4):331–344.

Fu, Z. F. (1997). Rabies and rabies research: Past, present and future. *Vaccine* **15**(Suppl.): S20–S24.

Fu, Z. F., Weihe, E., Zheng, Y. M., Schafer, M. K., Sheng, H., Corisdeo, S., Rauscher, F. J., 3rd, Koprowski, H., and Dietzschold, B. (1993). Differential effects of rabies and borna disease viruses on immediate-early- and late-response gene expression in brain tissues. *J. Virol.* **67**(11):6674–6681.

Fung-Leung, W. P., Kundig, T. M., Zinkernagel, R. M., and Mak, T. W. (1991). Immune response against lymphocytic choriomeningitis virus infection in mice without CD8 expression. *J. Exp. Med.* **174**(6):1425–1429.

Gale, L. M., and McColl, S. R. (1999). Chemokines: Extracellular messengers for all occasions? *Bioessays* **21**(1):17–28.

Gibson, S. J., Lindh, J. M., Riter, T. R., Gleason, R. M., Rogers, L. M., Fuller, A. E., Oesterich, J. L., Gorden, K. B., Qiu, X., McKane, S. W., Noelle, R. J., Miller, R. L., *et al.* (2002). Plasmacytoid dendritic cells produce cytokines and mature in response to the TLR7 agonists, imiquimod and resiquimod. *Cell. Immunol.* **218**(1–2):74–86.

Glabinski, A. R., and Ransohoff, R. M. (1999). Sentries at the gate: Chemokines and the blood-brain barrier. *J. Neurovirol.* **5**(6):623–634.

Glass, W. G., Hickey, M. J., Hardison, J. L., Liu, M. T., Manning, J. E., and Lane, T. E. (2004). Antibody targeting of the CC chemokine ligand 5 results in diminished leukocyte infiltration into the central nervous system and reduced neurologic disease in a viral model of multiple sclerosis. *J. Immunol.* **172**(7):4018–4025.

Glass, W. G., Lim, J. K., Cholera, R., Pletnev, A. G., Gao, J. L., and Murphy, P. M. (2005). Chemokine receptor CCR5 promotes leukocyte trafficking to the brain and survival in West Nile virus infection. *J. Exp. Med.* **202**(8):1087–1098.

Glass, W. G., McDermott, D. H., Lim, J. K., Lekhong, S., Yu, S. F., Frank, W. A., Pape, J., Cheshier, R. C., and Murphy, P. M. (2006). CCR5 deficiency increases risk of symptomatic West Nile virus infection. *J. Exp. Med.* **203**(1):35–40.

Godiska, R., Chantry, D., Raport, C. J., Sozzani, S., Allavena, P., Leviten, D., Mantovani, A., and Gray, P. W. (1997). Human macrophage-derived chemokine (MDC), a novel chemoattractant for monocytes, monocyte-derived dendritic cells, and natural killer cells. *J. Exp. Med.* **185**(9):1595–1604.

Hamilton, J. A., and Anderson, G. P. (2004). GM-CSF biology. *Growth Factors* **22**(4):225–231.

Han, Y. W., Aleyas, A. G., George, J. A., Kim, S. J., Kim, H. K., Yoo, D. J., Kang, S. H., and Eo, S. K. (2009). Genetic co-transfer of CCR7 ligands enhances immunity and prolongs survival against virulent challenge of pseudorabies virus. *Immunol. Cell Biol.* **87**(1):91–99.

Hofer, M. J., Carter, S. L., Muller, M., and Campbell, I. L. (2008). Unaltered neurological disease and mortality in CXCR3-deficient mice infected intracranially with lymphocytic choriomeningitis virus-Armstrong. *Viral Immunol.* **21**(4):425–433.

Holman, D. W., Klein, R. S., and Ransohoff, R. M. (2010). The blood-brain barrier, chemokines and multiple sclerosis. *Biochim. Biophys. Acta.* **1812**(2):220–230.

Hooper, D. C., Morimoto, K., Bette, M., Weihe, E., Koprowski, H., and Dietzschold, B. (1998). Collaboration of antibody and inflammation in clearance of rabies virus from the central nervous system. *J. Virol.* **72**(5):3711–3719.

Hooper, D. C., Phares, T. W., Fabis, M. J., and Roy, A. (2009). The production of antibody by invading B cells is required for the clearance of rabies virus from the central nervous system. *PLoS Negl. Trop. Dis.* **3**(10):e535.

Hosking, M. P., and Lane, T. E. (2010). The role of chemokines during viral infection of the CNS. *PLoS Pathog.* **6**(7):e1000937.

Iellem, A., Mariani, M., Lang, R., Recalde, H., Panina-Bordignon, P., Sinigaglia, F., and D'Ambrosio, D. (2001). Unique chemotactic response profile and specific expression of chemokine receptors CCR4 and CCR8 by CD4(+)CD25(+) regulatory T cells. *J. Exp. Med.* **194**(6):847–853.

Imai, T., Nagira, M., Takagi, S., Kakizaki, M., Nishimura, M., Wang, J., Gray, P. W., Matsushima, K., and Yoshie, O. (1999). Selective recruitment of CCR4-bearing Th2 cells toward antigen-presenting cells by the CC chemokines thymus and activation-regulated chemokine and macrophage-derived chemokine. *Int. Immunol.* **11**(1):81–88.

Kim, T. S., and Perlman, S. (2005). Viral expression of CCL2 is sufficient to induce demyelination in RAG1−/− mice infected with a neurotropic coronavirus. *J. Virol.* **79**(11):7113–7120.

Kim, J. V., Kang, S. S., Dustin, M. L., and McGavern, D. B. (2009). Myelomonocytic cell recruitment causes fatal CNS vascular injury during acute viral meningitis. *Nature* **457**(7226):191–195.

Kuang, Y., Lackay, S. N., Zhao, L., and Fu, Z. F. (2009). Role of chemokines in the enhancement of BBB permeability and inflammatory infiltration after rabies virus infection. *Virus Res.* **144**(1–2):18–26.

Kutzler, M. A., Kraynyak, K. A., Nagle, S. J., Parkinson, R. M., Zharikova, D., Chattergoon, M., Maguire, H., Muthumani, K., Ugen, K., and Weiner, D. B. (2010). Plasmids encoding the mucosal chemokines CCL27 and CCL28 are effective adjuvants in eliciting antigen-specific immunity in vivo. *Gene Ther.* **17**(1):72–82.

Lackay, S. N., Kuang, Y., and Fu, Z. F. (2008). Rabies in small animals. *Vet. Clin. North Am. Small Anim. Pract.* **38**(4):851–861, ix.

Lima, G. K., Zolini, G. P., Mansur, D. S., Freire Lima, B. H., Wischhoff, U., Astigarraga, R. G., Dias, M. F., Silva, M. D., Bela, S. R., do Valle Antonelli, L. R., Arantes, R. M., Gazzinelli, R. T., et al. (2010). Toll-like receptor (TLR) 2 and TLR9 expressed in trigeminal ganglia are critical to viral control during herpes simplex virus 1 infection. *Am. J. Pathol.* **177**(5):2433–2445.

Lin, A. A., Tripathi, P. K., Sholl, A., Jordan, M. B., and Hildeman, D. A. (2009). Gamma interferon signaling in macrophage lineage cells regulates central nervous system inflammation and chemokine production. *J. Virol.* **83**(17):8604–8615.

Liu, M. T., Keirstead, H. S., and Lane, T. E. (2001). Neutralization of the chemokine CXCL10 reduces inflammatory cell invasion and demyelination and improves neurological function in a viral model of multiple sclerosis. *J. Immunol.* **167**(7):4091–4097.

Mansfield, K. L., Johnson, N., Nunez, A., Hicks, D., Jackson, A. C., and Fooks, A. R. (2008). Up-regulation of chemokine gene transcripts and T-cell infiltration into the central nervous system and dorsal root ganglia are characteristics of experimental European bat lyssavirus type 2 infection of mice. *J. Neurovirol.* **14**(3):218–228.

Martinez, L. (2000). Global infectious disease surveillance. *Int. J. Infect. Dis.* **4**(4):222–228.

Masatani, T., Ito, N., Shimizu, K., Ito, Y., Nakagawa, K., Sawaki, Y., Koyama, H., and Sugiyama, M. (2010). Rabies virus nucleoprotein functions to evade activation of the RIG-I-mediated antiviral response. *J. Virol.* **84**(8):4002–4012.

Maurer, M., and von Stebut, E. (2004). Macrophage inflammatory protein-1. *Int. J. Biochem. Cell Biol.* **36**(10):1882–1886.

McKay, P. F., Barouch, D. H., Santra, S., Sumida, S. M., Jackson, S. S., Gorgone, D. A., Lifton, M. A., and Letvin, N. L. (2004). Recruitment of different subsets of antigen-presenting cells selectively modulates DNA vaccine-elicited CD4(+) and CD8(+) T lymphocyte responses. *Eur. J. Immunol.* **34**(4):1011–1020.

Meslin, F. X., Fishbein, D. B., and Matter, H. C. (1994). Rationale and prospects for rabies elimination in developing countries. *Curr. Top. Microbiol. Immunol.* **187**:1–26.

Metcalf, D. (2008). Hematopoietic cytokines. *Blood* **111**(2):485–491.

Miyamoto, K., and Matsumoto, S. (1967). Comparative studies between pathogenesis of street and fixed rabies infection. *J. Exp. Med.* **125**(3):447–456.

Morimoto, K., Patel, M., Corisdeo, S., Hooper, D. C., Fu, Z. F., Rupprecht, C. E., Koprowski, H., and Dietzschold, B. (1996). Characterization of a unique variant of bat rabies virus responsible for newly emerging human cases in North America. *Proc. Natl. Acad. Sci. USA* **93**(11):5653–5658.

Moser, B., and Loetscher, P. (2001). Lymphocyte traffic control by chemokines. *Nat. Immunol.* **2**(2):123–128.

Murphy, F. A. (1977). Rabies pathogenesis. *Arch. Virol.* **54**(4):279–297.

Nakamichi, K., Inoue, S., Takasaki, T., Morimoto, K., and Kurane, I. (2004). Rabies virus stimulates nitric oxide production and CXC chemokine ligand 10 expression in macrophages through activation of extracellular signal-regulated kinases 1 and 2. *J. Virol.* **78** (17):9376–9388.

Nakamichi, K., Saiki, M., Sawada, M., Takayama-Ito, M., Yamamuro, Y., Morimoto, K., and Kurane, I. (2005). Rabies virus-induced activation of mitogen-activated protein kinase and NF-kappaB signaling pathways regulates expression of CXC and CC chemokine ligands in microglia. *J. Virol.* **79**(18):11801–11812.

Pachter, J. S., de Vries, H. E., and Fabry, Z. (2003). The blood-brain barrier and its role in immune privilege in the central nervous system. *J. Neuropathol. Exp. Neurol.* **62** (6):593–604.

Patterson, C. E., Daley, J. K., Echols, L. A., Lane, T. E., and Rall, G. F. (2003). Measles virus infection induces chemokine synthesis by neurons. *J. Immunol.* **171**(6):3102–3109.

Phares, T. W., Kean, R. B., Mikheeva, T., and Hooper, D. C. (2006). Regional differences in blood-brain barrier permeability changes and inflammation in the apathogenic clearance of virus from the central nervous system. *J. Immunol.* **176**(12):7666–7675.

Pinto, A. R., Reyes-Sandoval, A., and Ertl, H. C. (2003). Chemokines and TRANCE as genetic adjuvants for a DNA vaccine to rabies virus. *Cell. Immunol.* **224**(2):106–113.

Prehaud, C., Megret, F., Lafage, M., and Lafon, M. (2005). Virus infection switches TLR-3-positive human neurons to become strong producers of beta interferon. *J. Virol.* **79** (20):12893–12904.

Rossi, D., and Zlotnik, A. (2000). The biology of chemokines and their receptors. *Annu. Rev. Immunol.* **18**:217–242.

Roy, A., and Hooper, D. C. (2007). Lethal silver-haired bat rabies virus infection can be prevented by opening the blood-brain barrier. *J. Virol.* **81**(15):7993–7998.

Roy, A., Phares, T. W., Koprowski, H., and Hooper, D. C. (2007). Failure to open the blood-brain barrier and deliver immune effectors to central nervous system tissues leads to the lethal outcome of silver-haired bat rabies virus infection. *J. Virol.* **81**(3):1110–1118.

Sallusto, F., Palermo, B., Lenig, D., Miettinen, M., Matikainen, S., Julkunen, I., Forster, R., Burgstahler, R., Lipp, M., and Lanzavecchia, A. (1999). Distinct patterns and kinetics of chemokine production regulate dendritic cell function. *Eur. J. Immunol.* **29**(5):1617–1625.

Sarmento, L., Li, X. Q., Howerth, E., Jackson, A. C., and Fu, Z. F. (2005). Glycoprotein-mediated induction of apoptosis limits the spread of attenuated rabies viruses in the central nervous system of mice. *J. Neurovirol.* **11**(6):571–581.

Schaniel, C., Pardali, E., Sallusto, F., Speletas, M., Ruedl, C., Shimizu, T., Seidl, T., Andersson, J., Melchers, F., Rolink, A. G., and Sideras, P. (1998). Activated murine B lymphocytes and dendritic cells produce a novel CC chemokine which acts selectively on activated T cells. *J. Exp. Med.* **188**(3):451–463.

So, E. Y., and Kim, B. S. (2009). Theiler's virus infection induces TLR3-dependent upregulation of TLR2 critical for proinflammatory cytokine production. *Glia* **57**(11):1216–1226.

Stiles, L. N., Liu, M. T., Kane, J. A., and Lane, T. E. (2009). CXCL10 and trafficking of virus-specific T cells during coronavirus-induced demyelination. *Autoimmunity* **42**(6):484–491.

Thapa, M., and Carr, D. J. (2008). Herpes simplex virus type 2-induced mortality following genital infection is blocked by anti-tumor necrosis factor alpha antibody in CXCL10-deficient mice. *J. Virol.* **82**(20):10295–10301.

Thapa, M., Kuziel, W. A., and Carr, D. J. (2007). Susceptibility of CCR5-deficient mice to genital herpes simplex virus type 2 is linked to NK cell mobilization. *J. Virol.* **81**(8):3704–3713.

Ubogu, E. E., Cossoy, M. B., and Ransohoff, R. M. (2006). The expression and function of chemokines involved in CNS inflammation. *Trends Pharmacol. Sci.* **27**(1):48–55.

Vanguri, P., and Farber, J. M. (1994). IFN and virus-inducible expression of an immediate early gene, crg-2/IP-10, and a delayed gene, I-A alpha in astrocytes and microglia. *J. Immunol.* **152**(3):1411–1418.

Wang, Z. W., Sarmento, L., Wang, Y., Li, X. Q., Dhingra, V., Tseggai, T., Jiang, B., and Fu, Z. F. (2005). Attenuated rabies virus activates, while pathogenic rabies virus evades, the host innate immune responses in the central nervous system. *J. Virol.* **79**(19):12554–12565.

Wang, H. and Fu, Z. F. (unpublished data).

Wen, Y., Wang, H., Wu, H., Yang, F., Tripp, R. A., Hogan, R. J., Fu, Z. F. (2011). Rabies virus expressing dendritic cell-activating molecules enhances the innate and adaptive immune response to vaccination. *J. Virol.* **85**:1634–1644.

Wu, M., Fang, H., and Hwang, S. T. (2001). Cutting edge: CCR4 mediates antigen-primed T cell binding to activated dendritic cells. *J. Immunol.* **167**(9):4791–4795.

Yan, X., Prosniak, M., Curtis, M. T., Weiss, M. L., Faber, M., Dietzschold, B., and Fu, Z. F. (2001). Silver-haired bat rabies virus variant does not induce apoptosis in the brain of experimentally infected mice. *J. Neurovirol.* **7**(6):518–527.

Yoshie, O., Imai, T., and Nomiyama, H. (2001). Chemokines in immunity. *Adv. Immunol.* **78**:57–110.

Zhang, B., Chan, Y. K., Lu, B., Diamond, M. S., and Klein, R. S. (2008). CXCR3 mediates region-specific antiviral T cell trafficking within the central nervous system during West Nile virus encephalitis. *J. Immunol.* **180**(4):2641–2649.

Zhao, L., Toriumi, H., Kuang, Y., Chen, H., and Fu, Z. F. (2009). The roles of chemokines in rabies virus infection: Overexpression may not always be beneficial. *J. Virol.* **83**(22):11808–11818.

Zhao, L., Toriumi, H., Wang, H., Kuang, Y., Guo, X., Morimoto, K., and Fu, Z. F. (2010). Expression of MIP-1alpha (CCL3) by a recombinant rabies virus enhances its immunogenicity by inducing innate immunity and recruiting dendritic cells and B cells. *J. Virol.* **84**(18):9642–9648.

Zlotnik, A., and Yoshie, O. (2000). Chemokines: A new classification system and their role in immunity. *Immunity* **12**(2):121–127.

CHAPTER 6

Interferon in Rabies Virus Infection

Martina Rieder and Karl-Klaus Conzelmann

Abstract

Rabies is among the longest known and most dangerous and feared infectious diseases for humans and animals and still is responsible for tenth of thousands of human deaths per year. The rabies virus (RABV) is a rather atypical member of the *Rhabdoviridae* family as it has completely adapted during evolution to warm-blooded hosts and is directly transmitted between them, whereas most other rhabdoviruses are transmitted by insect vectors. The virus is also unique with respect to its extremely broad host species range and a very narrow host organ range, namely its strict neurotropism. It is becoming increasingly clear that the host innate immune system, particularly the type I interferon system, and the viral counter-actions profoundly shape this virus–host relationship. In the past few years, exciting new insight was obtained on how viruses are sensed by innate immune receptors, how the downstream signaling

Max von Pettenkofer Institute and Gene Center, Ludwig-Maximilians-University Munich, Munich, Germany

Advances in Virus Research, Volume 79
ISSN 0065-3527, DOI: 10.1016/B978-0-12-387040-7.00006-8

networks for activation of interferon are working, and how viruses can interfere with the system. While RABV 5'-triphosphate RNAs were identified as the major pathogen-associated molecular pattern sensed by cytoplasmic RIG-I-like receptors (RLR), the RABV phosphoprotein (P) has emerged as a potent multifunctional antagonist able to counteract the signaling cascades leading to transcriptional activation of interferon genes as well as interferon signaling pathways, thereby limiting expression of antiviral and immune-stimulatory genes.

I. INTRODUCTION

Rabies is a zoonotic disease known to mankind since more than 4 millenniums (Steele and Fernandez, 1991; Theodorides, 1986). The main causative agent is rabies virus (RABV), the prototype of the *Lyssavirus* genus in the *Rhabdoviridae* family (Fu, 2005), which is transmitted mainly by carnivores. RABV is highly immunogenic, and efficient inactivated virus vaccines for humans and live-attenuated vaccines for wildlife have enabled control of rabies in developed countries. Still, however, rabies encephalitis causes tens of thousands of human deaths each year in developing countries (Knobel *et al.*, 2005; Warrell and Warrell, 2004).

The *Rhabdoviridae* family belongs to the order of *Mononegavirales*, also known as nonsegmented negative-strand RNA viruses (NNSV), which also comprises the *Paramyxoviridae*, *Filoviridae*, and *Bornaviridae* families. The virions of *Mononegavirales* are made up of a highly stable, helical nucleocapsid, or ribonucleoprotein (RNP), comprising the negative sense genome RNA. The RNP is enwrapped with a lipid envelope containing glycoproteins that mediate entry into host cells by membrane fusion. The *Rhabdoviridae* [*rhabdos*; greek: rod] are further characterized by a typical rod- or bullet-shaped morphology (Ge *et al.*, 2010) and comprise viruses infecting a broad host range, including plants, insects, fish, and other vertebrates (Fu, 2005). Rhabdoviruses of mammals include economically important livestock pathogens such as vesicular stomatitis virus (VSV; *Vesiculovirus* genus). In general, mammalian rhabdoviruses are transmitted by insect vectors and for a long time were not thought to cause human disease, but sporadic outbreaks of encephalitis were recently caused by the sandfly-transmitted VSV-like Chandipura virus (Basak *et al.*, 2007). The outstanding exception is the *Lyssavirus* genus, which is probably the only mammalian rhabdovirus group that lacks an insect vector for transmission, and which represents a constant human threat. However, in terms of virus structure and shape, genome organization, expression strategy, and an exclusive cytoplasmic life cycle, RABV remains a typical member of vertebrate rhabdoviruses (Albertini *et al.*, 2008; Luo *et al.*, 2007; Whelan *et al.*, 2004).

A. RABV life cycle

RABV entry into cells involves receptor-mediated endocytosis, membrane fusion at acidic pH, and release of the virus RNP into the cytoplasm, involving its transition from a supercoiled state to a relaxed form which can serve as a template for the associated polymerase. The viral RNA appears to be completely shielded by the N protein and not accessible to small cellular compounds, including RNA-binding proteins like RNases or small (interfering) RNAs (Albertini *et al.*, 2006, 2008). The 12-kb negative-strand RNA has unmodified 5'-triphosphate (5'-ppp) and 3'-hydroxyl ends and comprises five genes in the conserved order 3'-N-P-M-G-L-5' encoding (1) the nucleoprotein (N), which encloses the RNA; (2) the phosphoprotein (P), which is a cofactor for the RNA polymerase and a chaperone for soluble N protein (N^0); (3) the matrix protein (M), which is critical for virus assembly and budding; (4) the transmembrane spike glycoprotein (G) responsible for attachment to target cells and membrane fusion; and (5) the "large" protein (L), which is the catalytic subunit of the viral RNA polymerase.

The tight N-RNA clamping appears to open exclusively and transiently during transcription and replication to grant specific access of the polymerase complex (L/P) to the RNA template (Albertini *et al.*, 2008), such that immune-stimulatory long dsRNAs are not typically produced (Weber *et al.*, 2006). Transcription of the genome RNA (RNP) starts exclusively at the 3'-end and, according to the widely acknowledged stop–restart mechanism of *Mononegavirales*, gives rise to a declining gradient of subgenomic, monocistronic mRNAs with a 5'-cap and 3'-poly(A) tail (Li *et al.*, 2006; Ogino and Banerjee, 2007), and which in this respect look like typical cellular mRNAs (see Whelan *et al.*, 2004 and Chapter 1 for details).

Replication of full-length RNPs critically involves concurrent elongation and encapsidation of the nascent RNA into N-RNA and can, therefore, occur only upon prior accumulation of high N protein levels. The synthesis of abundant amounts of a short 5'-ppp leader RNA from the 3'-end of the genome (Leppert *et al.*, 1979), which is partially found in complexes with N (Blumberg *et al.*, 1983), may represent abortive replication due to insufficient amounts of N protein for encapsidation. In this case, product control may cause the polymerase to release the leader RNA product and to switch to the transcription mode at the leader/N gene junction (Vidal and Kolakofsky, 1989). Leader RNA synthesis was originally thought to be required for transcription of the downstream genes, but recent data from several virus systems argue in favor of independent transcription initiation mechanisms (Banerjee, 2008; Curran and Kolakofsky, 2008; Whelan, 2008). The full-length antigenome RNP is exclusively a template for replicative amplification of genome RNPs, which may serve for secondary transcription or assembly of novel virions at the plasma membrane.

While *in vitro* RABV is able to enter virtually any cell type, including nonneuronal cells, infection *in vivo* is characterized by a high neurotropism. Infection of neurons is in fact essential for the virus to gain access to the CNS. The long-range retrograde transport involves microtubule-mediated passage of membrane vesicles containing complete, enveloped virus particles, and the selection of the type of vesicle to take (as a taxi) appears to largely depend on the G protein (Klingen *et al.*, 2008). After membrane fusion and virus replication in the cell body, new viruses are formed which are transmitted exclusively via synaptic connections to presynaptic neurons (Astic *et al.*, 1993; Ugolini, 1995). In this respect, RABV is unique among all viruses. Both natural and recombinant RABV tracers, therefore, represent unique tools for mapping synaptic connections and neuronal circuits (Ugolini, 2008; Wickersham *et al.*, 2007a,b).

The ability to reach the CNS from a peripheral infection site, referred to as "neuroinvasiveness," largely determines the virulence of the virus. A key strategy of the virus must therefore be to avoid direct cytotoxicity, innate immunity, and inflammation to conserve the integrity of the neuronal network and to gain time to reach the CNS (Dietzschold *et al.*, 2008; Finke and Conzelmann, 2005; Lafon, 2008; Nadin-Davis and Fehlner-Gardiner, 2008; Schnell *et al.*, 2010) (see also Chapter 3). Indeed, compared to other viral encephalitides, little inflammation is observed in rabies and symptoms appear to arise from neuronal dysfunction rather than damage (Fu and Jackson, 2005). Multiple viral genes are critical in this respect. Mutations in any of the genes were shown to affect virulence and neuroinvasiveness. Particularly, the G proteins from different RABV strains and isolates differ in sequence and receptor use (Dietzschold *et al.*, 2008), induction of cellular apoptosis (Lafon, 2008), and neuroprotective activities (Prehaud *et al.*, 2010).

B. The interferon system

Host defense against viruses relies on the recognition of "nonself" structures, so-called pathogen-associated molecular patterns (PAMPs), by pattern recognition receptors (PRRs; Janeway and Medzhitov, 2002), which induce the production of the potent antiviral type I interferons (IFN-α/β), type III IFNs (IFN-λ), and proinflammatory cytokines like TNF and IL12 (Kawai and Akira, 2010; Pichlmair and Reis e Sousa, 2007; Yoneyama and Fujita, 2010). Type I IFNs, including the single IFN-β and the IFN-α family comprising a dozen of partially homologous proteins (Calam, 1980), are long known as antiviral cytokines (Isaacs and Lindenmann, 1957). However, type I IFNs also stimulate adaptive immunity by induction of immune-modulatory genes, supporting activation of dendritic cells (DCs), stimulating macrophages, increasing major histocompatibility complex class-I expression, stimulating antibody secretion, and thereby support a Th1-biased immune response, thus integrating innate and adaptive immunity (Goodbourn *et al.*, 2000; Le and Tough, 2002; Theofilopoulos *et al.*, 2005). IFN-α/β can be expressed almost ubiquitously and acts in an auto- and paracrine fashion by binding to the also ubiquitously expressed IFN-α receptor (IFNAR). Binding triggers the canonical JAK/STAT signal transduction pathways, which activate hundreds of interferon-stimulated genes (ISG), several of which have direct antiviral and antiproliferative activities that contribute to the establishment of an antiviral state. Importantly, many components of the IFN-inducing pathways are ISGs, hence providing a positive feedback loop and increasing the magnitude of virus sensing and IFN response. The more recently described type III IFNs (IFN-λ1,2,3) also have antiviral and immune-modulatory functions, but expression of the specific IFN-λ receptors is restricted to certain cell types, including epithelial cells and plasmacytoid DCs. The activation pathways inducing IFN-λ transcription seem to parallel those of IFN-α/β (Li *et al.*, 2009a). Type II IFN (IFN-γ) is not induced by virus infection itself but is produced by activated immune cells.

Although dsRNA, and synthetic dsRNA analogs like poly(I:C) are long known as potent inducers of type I IFN (Field *et al.*, 1967; Kerr *et al.*, 1974), details on the identity of the PRRs that can trigger an IFN response upon virus infection, the exact nature of their ligands, the signaling cascades activated, and the transcription factors involved have been revealed only during the past 10 years. The major viral PAMPs are indeed nucleic acids, and two PRRs families have been identified which specifically recognize nonself viral RNA. These include the endosomal transmembrane Toll-like receptors (TLRs) 3 and 7/8, and the cytoplasmic retinoic acid inducible gene I-(RIG-I)-like helicases (RLR) RIG-I and MDA5 (melanoma differentiation-associated gene 5; for review, see Kawai and Akira, 2010; Yoneyama and Fujita, 2010). In common, these receptors activate both IFN and proinflammatory cytokines, although different signaling cascades are triggered by TLR and RLR. The pathways for IFN induction merge in the activation of interferon regulatory factors (IRFs) 3 and IRF7, which are the major transcription factors controlling transcription of type I and type III IFN genes (Honda and Taniguchi, 2006). The pathways for induction of proinflammatory cytokines lead to canonical activation of NF-κB, which is not only the major transcription factor controlling a variety of proinflammatory cytokines, such as TNF-α and interleukins, but also supports transcription of the early IFNs (IFN-β, IFN-α4) (Perkins, 2007).

II. RABIES AND INTERFERON

A. Host type I IFN is able to limit RABV infection

Probably all RABVs and other lyssaviruses induce at least little IFN and thereby upregulate ISGs in the brain (Johnson *et al.*, 2006; Marcovistz *et al.*, 1994; Sodja, 1975; Stewart and Sulkin, 1966), although RABV is long known to be "sensitive" to IFN in the sense that it cannot replicate in cells in which an antiviral state has been induced before infection is established. This is illustrated by early experiments in which animals were treated before or simultaneous with RABV infection with IFN, IFN-inducing poly(I:C), or viruses that strongly induce IFN in mammalian cells, such as Newcastle disease virus, and in which the exogenous or the induced endogenous IFN could control RABV infection (Marcovistz *et al.*, 1987; Postic and Fenje, 1971; Weinmann *et al.*, 1979). Early direct evidence for a protective role of IFN *in vivo* has also been obtained in experiments in which IFN was neutralized (Marcovistz *et al.*, 1986). The availability of transgenic mice genetically deficient for a functional IFN receptor (IFNAR-KO mice) illustrated that (as for viruses in general) IFN-mediated mechanisms are major factors restricting RABV replication *in vivo*. These mice revealed a significantly higher susceptibility to RABV than wild-type mice and were even highly susceptible to RABV mutants, which could not cause disease in mice having an intact IFN system (Faul *et al.*, 2008; Marschalek *et al.*, 2009). The observation that attenuated strains induce more IFN than virulent strains, however, first indicated differential ability of viruses to counteract the mammalian IFN system and a correlation with virulence (Wang *et al.*, 2005).

B. Recognition of RABV RNAs by PRRs

The recently described RLRs RIG-I (also known as Ddx58) and MDA5 (also known as Ifih1 or helicard; Andrejeva *et al.*, 2004; Yoneyama *et al.*, 2004, 2005) are emerging as the major PRRs for activating an IFN response upon RNA virus infection (Yoneyama and Fujita, 2010). They are composed of two N-terminal caspase activation and recruitment domains (CARDs) that mediate downstream signaling events, a central ATP-dependent helicase domain, and a short C-terminal domain known as regulatory domain (RD). A third member of the RLR family, Lgp2, lacks a CARD and appears to have regulatory functions.

Notably, the closely related RNA helicases were found to respond to distinct RNA virus types (Gitlin *et al.*, 2006; Yoneyama *et al.*, 2004). Whereas MDA5 seemed to only recognize positive-stranded picornaviruses like encephalomyocarditis virus (Kato *et al.*, 2006; Loo *et al.*, 2008), RIG-I responded to a variety of positive- and negative-strand

RNA viruses, including VSV (Gitlin *et al.*, 2006; Kato *et al.*, 2005, 2006). Indeed, our own experiments using RIG-I siRNA knockdown suggested RIG-I as the major PRR for IFN induction in RABV-infected cells. In addition, RNA isolated from RABV-infected cells did induce IFN transcription in transfected 293 cells, whereas RNA from noninfected cells did not, indicating that some pattern present in RABV RNA is specifically recognized as nonself by RIG-I. Notably, purified RNA from virions containing the full-length 5′-ppp RNA, as well as an *in vitro* transcribed T7 RNA polymerase transcript corresponding to the RABV leader RNA and containing a 5′-ppp potently activated RIG-I, but not MDA5. Enzymatic removal of the 5′-ppp, however, abolished RIG-I activation completely. This demonstrated that viral 5′-ppp RNA is a specific ligand for RIG-I (Hornung *et al.*, 2006), which was confirmed by parallel work on influenza virus RNA (Pichlmair *et al.*, 2006). The most potent activators of RIG-I are 5′-ppp dsRNAs and -hairpin RNAs (Schlee *et al.*, 2009; Schmidt *et al.*, 2009), but nonphosphorylated dsRNA and poly(I:C) can also activate RIG-I (Wilkins and Gale, 2010). Further biochemical and structural analyses revealed the C-terminal RLR RD domains as the specific binding partners for 5′-ppp RNAs (Cui *et al.*, 2008), whereas the RDs of MDA5 or Lgp2 can accommodate blunt dsRNA ends (Li *et al.*, 2009b; Pippig *et al.*, 2009), and suggested a model in which nonactivated RLRs are present in a closed conformation, but upon ligand binding to the RD and dsRNA binding to the helicase domain an ATP-dependent conformational change occurs allowing the CARDs to interact with the downstream adapter IPS-1 (Cui *et al.*, 2008).

MDA5 recognizes dsRNAs lacking 5′-terminal phosphates (Gitlin *et al.*, 2006; Kato *et al.*, 2006; Yoneyama *et al.*, 2005) and in contrast to RIG-I appears to prefer longer dsRNAs (Kato *et al.*, 2008). While MDA5 was initially involved only in recognition of picornavirus infection, recent data indicate that, in immune cells, MDA5 may contribute to recognition of various virus types of RNA viruses and to sustain IFN induction, including paramyxoviruses like Sendai virus (Gitlin *et al.*, 2010) and measles virus (Ikegame *et al.*, 2010). Similarly, RABV was recently seen to induce IFN in DC of RIG-I knockout mice (Faul *et al.*, 2010).

Though specific purified and synthetic RNAs have been identified to activate RIG-I and MDA5 *in vitro* and *in vivo*, the natural virus RNAs sensed by these RLRs in infection remain vague. As in other *Mononegavirales*, long dsRNA intermediates are not typically produced during RABV replication (Weber *et al.*, 2006). The subgenomic mRNAs are not expected to provide PAMPs because they contain 5′-cap and 3′-poly(A) modifications, just like cellular mRNA. While the genome and antigenome RNAs do contain triphosphates, they are tightly encapsidated by N protein shielding the RNA from access by cellular proteins (Albertini *et al.*, 2006), which makes them an unlikely candidate for recognition by

RLRs. Only the leader and trailer RNAs, which may be encapsidated only partially, or aberrant replicative RNAs like DI RNAs appear to be accessible by RIG-I. Indeed, the levels of DI RNA in VSV and paramyxovirus preparations were shown to correlate with the degree of IFN induction (Panda *et al.*, 2010; Strahle *et al.*, 2006). In addition, VSV Pol mutants were identified which overproduce dsRNA and thereby induce a host response (Ostertag *et al.*, 2007).

While TLR3 can detect dsRNA and was shown to be involved in the recognition of various viruses, including respiratory syncytial virus (Rudd *et al.*, 2006), the physiological role of TLR3 in antiviral immunity is controversial (Edelmann *et al.*, 2004). As seen recently, during RABV infections of TLR3 knockout mice, TLR3 did not contribute to IFN production in DC or in DC activation (Faul *et al.*, 2010). However, RABV infection and treatment with the TLR3 agonist poly(I:C) generated similar cytokine profiles, and TLR3 was upregulated after RABV infection of mice and in the human cerebellar cortex tissues (Jackson *et al.*, 2006; Lafon *et al.*, 2006; Prehaud *et al.*, 2005) indicating an important link. Notably, TLR3 was found to be involved in the generation of RABV Negri bodies (Menager *et al.*, 2009), supporting previous observations in other virus systems that TLR3 may have rather proviral roles (Le Goffic *et al.*, 2006; Wang *et al.*, 2004).

TLR7, which is expressed mainly in pDC, the major producers of systemic IFN-α after pathogen infection, is an important receptor for both extra- and intracellular virus RNAs, which gain access to the endosomal receptor by autophagy, as well as self-RNAs in RNP complexes (Kawai and Akira, 2010). While VSV RNA appears to be recognized readily by mouse TLR7 (Lund *et al.*, 2004), we did not observe TLR7-dependent activation of IFN expression by RABV in isolated human pDC (Hornung *et al.*, 2004). Also in RABV-infected mouse DC, the lack of TLR7 did not alter IFN expression (Faul *et al.*, 2010).

C. RABV countermeasures to IFN system

1. The RABV P protein

In the past few years, the RABV phosphoprotein P was identified as a major and multifunctional IFN antagonist, with important roles in counteracting specific steps in IFN gene expression, IFN-induced STAT signaling, and the functions of antiviral proteins. Generally, the P proteins of *Mononegavirales* are proteins critically involved in RNA synthesis, by acting as a noncatalytic factor of the polymerase complex L–P. In addition, RABV P protein binds to soluble N protein (N^0), thereby aiding specific encapsidation of viral RNA. Moreover, RABV is a binding partner of various cellular proteins, including dynein light chain, indicating a role in intracellular transport of viral components. Such plethora of functions and binding partners define P as a "hub" protein central to the virus life cycle.

RABV P is a 299 aa phosphoprotein containing three structured domains located at the N-terminus (P_{NTD}), the center of the protein (P_{CED}), and the C-terminus (P_{CTD}), which are separated by two intrinsically disordered domains providing flexibility. P_{NTD} comprises the binding sites for L and N^0 and is, therefore, important for polymerase cofunction and RNA encapsidation. The central P_{CED} harbors a self-association domain leading to the formation of elongated P homodimers *in vitro* and *in vivo* (Gerard *et al.*, 2009; Ivanov *et al.*, 2010; Jacob *et al.*, 2001) (Fig. 1). A strong dynein light chain 8 (DLC; LC8) binding site is located in the downstream disordered domain of P (Jacob *et al.*, 2000; Raux *et al.*, 2000). RABV mutants lacking the DLC binding site appear to have defects in efficient virus transcription in neurons (Tan *et al.*, 2007) rather than in axonal transport (Rasalingam *et al.*, 2005) or subcellular location of P forms (Moseley *et al.*, 2007b). The large P_{CTD} mediates binding to the N-RNA complex and is, therefore, probably important for linking the polymerase P–L complex to the template (Gerard *et al.*, 2009; Mavrakis *et al.*, 2004, 2006; Ribeiro *et al.*, 2008; Schoehn *et al.*, 2001). In contrast to VSV P, phosphorylation of RABV P is not required for transcription. The N-terminal residue S63, which is phosphorylated by a so far unidentified cellular RABV-specific kinase (Gupta *et al.*, 2000), did not reveal a functional relevance yet (Gigant *et al.*, 2000). Phosphorylation of C-terminal residues (S162, S210, and S271) by

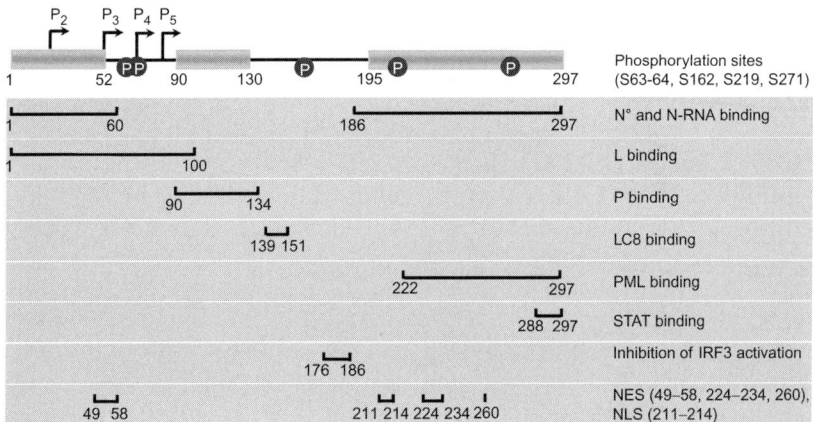

FIGURE 1   Schematic overview of the RABV phosphoprotein domains. Depicted are the three structured domains, the N-terminus (P_{NTD}), the center of the protein (P_{CED}), and the C-terminus (P_{CTD}), separated by two intrinsically disordered domains. Truncated P forms and their respective transcription start sites are indicated by arrows. Phosphorylation sites, interacting domains, NLS and NES, and the aa that antagonize IRF3 activation are shown.

protein kinase C (PKC) was found to influence the nucleocytoplasmic distribution of P (Moseley *et al.*, 2007a).

Full-length P is the major product from P mRNA, but truncated P proteins are generated in virus-infected cells by ribosomal leaky scanning from downstream in-frame AUG initiation codons located at aa 20 (P_2), 53 (P_3), 69(P_4), and 83(P_5) (Chenik *et al.*, 1995). While P is located in the cytoplasm, the lack of an N-terminal NES in P_3 and shorter P forms can result in a nuclear localization (Moseley *et al.*, 2007a; Pasdeloup *et al.*, 2005; Vidy *et al.*, 2007).

2. Inhibition of RLR-mediated IFN induction by the RABV P protein

Though RABV RNAs obviously activate RLR signaling, natural RABVs are poor inducers of IFN, indicating that the virus must have the means to counteract the signaling cascades triggered. Activation of RIG-I and MDA5 results in association of their CARDs with the CARD of the common adaptor protein IPS-1 (Kawai *et al.*, 2005) also named MAVS, VISA, or Cardif, which is located in the outer mitochondrial membrane (Loo *et al.*, 2006; Seth *et al.*, 2005). Subsequently, TRAF3 associates to the C-terminal region of IPS-1, and further complex formation with TRADD, TANK (Michallet *et al.*, 2008; Pomerantz and Baltimore, 1999), Nap1 (Fujita *et al.*, 2003; Sasai *et al.*, 2005), and TBKBP1 (Ryzhakov and Randow, 2007) takes place. Formation of this complex is a prerequisite for activation of the ubiquitous kinase TBK-1, and the related IKK-i (or IKK-ε), which is mainly expressed in immune cells. These kinases phosphorylate and thus activate the latent ubiquitous transcription factor IRF3 and the IFN-inducible IRF7. In addition, FADD1 and RIP1are recruited to the IPS-1 complex via the adapter protein TRADD (Balachandran *et al.*, 2004; Michallet *et al.*, 2008), leading to canonical NF-κB activation through the IKK-α/β/γ complex (see Fig. 1). A protein named MITA, also called STING or MPYS, which interacts with RIG-I, IPS-1, and possibly IRF3, is required for RIG-I downstream signaling (Bowzard *et al.*, 2009). Phosphorylated IRF3 forms dimers and translocates to the nucleus where it activates the IFN-β promoter, together with NF-κB and AP1 transcription factors, leading to the production of IFN-β (Panne *et al.*, 2007; Thanos and Maniatis, 1995).

The ability of RABV to counteract IFN induction was indicated in studies in which mice infected with attenuated RABV induced stronger inflammatory reactions and upregulation of various ISGs than mice infected with wt RABV (Wang *et al.*, 2005), although the proteins involved were not demonstrated. A first hint on the involvement of the RABV P protein was obtained in studies on recombinant viruses expressing an eGFP-P fusion protein (Finke *et al.*, 2004). While this virus replicated well in BSR cells, which cannot express IFN, infection of interferon competent cells resulted in induction of IFN and elimination of the virus, indicating P protein-related defects in counteracting IFN induction. Indeed, as revealed by P cDNA transfection experiments, the presence of RABV P specifically blocks phosphorylation of IRF3 and IRF7 by the kinases TBK-1 and IKK-i and, therefore, prevents transcription of *IFN-α/β* genes (Brzózka *et al.*, 2005). The activation of NF-κB, however, is not disturbed. Attempts to unravel the binding partners and exact mechanisms employed by P are in progress. We assume that the assembly of the IPS-1-linked TRAF6/NAP1/TBKBP1/TANK-complex necessary for TBK-1 to phosphorylate IRF3 and IRF7 is hampered in the presence of P (Rieder, unpublished data) (Fig. 2).

An important role of P in the virus context was readily verified by recombinant viruses expressing reduced amounts of P, through P gene shift experiments (Brzózka *et al.*, 2005), or IRES-dependent reduction of P protein expression (Marschalek *et al.*, 2009). Whereas in cells infected with a wt RABV (SAD L16) activation of IRF3 was hardly detectable, the former viruses led to strong activation of IRF3 and IFN induction. Transfection experiments showed that both P and truncated P constructs were equally effective in preventing IRF3 activation when expressed at equal levels. Indeed, in the natural virus context the abundantly expressed P2 seems to contribute considerably to preventing an IFN response, as indicated by the analysis of recombinant viruses expressing distinct amounts of P1 and P2 (Marschalek *et al.*, 2011). However, recombinant viruses able to express only full-length P, by mutation of downstream AUG codons, still effectively counteracted induction of IFN (Brzózka *et al.*, 2005).

Importantly, the recombinant viruses expressing low amounts of P were attenuated in mice after intracerebral injection, illustrating a crucial role of the IFN antagonistic functions of P to survival of RABV in the host. However, as P also inhibits STAT signaling (see below), the individual contribution of the IRF and STAT inhibitory mechanisms of P could not be appreciated in these experiments. Recent mutagenesis approaches, however, identified P proteins specifically defective in preventing IRF3 activation, while STAT inhibition was unaffected. A region relevant (aa 176–186) was located immediately upstream of the P_{CTD} in the disordered region (Fig. 1). A virus carrying a deletion of P aa 176–181 (SAD ΔInd1) has lost the ability to prevent IRF3 activation and IFN induction and was considerably attenuated after intracerebral injection into mouse brains (Rieder *et al.*, 2011). This is the first direct evidence that the ability of RABV P to prevent IFN induction contributes to RABV pathogenicity *in vivo*. Notably, while P is perfect in preventing the canonical activation of IRF3/7 by the TBK-1/IKK-i complex and, therefore, inhibits activation of cells by RLR and TLR3, which merge in this complex, it is not able to prevent IFN induction in pDC, where IRF7 is activated via

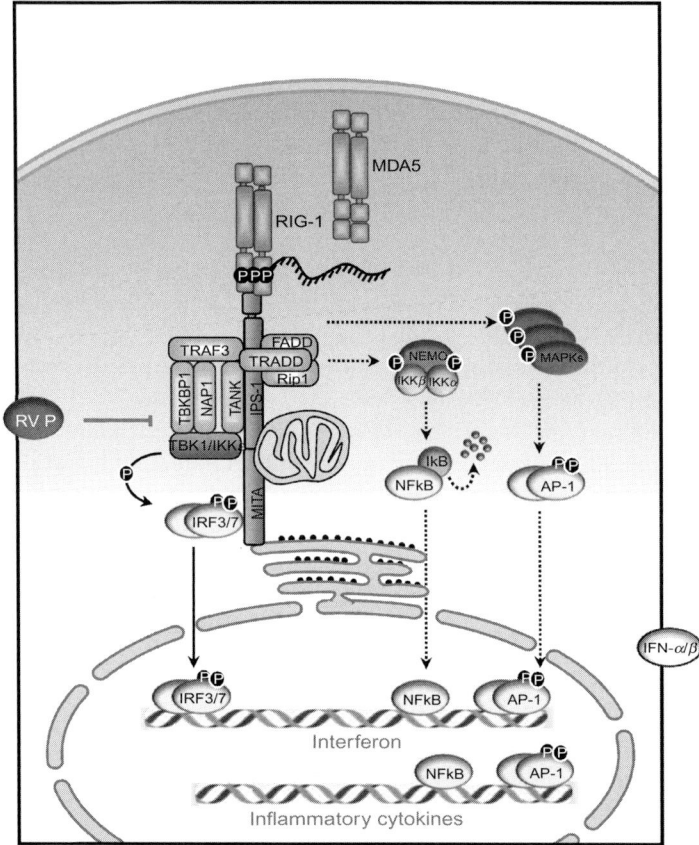

FIGURE 2 Recognition of RABV 5′-ppp RNAs by RIG-I leads to association of the RIG-I CARD to the CARD of the adaptor protein IPS-1. A complex forms on IPS-1, including the proteins TRAF3, TBKBP1, NAP1, TANK, TRADD, RIP1, and FADD in which IRF3 or IRF7 is phosphorylated by TBK-1 or IKK-i. Phosphorylation initiates homodimerization of IRF3/7, import into the nucleus, and transcriptional activation of the *IFN-α/β* genes. Simultaneously, the IKK-α/β/γ complex is activated, which induces the ubiquitination of IκB and thus allows the translocation of NF-κB to the nucleus. NF-κB and AP-1 also associate to the IFN-α/β promoter, allowing the full capacity of IFN-α/β transcription.

TLR7/9-mediated signaling cascades resulting in IKKα-mediated phosphorylation of IRF7 (Pfaller and Conzelmann, 2008).

3. Inhibition of STAT signaling by the RABV P protein

IFN-α/β and IFN-γ exert their antiviral and biological effects by binding to their respective heterodimeric receptors IFNAR or IFNGR. Upon binding, the intracellular moieties of the receptors are subject to tyrosine phosphorylation by the Janus kinases (JAKs) JAK1/TYK2 and JAK1/

JAK2, respectively. STAT1 and STAT2 dock to the phosphorylated IFNAR chains and are phosphorylated by the JAKs. IRF9 (p48) is recruited to the STAT dimer forming a heteromeric complex referred to as IFN-stimulated gene factor 3 (ISGF3). In case of IFNGR, only STAT1 is phosphorylated to form the homodimeric γ-activated factor (GAF). ISGF3 and GAF translocate to the nucleus and bind to DNA sequences called interferon-stimulated response element (ISRE) and IFN-γ-activated sequences (GAS), respectively, which are present in the promoters of ISG to promote their transcription (Platanias, 2005).

As for most viruses, IFN treatment of cells in which an infection has been established previously does not have major inhibitory effects on RABV replication, indicating viral means to effectively prevent expression of IFN-induced antiviral proteins. Indeed, RABV P was found to interact in yeast-two-hybrid experiments with STAT1 and to prevent STAT1-mediated reporter ISG expression in mammalian cells (Vidy et al., 2005). In independent work, we showed that the above described recombinant RABVs expressing low P levels were sensitive to exogenous IFN and had lost the ability to prevent IFN-α/β and IFN-γ signaling (Brzózka et al., 2006). Activation of STAT1 and STAT2 involves phosphorylation of the residues Y701 and Y689, respectively, leading to dimerization and trans-location to the nucleus. Although the above yeast-two-hybrid experiments indicated a general affinity of P and STAT1, we found that in mammalian cells P binds almost exclusively to tyrosine-phosphorylated STAT1 and STAT2, whereas in nonactivated cells the association of P with STATs was not indicated (Brzózka et al., 2006). In the presence of P, the activated STATs are unable to accumulate in the nucleus (Fig. 3). Such conditional, purposive activity only on demand may stem from the busy nature of P, allowing P to perform its many other functions in virus replication.

For binding STAT1 and STAT2 and their retention in the cytoplasm, the P_{CTD} is required. Deletion of the 10 C-terminal aa residues abolishes binding completely (Brzózka et al., 2006; Vidy et al., 2005). In addition to full-length P, also N-terminally truncated constructs are able to bind and retain STATs in the cytoplasm, including the natural shorter forms of P. Interestingly, though representing a minor fraction of total P products, the nuclear forms of P were found to block an intranuclear step in that they prevent STAT1 binding to the promoter of the ISGs (Vidy et al., 2007). In this respect, the intriguing observation was made that monomeric P_3 localizes to the nucleus and interacts with nuclear STAT, whereas dimeric P_3 associates with microtubules in the cytoplasm and there prevents STAT nuclear import (Moseley et al., 2009). While dimerization is essential for the stable association of P_3 with microtubules, it was shown to be dispensable for P-supported transcription (Jacob et al., 2001).

It is obvious that the ability to potently counteract signaling by IFN, induced by the virus itself, through infections with other pathogens, or

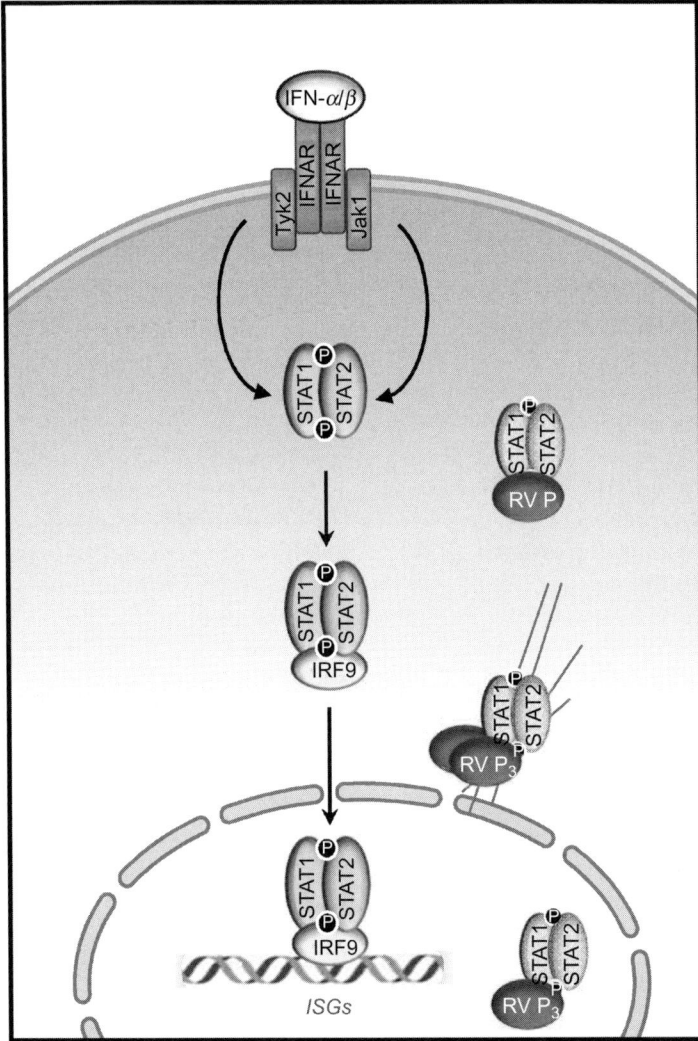

FIGURE 3 IFN-α/β acts in an auto- and paracrine fashion by binding to cell surface IFNAR1/2, inducing phosphorylation of STAT1 and STAT2 by receptor-associated kinases JAK1/TYK2. Subsequent STAT1/2 dimerization and recruitment of IRF9 (to form ISGF3) lead to nuclear translocation and transcriptional activation of *ISRE* genes. Inhibition of IFN signaling is accomplished by RABV P binding to phosphorylated STAT1 and STAT2 to block nuclear import and transcription of ISGs. The dimerized P_3 associates to microtubules where it sequesters STATs away from nuclear import; however, in its monomeric form, it is located in the nucleus, inhibiting STAT binding to ISGs.

other inflammatory reactions, is crucial for replication and virulence of RABV *in vivo*. This is supported by the complete attenuation of recombinant viruses expressing low amounts of P, although these are defective in counteracting IFN induction as well (Marschalek *et al.*, 2009). Moreover, the high attenuation of a vaccine RABV (Ni-CE) could be attributed partially to a defect of the P protein in preventing STAT signaling (Ito *et al.*, 2010). The importance of cytoplasmic localization of the P protein was emphasized in this study, as the defect of P in counteracting STAT signaling could be assigned to a mutated NES such that the protein could not prevent STAT nuclear import. Introduction of this P gene into the parental highly virulent Ni strain led to an intermediate attenuation phenotype in the resulting chimeric virus (Ito *et al.*, 2010).

4. Interplay of RABV and antiviral ISGs

ISG-encoded proteins include molecules with direct antiviral roles, such as protein kinase R (PKR), 2'-5'OAS and RNaseL, or Mx proteins (Haller *et al.*, 2007; Silverman, 2007; Williams, 1999). While the 2'-5'OAS/RNase L system, which degrades viral and cellular RNAs, appears not to have negative effects on rhabdovirus replication (Silverman, 2007), PKR emerged as a key component of IFN-induced resistance to VSV (Balachandran *et al.*, 2000; Lee *et al.*, 1996; Stojdl *et al.*, 2000). PKR is activated by dsRNA (Kerr *et al.*, 1974; Lebleu *et al.*, 1976) or by proteins like PACT (Sen and Peters, 2007) and limits viral translation by phosphorylating the initiation factor eIF-2. However, PKR seems not to be involved in restricting RABV infection (Blondel *et al.*, 2010). Mx proteins are dynamin-like GTPases and are effective against a broad variety of positive- and negative-strand RNA viruses, including VSV (for review, see Haller *et al.*, 2007). Although a general inhibition of RABV and lyssaviruses by Mx proteins is not observed, IFN-α/β induced bovine, but not human MxA, was identified to inhibit specific strains of RABV (Leroy *et al.*, 2006; Sandrock *et al.*, 2001).

However, data accumulate indicating that promyelocytic leukemia (PML) protein, also known as the tripartite motif protein 19 (TRIM19), may play a role in IFN-induced antiviral activities against RABV. PML is induced by type I and type II IFNs and is a component of nuclear multiprotein complexes named PML nuclear bodies (NBs). Infectious titers of the RABV strain CVS were 10- to 20-fold increased in PML$^{-/-}$ MEFs (Blondel *et al.*, 2002). Moreover, overexpressing the PML isoforms IV and IVa, but not other isoforms, led to reduction of RABV replication, indicating specific antiviral activities (Blondel *et al.*, 2010). Notably, P of the RABV strain CVS binds to PML and retains it in the cytoplasm, suggesting that P is an antagonist of the antiviral PML function (Blondel *et al.*, 2002; Chelbi-Alix *et al.*, 1998; Everett and Chelbi-Alix, 2007). Notably, this interaction occurs via the P$_{CTD}$ which is also engaged in STAT binding.

III. CONCLUSIONS AND FUTURE OUTLOOK

RABV is effectively recognized by RLR, but it has coevolved means to limit the host response as far as possible. These means include multiple "active" functions like those performed by the P protein, which counteracts IFN-inducing signaling pathways, expression of IFN-induced genes, and the function of antiviral proteins. However, P is not an all-rounder, as it completely fails in counteracting specific IFN induction pathways active in hematopoietic cells like pDC (Pfaller and Conzelmann, 2008). In addition, P needs to be expressed in reasonable amounts for exerting its multiple anti-IFN activities. As for other viruses, the phase of initial virus infection where protein expression just commences but RNAs are recognized is the Achilles' heel (Brzózka and Conzelmann, 2009; Randall and Goodbourn, 2008). This critical phase is longer in cells that do not well support RABV replication and P gene expression, and obviously, interference with the IFN system will be ineffective until enough P is present. This phase may be more critical in cells that are more professional in sensing RNA and faster in activating a strong response. Both parameters, a slower virus replication and a faster strong IFN response, may apply in mouse cDCs, which can be infected by RABV, do not support virus growth, and rather produce IFN (Faul et al., 2010). Neuronal cells, however, do support RABV replication very well, and though they can express and respond well to IFN (Delhaye et al., 2006), RABV can establish the infection. What makes RABV a RABV seems to be a combination of what the virus can achieve and what the host allows for.

Though RABV P has the major active role in counteracting IFN, other viral factors certainly facilitate this mission of P. The physical and constant nature of the RNP and controlled RNA synthesis are critical in preventing recognition of RNAs by PRR. Indeed, a mutation in the N protein of an attenuated RABV strain (Ni-CE) was shown to cause enhanced IFN induction, indicating defects in packaging and better recognition of viral RNA. In addition, recombinant viruses with certain mutations in the M protein, which is involved in the regulation of RABV transcription and replication (Finke et al., 2003), were found to be better IFN inducers than the isogenic parental virus. Detailed analysis of the RNAs produced by these viruses may finally provide hints of the natural RNAs activating RLRs.

The further study of the structure of immune-stimulating RNAs, and how these activate distinct cell types, and the viral inhibitory mechanisms will not only provide strategies to generate immune-stimulatory and attenuated RABV vaccines but also provide targets for therapeutic intervention.

ACKNOWLEDGMENTS

Work in the authors' laboratory is funded by the Deutsche Forschungsgemeinschaft through SFB455, SFB870, GraKo1202, and SPP1175 and by the BMBF Lyssavirus Network.

REFERENCES

Albertini, A. A., Wernimont, A. K., Muziol, T., Ravelli, R. B., Clapier, C. R., Schoehn, G., Weissenhorn, W., and Ruigrok, R. W. (2006). Crystal structure of the rabies virus nucleoprotein-RNA complex. *Science* **313**:360–363.

Albertini, A. A., Schoehn, G., Weissenhorn, W., and Ruigrok, R. W. (2008). Structural aspects of rabies virus replication. *Cell. Mol. Life Sci.* **65**:282–294.

Andrejeva, J., Childs, K. S., Young, D. F., Carlos, T. S., Stock, N., Goodbourn, S., and Randall, R. E. (2004). The V proteins of paramyxoviruses bind the IFN-inducible RNA helicase, mda-5, and inhibit its activation of the IFN-beta promoter. *Proc. Natl. Acad. Sci. USA* **101**:17264–17269.

Astic, L., Saucier, D., Coulon, P., Lafay, F., and Flamand, A. (1993). The CVS strain of rabies virus as transneuronal tracer in the olfactory system of mice. *Brain Res.* **619**:146–156.

Balachandran, S., Roberts, P. C., Brown, L. E., Truong, H., Pattnaik, A. K., Archer, D. R., and Barber, G. N. (2000). Essential role for the dsRNA-dependent protein kinase PKR in innate immunity to viral infection. *Immunity* **13**:129–141.

Balachandran, S., Thomas, E., and Barber, G. N. (2004). A FADD-dependent innate immune mechanism in mammalian cells. *Nature* **432**:401–405.

Banerjee, A. K. (2008). Response to "Non-segmented negative-strand RNA virus RNA synthesis in vivo" *Virology* **371**:231–233.

Basak, S., Mondal, A., Polley, S., Mukhopadhyay, S., and Chattopadhyay, D. (2007). Reviewing Chandipura: A vesiculovirus in human epidemics. *Biosci. Rep.* **27**:275–298.

Blondel, D., Regad, T., Poisson, N., Pavie, B., Harper, F., Pandolfi, P. P., De The, H., and Chelbi-Alix, M. K. (2002). Rabies virus P and small P products interact directly with PML and reorganize PML nuclear bodies. *Oncogene* **21**:7957–7970.

Blondel, D., Kheddache, S., Lahaye, X., Dianoux, L., and Chelbi-Alix, M. K. (2010). Resistance to rabies virus infection conferred by the PMLIV isoform. *J. Virol.* **84**:10719–10726.

Blumberg, B. M., Giorgi, C., and Kolakofsky, D. (1983). N protein of vesicular stomatitis virus selectively encapsidates leader RNA in vitro. *Cell* **32**:559–567.

Bowzard, J. B., Ranjan, P., Sambhara, S., and Fujita, T. (2009). Antiviral defense: RIG-Ing the immune system to STING. *Cytokine Growth Factor Rev.* **20**:1–5.

Brzózka, K., and Conzelmann, K. K. (2009). IFN escape of Rhabdoviruses. *In* "Cellular Signaling and Innate Immune Responses to RNA Virus Infections" (A. Brasier and A. Garcia-Sastre, eds.). ASM Press, Washington.

Brzózka, K., Finke, S., and Conzelmann, K. K. (2005). Identification of the rabies virus alpha/beta interferon antagonist: Phosphoprotein P interferes with phosphorylation of interferon regulatory factor 3. *J. Virol.* **79**:7673–7681.

Brzózka, K., Finke, S., and Conzelmann, K. K. (2006). Inhibition of interferon signaling by rabies virus phosphoprotein P: Activation-dependent binding of STAT1 and STAT2. *J. Virol.* **80**:2675–2683.

Calam, D. H. (1980). Nomenclature of interferons. *Lancet* **2**:259.

Chelbi-Alix, M. K., Quignon, F., Pelicano, L., Koken, M. H., and De The, H. (1998). Resistance to virus infection conferred by the interferon-induced promyelocytic leukemia protein. *J. Virol.* **72**:1043–1051.

Chenik, M., Chebli, K., and Blondel, D. (1995). Translation initiation at alternate in-frame AUG codons in the rabies virus phosphoprotein mRNA is mediated by a ribosomal leaky scanning mechanism. *J. Virol.* **69:**707–712.

Cui, S., Eisenacher, K., Kirchhofer, A., Brzózka, K., Lammens, A., Lammens, K., Fujita, T., Conzelmann, K. K., Krug, A., and Hopfner, K. P. (2008). The C-terminal regulatory domain is the RNA 5′-triphosphate sensor of RIG-I. *Mol. Cell* **29:**169–179.

Curran, J., and Kolakofsky, D. (2008). Nonsegmented negative-strand RNA virus RNA synthesis in vivo. *Virology* **371:**227–230.

Delhaye, S., Paul, S., Blakqori, G., Minet, M., Weber, F., Staeheli, P., and Michiels, T. (2006). Neurons produce type I interferon during viral encephalitis. *Proc. Natl. Acad. Sci. USA* **103:**7835–7840.

Dietzschold, B., Li, J., Faber, M., and Schnell, M. (2008). Concepts in the pathogenesis of rabies. *Future Virol.* **3:**481–490.

Edelmann, K. H., Richardson-Burns, S., Alexopoulou, L., Tyler, K. L., Flavell, R. A., and Oldstone, M. B. (2004). Does Toll-like receptor 3 play a biological role in virus infections? *Virology* **322:**231–238.

Everett, R. D., and Chelbi-Alix, M. K. (2007). PML and PML nuclear bodies: Implications in antiviral defence. *Biochimie* **89:**819–830.

Faul, E. J., Wanjalla, C. N., McGettigan, J. P., and Schnell, M. J. (2008). Interferon-beta expressed by a rabies virus-based HIV-1 vaccine vector serves as a molecular adjuvant and decreases pathogenicity. *Virology* **382:**226–238.

Faul, E. J., Wanjalla, C. N., Suthar, M. S., Gale, M., Wirblich, C., and Schnell, M. J. (2010). Rabies virus infection induces type I interferon production in an IPS-1 dependent manner while dendritic cell activation relies on IFNAR signaling. *PLoS Pathog.* **6:**e1001016.

Field, A. K., Tytell, A. A., Lampson, G. P., and Hilleman, M. R. (1967). Inducers of interferon and host resistance. II. Multistranded synthetic polynucleotide complexes. *Proc. Natl. Acad. Sci. USA* **58:**1004–1010.

Finke, S., and Conzelmann, K. K. (2005). Replication strategies of rabies virus. *Virus Res.* **111:**120–131.

Finke, S., Mueller-Waldeck, R., and Conzelmann, K. K. (2003). Rabies virus matrix protein regulates the balance of virus transcription and replication. *J. Gen. Virol.* **84:**1613–1621.

Finke, S., Brzózka, K., and Conzelmann, K. K. (2004). Tracking fluorescence-labeled rabies virus: Enhanced green fluorescent protein-tagged phosphoprotein P supports virus gene expression and formation of infectious particles. *J. Virol.* **78:**12333–12343.

Fu, Z. F. (2005). Genetic comparison of the rhabdoviruses from animals and plants. *Curr. Top. Microbiol. Immunol.* **292:**1–24.

Fu, Z. F., and Jackson, A. C. (2005). Neuronal dysfunction and death in rabies virus infection. *J. Neurovirol.* **11:**101–106.

Fujita, F., Taniguchi, Y., Kato, T., Narita, Y., Furuya, A., Ogawa, T., Sakurai, H., Joh, T., Itoh, M., Delhase, M., Karin, M., and Nakanishi, M. (2003). Identification of NAP1, a regulatory subunit of IkappaB kinase-related kinases that potentiates NF-kappaB signaling. *Mol. Cell. Biol.* **23:**7780–7793.

Ge, P., Tsao, J., Schein, S., Green, T. J., Luo, M., and Zhou, Z. H. (2010). Cryo-EM model of the bullet-shaped vesicular stomatitis virus. *Science* **327:**689–693.

Gerard, F. C., Ribeiro, E. A., Jr., Leyrat, C., Ivanov, I., Blondel, D., Longhi, S., Ruigrok, R. W., and Jamin, M. (2009). Modular organization of rabies virus phosphoprotein. *J. Mol. Biol.* **388:**978–996.

Gigant, B., Iseni, F., Gaudin, Y., Knossow, M., and Blondel, D. (2000). Neither phosphorylation nor the amino-terminal part of rabies virus phosphoprotein is required for its oligomerization. *J. Gen. Virol.* **81:**1757–1761.

Gitlin, L., Barchet, W., Gilfillan, S., Cella, M., Beutler, B., Flavell, R. A., Diamond, M. S., and Colonna, M. (2006). Essential role of mda-5 in type I IFN responses to polyriboinosinic:

polyribocytidylic acid and encephalomyocarditis picornavirus. *Proc. Natl. Acad. Sci. USA* **103:**8459–8464.

Gitlin, L., Benoit, L., Song, C., Cella, M., Gilfillan, S., Holtzman, M. J., and Colonna, M. (2010). Melanoma differentiation-associated gene 5 (MDA5) is involved in the innate immune response to Paramyxoviridae infection in vivo. *PLoS Pathog.* **6:**e1000734.

Goodbourn, S., Didcock, L., and Randall, R. E. (2000). Interferons: Cell signalling, immune modulation, antiviral response and virus countermeasures. *J. Gen. Virol.* **81:**2341–2364.

Gupta, A. K., Blondel, D., Choudhary, S., and Banerjee, A. K. (2000). The phosphoprotein of rabies virus is phosphorylated by a unique cellular protein kinase and specific isomers of protein kinase C. *J. Virol.* **74:**91–98.

Haller, O., Staeheli, P., and Kochs, G. (2007). Interferon-induced Mx proteins in antiviral host defense. *Biochimie* **89:**812–818.

Honda, K., and Taniguchi, T. (2006). IRFs: Master regulators of signalling by Toll-like receptors and cytosolic pattern-recognition receptors. *Nat. Rev. Immunol.* **6:**644–658.

Hornung, V., Schlender, J., Guenthner-Biller, M., Rothenfusser, S., Endres, S., Conzelmann, K. K., and Hartmann, G. (2004). Replication-dependent potent IFN-alpha induction in human plasmacytoid dendritic cells by a single-stranded RNA virus. *J. Immunol.* **173:**5935–5943.

Hornung, V., Ellegast, J., Kim, S., Brzózka, K., Jung, A., Kato, H., Poeck, H., Akira, S., Conzelmann, K. K., Schlee, M., Endres, S., and Hartmann, G. (2006). 5′-Triphosphate RNA is the ligand for RIG-I. *Science* **314:**994–997.

Ikegame, S., Takeda, M., Ohno, S., Nakatsu, Y., Nakanishi, Y., and Yanagi, Y. (2010). Both RIG-I and MDA5 RNA helicases contribute to the induction of alpha/beta interferon in measles virus-infected human cells. *J. Virol.* **84:**372–379.

Isaacs, A., and Lindenmann, J. (1957). Virus interference. I. The interferon. *Proc. R. Soc. Lond. B Biol. Sci.* **147:**258–267.

Ito, N., Moseley, G. W., Blondel, D., Shimizu, K., Rowe, C. L., Ito, Y., Masatani, T., Nakagawa, K., Jans, D. A., and Sugiyama, M. (2010). The role of interferon-antagonist activity of rabies virus phosphoprotein in viral pathogenicity. *J. Virol.* **84:**6699–6710.

Ivanov, I., Crepin, T., Jamin, M., and Ruigrok, R. W. (2010). Structure of the dimerization domain of the rabies virus phosphoprotein. *J. Virol.* **84:**3707–3710.

Jackson, A. C., Rossiter, J. P., and Lafon, M. (2006). Expression of toll-like receptor 3 in the human cerebellar cortex in rabies, herpes simplex encephalitis, and other neurological diseases. *J. Neurovirol.* **12:**229–234.

Jacob, Y., Badrane, H., Ceccaldi, P. E., and Tordo, N. (2000). Cytoplasmic dynein LC8 interacts with lyssavirus phosphoprotein. *J. Virol.* **74:**10217–10222.

Jacob, Y., Real, E., and Tordo, N. (2001). Functional interaction map of lyssavirus phospho-protein: Identification of the minimal transcription domains. *J. Virol.* **75:**9613–9622.

Janeway, C. A., Jr., and Medzhitov, R. (2002). Innate immune recognition. *Annu. Rev. Immunol.* **20:**197–216.

Johnson, N., McKimmie, C. S., Mansfield, K. L., Wakeley, P. R., Brookes, S. M., Fazakerley, J. K., and Fooks, A. R. (2006). Lyssavirus infection activates interferon gene expression in the brain. *J. Gen. Virol.* **87:**2663–2667.

Kato, H., Sato, S., Yoneyama, M., Yamamoto, M., Uematsu, S., Matsui, K., Tsujimura, T., Takeda, K., Fujita, T., Takeuchi, O., and Akira, S. (2005). Cell type-specific involvement of RIG-I in antiviral response. *Immunity* **23:**19–28.

Kato, H., Takeuchi, O., Sato, S., Yoneyama, M., Yamamoto, M., Matsui, K., Uematsu, S., Jung, A., Kawai, T., Ishii, K. J., Yamaguchi, O., Otsu, K., *et al.* (2006). Differential roles of MDA5 and RIG-I helicases in the recognition of RNA viruses. *Nature* **441:**101–105.

Kato, H., Takeuchi, O., Mikamo-Satoh, E., Hirai, R., Kawai, T., Matsushita, K., Hiiragi, A., Dermody, T. S., Fujita, T., and Akira, S. (2008). Length-dependent recognition of double-stranded ribonucleic acids by retinoic acid-inducible gene-I and melanoma differentiation-associated gene 5. *J. Exp. Med.* **205**:1601–1610.

Kawai, T., and Akira, S. (2010). The role of pattern-recognition receptors in innate immunity: Update on Toll-like receptors. *Nat. Immunol.* **11**:373–384.

Kawai, T., Takahashi, K., Sato, S., Coban, C., Kumar, H., Kato, H., Ishii, K. J., Takeuchi, O., and Akira, S. (2005). IPS-1, an adaptor triggering RIG-I- and Mda5-mediated type I interferon induction. *Nat. Immunol.* **6**:981–988.

Kerr, I. M., Brown, R. E., and Ball, L. A. (1974). Increased sensitivity of cell-free protein synthesis to double-stranded RNA after interferon treatment. *Nature* **250**:57–59.

Klingen, Y., Conzelmann, K. K., and Finke, S. (2008). Double-labeled rabies virus live tracking of enveloped virus transport. *J. Virol* **82**:237–245.

Knobel, D. L., Cleaveland, S., Coleman, P. G., Fevre, E. M., Meltzer, M. I., Miranda, M. E., Shaw, A., Zinsstag, J., and Meslin, F. X. (2005). Re-evaluating the burden of rabies in Africa and Asia. *Bull. World Health Organ.* **83**:360–368.

Lafon, M. (2008). Immune evasion, a critical strategy for rabies virus. *Dev. Biol. (Basel)* **131**:413–419.

Lafon, M., Megret, F., Lafage, M., and Prehaud, C. (2006). The innate immune facet of brain: Human neurons express TLR-3 and sense viral dsRNA. *J. Mol. Neurosci.* **29**:185–194.

Le Goffic, R., Balloy, V., Lagranderie, M., Alexopoulou, L., Escriou, N., Flavell, R., Chignard, M., and Si-Tahar, M. (2006). Detrimental contribution of the toll-like receptor (TLR)3 to influenza A virus-induced acute pneumonia. *PLoS Pathog.* **2**:e53.

Le, B. A., and Tough, D. F. (2002). Links between innate and adaptive immunity via type I interferon. *Curr. Opin. Immunol.* **14**:432–436.

Lebleu, B., Sen, G. C., Shaila, S., Cabrer, B., and Lengyel, P. (1976). Interferon, double-stranded RNA, and protein phosphorylation. *Proc. Natl. Acad. Sci. USA* **73**:3107–3111.

Lee, S. B., Bablanian, R., and Esteban, M. (1996). Regulated expression of the interferon-induced protein kinase p68 (PKR) by vaccinia virus recombinants inhibits the replication of vesicular stomatitis virus but not that of poliovirus. *J. Interferon Cytokine Res.* **16**:1073–1078.

Leppert, M., Rittenhouse, L., Perrault, J., Summers, D. F., and Kolakofsky, D. (1979). Plus and minus strand leader RNAs in negative strand virus-infected cells. *Cell* **18**:735–747.

Leroy, M., Pire, G., Baise, E., and Desmecht, D. (2006). Expression of the interferon-alpha/beta-inducible bovine Mx1 dynamin interferes with replication of rabies virus. *Neurobiol. Dis.* **21**:515–521.

Li, J., Wang, J. T., and Whelan, S. P. (2006). A unique strategy for mRNA cap methylation used by vesicular stomatitis virus. *Proc. Natl. Acad. Sci. USA* **103**:8493–8498.

Li, M., Liu, X., Zhou, Y., and Su, S. B. (2009a). Interferon-lambdas: The modulators of antivirus, antitumor, and immune responses. *J. Leukoc. Biol.* **86**:23–32.

Li, X., Lu, C., Stewart, M., Xu, H., Strong, R. K., Igumenova, T., and Li, P. (2009b). Structural basis of double-stranded RNA recognition by the RIG-I like receptor MDA5. *Arch. Biochem. Biophys.* **488**:23–33.

Loo, Y. M., Owen, D. M., Li, K., Erickson, A. K., Johnson, C. L., Fish, P. M., Carney, D. S., Wang, T., Ishida, H., Yoneyama, M., Fujita, T., Saito, T., *et al.* (2006). Viral and therapeutic control of IFN-beta promoter stimulator 1 during hepatitis C virus infection. *Proc. Natl. Acad. Sci. USA* **103**:6001–6006.

Loo, Y. M., Fornek, J., Crochet, N., Bajwa, G., Perwitasari, O., Martinez-Sobrido, L., Akira, S., Gill, M. A., Garcia-Sastre, A., Katze, M. G., and Gale, M., Jr. (2008). Distinct RIG-I and MDA5 signaling by RNA viruses in innate immunity. *J Virol.* **82**:335–345.

Lund, J. M., Alexopoulou, L., Sato, A., Karow, M., Adams, N. C., Gale, N. W., Iwasaki, A., and Flavell, R. A. (2004). Recognition of single-stranded RNA viruses by Toll-like receptor 7. *Proc. Natl. Acad. Sci. USA* **101**:5598–5603.

Luo, M., Green, T. J., Zhang, X., Tsao, J., and Qiu, S. (2007). Conserved characteristics of the rhabdovirus nucleoprotein. *Virus Res.* **129:**246–251.

Marcovistz, R., Galabru, J., Tsiang, H., and Hovanessian, A. G. (1986). Neutralization of interferon produced early during rabies virus infection in mice. *J. Gen. Virol.* **67**(Pt. 2)**:**387–390.

Marcovistz, R., Germano, P. M., Riviere, Y., Tsiang, H., and Hovanessian, A. G. (1987). The effect of interferon treatment in rabies prophylaxis in immunocompetent, immunosuppressed, and immunodeficient mice. *J. Interferon Res.* **7:**17–27.

Marcovistz, R., Leal, E. C., Matos, D. C., and Tsiang, H. (1994). Interferon production and immune response induction in apathogenic rabies virus-infected mice. *Acta Virol.* **38:**193–197.

Marschalek, A., Finke, S., Schwemmle, M., Mayer, D., Heimrich, B., Stitz, L., and Conzelmann, K. K. (2009). Attenuation of rabies virus replication and virulence by picornavirus internal ribosome entry site elements. *J. Virol.* **83:**1911–1919.

Marschalek, A., Drechsel, L., and Conzelmann, K. K. (2011). The importance of being short: The role of rabies virus phosphoprotein isoforms assessed by differential IRES translation initiation. *Eur. J. Cell Biol.* doi: 10.1016/j.ejcb.2011.01.009.

Mavrakis, M., McCarthy, A. A., Roche, S., Blondel, D., and Ruigrok, R. W. (2004). Structure and function of the C-terminal domain of the polymerase cofactor of rabies virus. *J. Mol. Biol.* **343:**819–831.

Mavrakis, M., Mehouas, S., Real, E., Iseni, F., Blondel, D., Tordo, N., and Ruigrok, R. W. (2006). Rabies virus chaperone: Identification of the phosphoprotein peptide that keeps nucleoprotein soluble and free from non-specific RNA. *Virology* **349:**422–429.

Menager, P., Roux, P., Megret, F., Bourgeois, J. P., Le Sourd, A. M., Danckaert, A., Lafage, M., Prehaud, C., and Lafon, M. (2009). Toll-like receptor 3 (TLR3) plays a major role in the formation of rabies virus Negri Bodies. *PLoS Pathog.* **5:**e1000315.

Michallet, M. C., Meylan, E., Ermolaeva, M. A., Vazquez, J., Rebsamen, M., Curran, J., Poeck, H., Bscheider, M., Hartmann, G., Konig, M., Kalinke, U., Pasparakis, M., *et al.* (2008). TRADD protein is an essential component of the RIG-like helicase antiviral pathway. *Immunity* **28:**651–661.

Moseley, G. W., Filmer, R. P., Dejesus, M. A., and Jans, D. A. (2007a). Nucleocytoplasmic distribution of rabies virus p-protein is regulated by phosphorylation adjacent to C-terminal nuclear import and export signals. *Biochemistry.* **46:**12053–12061.

Moseley, G. W., Roth, D. M., Dejesus, M. A., Leyton, D. L., Filmer, R. P., Pouton, C. W., and Jans, D. A. (2007b). Dynein light chain association sequences can facilitate nuclear protein import. *Mol. Biol. Cell* **18:**3204–3213.

Moseley, G. W., Lahaye, X., Roth, D. M., Oksayan, S., Filmer, R. P., Rowe, C. L., Blondel, D., and Jans, D. A. (2009). Dual modes of rabies P-protein association with microtubules: A novel strategy to suppress the antiviral response. *J. Cell Sci.* **122:**3652–3662.

Nadin-Davis, S. A., and Fehlner-Gardiner, C. (2008). Lyssaviruses: Current trends. *Adv. Virus Res.* **71:**207–250.

Ogino, T., and Banerjee, A. K. (2007). Unconventional mechanism of mRNA capping by the RNA-dependent RNA polymerase of vesicular stomatitis virus. *Mol. Cell* **25:**85–97.

Ostertag, D., Hoblitzell-Ostertag, T. M., and Perrault, J. (2007). Overproduction of double-stranded RNA in vesicular stomatitis virus-infected cells activates a constitutive cell-type-specific antiviral response. *J. Virol.* **81:**503–513.

Panda, D., Dinh, P. X., Beura, L. K., and Pattnaik, A. K. (2010). Induction of interferon and interferon signaling pathways by replication of defective interfering particle RNA in cells constitutively expressing vesicular stomatitis virus replication proteins. *J. Virol.* **84:**4826–4831.

Panne, D., Maniatis, T., and Harrison, S. C. (2007). An atomic model of the interferon-beta enhanceosome. *Cell* **129:**1111–1123.

Pasdeloup, D., Poisson, N., Raux, H., Gaudin, Y., Ruigrok, R. W., and Blondel, D. (2005). Nucleocytoplasmic shuttling of the rabies virus P protein requires a nuclear localization signal and a CRM1-dependent nuclear export signal. *Virology* **334**:284–293.

Perkins, N. D. (2007). Integrating cell-signalling pathways with NF-kappaB and IKK function. *Nat. Rev. Mol. Cell Biol.* **8**:49–62.

Pfaller, C. K., and Conzelmann, K. K. (2008). Measles virus V protein is a decoy substrate for IkappaB kinase alpha and prevents Toll-like receptor 7/9-mediated interferon induction. *J. Virol.* **82**:12365–12373.

Pichlmair, A., and Reis e Sousa, C. (2007). Innate recognition of viruses. *Immunity* **27**:370–383.

Pichlmair, A., Schulz, O., Tan, C. P., Naslund, T. I., Liljestrom, P., Weber, F., and Reis e Sousa, C. (2006). RIG-I-mediated antiviral responses to single-stranded RNA bearing 5′-phosphates. *Science* **314**:997–1001.

Pippig, D. A., Hellmuth, J. C., Cui, S., Kirchhofer, A., Lammens, K., Lammens, A., Schmidt, A., Rothenfusser, S., and Hopfner, K. P. (2009). The regulatory domain of the RIG-I family ATPase LGP2 senses double-stranded RNA. *Nucleic Acids Res.* **37**:2014–2025.

Platanias, L. C. (2005). Mechanisms of type-I- and type-II-interferon-mediated signalling. *Nat. Rev. Immunol.* **5**:375–386.

Pomerantz, J. L., and Baltimore, D. (1999). NF-kappaB activation by a signaling complex containing TRAF2, TANK and TBK1, a novel IKK-related kinase. *EMBO J.* **18**:6694–6704.

Postic, B., and Fenje, P. (1971). Effect of administered interferon on rabies in rabbits. *Appl. Microbiol.* **22**:428–431.

Prehaud, C., Megret, F., Lafage, M., and Lafon, M. (2005). Virus infection switches TLR-3-positive human neurons to become strong producers of beta interferon. *J. Virol.* **79**:12893–12904.

Prehaud, C., Wolff, N., Terrien, E., Lafage, M., Megret, F., Babault, N., Cordier, F., Tan, G. S., Maitrepierre, E., Menager, P., Chopy, D., Hoos, S., *et al.* (2010). Attenuation of rabies virulence: Takeover by the cytoplasmic domain of its envelope protein. *Sci. Signal.* **3**:ra5.

Randall, R. E., and Goodbourn, S. (2008). Interferons and viruses: An interplay between induction, signalling, antiviral responses and virus countermeasures. *J. Gen. Virol.* **89**:1–47.

Rasalingam, P., Rossiter, J. P., Mebatsion, T., and Jackson, A. C. (2005). Comparative pathogenesis of the SAD-L16 strain of rabies virus and a mutant modifying the dynein light chain binding site of the rabies virus phosphoprotein in young mice. *Virus Res.* **111**:55–60.

Raux, H., Flamand, A., and Blondel, D. (2000). Interaction of the rabies virus P protein with the LC8 dynein light chain. *J. Virol.* **74**:10212–10216.

Ribeiro, E. A., Jr., Favier, A., Gerard, F. C., Leyrat, C., Brutscher, B., Blondel, D., Ruigrok, R. W., Blackledge, M., and Jamin, M. (2008). Solution structure of the C-terminal nucleoprotein-RNA binding domain of the vesicular stomatitis virus phosphoprotein. *J. Mol. Biol.* **382**:525–538.

Rieder, M., Brzózka, K., Pfaller, C. K., Cox, J. H., Stitz, L., and Conzelmann, K. K. (2011). Genetic dissection of interferon antagonistic functions of rabies virusphosphoprotein: Inhibition of interferon regulatory factor 3 activation is important for pathogenicity. *J. Virol.* **85**:842–852.

Rudd, B. D., Smit, J. J., Flavell, R. A., Alexopoulou, L., Schaller, M. A., Gruber, A., Berlin, A. A., and Lukacs, N. W. (2006). Deletion of TLR3 alters the pulmonary immune environment and mucus production during respiratory syncytial virus infection. *J. Immunol.* **176**:1937–1942.

Ryzhakov, G., and Randow, F. (2007). SINTBAD, a novel component of innate antiviral immunity, shares a TBK1-binding domain with NAP1 and TANK. *EMBO J.* **26**:3180–3190.

Sandrock, M., Frese, M., Haller, O., and Kochs, G. (2001). Interferon-induced rat Mx proteins confer resistance to Rift Valley fever virus and other arthropod-borne viruses. *J. Interferon Cytokine Res.* **21**:663–668.

Sasai, M., Oshiumi, H., Matsumoto, M., Inoue, N., Fujita, F., Nakanishi, M., and Seya, T. (2005). Cutting edge: NF-kappaB-activating kinase-associated protein 1 participates in TLR3/Toll-IL-1 homology domain-containing adapter molecule-1-mediated IFN regulatory factor 3 activation. *J. Immunol.* **174**:27–30.

Schlee, M., Roth, A., Hornung, V., Hagmann, C. A., Wimmenauer, V., Barchet, W., Coch, C., Janke, M., Mihailovic, A., Wardle, G., Juranek, S., Kato, H., *et al.* (2009). Recognition of 5′ triphosphate by RIG-I helicase requires short blunt double-stranded RNA as contained in panhandle of negative-strand virus. *Immunity* **31**:25–34.

Schmidt, A., Schwerd, T., Hamm, W., Hellmuth, J. C., Cui, S., Wenzel, M., Hoffmann, F. S., Michallet, M. C., Besch, R., Hopfner, K. P., Endres, S., and Rothenfusser, S. (2009). 5′-triphosphate RNA requires base-paired structures to activate antiviral signaling via RIG-I. *Proc Natl. Acad. Sci. USA.* **106**:12067–12072.

Schnell, M. J., McGettigan, J. P., Wirblich, C., and Papaneri, A. (2010). The cell biology of rabies virus: Using stealth to reach the brain. *Nat. Rev. Microbiol.* **8**:51–61.

Schoehn, G., Iseni, F., Mavrakis, M., Blondel, D., and Ruigrok, R. W. (2001). Structure of recombinant rabies virus nucleoprotein-RNA complex and identification of the phosphoprotein binding site. *J. Virol.* **75**:490–498.

Sen, G. C., and Peters, G. A. (2007). Viral stress-inducible genes. Adv. Virus Res. **70**:233–263.

Seth, R. B., Sun, L., Ea, C. K., and Chen, Z. J. (2005). Identification and characterization of MAVS, a mitochondrial antiviral signaling protein that activates NF-kappaB and IRF 3. *Cell* **122**:669–682.

Silverman, R. H. (2007). Viral encounters with OAS and RNase L during the IFN antiviral response. *J. Virol.* **81**:12720–12729.

Sodja, I. (1975). Interferon production by rabies strains isolated from wild rodents. *Acta Virol.* **19**:84–87.

Steele, J. H., and Fernandez, P. J. (1991). History of rabies and global aspects. *In* "The Natural History of Rabies" (G. M. Baer, ed.), pp. 1–26. CRC Press, Boca Raton, USA.

Stewart, W. E., and Sulkin, S. E. (1966). Interferon production in hamsters experimentally infected with rabies virus. *Proc. Soc. Exp. Biol. Med.* **123**:650–654.

Stojdl, D. F., Abraham, N., Knowles, S., Marius, R., Brasey, A., Lichty, B. D., Brown, E. G., Sonenberg, N., and Bell, J. C. (2000). The murine double-stranded RNA-dependent protein kinase PKR is required for resistance to vesicular stomatitis virus. *J. Virol.* **74**:9580–9585.

Strahle, L., Garcin, D., and Kolakofsky, D. (2006). Sendai virus defective-interfering genomes and the activation of interferon-beta. *Virology* **351**:101–111.

Tan, G. S., Preuss, M. A., Williams, J. C., and Schnell, M. J. (2007). The dynein light chain 8 binding motif of rabies virus phosphoprotein promotes efficient viral transcription. *Proc. Natl. Acad. Sci. USA* **104**:7229–7234.

Thanos, D., and Maniatis, T. (1995). Virus induction of human IFN beta gene expression requires the assembly of an enhanceosome. *Cell* **83**:1091–1100.

Theodorides, J. (1986). Histoire de la rage. Paris: Masson, p. 289.

Theofilopoulos, A. N., Baccala, R., Beutler, B., and Kono, D. H. (2005). Type I interferons (α/β) in immunity and autoimmunity. *Annu. Rev. Immunol.* **23**:307–335.

Ugolini, G. (1995). Specificity of rabies virus as a transneuronal tracer of motor networks: Transfer from hypoglossal motoneurons to connected second-order and higher order central nervous system cell groups. *J. Comp. Neurol.* **356**:457–480.

Ugolini, G. (2008). Use of rabies virus as a transneuronal tracer of neuronal connections: Implications for the understanding of rabies pathogenesis. *Dev. Biol (Basel)* **131**:493–506.

Vidal, S., and Kolakofsky, D. (1989). Modified model for the switch from Sendai virus transcription to replication. *J. Virol.* **63**:1951–1958.

Vidy, A., Chelbi-Alix, M., and Blondel, D. (2005). Rabies virus P protein interacts with STAT1 and inhibits interferon signal transduction pathways. *J. Virol.* **79**:14411–14420.

Vidy, A., El Bougrini, J., Chelbi-Alix, M. K., and Blondel, D. (2007). The nucleocytoplasmic rabies virus P protein counteracts interferon signaling by inhibiting both nuclear accumulation and DNA binding of STAT1. *J. Virol.* **81:**4255–4263.

Wang, T., Town, T., Alexopoulou, L., Anderson, J. F., Fikrig, E., and Flavell, R. A. (2004). Toll-like receptor 3 mediates West Nile virus entry into the brain causing lethal encephalitis. *Nat. Med.* **10:**1366–1373.

Wang, Z. W., Sarmento, L., Wang, Y., Li, X. Q., Dhingra, V., Tseggai, T., Jiang, B., and Fu, Z. F. (2005). Attenuated rabies virus activates, while pathogenic rabies virus evades, the host innate immune responses in the central nervous system. *J. Virol.* **79:**12554–12565.

Warrell, M. J., and Warrell, D. A. (2004). Rabies and other lyssavirus diseases. *Lancet* **363:**959–969.

Weber, F., Wagner, V., Rasmussen, S. B., Hartmann, R., and Paludan, S. R. (2006). Double-stranded RNA is produced by positive-strand RNA viruses and DNA viruses but not in detectable amounts by negative-strand RNA viruses. *J. Virol.* **80:**5059–5064.

Weinmann, E., Majer, M., and Hilfenhaus, J. (1979). Intramuscular and/or intralumbar postexposure treatment of rabies virus-infected cynomolgus monkeys with human interferon. *Infect. Immun.* **24:**24–31.

Whelan, S. P. (2008). Response to "Non-segmented negative-strand RNA virus RNA synthesis in vivo" *Virology* **371:**234–237.

Whelan, S. P., Barr, J. N., and Wertz, G. W. (2004). Transcription and replication of non-segmented negative-strand RNA viruses. *Curr. Top. Microbiol. Immunol.* **283:**61–119.

Wickersham, I. R., Finke, S., Conzelmann, K. K., and Callaway, E. M. (2007a). Retrograde neuronal tracing with a deletion-mutant rabies virus. *Nat. Methods* **4:**47–49.

Wickersham, I. R., Lyon, D. C., Barnard, R. J., Mori, T., Finke, S., Conzelmann, K. K., Young, J. A., and Callaway, E. M. (2007b). Monosynaptic restriction of transsynaptic tracing from single, genetically targeted neurons. *Neuron* **53:**639–647.

Wilkins, C., and Gale, M., Jr. (2010). Recognition of viruses by cytoplasmic sensors. *Curr. Opin. Immunol.* **22:**41–47.

Williams, B. R. (1999). PKR; a sentinel kinase for cellular stress. *Oncogene* **18:**6112–6120.

Yoneyama, M., and Fujita, T. (2010). Recognition of viral nucleic acids in innate immunity. *Rev. Med. Virol.* **20:**4–22.

Yoneyama, M., Kikuchi, M., Natsukawa, T., Shinobu, N., Imaizumi, T., Miyagishi, M., Taira, K., Akira, S., and Fujita, T. (2004). The RNA helicase RIG-I has an essential function in double-stranded RNA-induced innate antiviral responses. *Nat. Immunol.* **5:**730–737.

Yoneyama, M., Kikuchi, M., Matsumoto, K., Imaizumi, T., Miyagishi, M., Taira, K., Foy, E., Loo, Y. M., Gale, M., Jr., Akira, S., Yonehara, S., Kato, A., *et al.* (2005). Shared and unique functions of the DExD/H-box helicases RIG-I, MDA5, and LGP2 in antiviral innate immunity. *J. Immunol.* **175:**2851–2858.

CHAPTER 7

The Role of Toll-Like Receptors in the Induction of Immune Responses During Rabies Virus Infection

Jianwei Li,* Milosz Faber,[†] Bernhard Dietzschold,[†] and D. Craig Hooper*,[‡]

Contents

* Center for Neurovirology, Department of Cancer Biology, Thomas Jefferson University, Philadelphia, Pennsylvania, USA
[†] Center for Neurovirology, Department of Microbiology and Immunology, Thomas Jefferson University, Philadelphia, Pennsylvania, USA
[‡] Center for Neurovirology, Department of Neurological Surgery, Thomas Jefferson University, Philadelphia, Pennsylvania, USA

Advances in Virus Research, Volume 79
ISSN 0065-3527, DOI: 10.1016/B978-0-12-387040-7.00007-X

Abstract   The host response to infection generally begins with interactions
between pathogen-associated molecular patterns common to a
variety of infectious agents and reciprocal pattern-recognition
receptors (PRRs) expressed by cells of the innate immune system.
The innate responses triggered by these interactions contribute to
the early, innate control of infection as well as the induction of
pathogen-specific adaptive immunity. The outcome of infection
with wild-type rabies virus is particularly dependent upon the rapid
induction of innate and adaptive immune mechanisms that can
prevent the virus from reaching central nervous system (CNS)
tissues, where it can evade immune clearance. However, laboratory
strains that reach the CNS can be cleared, and this has evidently
occurred in individuals with rabies. Therefore, PRRs may be active in
the periphery and the CNS during rabies virus infection, possibly
depending upon the nature of the infecting virus. To investigate
these possibilities, we first examined the outcome of infection with
attenuated rabies virus in mice lacking MyD88, an adaptor protein
that is used to activate the transcription factor NF-κB by a number
of PRRs including all of the Toll-like receptors (TLRs) except for
TLR3. Finding that attenuated rabies virus mediates lethal disease in
the absence of MyD88, we then examined the effects of the
deletion of receptors using MyD88 including TLRs 2, 4, 7, and 9 as
well as IL-1-receptor 1, and IFN-αβR on infection. Only mice lacking
TLR7 exhibited a phenotype, with mortality intermediate between
MyD88$^{-/-}$ and control mice with deficits in both the development
of peripheral immunity and rabies virus clearance from the CNS.

I. TOLL-LIKE RECEPTORS

Toll-like receptors (TLRs) are transmembrane receptor proteins that bind
pathogen-associated molecular patterns (PAMPs), conserved structures
expressed by various pathogens. Expressed either at the surface or in cell
compartments, primarily of cells relevant to antigen presentation including monocytes, dendritic cells, and B cells, TLRs are important sensors of
infection that are responsible for the induction of innate responses that
contribute to both the early control of infection and stimulation of adaptive immunity. While each TLR binds to a different conserved structural
element of a pathogen, the patterns of genes activated often overlap due
to the involvement of shared signaling pathways. For example, signaling
through most TLRs is mediated by the adapter proteins MyD88, TRIF,
TRAM, and Mal/TIRAP with TLRs 1, 2, 4, 5, 6, 7, 8, 9, 11 requiring the

MyD88 adapter molecule with or without other adapter molecules (Yamamoto *et al.*, 2002a, 2003). TLR3 is unique in utilizing TRIF without MyD88 (Yamamoto *et al.*, 2002b). TLR binding to its ligand leads, through the adaptor molecules, to the activation of a variety of kinases and subsequently to the activity of transcription factors such as NF-κB and IRF3. These transcription factors promote the expression by the cells of costimulatory molecules and factors that contribute to innate immune mechanisms and the induction of adaptive immunity.

Depending on the nature of the infecting virus, different TLRs are involved in triggering innate antiviral immunity. In both mice and humans, TLR3, which is expressed in the endoplasmic reticulum and endosomes, binds double-stranded RNA (dsRNA; Alexopoulou *et al.*, 2001) and the endosomal TLR7 binds single-stranded RNA (Diebold *et al.*, 2004). Also endosomal, TLR8 in humans recognizes single-stranded RNA but in mice, where TLR8 was initially thought to be inactive (Heil *et al.*, 2004), there is recent evidence that it is activated by poly(A)/T rich DNA sequences such as the vaccinia virus genome (Martinez *et al.*, 2010). Expressed on the cell surface, TLRs 2 and 4 can participate in antiviral responses by binding the products of infected cells such as heat shock proteins (Asea *et al.*, 2002; Vabulas *et al.*, 2001).

The role of TLRs in rabies virus infection has only recently come under investigation. The initial findings were that a TLR3-positive human neuronal cell line upregulates genes associated with innate immunity when infected with rabies virus *in vitro* (Prehaud *et al.*, 2005) and that TLR3 expression is elevated in Purkinje cells during human rabies virus infection (Jackson *et al.*, 2006). Recently, TLR3 was identified as a component of Negri bodies, the cell inclusions characteristic of rabies (Menager *et al.*, 2009). Observations with TLR3$^{-/-}$ mice have led to the suggestion that TLR3 may promote rabies pathogenesis (Menager *et al.*, 2009). From the perspective of the induction of protective antiviral immunity, it is unlikely that TLR3 is active as a dsRNA sensor in a rabies virus infection. The virus uses a protein-coated template to generate mRNAs or protein-stabilized genomic RNAs from its negative, single-stranded RNA genome, thereby preventing the formation of dsRNAs. However hand, TLR7 in mice and TLR7 and 8 in humans are more likely to be activated during rabies virus infection through the binding of single strand viral RNA, possibly targeted to endosomes via the autophagy pathway (Delgado *et al.*, 2009). In addition, TLRs 2 and 4 may contribute to the induction of antirabies viral immunity through recognition of host cell components, such as heat shock proteins that are expressed during rabies infection (Prosniak *et al.*, 2001).

II. RABIES IN MYD88-DEFICIENT MICE

Mice without MyD88, an adaptor protein involved in the signaling of all TLRs with the exception of TLR3 (Kopp and Medzhitov, 2003; Akira and Takeda, 2004), have an established immune defect that manifests as the inability to mediate a Th1-biased response (Akira, 2000; Scanga et al., 2004). As a result, their response to infection with attenuated rabies virus is characterized by the production of IgG1 and IgG2b VNA as opposed to the IgG2a and IgG2b VNA seen in normal mice. $MyD88^{-/-}$ mice survive intracranial (i.c.) infection with TriGAS, a highly attenuated vaccine variant of rabies virus that expresses three copies of the viral glycoprotein gene and is nonpathogenic for 5-day-old mice (Faber et al., 2009). However, unlike control animals, $MyD88^{-/-}$ mice succumb to i.c. administration of a mixture of TriGAS and virulent Dog4 rabies virus (Faber et al., 2009). To examine whether the likely cause of this reduced capacity to clear the mixed infection may be a consequence of the Th2 bias of the response or the absence of TLR signaling, we compared the outcome of infection of $Tbet^{-/-}$ mice which have a defect in the generation of Th1 cells, but no known deficit in TLR signaling. $Tbet^{-/-}$ mice proved to be as susceptible to a lethal outcome following i.c. administration of a mixture of TriGAS and virulent Dog4 rabies virus (Table I). However, $Tbet^{-/-}$ mice recover from intramuscular (gastrocnemius) infection with the recombinant rabies virus SNBG that is lethal for $MyD88^{-/-}$ mice (Table I). SNBG has an SN backbone and the glycoprotein gene from a virulent silver-haired bat-associated rabies virus resulting in a variant with moderate pathogenicity as defined by the capacity to mediate a lethal infection in a small percentage (20%) of Swiss-Webster mice following intramuscular inoculation (Pulmanausahakul et al., 2008). These results suggest that the absence of MyD88-dependent signaling may result in a more profound deficit in the capacity in the host response to rabies than the inability to mediate a Th1-centered response.

TABLE I Survival of $MyD88^{-/-}$ and $Tbet^{-/-}$ mice infected with different rabies viruses

Mouse strain	Survival following infection with[a]	
	TriGAS + Dog4 (%)	SNBG (%)
$MyD88^{-/-}$	0	0
$Tbet^{-/-}$	0	100
C57BL/6	100	100

[a] Mice were infected intracranially with the mixture of 10^7 focus-forming units (f.f.u.) of TriGAS and 10^2 f.f.u. of Dog4, or intramuscularly in the gastrocnemius with 10^5 f.f.u. of SNBG.

III. THE HOST RESPONSE TO RABIES INFECTION INVOLVES TLR7

The MyD88-dependent TLR that is most likely to recognize rabies viral RNA is TLR7, which would recognize single-stranded RNA translocated into endosomes. In addition, TLRs 2 and 4 may contribute to the host response to rabies through recognition of products of infected cells, such as heat shock proteins. To establish whether these TLRs contribute to the host response to rabies, either from a protective or from a pathological perspective, we intramuscularly (gastrocnemius) infected mice lacking TLR7, TLRs 2 and 4, or TLRs 2 and 9 with SNBG which is pathogenic for MyD88 knockout mice, but not for normal mice. Only TLR7$^{-/-}$ mice exhibited a phenotype different from normal animals with mortality ranging around 60% (Table II). In addition, we found that mice lacking IL-1 receptor type 1, which is also dependent upon MyD88 for signaling, do not have increased susceptibility to SNBG infection, nor do mice without IFN-$\alpha\beta$ receptors (Table II). These observations suggest that the activity of TLRs 2, 4, and 9 in rabies virus infection, if any, cannot overcome the lack of TLR7-signaling and that the deficit in controlling rabies virus infection due to the absence of TLR7 is unlikely to be entirely due to a reduction in the production of either IL-1 or type 1 interferon. To provide insight into whether the intermediate susceptibility of TLR7$^{-/-}$ mice between normal and MyD88$^{-/-}$ mice to infection with SNBG is more likely to be due to a partial Th2 bias or a deficit in the early detection of virus, we compared the development of the circulating antibody response in SNBG-infected TLR7$^{-/-}$ and normal congenic C57BL/6 mice. The onset of the rabies virus-neutralizing humoral response is delayed in TLR7$^{-/-}$ mice by comparison with normal controls (Fig. 1). When the humoral response appears, it differs from that of normal mice

TABLE II Survival of mice deficient in MyD88, MyD88-dependent TLRs, and receptors for IL-1 and type 1 interferons following intramuscular infection with SNBG

Mouse strain	Survival following SNBG infection (%)[a]
MyD88$^{-/-}$	0
TLR2x4$^{-/-}$	100
TLR2x9$^{-/-}$	100
TLR7$^{-/-}$	40
IL-1R$^{-/-}$	100
IFN-$\alpha\beta$R$^{-/-}$	100

[a] Mice were infected in the gastrocnemius with 10^5 f.f.u. of SNBG.

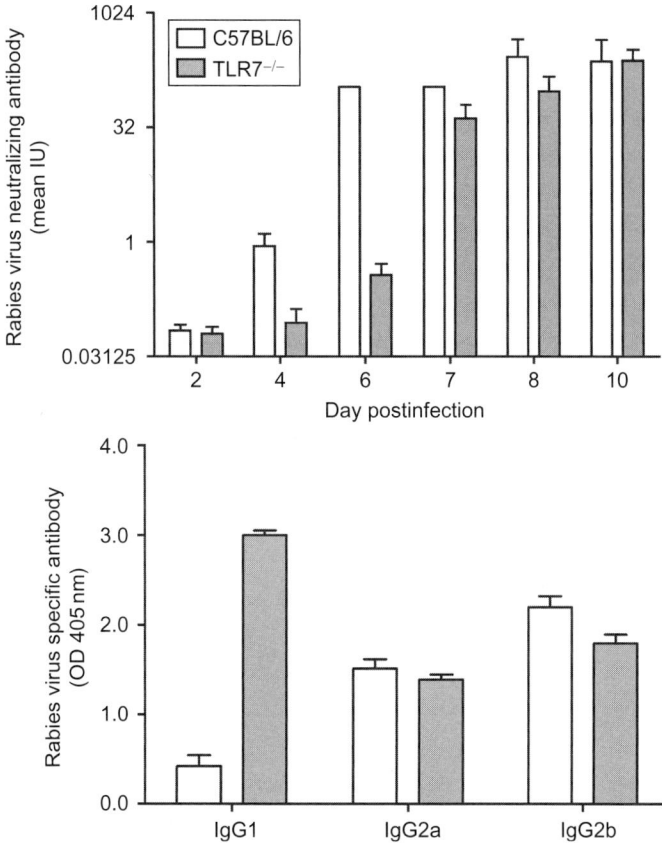

FIGURE 1   The rabies virus-neutralizing antibody response in SNBG-infected TLR7$^{-/-}$ mice is delayed and exhibits a Th2 bias. TLR7$^{-/-}$ and congenic C57BL/6 mice were infected in the gastrocnemius with 10^5 f.f.u. of SNBG and sera obtained 2, 4, 6, 7, 8, and 10 days after infection. Shown in the upper panel, serum VNA titers were determined by the rapid fluorescence inhibition test (Hooper, 2006). The lower panel shows the IgG isotypes of mouse serum rabies virus-specific antibodies at 10 days after infection, determined by ELISA as previously described (Roy *et al.*, 2007).

by having a considerably higher level of rabies virus-specific antibodies of the IgG1 isotype, indicating a more Th2 biased response. However, by day 10 postinfection, the TLR7$^{-/-}$ mice are producing levels of rabies virus-specific antibodies of the IgG2a and IgG2b isotypes that are approaching those of controls. Consequently, we speculate that TLR7 engagement is important for the timely induction of processes leading to the development of rabies virus-specific immunity and that the delay due to the absence of TLR7 leads to greater virus spread to the CNS and enhanced pathogenicity.

IV. THE CONTRIBUTION OF TLR7 SIGNALING TO THE CONTROL OF RABIES VIRUS SPREAD TO THE CNS AND CLEARANCE FROM CNS TISSUES

The primary objective of a therapeutic rabies virus-specific immune response is to prevent the virus from spreading to the CNS. A delay in the induction of innate and adaptive immunity in the periphery may be expected to result in more rabies virus reaching the CNS. Once the virus has entered CNS tissues, additional innate and adaptive immune mechanisms are required for its clearance. These include the production of proinflammatory cytokines and chemokines by infected tissues (Phares *et al.*, 2006), innate and CD4 T cell-mediated alterations in blood–brain barrier (BBB) function that facilitate immune effector infiltration into the tissues (Hooper *et al.*, 2009; Roy and Hooper, 2008), and production of antibody in the CNS parenchyma (Hooper *et al.*, 2009). As a consequence of their slow development of rabies virus-specific immunity in the periphery, it may be expected that the spread of rabies virus from the periphery to the CNS may be increased in TLR7$^{-/-}$ mice. However, it is also possible that TLR7 signaling is involved in the detection of virus in the CNS and the induction of the innate immune mechanisms that contribute to virus clearance from CNS tissues. At 14 days following SNBG infection, rabies viral nucleoprotein mRNA levels are substantially higher in the CNS tissues of TLR7$^{-/-}$ than C57BL/6 mice suggesting that the spread to, or replication in, CNS tissues is better controlled in the later (Fig. 2). At the same time, levels of IFN-γ mRNA are considerably higher in the CNS of the TLR7$^{-/-}$ mice (Fig. 2), suggesting that the processes responsible for immune effector accumulation in CNS tissues may not be compromised. However, the possibility that there is a subtle deficit or delay in the CNS immune response to rabies virus in TLR7$^{-/-}$ mice is raised by the fact that only one-third survive intracranial infection with a mixture of TriGAS and Dog4, which is not lethal for congenic controls, and by the differential response of rabies-vaccinated TLR7$^{-/-}$ mice to intramuscular versus intracranial challenge with virulent rabies virus. Intramuscular administration of the live-attenuated SPBNGAS-GAS rabies virus vaccine variant has no overt effect on either C57BL/6 or TLR7$^{-/-}$ mice and protects the majority of the latter and all of the congenic controls from a lethal dose of Dog4 given intramuscularly (gastrocnemius) 14 days later (Table III). When vaccinated mice surviving a lethal intramuscular challenge are rechallenged intracranially with Dog4, a different pattern emerges. While all C57BL/6 mice survive, approximately 40% of the TLR7$^{-/-}$ mice succumb to intracranial challenge. Thus, the presence of an immune response that is sufficient to protect against peripheral Dog4 challenge does not dictate that TLR7$^{-/-}$ mice will be protected from an intracranial

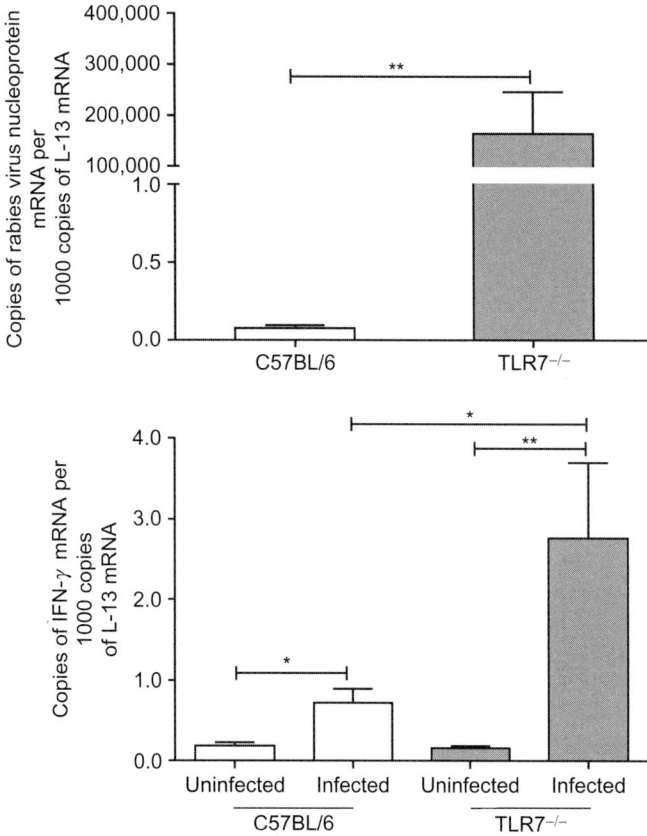

FIGURE 2 Spread of rabies SNBG virus from the periphery to the CNS is extensive in TLR7$^{-/-}$ mice and leads to an exaggerated interferon-γ response in CNS tissues. Mice were either left uninfected (control) or infected in the gastrocnemius with 10^5 f.f.u. of SNBG and cerebral cortices were collected at 14 days after infection. Quantification of rabies viral nucleoprotein and IFN-γ mRNAs in the cortices were performed by real-time PCR as described elsewhere (Faber *et al.*, 2009; Phares *et al.*, 2006). Data are presented as the copy number of rabies virus nucleoprotein (upper panel) or IFN-γ (lower panel) mRNA per 1000 copies of L-13 mRNA. Statistically significant differences in the results between the groups of mice indicated by bars, determined by the Mann–Whitney test, are denoted by * $p < 0.05$ and ** $p < 0.01$.

challenge. This suggests that a TLR7-mediated process may contribute to the delivery of immune effectors to the CNS. TLR7 is known to be expressed by CNS resident cells including astrocytes, microglia, and neurons (Butchi *et al.*, 2008, 2010), and administration of the TLR7 agonist imiquimod to the neonatal mouse brain induces the expression of IFN-β, TNFα, and the proinflammatory cytokines CXCL10 (IP-10) and CCL2

TABLE III   Survival of rabies-vaccinated TLR7$^{-/-}$ mice intramuscularly and then intracranially challenged with wild-type rabies virus[a]

Immunization	Initial challenge—intramuscular	Second challenge—intracranial
8/8	7/8	4/7

[a] Eight TLR7$^{-/-}$ mice were intramuscularly immunized with 10^5 f.f.u. of the live-attenuated rabies vaccine strain SPBNGAS-GAS which is characterized in detail elsewhere (Li *et al.*, 2008). Fourteen days later, the mice were challenged with 10^5 f.f.u. of Dog4 in the gastrocnemius muscle, which is lethal for nonimmune animals but not for vaccinated normal controls. The surviving mice were then (31 days) challenged intracranially with 10^3 f.f.u. of Dog4 which is lethal for nonimmune animals. The numbers of survivors out of the challenged group of mice are shown.

(MCP-1; Butchi *et al.*, 2008). We speculate that TLR7 recognition of viral RNA contributes to protective CNS immune mechanisms during rabies virus infection through antiviral effects mediated by type 1 interferons and through triggering the production of factors that facilitate immune effector infiltration into the infected tissues.

V. TLR7 AND THE DIVERSE PATHOGENICITIES OF RABIES VIRUS VARIANTS

In the absence of TLR7, certain rabies variants are more pathogenic, and rabies vaccination protocols are less effective. The concept that TLR7 is an important sensor of rabies virus infection is supported by these observations as is the possibility that more pathogenic rabies viruses may not trigger TLR7 as efficiently as attenuated strains. There are several aspects of pathogenic rabies virus infection that may have relevance to reduced TLR7 signaling. The low replication rate common to most pathogenic rabies viruses (Yan *et al.*, 2001) may be expected to limit TLR7 recognition. In addition, there is likely to be variability in the cells infected by different rabies viruses (Morimoto *et al.*, 1996) and in TLR7 expression by different CNS resident cell types (Butchi *et al.*, 2008) such that the nature of the cells infected may contribute to the level of TLR7 activation.

A well-known but not entirely understood phenomenon in rabies is that viruses expressing high levels of glycoprotein are cytotoxic, but more immunogenic and less pathogenic for the host. We hypothesize that this is in part a consequence of a forward loop involving autophagy and TLR7 activation. In our model, the overexpression of rabies virus glycoprotein during infection with attenuated rabies viruses causes ER stress and autophagy that, in antigen-presenting cells such as dendritic cells, delivers single-stranded rabies viral RNA to the endosome activating the TLR7 signaling cascade which, in turn, further activates autophagy.

This would result in the infection of the target cell being self-limiting, leading to programmed cell death in certain cell types but with heightened activation of innate immune functions and antigen presentation in others. Differences in the capacity of TLR7 to detect infection with pathogenic versus attenuated rabies viruses would be expected to be reflected in the nature or magnitude of the CNS innate response, as has been reported. Lower levels of the production of certain chemokines in the CNS tissues of mice infected with pathogenic by comparison with attenuated rabies viruses have been detected (Kuang *et al.*, 2009). In addition, the BBB functions required for immune effector entry into the CNS tissues are induced by infection with attenuated, but not pathogenic rabies viruses (Roy *et al.*, 2007). We speculate that differential induction of TLR7-signaling may contribute to this variability in the innate response to rabies viruses.

VI. CONCLUSIONS AND RELEVANCE TO THERAPEUTIC IMMUNIZATION

The finding that TLR7 plays an important role in the timing and Th1 bias of the immune response to rabies virus has implications for vaccination. TLR7 engagement is dependent upon the delivery of rabies viral RNA to the endosomal compartment. This is unlikely to happen with inactivated vaccines in which rabies virus RNA is protein coated. Therefore, our finding that TLR7 recognition is required for the timely development of protective immunity suggests that infection of antigen-presenting cells, which has been demonstrated for dendritic cells and monocytes for SPBNGAS-GAS and Dog4 (Li *et al.*, 2008), may contribute to this process. In fact, immunization of normal mice with live-attenuated CVS-F3 rabies virus elicits antibodies characteristic of a Th1 response whereas vaccination with inactivated CVS-F3 induces a Th2 antibody profile (Hooper *et al.*, 2011). As it initially develops, the immune response to attenuated rabies virus infection in TLR7$^{-/-}$ mice exhibits a Th2 bias. We have previously demonstrated that rabies virus clearance from the CNS involves Th1 activity (Hooper *et al.*, 1998; Phares *et al.*, 2006). We conclude that TLR7 signaling is key to the timely induction of an immune response with the capacity to clear rabies virus from CNS tissues and that this is unlikely to be accomplished with inactivated vaccines.

ACKNOWLEDGMENTS

This work was supported by National Institutes of Health Grants AI 077033, AI 060005, AI083046 (to D. C. H.), and AI060686 (to B. D.).

REFERENCES

Akira, S. (2000). The role of IL-18 in innate immunity. *Curr. Opin. Immunol.* **12:**59–63.

Akira, S., and Takeda, K. (2004). Toll-like receptor signalling. *Nat. Rev. Immunol.* **4:**499–511.

Alexopoulou, L., Holt, A. C., Medzhitov, R., and Flavell, R. A. (2001). Recognition of double-stranded RNA and activation of NF-kappaB by Toll-like receptor 3. *Nature* **413:**732–738.

Asea, A., Rehli, M., Kabingu, E., Boch, J. A., Bare, O., Auron, P. E., Stevenson, M. A., and Calderwood, S. K. (2002). Novel signal transduction pathway utilized by extracellular HSP70: Role of toll-like receptor (TLR) 2 and TLR4. *J. Biol. Chem.* **277:**15028–15034.

Butchi, N. B., Pourciau, S., Du, M., Morgan, T. W., and Peterson, K. E. (2008). Analysis of the neuroinflammatory response to TLR7 stimulation in the brain: Comparison of multiple TLR7 and/or TLR8 agonists. *J. Immunol.* **180:**7604–7612.

Butchi, N. B., Du, M., and Peterson, K. E. (2010). Interactions between TLR7 and TLR9 agonists and receptors regulate innate immune responses by astrocytes and microglia. *Glia* **58:**650–664.

Delgado, M., Singh, S., DeHaro, S., Master, S., Ponpuak, M., Dinkins, C., Ornatowski, W., Vergne, I., and Deretic, V. (2009). Autophagy and pattern recognition receptors in innate immunity. *Immunol. Rev.* **229:**189–202.

Diebold, S. S., Kaisho, T., Hemmi, H., Akira, S., and Reis e Sousa, C. (2004). Innate antiviral responses by means of TLR7-mediated recognition of single-stranded RNA. *Science* **303:**1529–1531.

Faber, M., Li, J., Kean, R. B., Hooper, D. C., Alugupalli, K. R., and Dietzschold, B. (2009). Effective preexposure and postexposure prophylaxis of rabies with a highly attenuated recombinant rabies virus. *Proc. Natl. Acad. Sci. USA* **106:**11300–11305.

Heil, F., Hemmi, H., Hochrein, H., Ampenberger, F., Kirschning, C., Akira, S., Lipford, G., Wagner, H., and Bauer, S. (2004). Species-specific recognition of single-stranded RNA via toll-like receptor 7 and 8. *Science* **303:**1526–1529.

Hooper, D. C., Morimoto, K., Bette, M., Weihe, E., Koprowski, H., and Dietzschold, B. (1998). Collaboration of antibody and inflammation in clearance of rabies virus from the central nervous system. *J. Virol.* **72:**3711–3719.

Hooper, D. C. (2006). Rabies virus. *In* "Manual of Molecular and Clinical Laboratory Immunology" (B. Detrick, R. G. Hamilton, and J. D. Folds, eds.), 7th edn. pp. 791–797. ASM Press, Washington, DC.

Hooper, D. C., Phares, T. W., Fabis, M. J., and Roy, A. (2009). The production of antibody by invading B cells is required for the clearance of rabies virus from the central nervous system. *PLoS Negl. Trop. Dis.* **3:**e535.

Hooper, D. C., Roy, A., Barkhouse, D.A., Li, J., Kean, R. B. (2011) Chapter 4. Rabies virus clearance from the central nervous system. *In* "Research Advances in Rabies" (A. C. Jackson, Ed.). pp. 55-71. Elsevier.

Jackson, A. C., Rossiter, J. P., and Lafon, M. (2006). Expression of Toll-like receptor 3 in the human cerebellar cortex in rabies, herpes simplex encephalitis, and other neurological diseases. *J. Neurovirol.* **12:**229–234.

Kopp, Z., and Medzhitov, R. (2003). Recognition of microbial infection by Toll-like receptors. *Curr. Opin. Immunol.* **15:**396–401.

Kuang, Y., Lackay, S. N., Zhao, L., and Fu, Z. F. (2009). Role of chemokines in the enhancement of BBB permeability and inflammatory infiltration after rabies virus infection. *Virus Res.* **144:**18–26.

Li, J., McGettigan, J. P., Faber, M., Schnell, M. J., and Dietzschold, B. (2008). Infection of monocytes or immature dendritic cells (DCs) with an attenuated rabies virus results in DC maturation and a strong activation of the NFkappaB signaling pathway. *Vaccine* **26:**419–426.

Martinez, J., Huang, X., and Yang, Y. (2010). Toll-like receptor 8-mediated activation of murine plasmacytoid dendritic cells by vaccinia viral DNA. *Proc. Natl. Acad. Sci. USA* **107:**6442–6447.

Menager, P., Roux, P., Megret, F., Bourgeois, J. P., Le Sourd, A. M., Danckaert, A., Lafage, M., Prehaud, C., and Lafon, M. (2009). Toll-like receptor 3 (TLR3) plays a major role in the formation of rabies virus Negri bodies. *PLoS Pathog.* **5:**e1000315.

Morimoto, K., Patel, M., Corisdeo, S., Hooper, D. C., Fu, Z. F., Rupprecht, C. E., Koprowski, H., and Dietzschold, B. (1996). Characterization of a unique variant of bat rabies virus responsible for newly emerging human cases in North America. *Proc. Natl. Acad. Sci. USA* **93:**5653–5658.

Phares, T. W., Kean, R. B., Mikheeva, T., and Hooper, D. C. (2006). Regional differences in blood–brain barrier permeability changes and inflammation in the apathogenic clearance of virus from the central nervous system. *J. Immunol.* **176:**7666–7675.

Prehaud, C., Megret, F., Lafage, M., and Lafon, M. (2005). Virus infection switches TLR-3-positive human neurons to become strong producers of beta interferon. *J. Virol.* **79:**12893–12904.

Prosniak, M., Hooper, D. C., Dietzschold, B., and Koprowski, H. (2001). Effect of rabies virus infection on gene expression in mouse brain. *Proc. Natl. Acad. Sci. USA* **98:**2758–2763.

Pulmanausahakul, R., Li, J., Schnell, M. J., and Dietzschold, B. (2008). The glycoprotein and the matrix protein of rabies virus affect pathogenicity by regulating viral replication and facilitating cell-to-cell spread. *J. Virol.* **82:**2330–2338.

Roy, A., and Hooper, D. C. (2008). Immune evasion by rabies viruses through the maintenance of blood–brain barrier integrity. *J. Neurovirol.* **14:**401–411.

Roy, A., Phares, T. W., Koprowski, H., and Hooper, D. C. (2007). Failure to open the blood–brain barrier and deliver immune effectors to central nervous system tissues leads to the lethal outcome of silver-haired bat rabies virus infection. *J. Virol.* **81:**1110–1118.

Scanga, C. A., Bafica, A., Feng, C. G., Cheever, A. W., Hieny, S., and Sher, A. (2004). MyD88-deficient mice display a profound loss in resistance to *Mycobacterium tuberculosis* associated with partially impaired Th1 cytokine and nitric oxide synthase 2 expression. *Infect. Immun.* **72:**2400–2404.

Vabulas, R. M., Ahmad-Nejad, P., da Costa, C., Miethke, T., Kirschning, C. J., Hacker, H., and Wagner, H. (2001). Endocytosed HSP60s use toll-like receptor 2 (TLR2) and TLR4 to activate the toll/interleukin-1 receptor signaling pathway in innate immune cells. *J. Biol. Chem.* **276:**31332–31339.

Yamamoto, M., Sato, S., Hemmi, H., Sanjo, H., Uematsu, S., Kaisho, T., Hoshino, K., Takeuchi, O., Kobayashi, M., Fujita, T., Takeda, K., and Akira, S. (2002a). Essential role for TIRAP in activation of the signalling cascade shared by TLR2 and TLR4. *Nature* **420:**324–329.

Yamamoto, M., Sato, S., Mori, K., Hoshino, K., Takeuchi, O., Takeda, K., and Akira, S. (2002b). Cutting edge: A novel Toll/IL-1 receptor domain-containing adapter that preferentially activates the IFN-beta promoter in the Toll-like receptor signaling. *J. Immunol.* **169:**6668–6672.

Yamamoto, M., Sato, S., Hemmi, H., Uematsu, S., Hoshino, K., Kaisho, T., Takeuchi, O., Takeda, K., and Akira, S. (2003). TRAM is specifically involved in the Toll-like receptor 4-mediated MyD88-independent signaling pathway. *Nat. Immunol.* **4:**1144–1150.

Yan, X., Prosniak, M., Curtis, M. T., Weiss, M. L., Faber, M., Dietzschold, B., and Fu, Z. F. (2001). Silver-haired bat rabies virus variant does not induce apoptosis in the brain of experimentally infected mice. *J. Neurovirol.* **7:**518–527.

CHAPTER 8

Role of Oxidative Stress in Rabies Virus Infection

Alan C. Jackson,[*,†] **Wafa Kammouni,**[*] and
Paul Fernyhough[‡,§]

Contents		

Abstract   Recent studies in an experimental model of rabies indicated that there are major structural changes in the brain involving neuronal processes that are associated with severe clinical disease. Cultured adult mouse dorsal root ganglion (DRG) neurons are a good *in vitro* model for studying the mechanisms involved in rabies virus-induced degeneration of neurites (axons) because, unlike other neuronal cell types, these neurons are fairly permissive to rabies virus infection. DRG neurons infected with the challenge virus standard-11 (CVS) strain of rabies virus show axonal swellings and immunostaining for 4-hydroxy-2-nonenal (4-HNE), indicating evidence of lipid

[*] Department of Internal Medicine (Neurology), University of Manitoba, Winnipeg, Manitoba, Canada
[†] Department of Medical Microbiology, University of Manitoba, Winnipeg, Manitoba, Canada
[‡] Division of Neurodegenerative Disorders, St. Boniface Hospital Research Centre, Winnipeg, Manitoba, Canada
[§] Department of Pharmacology and Therapeutics, University of Manitoba, Winnipeg, Manitoba, Canada

Advances in Virus Research, Volume 79
ISSN 0065-3527, DOI: 10.1016/B978-0-12-387040-7.00008-1

peroxidation associated with oxidative stress, and also reduced axonal growth in comparison with mock-infected DRG neurons. Treatment with the antioxidant *N*-acetyl cysteine prevented the reduction in axonal outgrowth that occurred with CVS infection. The axonal swellings with 4-HNE-labeled puncta were found to be associated with aggregations of actively respiring mitochondria. We postulate that rabies virus infection likely induces mitochondrial dysfunction resulting in oxidative stress and degenerative changes involving neuronal processes. This mitochondrial dysfunction may be the result of either direct or indirect effects of the virus on the mitochondrial electron-transport chain or it may occur through other mechanisms. Further investigations are needed to gain a better understanding of the basic mechanisms involved in the oxidative damage associated with rabies virus infection. This information may prove helpful in the design of future therapeutic effects for this dreaded ancient disease.

I. INTRODUCTION

Rabies remains an important public health problem with at least 55,000 human cases per year, mostly in Asia and Africa (World Health Organization, 2005). Although human rabies is a preventable disease after recognized exposures, the disease is virtually always fatal once clinical features develop. Unfortunately, there is no effective therapy for human rabies (Jackson, 2009). Rare survivors have occurred, and in most of these cases, doses of rabies vaccine were administered prior to the onset of the disease. Gaps in our understanding of pathogenetic mechanisms involved in producing the neurological disease in rabies have been an important barrier in the development of novel therapeutic approaches (Jackson, 2007). Hence, there is an important need to gain a better understanding of basic mechanisms underlying the disease, which should put us in a much better position for the design of effective new therapeutic approaches in the future.

II. DEGENERATION OF NEURONAL PROCESSES IN EXPERIMENTAL RABIES

Although rabies is a highly lethal infectious disease of the central nervous system (CNS), relatively few degenerative neuronal changes are usually observed in the CNS using routine methods both in natural disease and in most experimental models using a peripheral route of inoculation (Iwasaki and Tobita, 2002; Rossiter and Jackson, 2007). Recently, detailed studies in experimental rabies using a transgenic mouse model that expresses the yellow fluorescent protein in a subpopulation of neurons have shown extensive degenerative changes involving neuronal processes, including both dendrites and axons, whereas conventional histopathology showed inflammatory changes without apparent degenerative neuronal changes (Scott *et al.*, 2008). With the development of severe clinical neurological disease, fluorescence microscopy showed marked structural abnormalities, especially beading and/or swelling, in dendrites and axons of layer V cortical pyramidal neurons and with severe involvement of axons in the brainstem, inferior cerebellar peduncle, and cerebellar mossy fibers (Fig. 1). Toluidine blue-stained resin sections and electron microscopy showed vacuolation in cortical neurons that corresponded to swollen mitochondria and vacuolation in the neuropil of the cerebral cortex. Axonal swellings were observed. Vacuolation was also observed ultrastructurally in axons and in presynaptic nerve endings. The involvement of axons has a striking morphologic similarity to the degenerative changes that occur in diabetic sensory and autonomic neuropathy, in which a key feature is the presence of axonal swellings that are composed of accumulations of mitochondria and cytoskeletal proteins (e.g., neurofilaments) (Lauria *et al.*, 2003; Schmidt *et al.*, 1997). Diabetes-induced oxidative stress in sensory neurons and peripheral nerves is demonstrated by increased production of reactive oxygen species (ROS; Nishikawa *et al.*, 2000; Russell *et al.*, 2002; Zherebitskaya *et al.*, 2009), lipid peroxidation (Obrosova *et al.*, 2002; Zherebitskaya *et al.*, 2009), and protein nitrosylation (Obrosova *et al.*, 2005). Because of morphological similarities with diabetic neuropathy, we have hypothesized that oxidative stress may play an important etiological role in axonal swelling formation and subsequent neuronal process degeneration that has been observed in experimental rabies in mice (Scott *et al.*, 2008), and may also be important in natural rabies in humans and animals.

III. CULTURED DORSAL ROOT GANGLION NEURONS FOR STUDYING NEURONAL PROCESS DEGENERATION

We have studied cultured adult mouse dorsal root ganglion (DRG) (sensory) neurons infected with the challenge virus standard-11 (CVS) strain of fixed rabies virus and also mock-infected DRG neurons as an uninfected control in order to evaluate the role of oxidative stress in CVS-infected DRG neurons and their neurites (axons). We have used cultured DRG neurons because these neurons are known to be relatively permissive to rabies virus infection (Castellanos *et al.*, 2000; Martinez-Gutierrez and Castellanos, 2007; Tsiang *et al.*, 1989, 1991; Tuffereau *et al.*, 2007), which facilitates evaluation of mechanisms of disease involving axons.

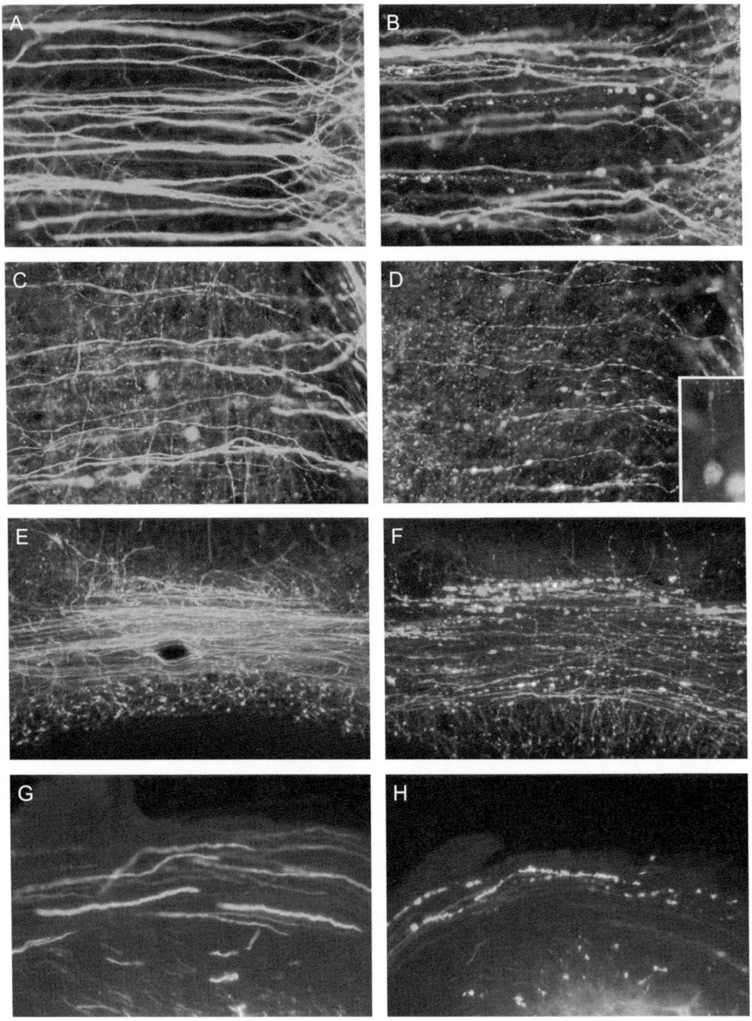

FIGURE 1 Fluorescence microscopy showing dendrites (A and B) and axons (C and D) of layer V pyramidal neurons in the cerebral cortex of mock-infected (A and C) and moribund CVS-infected (B, D, and D inset) YFP mice. In infected mice, beading is observed in a minority of dendrites (B), while more axons are involved (D). There are no abnormalities in the dendrites (A) or axons (C) of mock-infected mice. Axons in mock-infected mice are slightly varicose (C), which is characteristic of these fibers. Fluorescence microscopy shows rabies virus antigen (red) in the perikaryon and dendrite of an YFP-expressing neuron (D inset). Morphology of the cerebellar mossy fibers of mock-infected (E) and moribund CVS-infected YFP mice (F). Mossy fiber axons in the cerebellar commissure of moribund mice show severe beading (F), whereas no abnormalities were observed in mock-infected mice (E). Axons in the inferior cerebellar peduncles are normal in mock-infected mice (G) and show marked beading in CVS-infected moribund mice (H). (A–D) × 235; (D inset) × 225; (E, F) × 80; and (G, H) × 220. Adapted with permission from Scott *et al.* (2008). (See Page 5 in Color Section at the back of the book.)

DRG neurons from adult rodents are most suitable for the evaluation of neurites (axons). CVS infects up to about half of the cultured DRG neurons (Jackson et al., 2010), similar to the findings of other investigators. The basis for this selectivity is unknown. In order to establish that CVS was not killing infected neurons, we evaluated neuronal viability by assessing the ability of DRG neurons to exclude the "vital" dye trypan blue and observed a similar percentage of nonviable neurons in CVS- and mock-infected DRG cultures (Jackson et al., 2010). With a similar approach, we evaluated the cultures for evidence of neuronal apoptosis with terminal deoxynucleotidyl transferase-mediated dUTP nick end-labeling (TUNEL) staining and found a similar low percentage of TUNEL-staining neurons in CVS- and mock-infected DRG neuron cultures (Jackson et al., 2010).

We observed immunostaining for rabies virus antigen in a subpopulation of neuronal cell bodies with associated staining of axons at 24 h after viral adsorption (Fig. 2). By 48 h postinfection, swellings were observed in infected axons, and these became larger at 72 h postinfection (Fig. 2B); these axonal swellings were associated with the intense expression of rabies virus antigen (Fig. 2D, F).

IV. OXIDATIVE STRESS

In the nervous system, excessive production of ROS and reactive nitrogen species (RNS) is thought to be a mechanism for neurodegeneration associated with a variety of insults to neurons and also play an important role in a variety of neurodegenerative disorders, including Alzheimer's disease, Parkinson's disease, and amyotrophic lateral sclerosis (Andersen, 2004; Dexter et al., 1989; Giasson et al., 2000; Lin and Beal, 2006; Pedersen et al., 1998; Sayre et al., 1997). Aging is an important risk factor for these neurodegenerative diseases, and mitochondria are thought to contribute to aging by the accumulation of mutations in mitochondrial DNA, resulting in a net production of ROS (Lin and Beal, 2006). Oxidative stress is caused by an imbalance between the generation and detoxification of ROS/RNS, which leads to oxidative modification and dysfunction of nucleic acids, proteins, and lipids (Wang and Michaelis, 2010) and may result in pathological processes, including cellular dysfunction and cell death.

It has been recognized for over a decade that oxidative stress is a feature of many viral infections (Schwarz, 1996), but its importance has likely not yet been fully appreciated. ROS, often generated by mitochondria, modulate the permissiveness of cells to viral replication, regulate host inflammatory and immune responses, and cause oxidative damage to both host tissues and progeny virus (Valyi-Nagy and Dermody, 2005).

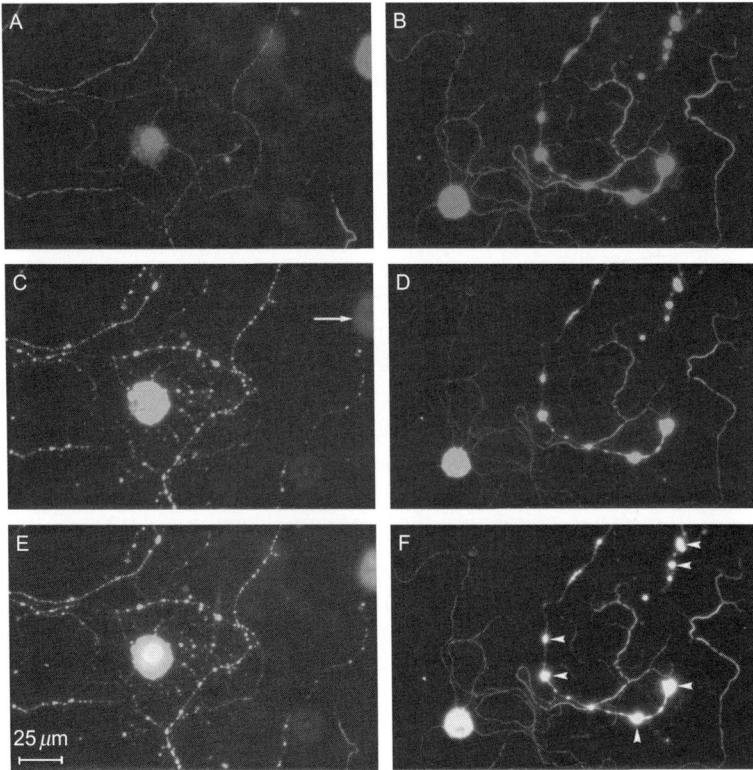

FIGURE 2 CVS infection causes formation of axonal swellings in DRG cultures. Fluorescence microscopy showing CVS-infected DRG neurons at 24 h (A, C, and E) and at 72 h (B, D, and F) postinfection (p.i.) Staining for β-tubulin III (A and B) shows two neuronal cell bodies at 24 h postinfection (p.i.) (A) and one (large spherical body) at 72 h p.i. (B). There is strong rabies virus antigen staining of one of the two neuronal cells bodies at 24 h p.i., but not of the other (arrow), demonstrating that CVS infects only a subpopulation of DRG neurons (C). Definite axonal swellings are not yet present at 24 h p.i. (A, C, and E), but axonal swellings are well established at 72 h p.i. (B, D, and F; indicated by arrowheads in F). Rabies virus antigen is strongly expressed in the neuronal cell bodies and axons at 24 and 72 h p.i. (C–F) and also in axonal swellings at 72 h p.i. (D and F). Adapted with permission from Jackson *et al.* (2010). (See Page 6 in Color Section at the back of the book.)

Oxidative injury has been shown to be an important component of experimental acute encephalitis caused by herpes simplex virus type 1 in mice (Milatovic *et al.*, 2002; Schachtele *et al.*, 2010; Valyi-Nagy *et al.*, 2000). Oxidative injury has also been shown to be an important component in human immunodeficiency virus (HIV) infection, particularly in HIV dementia (Hahn *et al.*, 2008; Williams *et al.*, 2010). It is likely that oxidative stress plays an important etiological role in diverse viral diseases.

V. OXIDATIVE STRESS IN RABIES VIRUS INFECTION

We have evaluated the role of oxidative stress in rabies virus infection in cultured DRG neurons. We assessed immunostaining in CVS- and mock-infected cultures of DRG neurons for neuron-specific β-tubulin, rabies virus antigen, and amino acid adducts of 4-hydroxy-2-nonenal (4-HNE), which is a marker of lipid peroxidation and, hence, oxidative stress (Jackson *et al.*, 2010). There were significantly more 4-HNE-labeled puncta at 2 and 3 days postinfection in CVS-infected cultures than in mock infection (Fig. 3). Axonal outgrowth was also reduced at these time points in CVS infection in comparison with mock-infected cultures. Treatment with the antioxidant *N*-acetyl cysteine at 1 mM in the culture media for 72 h beginning immediately after viral adsorption markedly reduced the expression of 4-HNE in axons and prevented the reduction in axonal outgrowth that occurred in CVS infection in comparison with mock infection ($p < 0.005$), although no "neuroprotective" effect was observed in preventing the development of axonal swellings in CVS-infected cultures (data not shown).

Axonal swellings with 4-HNE-labeled puncta were found to be associated with aggregations of actively respiring mitochondria (Jackson *et al.*, 2010), and recently, it has been shown that 4-HNE directly impairs mitochondrial function in cultured DRG neurons (Akude *et al.*, 2010). Mitochondrial dysfunction can play a key role in producing oxidative stress. Mitochondria consume oxygen in cells and contain many redox enzymes capable of transferring single electrons to oxygen generating the ROS superoxide, including the tricarboxylic acid cycle enzymes aconitase and α-ketoglutarate dehydrogenase; the electron-transport chain complexes I, II, and III; pyruvate dehydrogenase and glycerol-3-phosphate dehydrogenase; dihydroorotate dehydrogenase; the monoamine oxidases A and B; and cytochrome *b*5 reductase (Lin and Beal, 2006). Mitochondria also contain an extensive antioxidant defense system to detoxify ROS, including the enzymes manganese superoxide dismutase, catalase, glutathione peroxidase, phospholipid hydroperoxide glutathione peroxidase, glutathione reductase; peroxiredoxins, glutaredoxin, thioredoxin, and thioredoxin reductase as well as nonenzymatic components, including α-tocopherol, coenzyme Q10, cytochrome *c*, and glutathione (Lin and Beal, 2006). Mitochondrial damage with a decrease in the antioxidant defense capacity may result in net ROS production.

It is known that viral proteins from different viral families may target mitochondria, alter mitochondrial membrane permeabilization, and disrupt mitochondrial morphology (Boya *et al.*, 2003, 2004; Li *et al.*, 2004, 2007; Lichty *et al.*, 2006). For example, oxidative stress and ROS production in hepatitis C infection are related, at least in part, to stimulation of

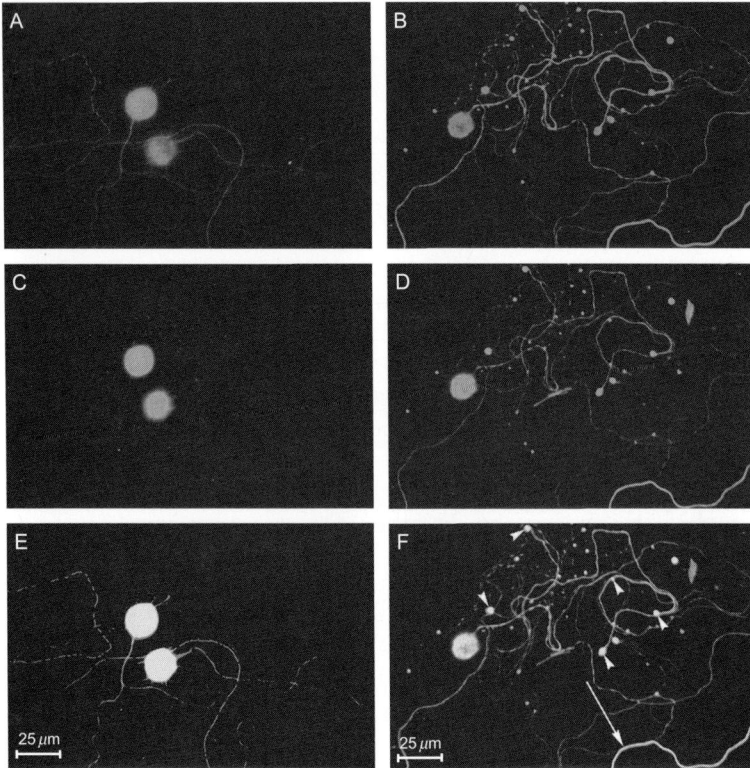

FIGURE 3 CVS infection, but not mock infection, induces formation of 4-hydroxy-2-nonenal (4-HNE)-labeled axonal swellings. Fluorescence microscopy showing mock-(A, C, and E) and CVS-infected (B, D, and F) DRG neurons at 72 h p.i. β-Tubulin (A and B) is a marker of DRG neuronal cell bodies and axons (red) and expression of β-tubulin in CVS-infected neurons (B) showed multiple axonal swellings, but a lack of axonal swellings in mock-infected neurons (A). 4-HNE (green) was poorly expressed in the axons of mock-infected DRG neurons (C) but showed greater expression in the axons of CVS-infected neurons (D) and showed accumulation in regions with axonal swellings (D). In CVS-infected neurons, merging of signals for β-tubulin and 4-HNE (yellow) showed there was strong expression of these elements in axons, both with axonal swellings (arrowheads) and without axonal swellings (arrow) (F) but not in mock-infected neurons (E). Reproduced with permission from Jackson *et al.* (2010). (See Page 7 in Color Section at the back of the book.)

the mitochondrial Ca^{2+} uniporter activity (Li *et al.*, 2007). We hypothesize that rabies virus-induced oxidative stress may be a direct consequence of mitochondrial dysfunction in virus-infected neurons. Exactly how rabies virus infection results in this dysfunction remains unknown, but there are a number of probable mechanisms that require investigation. Mokola virus is a member of genotype 3 lyssaviruses, which is less pathogenic than genotype 1 lyssaviruses that include wild-type (street) and laboratory (e.g., CVS) strains of rabies virus. Bourhy and coworkers have recently found evidence that there is reduction of the mitochondrial electron-transport system during Mokola virus infection (Gholami *et al.*, 2008). Studies using a yeast two-hybrid screening system indicate that the Mokola matrix protein interacts with subunit I of the cytochrome *c* oxidase [complex IV] of the mitochondrial respiratory chain. The mechanism of transport of the viral matrix protein into mitochondria is uncertain; it has been speculated that an α-helix in the viral matrix protein at position 69–82 may act as a mitochondrial import signal and also that heat shock protein-70, which rabies virus is known to incorporate (Sagara and Kawai, 1992), may act as a cytoplasmic chaperone to help maintain the viral matrix protein in an import-competent state (Gholami *et al.*, 2008; Stojanovski *et al.*, 2003; Young *et al.*, 2003). Further, a 20 amino acid fragment (positions 67–86) of the matrix protein inhibited cytochrome *c* oxidase activity and directed mutagenesis demonstrated that position 77 affected cytochrome *c* oxidase activity (Larrous *et al.*, 2010). Hence, rabies virus may directly or indirectly interact with one or more of the complexes of the mitochondrial electron-transport chain producing mitochondrial dysfunction and resulting in oxidative stress with structural changes in neuronal processes, which would explain what we have observed in an experimental mouse model of rabies.

VI. CONCLUSIONS

In rabies, there have been recent new insights in understanding the basic mechanisms involved in the brain resulting in the severe neurological disease and a fatal outcome. Recognition of degeneration of neuronal processes in an experimental model of rabies has recently provided a neuroanatomical explanation for the severe clinical disease with a fatal outcome (Scott *et al.*, 2008). Cultured DRG neurons are an excellent *in vitro* model for studying the mechanisms involved in CVS-induced degeneration of neurites (axons). In this model, CVS-infected neurons show reduced axonal growth, which is inhibited by the antioxidant *N*-acetyl cysteine, and axonal swellings and immunostaining for 4-HNE, which is a marker of oxidative stress. We postulate that rabies virus infection likely induces mitochondrial dysfunction, which may be caused by either direct or indirect effects of rabies virus on the mitochondrial electron-transport chain, resulting in oxidative stress and the observed structural changes involving neuronal processes. Further investigations are needed to gain a better understanding of the basic mechanisms involved in producing oxidative damage associated with rabies virus infection. This information should prove to be helpful in the design of future therapeutic effects for this dreaded ancient disease.

ACKNOWLEDGMENTS

This work was supported by Canadian Institutes of Health Research operating grant III-94590 (to A. C. J. and P. F.) and the St. Boniface General Hospital Research Foundation.

REFERENCES

Akude, E., Zherebitskaya, E., Chowdhury, S. K. R., Girling, K., and Fernyhough, P. (2010). 4-Hydroxy-2-nonenal induces mitochondrial dysfunction and aberrant axonal outgrowth in adult sensory neurons that mimics features of diabetic neuropathy. *Neurotox. Res.* **17:**28–38.

Andersen, J. K. (2004). Oxidative stress in neurodegeneration: Cause or consequence? *Nat. Med.* **10**(Suppl.):S18–S25.

Boya, P., Roumier, T., Andreau, K., Gonzalez-Polo, R. A., Zamzami, N., Castedo, M., and Kroemer, G. (2003). Mitochondrion-targeted apoptosis regulators of viral origin. *Biochem. Biophys. Res. Commun.* **304:**575–581.

Boya, P., Pauleau, A. L., Poncet, D., Gonzalez-Polo, R. A., Zamzami, N., and Kroemer, G. (2004). Viral proteins targeting mitochondria: Controlling cell death. *Biochim. Biophys. Acta* **1659:**178–189.

Castellanos, J. E., Martinez, M., Acosta, O., and Hurtado, H. (2000). Nerve growth factor and neurotrophin-3 modulate the rabies infection of adult sensory neurons in primary cultures. *Brain Res.* **871:**120–126.

Dexter, D. T., Carter, C. J., Wells, F. R., Javoy-Agid, F., Agid, Y., Lees, A., Jenner, P., and Marsden, C. D. (1989). Basal lipid peroxidation in substantia nigra is increased in Parkinson's disease. *J. Neurochem.* **52:**381–389.

Gholami, A., Kassis, R., Real, E., Delmas, O., Guadagnini, S., Larrous, F., Obach, D., Prevost, M. C., Jacob, Y., and Bourhy, H. (2008). Mitochondrial dysfunction in lyssavirus-induced apoptosis. *J. Virol.* **82:**4774–4784.

Giasson, B. I., Duda, J. E., Murray, I. V., Chen, Q., Souza, J. M., Hurtig, H. I., Ischiropoulos, H., Trojanowski, J. Q., and Lee, V. M. (2000). Oxidative damage linked to neurodegeneration by selective alpha-synuclein nitration in synucleinopathy lesions. *Science* **290:**985–989.

Hahn, K., Robinson, B., Anderson, C., Li, W., Pardo, C. A., Morgello, S., Simpson, D., and Nath, A. (2008). Differential effects of HIV infected macrophages on dorsal root ganglia neurons and axons. *Exp. Neurol.* **210:**30–40.

Iwasaki, Y., and Tobita, M. (2002). Pathology. *In* "Rabies" (A. C. Jackson and W. H. Wunner, eds.), pp. 283–306. Academic Press, San Diego.

Jackson, A. C. (2007). Pathogenesis. *In* "Rabies" (A. C. Jackson and W. H. Wunner, eds.), pp. 341–381. Elsevier Academic Press, London.

Jackson, A. C. (2009). Update on rabies diagnosis and treatment. *Curr. Infect. Dis. Rep.* **11:**296–301.

Jackson, A. C., Kammouni, W., Zherebitskaya, E., and Fernyhough, P. (2010). Role of oxidative stress in rabies virus infection of adult mouse dorsal root ganglion neurons. *J. Virol.* **84:**4697–4705.

Larrous, F., Gholami, A., Mouhamad, S., Estaquier, J., and Bourhy, H. (2010). Two overlapping domains of lyssavirus matrix protein acting on different cell death pathways. *J. Virol.* **84:**9897–9906.

Lauria, G., Morbin, M., Lombardi, R., Borgna, M., Mazzoleni, G., Sghirlanzoni, A., and Pareyson, D. (2003). Axonal swellings predict the degeneration of epidermal nerve fibers in painful neuropathies. *Neurology* **61:**631–636.

Li, D., Wang, X. Z., Yu, J. P., Chen, Z. X., Huang, Y. H., and Tao, Q. M. (2004). Cytochrome C oxidase III interacts with hepatitis B virus X protein *in vivo* by yeast two-hybrid system. *World J. Gastroenterol.* **10**:2805–2808.

Li, Y., Boehning, D. F., Qian, T., Popov, V. L., and Weinman, S. A. (2007). Hepatitis C virus core protein increases mitochondrial ROS production by stimulation of Ca^{2+} uniporter activity. *FASEB J.* **21**:2474–2485.

Lichty, B. D., McBride, H., Hanson, S., and Bell, J. C. (2006). Matrix protein of Vesicular stomatitis virus harbours a cryptic mitochondrial-targeting motif. *J. Gen. Virol.* **87**:3379–3384.

Lin, M. T., and Beal, M. F. (2006). Mitochondrial dysfunction and oxidative stress in neuro-degenerative diseases. *Nature* **443**:787–795.

Martinez-Gutierrez, M., and Castellanos, J. E. (2007). Morphological and biochemical char-acterisation of sensory neurons infected *in vitro* with rabies virus. *Acta Neuropathol. (Berlin)* **114**:263–269.

Milatovic, D., Zhang, Y., Olson, S. J., Montine, K. S., Roberts, L. J., Morrow, J. D., Montine, T. J., Dermody, T. S., and Valyi-Nagy, T. (2002). Herpes simplex virus type 1 encephalitis is associated with elevated levels of F2-isoprostanes and F4-neuroprostanes. *J. Neurovirol.* **8**:295–305.

Nishikawa, T., Edelstein, D., Du, X. L., Yamagishi, S., Matsumura, T., Kaneda, Y., Yorek, M. A., Beebe, D., Oates, P. J., Hammes, H. P., Giardino, I., and Brownlee, M. (2000). Normalizing mitochondrial superoxide production blocks three pathways of hyperglycaemic damage. *Nature* **404**:787–790.

Obrosova, I. G., Van, H. C., Fathallah, L., Cao, X. C., Greene, D. A., and Stevens, M. J. (2002). An aldose reductase inhibitor reverses early diabetes-induced changes in peripheral nerve function, metabolism, and antioxidative defense. *FASEB J.* **16**:123–125.

Obrosova, I. G., Pacher, P., Szabo, C., Zsengeller, Z., Hirooka, H., Stevens, M. J., and Yorek, M. A. (2005). Aldose reductase inhibition counteracts oxidative-nitrosative stress and poly(ADP-ribose) polymerase activation in tissue sites for diabetes complications. *Diabetes* **54**:234–242.

Pedersen, W. A., Fu, W., Keller, J. N., Markesbery, W. R., Appel, S., Smith, R. G., Kasarskis, E., and Mattson, M. P. (1998). Protein modification by the lipid peroxidation product 4-hydroxynonenal in the spinal cords of amyotrophic lateral sclerosis patients. *Ann. Neurol.* **44**:819–824.

Rossiter, J. P., and Jackson, A. C. (2007). Pathology. *In* "Rabies" (A. C. Jackson and W. H. Wunner, eds.), pp. 383–409. Elsevier Academic Press, London.

Russell, J. W., Golovoy, D., Vincent, A. M., Mahendru, P., Olzmann, J. A., Mentzer, A., and Feldman, E. L. (2002). High glucose-induced oxidative stress and mitochondrial dysfunc-tion in neurons. *FASEB J.* **16**:1738–1748.

Sagara, J., and Kawai, A. (1992). Identification of heat shock protein 70 in the rabies virion. *Virology* **190**:845–848.

Sayre, L. M., Zelasko, D. A., Harris, P. L., Perry, G., Salomon, R. G., and Smith, M. A. (1997). 4-Hydroxynonenal-derived advanced lipid peroxidation end products are increased in Alzheimer's disease. *J. Neurochem.* **68**:2092–2097.

Schachtele, S. J., Hu, S., Little, M. R., and Lokensgard, J. R. (2010). Herpes simplex virus induces neural oxidative damage via microglial cell Toll-like receptor-2. *J. Neuroinflamm.* **7**:35.

Schmidt, R. E., Dorsey, D., Parvin, C. A., Beaudet, L. N., Plurad, S. B., and Roth, K. A. (1997). Dystrophic axonal swellings develop as a function of age and diabetes in human dorsal root ganglia. *J. Neuropathol. Exp. Neurol.* **56**:1028–1043.

Schwarz, K. B. (1996). Oxidative stress during viral infection: A review. *Free Radic. Biol. Med.* **21**:641–649.

Scott, C. A., Rossiter, J. P., Andrew, R. D., and Jackson, A. C. (2008). Structural abnormalities in neurons are sufficient to explain the clinical disease and fatal outcome in experimental rabies in yellow fluorescent protein-expressing transgenic mice. *J. Virol.* **82:**513–521.

Stojanovski, D., Johnston, A. J., Streimann, I., Hoogenraad, N. J., and Ryan, M. T. (2003). Import of nuclear-encoded proteins into mitochondria. *Exp. Physiol.* **88:**57–64.

Tsiang, H., Lycke, E., Ceccaldi, P.-E., Ermine, A., and Hirardot, X. (1989). The anterograde transport of rabies virus in rat sensory dorsal root ganglia neurons. *J. Gen. Virol.* **70:**2075–2085.

Tsiang, H., Ceccaldi, P. E., and Lycke, E. (1991). Rabies virus infection and transport in human sensory dorsal root ganglia neurons. *J. Gen. Virol.* **72:**1191–1194.

Tuffereau, C., Schmidt, K., Langevin, C., Lafay, F., Dechant, G., and Koltzenburg, M. (2007). The rabies virus glycoprotein receptor p75NTR is not essential for rabies virus infection. *J. Virol.* **81:**13622–13630.

Valyi-Nagy, T., and Dermody, T. S. (2005). Role of oxidative damage in the pathogenesis of viral infections of the nervous system. *Histol. Histopathol.* **20:**957–967.

Valyi-Nagy, T., Olson, S. J., Valyi-Nagy, K., Montine, T. J., and Dermody, T. S. (2000). Herpes simplex virus type 1 latency in the murine nervous system is associated with oxidative damage to neurons. *Virology* **278:**309–321.

Wang, X., and Michaelis, E. K. (2010). Selective neuronal vulnerability to oxidative stress in the brain. *Front. Aging Neurosci.* **2**(12)**:**12.

Williams, R., Yao, H., Peng, F., Yang, Y., Bethel-Brown, C., and Buch, S. (2010). Cooperative induction of CXCL10 involves NADPH oxidase: Implications for HIV dementia. *Glia* **58:**611–621.

World Health Organization (2005). WHO Expert Consultation on Rabies: First Report. World Health Organization, Geneva.

Young, J. C., Hoogenraad, N. J., and Hartl, F. U. (2003). Molecular chaperones Hsp90 and Hsp70 deliver preproteins to the mitochondrial import receptor Tom70. *Cell* **112:**41–50.

Zherebitskaya, E., Akude, E., Smith, D. R., and Fernyhough, P. (2009). Development of selective axonopathy in adult sensory neurons isolated from diabetic rats: Role of glucose-induced oxidative stress. *Diabetes* **58:**1356–1364.

CHAPTER 9

Rabies Virus as a Research Tool and Viral Vaccine Vector

Emily A. Gomme,*,‡ Celestine N. Wanjalla,*,‡
Christoph Wirblich,*,‡ and Matthias J. Schnell*,†,1

Contents

* Department of Microbiology and Immunology, Jefferson Medical College, Thomas Jefferson University, Philadelphia, Pennsylvania, USA
† Jefferson Vaccine Center, Jefferson Medical College, Thomas Jefferson University, Philadelphia, Pennsylvania, USA
‡ First three authors contributed equally to this work
1 Corresponding author: Matthias.schnell@jefferson.edu

Advances in Virus Research, Volume 79
ISSN 0065-3527, DOI: 10.1016/B978-0-12-387040-7.00009-3

Abstract   Until recently, single-stranded negative sense RNA viruses (ssNSVs) were one of only a few important human viral pathogens, which could not be created from cDNA. The inability to manipulate their genomes hindered their detailed genetic analysis. A key paper from Conzelmann's laboratory in 1994 changed this with the publication of a method to recover rabies virus (RABV) from cDNA. This discovery not only dramatically changed the broader field of ssNSV biology but also opened a whole new avenue for studying RABV pathogenicity, developing novel RABV vaccines as well a new generation of RABV-based vaccine vectors, and creating research tools important in neuroscience such as neuronal tracing.

I. RABIES VIRUS AS A RESEARCH TOOL

Neurotropic viruses have become an invaluable tool for neuroscientists in their quest to elucidate the architecture of neuronal networks (Callaway, 2008; Taber *et al.*, 2005; Ugolini, 1995, 2010). Compared to conventional methods of neurotracing, viruses offer the advantage of self-amplification, which ensures equally strong labeling of each cell as the virus passes from one neuron to the next. In addition, viral tracers allow a more specific targeting of cell types. Although numerous neurotropic viruses are known, mostly rabies virus (RABV) and several members of the alphaherpesvirus family have been employed for neuronal tracer studies to date. RABV is particularly suited for this purpose because it is transported in a strictly transsynaptical way with very little spread to nonneuronal cells, at least at early times of the infection. In addition, RABV exhibits exceptionally low cytopathogenicity in infected neurons. In both respects, RABV is on par with or even superior to alphaherpesviruses, including the PRV Bharta isolate. RABV does, however, also have disadvantages compared to herpesviruses. Unlike PRV, RABV is pathogenic to humans and therefore necessitates special safety measures. Also, as RABV is an RNA virus with a strictly cytoplasmic replication cycle, it does not permit the use of cell type-specific promoters to limit marker gene expression to certain cell types. Notwithstanding those limitations, RABV has gained increasing popularity as a tool for neuronal circuit analysis. Here, we present an overview of studies that have employed recombinant and nonrecombinant RABV as neuronal tracers highlighting the technical advancements that have been made in recent years.

Early studies of RABV spread in the central nervous system (CNS) have utilized fixed and street viruses in different animal models mainly to study the basis for differences in viral pathogenesis (Coulon *et al.*, 1989; Gillet *et al.*, 1986; Kucera *et al.*, 1985; Lafay *et al.*, 1991; Smart and Charlton, 1992; Tsiang *et al.*, 1983). These studies clearly showed the strong tropism of RABV for neuronal cells. They also revealed that different types of neurons are not equally infected. Refractiveness to infection is in part explained by the strength of innervation and receptor density at the presynaptic membrane. Marked differences in cell tropism were observed not only between the pathogenic and attenuated mutant strains of CVS but also between pathogenic street and fixed viruses. These data strongly suggest the preferential use of different receptors by different RABV strains. In fact, several receptors have been reported in the literature, but their relative importance is unclear (Coulon *et al.*, 1998; Jacotot *et al.*, 1999; Lentz *et al.*, 1983; Superti *et al.*, 1986; Thoulouze *et al.*, 1998; Tuffereau *et al.*, 1998). Whether the absence of one or several of these receptors from certain types of neurons renders them refractive to infection by RABV remains to be determined.

The general suitability of RABV as a neuronal tracer was demonstrated in several detailed time-course studies of viral spread in rodent and primate models (Astic *et al.*, 1993; Kelly and Strick, 2000; Ugolini, 1995). These studies noted the exceptional low cytotoxicity of RABV, the strict time-dependence of viral spread to higher order neurons, and the limited spread to nonneuronal cells. Kelly and Strick also carried out a rigorous comparison of different RABV strains, which revealed significant differences in the kinetics of viral spread. The pioneering work carried out by Ugolini and Kelly laid the groundwork for a large number of similar studies that mostly employed CVS-11 alone or in combination with conventional tracers to elucidate the architecture of different neural circuits in monkeys, rats, guinea pigs, and cats (Buttner-Ennever *et al.*, 2002; Clower *et al.*, 2005; Graf *et al.*, 2002; Hashimoto *et al.*, 2010; Hoshi *et al.*, 2005; Iwata *et al.*, 2011; Kelly and Strick, 2003, 2004; Lois *et al.*, 2009; Morcuende *et al.*, 2002; Nassi and Callaway, 2006; Prevosto *et al.*, 2009; Rathelot and Strick, 2006; Rice *et al.*, 2009, 2010; Ugolini *et al.*, 2006; Viemari *et al.*, 2004a,b).

Low cytopathogenicity in neurons and "clockwork-like" kinetics of viral spread are the hallmarks that have made RABV such a widely used neurotracer. However, at least one study has highlighted some variability in both parameters (Ruigrok *et al.*, 2008). The reasons for this variability are not clear, but genetic variability of outbred animals and differences in the early innate and T-independent humoral immune responses among individual animals could play a role. Also, it should not be forgotten that RABV has an inherently higher spontaneous mutation rate and genetic variability than DNA viruses. This and the ability to form defective interfering particles if passaged at high multiplicity of infection (MOI) could easily result in phenotypic changes from the original virus isolate depending on the passage history of the particular virus stock in use. It will probably not be possible to completely eliminate the temporal dispersion in viral spread particularly once the virus has spread to higher order neurons, but it is generally advisable to use infectious doses as high as possible to synchronize timing of the infection and, therefore, increase reproducibility.

While attenuated strains of RABV are less suitable for neuronal tracer studies that require spread of RABV from peripheral nerve endings to higher order neurons in the CNS, they have proven quite useful for a different kind of neuronal tracer approach that aims to limit viral spread to monosynaptically connected neurons (Larsen *et al.*, 2007; Wickersham *et al.*, 2007a,b). This was achieved by deleting the glycoprotein (G) gene from a recombinant clone of the SAD-B19 strain. In addition, the virus was engineered to express GFP. Deletion of the RABV G prevents spread of the virus beyond initially infected cells, while insertion of the *GFP* gene ensures strong labeling of cell bodies, dendrites, and axons which obviates the need for histochemical staining methods to outline the infected neurons (Wickersham *et al.*, 2007a). In essence, this method prevents transsynaptic spread and limits labeling to first-order neurons. Wickersham and Wall then took this approach further and devised an ingenious strategy for targeting the initial infection in a cell-specific manner and limiting viral spread to monosynaptically connected neurons. Cell specificity was achieved by pseudotyping RABV with an avian virus glycoprotein and transfecting target neurons with an expression plasmid for the avian receptor protein TVA. To accomplish monosynaptic spread, the target cells also received an expression plasmid encoding the RABV G. The validity of the approach was first demonstrated *ex vivo* in brain slices transfected with the transcomplementing expression plasmids. In a further improvement of cell-specific targeting a recombinant AAV helper virus was used to express RABV G and TVA in a cre-dependent manner, which now opens a whole new avenue for targeting RABV infection to selected cell types by utilizing Cre-expressing transgenic mice (Wall *et al.*, 2010). This strategy holds great promise for labeling monosynaptic circuits in the mouse model. Unfortunately, such genome engineering approaches are only applicable to small mammals, as genome engineering of primates is impractical due to their long gestation period and high reproductive age.

Viral genome engineering was also instrumental in the first study that employed two different RABVs for dual tracing experiments (Ohara, 2009). To impart neuroinvasiveness and a stronger neurotropism onto an attenuated strain, the RABV G gene of CVS was used to replace the cognate G gene of the HEP-Flury strain. Beta-galactosidase (*β-Gal*) and GFP were then inserted between the nucleoprotein (N) and phosphoprotein (P) genes to generate two different marker viruses, which were utilized to detect neurons that project to two separate regions in the rat brain. Another elegant study utilized the monosynaptically restricted G-deleted viruses developed by the Callaway laboratory to double label premotor spinal interneurons after bilateral injection of two different marker viruses into the quadriceps muscles of newborn mice (Stepien *et al.*, 2010). As in other studies, little neurodegeneration was observed in infected neurons until 12 days postinfection. Interestingly, the authors also noted that the efficiency of infection declined dramatically in mice older than 10 days.

While the early pioneering neuronal tracer studies with RABV have utilized nonrecombinant fixed laboratory strains, the future of RABV neuronal tracers clearly lies in the use of recombinant clones. Several factors will have to be considered in these endeavors. The four main features that qualify RABV for neuronal tracer studies are its strong neurotropism, low cytopathogenicity, ability to invade the CNS from the periphery, and wide host range. Neurotropism of RABV is largely determined by the glycoprotein and its receptor specificity (Morimoto et al., 2000). The fact that rabies appears to utilize different cellular receptors and the marked differences in viral spread between different viral strains suggest that the specificity of neuronal labeling can be modified to some extent by constructing recombinant RABVs that express different glycoprotein genes. It is to be expected that this kind of approach will receive a significant boost once the three-dimensional structure of RABV G has been elucidated.

The other main feature that renders RABV suitable for neuronal tracer studies is its neuroinvasiveness. This is a multigenic trait and not solely determined by the RABV G (Faber et al., 2004; Shimizu et al., 2007; Yamada et al., 2006). Although the glycoprotein of a highly pathogenic virus can impart neuroinvasiveness onto an attenuated strain (Ohara et al., 2009b; Tan et al., 2007), the multigenic nature of neuroinvasiveness implies that recombinant viruses that utilize different viral backbones will differ markedly in the kinetics and extent of viral spread.

The glycoprotein also plays an important role in the cytopathogenicity of different RABVs. There is plenty of evidence for a direct relationship between RABV G expression level and cytopathogenicity, and it should be noted that the highly pathogenic CVS strains are considerably less cytopathic than attenuated strains (Morimoto et al., 1999). Cytopathogenicity is, for obvious reasons, of little concern in G-deleted viruses but might become an issue if foreign glycoproteins or other potentially proapoptotic proteins are used to replace the RABV glycoprotein.

With respect to host range, it needs to be kept in mind that different animals vary in their susceptibility to different RABV strains. CVS strains have been successfully used in different animals, but they are particularly suited for rodent models, as they have been developed by serial passaging in mouse brain.

RABV is readily amenable to genetic manipulation and insertions of additional transcription units due to the modular nature of its genome. This has been amply exploited for the expression of foreign antigens and marker genes like *GFP* and *beta-galactosidase*. Foreign genes up to 6.5 kb have been successfully inserted into the RABV genome (McGettigan et al., 2003a). The maximum coding capacity of RABV is likely considerably higher as the structure of the viral particle does not appear to pose a significant constraint on the size of foreign genes. Additional transcription cassettes can be placed at different positions, but they will affect genome replication and viral fitness to varying degrees. Insertions between N and P, for example, inhibit viral replication to a larger extent than insertions between G and L, and RABV does not tolerate the insertion of an additional transcription cassette upstream of the N gene. The positioning of foreign genes will also affect their expression level since there is a gradual decrease in transcription level from the N to the L gene (Schnell *et al.*, 2010). For the purpose of neuronal tracer studies, it is probably best to insert additional genes at more downstream positions where they exhibit less of an inhibiting effect on replication. Studies with recombinant variants of N2c (Wirblich and Schnell, 2011), which is characterized by a lower transcription level than attenuated viral strains, show that marker genes placed between G and L are sufficiently amplified to be readily detectable in neuronal cells (Wirblich and Schnell, unpublished). In any case, the effects of gene insertions on viral replication will have to be assessed in detailed time-course experiments for each virus. This is particularly the case if the viruses are to be employed in dual tracing experiments where the window for successful superinfection of neurons with two different viruses is potentially rather short (Ohara *et al.*, 2009a,b).

The technology for constructing and recovering recombinant RABV is still essentially the same as originally reported by Schnell *et al.* (1994). Notable improvements include the use of hammerhead ribozymes to generate an exact 5′-end of the antigenomic RNA and the use of CMV promoters to drive expression of the antigenomic RNA (Inoue *et al.*, 2003; Le Mercier *et al.*, 2002). Recovery has been performed in different cell lines, but 293T and mouse neuroblastoma cells appear to be particularly well suited for this purpose, as they are easily transfected and more permissive for neurotropic strains than baby hamster kidney (BHK) cells. A number of infectious full-length clones are now available, including two clones of bat RABV strains (Faber *et al.*, 2004; Orbanz and Finke, 2010), several clones of fixed attenuated viruses (Huang *et al.*, 2010; Inoue *et al.*, 2003; Ito *et al.*, 2001; Schnell *et al.*, 1994) and infectious clones of the pathogenic Nishigahara and N2c strains (Wirblich and Schnell, 2011; Yamada *et al.*, 2006). The latter should prove particularly valuable for neuronal tracer studies, as N2c is one of the most neurotropic, neuroinvasive strains available, while being one of the least cytopathic.

II. THE NEED FOR NOVEL VACCINES FOR RABV

World health reports estimate that RABV transmitted by infected animals is the cause of an estimated 55,000 human deaths annually (2005). One of the major goals for the treatment and control of RABV infections has focused on vaccine development. The first recorded vaccine against RABV was an attenuated form administered by Pasteur (1885). Since then, the field has accumulated more research with a better understanding of the pathogenicity of RABV and the immune biology of potential hosts.

Rabies is a disease affecting humans worldwide but its viral life cycle depends on a reservoir in other mammals (Dietzschold *et al.*, 2005; Schnell *et al.*, 2010). Both domestic and wildlife animals such as dogs, raccoons, skunks, mongoose, foxes, and bats can maintain the RABV cycle (Roseveare *et al.*, 2009; Schnell *et al.*, 2010); therefore, vaccine research has also targeted these groups to indirectly protect humans from this fatal disease.

Currently, whole killed (deactivated) RABV virions are used in both pre- and postexposure treatment of RABV in humans and domestic animals (for review, see McGettigan, 2010). As very safe killed RABV vaccines are available, replication-competent RABV vaccines are not considered for human use (McGettigan, 2010). However, the situation is different for the use in animals, especially for vaccination of wildlife. This is because killed virus administered in bait to wild wandering animals would be ineffective. However, orally administered, live-attenuated forms of RABV such as ERA, SAD-B19, SAG-1, and SAG-2 have been used widely in wildlife (more than 85 million doses) and have been successful at nearly eradiating RABV in Western Europe (Anonymous, 2006; Grimm, 2002). Despite their proven efficacy, replication-competent viruses retain the risk of reverting and causing disease (Faber *et al.*, 2005b). As such, research has focused on improving the safety of these vaccines even more while not compromising on their efficacy (see below). This has led to the development of novel vaccines for rabies in wildlife.

III. MODIFIED REPLICATION-COMPETENT RABV AS RABIES VACCINES FOR WILDLIFE

The success of live RABV vaccine regimens in the eradication of rabies in Western Europe indicates promise for this approach, but residual pathogenicity of these vaccines underlies the need to improve on RABV vectors. The reverse genetics technology of RABV (Schnell *et al.*, 1994) has provided the field with a new tool to manipulate the genome of RABV and therefore improve on both safety and efficacy of RABV vaccines (Dietzschold and Schnell, 2002; Dietzschold *et al.*, 2003; Faber *et al.*, 2002; McGettigan *et al.*, 2003b; Morimoto *et al.*, 2001; Pulmanausahakul *et al.*, 2001; Schnell *et al.*, 1994). These efforts include site-directed mutagenesis of viral genes, insertions of proapoptotic and antiviral genes, expression of inflammatory cytokines and chemokines, as well as gene deletions and duplication of the glycoprotein gene (Cenna *et al.*, 2009; Etessami *et al.*, 2000; Faber *et al.*, 2002, 2005a,b; Gomme *et al.*, 2010; Ito *et al.*, 2005; Kuang *et al.*, 2009; Morimoto *et al.*, 2005; Pulmanausahakul *et al.*, 2001; Shoji *et al.*, 2004; Wen *et al.*, 2010; Wirblich *et al.*, 2008; Zhao *et al.*, 2009, 2010).

RABV G is most often the target for attempted attenuation due to its known role in viral pathogenicity. RABV G is believed to be the main determinant of viral pathogenicity because it determines the viral tropism (for review, see Dietzschold *et al.*, 2008; Schnell *et al.*, 2010) and due to the fact that G is the primary target for virus-neutralizing antibodies (VNA) that prohibit cell-to-cell spread (Dietzschold *et al.*, 1983; Pulmanausahakul *et al.*, 2008). Despite the general success with conventional modified live viruses used to immunize against RABV, these vaccines were not as immunogenic in skunks and dogs. As such, further customized RABV vaccine constructs expressing G from different fixed and street strains of RABV were constructed and tested. Maximum protection in mice was achieved after vaccination with RABV expressing an identical RABV G (Morimoto *et al.*, 2001). Stemming from this, the findings gave credence for vaccine design custom made for groups of wildlife that do not respond to mainstream vaccines.

Several different factors have been employed to increase the immunogenicity of RABV vaccines. Enhanced apoptosis by overexpression of apoptotic genes has been shown to improve RABV immunogenicity (Faber *et al.*, 2002). RABV modified to overexpress cytochrome *c* showed increased apoptosis in primary neurons with a marked reduction in mortality when administered intranasally. Mouse survival had a direct correlation with the induction of VNA. In fact, compared to the control, RABV expressing cytochrome *c* had an effective dose 20-fold lower than the control, vastly improving the vaccine vector (Pulmanausahakul *et al.*, 2001).

Expression of multiple copies of RABV G has led to enhanced immunogenicity and viral attenuation. Neuronal cell lines and primary neurons infected with RABV expressing multiple G proteins showed evidence of increased apoptosis (Faber *et al.*, 2002). Immunogenicity studies with the same constructs resulted in higher antibody titers against RABV G and RABV N. Insertion of triple RABV G was shown to further attenuate the vaccine construct rendering the virus completely apathogenic when injected directly into the brains of immunocompromised and immune-sufficient mice (Faber *et al.*, 2009). RABV expressing triple G protected 5- and 10-day-old mice from intracranial (i.c.) challenge with a lethal RABV infection that killed 100% unvaccinated mice. Immune analysis showed induction of high VNA titers in these mice 21 days postimmunization. Further, postexposure immunization by RABV expressing triple G administered intracranially prevented lethal rabies encephalitis. Of note, the mechanism for viral attenuation secondary to expression of multiple G is not completely understood, and the presented data for the RABV expressing triple G actually showed that the G protein levels were less in the triple G construct compared to the control RABV at 24 h. However, there has to be some effect of the G protein expression levels on pathogenicity because the control virus (which encodes three G genes but only one with a functional start codon) was nearly as pathogenic as the construct containing only one G. Of note, if higher G expression levels are indeed responsible for the observed RABV attenuation, codon optimization (Wirblich and Schnell, 2011) might be a better approach to increase G levels. This is based on the fact that a single point mutation deleting the start codon of one or two G would result in virus with similar pathogenicity as the parental virus (Faber et al., 2009). However, caution is advised for strategies that are based solely on changes on the expression level of RABV G protein because changes in codon usage (and the resulting changes in G expression levels) do not suffice to render a pathogenic RABV apathogenic (Wirblich and Schnell, 2011).

Another practical way to improve on live RABV constructs is introduction of specific mutations, including those that abolish neurotropism of RABV (Dietzschold et al., 1983). As mentioned above, RABV G determines the tropism of the virus, albeit the spectrum of specific receptors absolutely necessary for infection remains elusive. Mutation of RABV G at position 333, replacing arginine with glutamic acid, attenuated the virus upon i.c. administration (McGettigan et al., 2003b). In addition, random mutations occurring at position 194 of G exchanging asparagine to lysine increased the pathogenicity of the attenuated RABV construct containing the 333 mutation (Faber et al., 2005b). This random mutation provided another residue that has been an excellent target for attenuation of RABV vaccine constructs (Faber et al., 2005b). An alternative approach tested by Mebatsion et al. showed that deletion of the conserved dynein light chain 8 (LC8)-binding motif in the RABV P in combination with the RABV G 333 mutation attenuated RABV 30-fold compared to the 333-mutation only RABV when administered in suckling mice (Mebatsion, 2001). Tan et al. (2007) confirmed these findings and showed that the deletion of LC8-binding motif in RABV P affects primary transcription of RABV. From these findings, the issue of custom made vaccines and the ability to use this mutation in conjunction with other mutations in specific strains of virus could be used to improve on the safety profile of these vaccines. Site-directed mutagenesis is an excellent method but based only on a very limited number of mutations (single or dual nucleotides) compared to wild-type RABV G; therefore, revertants are possible.

Another approach has taken advantage of immune components by expression of cytokines, chemokines, or hematopoietic factors to increase immunogenicity and decrease pathogenicity. Tumor necrosis factor-alpha, macrophage inflammatory protein 1-alpha, granulocyte macrophage cell stimulating factor, RANTES, and IP-10 have been expressed in RABV vectors and their pathogenicity and immunogenicity followed.

This is a modern and intriguing approach that has shown an increase in immunogenicity by manipulating arms of the innate and adaptive immune systems (Faber *et al.*, 2005a; Zhao *et al.*, 2009, 2010). Nevertheless, it also raises concerns about its application: cytokines/chemokines are species specific and the risk of their use in humans and animals is largely unknown, including toxicity and potential to trigger autoimmunity. RABV overexpressing RANTES or IP-10, for example, has been shown to increase the pathogenicity of RABV due to excessive inflammatory cells in the CNS (Zhao *et al.*, 2009). In addition, the same concern as indicated above for the expression of multiple copies of G exists; the exchange of one nucleotide within the ATG start codon of the inserted gene would revert the recombinant RABV to wild-type RABV.

In summary, many of these advancements have vastly improved the safety profile and immunogenicity of RABV vaccines. In addition, as more information is gathered on the interaction between RABV and the host, better-tailored vaccines can be designed.

IV. RABV-BASED VECTORS AS VACCINES AGAINST OTHER INFECTIOUS DISEASES

Vaccines have had and do have a great impact on human health and continue to be a mainstay in the prevention and treatment of disease. Scientific research has improved our understanding of the interactions between vaccines and the immune system. Of the different types of vaccine strategies available, viral vectors have been manipulated over the years and proved to be efficacious in the induction of both humoral and cellular immune responses.

This review focuses exclusively on RABV-based vaccines vectors. Of note, several important characteristics render RABV a favorable vaccine delivery platform. Virus recovery is conducted by the reverse genetics system using a cDNA copy of the RABV antigenome (Conzelmann and Schnell, 1994). RABV has a relatively simple genome organization that permits easy manipulation of cDNA by traditional cloning techniques. Foreign genes, such as a vaccine antigenic target, can be stably incorporated into the genome. Stability of a foreign, nonessential gene was exemplified by expression of the bacterial chloramphenicol acetyl-transferase (*CAT*) gene inserted into the RABV genome of recovered virus after 25 serial passages in cell culture (Mebatsion *et al.*, 1996a,b). Further, the viral vector sustains its replicative capacity after insertion of multiple, large genes. For instance, infectious virus was recovered after insertion of both the *HIV-1 Pr160* (Gag–Pol precursor) and *HIV-1 Env* genes; a 55% increase in genome size over wild type (McGettigan *et al.*, 2003a).

An important advantage of RABV is that, compared to other viral vectors such as adenovirus, preexisting RABV seropositivity is negligible in the general population. Further, RABV genetic and phenotypic similarity to fellow rhabdovirus, vesicular stomatitis virus (VSV), permits the exchange of the ectodomain of the RABV glycoprotein with that of VSV. This recombinant virus effectively boosts preimmunized individuals as part of a vaccine schedule (Foley *et al.*, 2000; Tan *et al.*, 2005).

Last, attenuation of RABV vectors effectively decreases pathogenicity while maintaining antigen-specific immunogenicity (McGettigan *et al.*, 2003b). This is critical, as vector-specific pathogenicity is a primary concern in live virus vectors. In addition to the use of a less pathogenic vaccine strain of RABV (see below), effective molecular attenuation techniques include gene mutation, deletion, insertion, and rearrangement (Gomme *et al.*, 2010; McGettigan *et al.*, 2003b). Further, the RABV life cycle is exclusively cytoplasmic, so recombination or integration is unlikely to occur.

The vaccine strain of RABV used for development of vaccines is derived from the attenuated SAD B19 strain used for oral immunization of foxes in Europe. SAD B19 was highly attenuated by successive passage in different cell types (Conzelmann *et al.*, 1990). Unlike pathogenic RABV strains, SAD B19 has no or limited ability to invade the CNS from a peripheral inoculation site (Conzelmann *et al.*, 1990). This limited invasion of the CNS by SAD B19 positively correlates with the immunogenicity of the virus. Perhaps the inability to sequester itself in the CNS allows it to be rapidly recognized by the immune system. This is beneficial for vaccine development in that it is both relatively safe and highly immunogenic when administered peripherally. However, even SAD B19 is pathogenic when administered directly to the brain via intranasal route (McGettigan *et al.*, 2003b). Thus, additional molecular strategies to further attenuate the virus have been developed (see below).

A. Human immunodeficiency virus-1

For the past 25 years, scientists have sought to develop a vaccine for human immunodeficiency virus-1 (HIV-1), but this goal remains unrealized. Although the correlates of protection are still uncertain, the current belief in the field is that an effective vaccine candidate should induce both arms of immunity: humoral and cellular (Haut and Ertl, 2009). Studies in monkeys immunized with live-attenuated simian immunodeficiency virus (SIV) showed protection from wild-type strains of homologous SIV (Koff *et al.*, 2006). This finding gave credence to the construction of live viral vaccines for the control of HIV. In recent years, several vaccine vector approaches capable of eliciting this type of immune response, such as DNA, Pox, and adenovirus vectors, have been evaluated preclinically (see Gomme *et al.*, 2010 and references within). RABV is one such vector with an intracellular life cycle and ability to stably express foreign antigens and, as such, is a probable candidate for an HIV vaccine.

An important study conducted in 2000 showed the immunogenicity of recombinant RABV vectors in animals for the first time. In this study, RABV was engineered to express HIV-1 gp160 envelope protein from either laboratory adapted (NL4-3) or dual-tropic isolate HIV-1 (89.6) (Schnell *et al.*, 2000). This recombinant virus was recovered on BHK cells, and the functionality of the foreign envelope protein was confirmed by a fusion assay in human T cell line, Sup-T1. Immunogenicity was evaluated by monitoring envelope-specific antibody responses in mice inoculated by footpad injection and left either unboosted or boosted with a recombinant gp120/gp41 protein. Only boosted mice seroconverted, and the recombinant virus expressing NL4-3 induced HIV-1 neutralizing antibodies. This demonstrated that RABV can efficiently prime B cells for robust humoral responses. A subsequent study showed that priming alone with these vectors could also induce cytotoxic T lymphocytes (CTL), which are cross-reactive to heterologous HIV-1 envelope proteins (McGettigan *et al.*, 2001a). Together these studies clearly demonstrated the potential RABV vectors have in eliciting a balanced humoral and cellular HIV-1-specific immune response.

As evidence in the field continued to promote the importance of cellular immune responses in controlling HIV-1 infection, RABV-based vectors were redesigned to incorporate structural, nonsurface proteins, such as HIV-1 Gag and Pol. Compared to the highly variable envelope protein, Gag is one of the most conserved proteins in HIV-1. In fact, Gag epitopes that are conserved among different HIV-1 clades have been found in individuals infected with HIV-1, suggesting their importance in viral fitness (Durali *et al.*, 1998; McAdam *et al.*, 1998; Rolland *et al.*, 2007). From the perspective of vaccine development, Gag is an attractive vaccine target antigen. McGettigan *et al.* (2001b) generated an RABV expressing HIV-1 Gag. Electron microscopy studies of infected HeLa cells showed that virus-encoded Gag protein manifested into HIV-1-like particles budding from both the plasma membrane and cytoplasmic vacuoles, as previously observed when expressed by other viruses (Karacostas *et al.*, 1989). *In vivo* immunogenicity studies demonstrated that the RABV HIV-1 Gag vector induced Gag-specific CD8+ T cells with MHC class I:Gag-specific T cell receptors, CTL activity, and IFN-γ-secretion (McGettigan *et al.*, 2001b).

Having shown that RABV vectors induce both humoral and cellular immune responses *in vivo*, research focus returned to that of vector safety. Besides efficacy, safety is a chief concern in vaccine development. Though the SAD B19 strain used for RABV-based vectors has substantially decreased   vector-associated   pathogenicity,   additional   attenuation techniques were employed. For this approach, RABV vectors expressing HIV-1 Gag were engineered to include either the R333E mutation or a deletion of 43 amino acids of the RABV G cytoplasmic domain, or a combination of both (McGettigan et al., 2003b). The engineered viruses were apathogenic following intracranial challenge in mice compared to the parental strain. Moreover, the Gag-specific cellular immune responses were not decreased by these changes to RABV G (McGettigan et al., 2003b). These immunogenicity studies were encouraging and, as such, the 333 mutation was introduced and tested in a RABV vector-encoding HIV-1 Pr160 (Gag–Pol precursor) and HIV-1 Env genes. Of note, this vector sustained replicative capacity and Gag-specific immunogenicity after a 55% increase in genome size over wild type (McGettigan et al., 2003a).

Vaccine research has also extended to the identification of adjuvants that can further improve or change the phenotype of the immune response to one that can deal with the target pathogen. In HIV vaccine research, live viral vectors have been manipulated to express inflammatory cytokines at the time of viral replication as a way to enhance the immune response. RABV vaccine studies have included IL-2, IL-4, and IFN-β as vaccine adjuvants (McGettigan et al., 2006). Both IL-4 and IL-2 can induce a Th2 response; in addition, IL-2 can stimulate proliferation of both T cells and B cells and, in general, stimulates a Th1 response. IFN-β, however, is an anti-inflammatory cytokine that is thought to skew the response to Th1 and may influence the expansion of CD8 T cells (Faul et al., 2008). RABV vaccine vector coexpressing HIV-1 Gag or Env and either murine IL-2 or IL-4 when tested in mice were highly attenuated. IL-4 expression reduced the cellular immune response to both Gag and Env, but did not significantly improve the humoral response. IL-2, however, did not reduce the cellular immune response but significantly improved the anti-Env humoral immune responses (McGettigan et al., 2006). More recently, it was shown that RABV expressing HIV-1 Gag and IFN-β was less pathogenic than controls. IFN-β expression resulted in 100-fold lower viral replication in vivo compared to controls. Even with lower viral replication, IFN-β expression seemed to increase the percentage of activated CD8+ T cells during the primary response (Faul et al., 2008, 2009a,b).

A more novel approach in vaccine design takes advantage of the antigen presentation capacity of dendritic cells (DCs). Earlier studies had shown that RABV could infect and mature human DCs with expression of proinflammatory cytokines via activation of the NF-κB pathway (Foley et al., 2002; Li et al., 2008). Immunization of mice with RABV-infected DCs stimulated cellular and humoral immune responses in mice. Further, it was shown that RABV-infected DCs, in contrast to inoculations with RABV-based vectors (McKenna et al., 2007; Tan et al., 2005), could be used in a homologous prime-boost approach leading to increased Gag-specific cellular immune responses (Wanjalla et al., 2010).

The final test of the effectiveness of such novel vaccine constructs requires a model in which protection from an AIDS-like infection could be monitored. For this approach, RABV backbone plasmids containing the R333E mutation or whose RABV G ectodomain was replaced with that of VSV were used to construct recombinant RABV expressing SIV Env and Gag or Gag–Pol proteins (Faul *et al.*, 2009a,b; McKenna *et al.*, 2007). These constructs allowed for a heterologous prime-boost vaccine regimen, an approach previously shown to increase the cellular response by about 4.5- to 5.5-fold higher than a prime-only approach (Tan *et al.*, 2005). In two independent monkey studies, rhesus macaques were primed and boosted with RABV constructs (SIV$_{mac239}$Gag, SIV$_{SHIV89.6}$Env) (McKenna *et al.*, 2007) or (SIV$_{mac239}$Gag–Pol and SIV$_{mac239}$Env) (Faul *et al.*, 2009a,b; McKenna *et al.*, 2007) and challenged with either SHIV-89.6 or the highly pathogenic SIV$_{mac251}$, respectively (Faul *et al.*, 2009a,b; McKenna *et al.*, 2007). Compared to vector controls, the vaccine groups seroconverted with induction of neutralizing antibodies and CD8+ T cells and the vaccines were protected from an AIDS-like disease. Specifically, the protection against the highly pathogenic SIV$_{mac251}$ strain combined with the lack of any vector-induced pathogenicity indicates great promise for RABV-based vectors as HIV-1 vaccines.

B. Hepatitis C virus

Hepatitis C virus (HCV) affects 120–170 million people worldwide and is the most common cause for liver disease requiring transplantation in adults (Tellinghuisen *et al.*, 2007). Most of these cases are chronically infected and 20% develop severe liver disease, including cirrhosis and hepatocellular carcinoma. A major obstacle in the treatment and control of HCV lies in the error-prone replicative machinery, which increases the genetic variability of HCV within an individual, resulting in quasispecies. Antiviral therapies have helped manage the disease; however, they have several disadvantages, including a low rate of response and toxicity. Similar to HIV, the correlates of protection against HCV are not well understood. There is, however, an appreciation of the need to induce neutralizing antibodies (nAb) and CD4+ and CD8+ T cells to multiple HCV antigens. However, for the humoral response, it remains largely unknown which epitopes are important for nAb to target leading to sterilizing immunity (Tellinghuisen *et al.*, 2007; von Hahn *et al.*, 2007).

RABV vaccine constructs against HCV were constructed and tested in mice and shown to induce both a humoral and cellular response. A recombinant RABV construct expressing chimeric E2 containing the CD4 transmembrane and RABV G cytoplasmic domain was shown to allow cell surface expression of E2. Moreover, the chimeric E2 was incorporated into RABV virions. For the humoral studies, these killed

RABV particles were administered to mice in a prime-boost regimen and shown to induce detectable antibodies against HCV-E2 after boost as measured by ELISA. Mice primed with live RABV construct cloned to express both HCV envelope proteins (E1 and E2), which upon expression interact in a noncovalent heterodimeric complex retained in the ER, were shown to mount a cellular immune response capable of lysing cells pulsed with an HCV-specific peptide (Siler *et al.*, 2002).

C. Severe acute respiratory syndrome

The global impact of emergent infectious diseases has become a topic of interest to vaccine developers and researchers (Faber *et al.*, 2005c). Severe acute respiratory syndrome (SARS) is one such disease whose causative agent is a coronavirus named SARS-CoV. From a vaccine standpoint, SARS-CoV may be an important pathogen despite the fast decline in SARS reported cases due to existence of animal reservoirs such as raccoon dogs and the Chinese ferret badger. It is thought that antibodies against SARS-CoV spike (S) protein are neutralizing and therefore a potential target for vaccines (see Faber *et al.*, 2005c and references within). For the vaccine studies, live-attenuated recombinant RABV containing the R333E mutation expressing SARS-CoV S protein was shown to induce high neutralizing antibodies in mice (Faber *et al.*, 2005c). The translation of these studies to wildlife reservoirs using live RABV may be possible based on the efficacy of live RABV vaccines in the eradication of RABV reservoirs in wildlife.

V. SAFETY: GENERATING SAFER RABV VACCINES AND VECTORS FOR USE IN HUMANS

Safety is a major concern in the development of vaccines, especially where live replication-competent vaccines are considered due to the likelihood of revertants or residual vector pathogenicity. There are several methods that have been used to improve the safety of RABV vaccines while maintaining their immunogenicity (see Wirblich and Schnell, 2011 and references within).

VI. REPLICATION-DEFICIENT OR SINGLE-CYCLE RABV

Despite the great improvements to replication-competent RABV, there are still potential safety concerns associated with the use of live viruses for widespread immunization of humans. Even highly attenuated RABV can be lethal following intracranial inoculation, at least in the immunodeficient host. In order to address such safety concerns, viruses have been further attenuated by complete genome deletion of an essential gene(s) that renders the vector unable to complete its viral life cycle. This attenuation strategy has been used on many viral backbones: adenovirus (Ad), vaccinia virus (VV), canarypox virus (CPV), herpes simplex virus (HSV), VSV, and RABV (Bozac *et al.*, 2006; Cenna *et al.*, 2008, 2009; Coulibaly *et al.*, 2005; Gomme *et al.*, 2010; Peng *et al.*, 2005; Publicover *et al.*, 2005; Russell *et al.*, 2007).

VII. POTENTIAL NOVEL HUMAN RABIES VACCINES BASED ON REPLICATION-DEFICIENT RABV

Deleting RABV genes *P* or *M* generated replication-deficient RABV (Cenna *et al.*, 2008, 2009), so termed because they lack viral components that are required for a complete viral life cycle. RABV P is a phosphoprotein cofactor to the viral RNA polymerase, and its deletion severely hinders intracellular replication (Cenna *et al.*, 2009). However, due to the role of M in assembly and budding, M-deleted virus is structurally impaired forming mainly cell-associated rod-shaped particles instead of the typical bullet-shaped particles. M also has a role in regulating the balance between transcription and replication, and as such, M-deleted virus may be impaired at the level of viral replication. These effects on virion formation reduce infectious titers as much as 500,000-fold (Mebatsion *et al.*, 1999). In addition, deletion of P and M may have additional, unknown effects on viral fitness that contribute to their immunogenicity. McGettigan *et al.* generated a P-deleted replication-deficient RABV for potential use in pre- or postexposure vaccine regimens for prevention of human rabies infections (Cenna *et al.*, 2008). A likely candidate would induce IgG2a antibodies for their potent antiviral effector functions. Current regimens use inactivated RABV particles that require several doses to be effective. In a head-to-head comparison of live P-deleted RABV and inactivated RABV, they found mice immunized with P-deleted had 10-fold greater survival and a proportionately greater IgG2a response after lethal challenge than mice immunized with inactivated virus (Cenna *et al.*, 2008). A later study showed M-deleted RABV is even more potent than P-deleted in mice, inducing greater IgG and VNA titers and protecting 100% of lethally challenged mice even at immunization titers as low as 10^3 foci-forming units (Cenna *et al.*, 2009). Notably, neither P- or M-deleted virus induced clinical signs of rabies, nor were they found in the brain or spinal cord following intramuscular injection of immunocompromised RAG2 knockout mice (Cenna *et al.*, 2008, 2009).

Replication impaired RABV vectors lacking RABV M, but expressing RABV G proteins, were shown to be safe and immunogenic in both mice and nonhuman primates. In fact, the M-deleted RABV had fourfold higher VNA titers 10 days after inoculation compared to a commercially available killed RABV vaccine. One hundred and eighty days later, the monkeys that received M-deleted RABV maintained higher VNA titers with antibodies shown to have a higher avidity than the killed HDCV (Cenna *et al.*, 2009). These data strongly demonstrate the potential for replication-deficient RABV to replace current pre- and postexposure RABV vaccines.

VIII. REPLICATION-DEFICIENT/SINGLE-CYCLE RABV AS VACCINE VECTOR

The G-deleted RABVs are termed "single-cycle" or "spread-deficient" because they lack viral components that are required for viral spread or infectivity. RABV G has a critical role in the attachment and entry of the virus into host cells, which makes G one of the most important determinants of viral pathogenicity (Dietzschold *et al.*, 1983, 2008; Pulmanausahakul *et al.*, 2008). Particles lacking G undergo one complete cycle of intracellular replication and produce progeny that are unable to spread (Mebatsion *et al.*, 1996a,b), as shown by infection of single neurons following intracranial inoculation of a G-deleted RABV (Etessami *et al.*, 2000; Wickersham *et al.*, 2007a). Virus particles lacking G are still capable of budding, although at a 30-fold lower efficiency (Mebatsion *et al.*, 1996a,b). These virions, however, are incapable of attachment and entry into a secondary host cell. Gomme *et al.* (2010) generated a G-deleted RABV-encoding HIV-1 Gag for development of an HIV-1 vaccine. Compared to the replication-competent parental virus, G-deleted RABV generated lower RABV-specific antibody responses but equivalent HIV-1 Gag-specific CD8+ T cell responses. Moreover, these responses were enhanced by a heterologous boost with a G-deleted RABV complemented with VSV glycoprotein. This shows that single-cycle RABV is a promising platform for safe, live viral vaccines and further studies will analyze if similar responses can be induced in nonhuman primates.

IX. KILLED RABV–RABV PROTEINS AS CARRIERS OF FOREIGN ANTIGENS

The simplicity and plasticity of the RABV genome is one of the many advantages as a vaccine vector. The genome is amenable to inclusion of whole foreign antigens as RABV protein chimeras. Both RABV G and N proteins have been tested as carriers of foreign antigens and proven to be immunogenic when applied as live or killed vaccines (Koser *et al.*, 2004;

Langley *et al.*, 2010; Smith *et al.*, 2006). There are several possible advantages to using RABV proteins as carriers: (i) RABV G as a carrier expressing a foreign envelope protein combined with the RABV-CD allows insertion of the foreign gene into the RABV virion (Mebatsion and Conzelmann, 1996; Mebatsion *et al.*, 1997; Smith *et al.*, 2006); (ii) in this setting, immunogenic epitopes may be presented in an organized structure which may increase their immunogenicity; and (iii) depending on the carrier (RABV N) and foreign antigen, forming the chimera could stabilize the antigen allowing longer expression and having an impact on the immunogenicity (Koser *et al.*, 2004).

The viability and immunogenicity of RABV constructs containing G or N fusion proteins have been extensively studied (Koser *et al.*, 2004; Siler *et al.*, 2002; Smith *et al.*, 2006). RNPs obtained from recombinant RABV constructs with GFP fused to RABV N were used to immunize mice in a prime-boost regimen. In comparison to the controls that were immunized with GFP, mice immunized with RNP had significantly higher antibodies against GFP, which seemed dependent on CD4+ T cell response, because no GFP-specific antibodies were detected after depletion of CD4+ T cells (Koser *et al.*, 2004).

RABV G protein as a carrier for foreign antigen has also been shown to be efficacious in inducing immune responses in mice and monkeys (McKenna *et al.*, 2003, 2004; Smith *et al.*, 2006). As a vaccine strategy, it is employed where a substantial humoral response is known to be a good correlate of protection. RABV G chimeras carrying the *Bacillus anthracis* protective antigen (PA) had sufficient incorporation of PA in the virions. Both live and killed viral particles induced anti-PA antibodies in mice that were detectable postprime and increased after boost (Smith *et al.*, 2006).

Potential conflicts of interest: M. J. S. is a consultant to Molecular Targeting Technologies, Inc., and is an inventor and coinventor of several patents on RABV-based vaccines and vaccine-based vector.

REFERENCES

Anonymous (2006). The prevention, control and eradication of rabies in Europe . *Dev. Biol. (Basel)* **125:**291–296.

Astic, L., Saucier, D., Coulon, P., Lafay, F., and Flamand, A. (1993). The CVS strain of rabies virus as transneuronal tracer in the olfactory system of mice. *Brain Res.* **619**(1–2):146–156.

Bozac, A., Berto, E., Vasquez, F., Grandi, P., Caputo, A., Manservigi, R., Ensoli, B., and Marconi, P. (2006). Expression of human immunodeficiency virus type 1 tat from a replication-deficient herpes simplex type 1 vector induces antigen-specific T cell responses. *Vaccine* **24**(49–50):7148–7158.

Buttner-Ennever, J. A., Horn, A. K., Graf, W., and Ugolini, G. (2002). Modern concepts of brainstem anatomy: From extraocular motoneurons to proprioceptive pathways. *Ann. NY Acad. Sci.* **956:**75–84.

Callaway, E. M. (2008). Transneuronal circuit tracing with neurotropic viruses. *Curr. Opin. Neurobiol.* **18**(6):617–623.

Cenna, J., Tan, G. S., Papaneri, A. B., Dietzschold, B., Schnell, M. J., and McGettigan, J. P. (2008). Immune modulating effect by a phosphoprotein-deleted rabies virus vaccine vector expressing two copies of the rabies virus glycoprotein gene. *Vaccine* **26** (50):6405–6414.

Cenna, J., Hunter, M., Tan, G. S., Papaneri, A. B., Ribka, E. P., Schnell, M. J., Marx, P. A., and McGettigan, J. P. (2009). Replication-deficient rabies virus-based vaccines are safe and immunogenic in mice and nonhuman primates. *J. Infect. Dis.* **200**(8):1251–1260.

Clower, D. M., Dum, R. P., and Strick, P. L. (2005). Basal ganglia and cerebellar inputs to 'AIP'. *Cereb. Cortex* **15**(7):913–920.

Conzelmann, K. K., and Schnell, M. (1994). Rescue of synthetic genomic RNA analogs of rabies virus by plasmid-encoded proteins. *J. Virol.* **68**(2):713–719.

Conzelmann, K. K., Cox, J. H., Schneider, L. G., and Thiel, H. J. (1990). Molecular cloning and complete nucleotide sequence of the attenuated rabies virus SAD B19. *Virology* **175** (2):485–499.

Coulibaly, S., Bruhl, P., Mayrhofer, J., Schmid, K., Gerencer, M., and Falkner, F. G. (2005). The nonreplicating smallpox candidate vaccines defective vaccinia Lister (dVV-L) and modified vaccinia Ankara (MVA) elicit robust long-term protection. *Virology* **341**(1):91–101.

Coulon, P., Derbin, C., Kucera, P., Lafay, F., Prehaud, C., and Flamand, A. (1989). Invasion of the peripheral nervous systems of adult mice by the CVS strain of rabies virus and its avirulent derivative AvO1. *J. Virol.* **63**(8):3550–3554.

Coulon, P., Ternaux, J. P., Flamand, A., and Tuffereau, C. (1998). An avirulent mutant of rabies virus is unable to infect motoneurons *in vivo* and *in vitro*. *J. Virol.* **72**(1):273–278.

Dietzschold, B., and Schnell, M. J. (2002). New approaches to the development of live attenuated rabies vaccines. *Hybrid. Hybridomics* **21**(2):129–134.

Dietzschold, B., Wunner, W. H., Wiktor, T. J., Lopes, A. D., Lafon, M., Smith, C. L., and Koprowski, H. (1983). Characterization of an antigenic determinant of the glycoprotein that correlates with pathogenicity of rabies virus. *Proc. Natl. Acad. Sci. USA* **80**(1):70–74.

Dietzschold, B., Faber, M., and Schnell, M. J. (2003). New approaches to the prevention and eradication of rabies. *Expert Rev. Vaccines* **2**(3):399–406.

Dietzschold, B., Schnell, M., and Koprowski, H. (2005). Pathogenesis of rabies. *Curr. Top. Microbiol. Immunol.* **292**:45–56.

Dietzschold, B., Li, J., Faber, M., and Schnell, M. (2008). Concepts in the pathogenesis of rabies. *Future Virol.* **3**(5):481–490.

Durali, D., Morvan, J., Letourneur, F., Schmitt, D., Guegan, N., Dalod, M., Saragosti, S., Sicard, D., Levy, J. P., and Gomard, E. (1998). Cross-reactions between the cytotoxic T-lymphocyte responses of human immunodeficiency virus-infected African and European patients. *J. Virol.* **72**(5):3547–3553.

Etessami, R., Conzelmann, K. K., Fadai-Ghotbi, B., Natelson, B., Tsiang, H., and Ceccaldi, P. E. (2000). Spread and pathogenic characteristics of a G-deficient rabies virus recombinant: An *in vitro* and *in vivo* study. *J. Gen. Virol.* **81**(Pt 9):2147–2153.

Faber, M., Pulmanausahakul, R., Hodawadekar, S. S., Spitsin, S., McGettigan, J. P., Schnell, M. J., and Dietzschold, B. (2002). Overexpression of the rabies virus glycoprotein results in enhancement of apoptosis and antiviral immune response. *J. Virol.* **76** (7):3374–3381.

Faber, M., Pulmanausahakul, R., Nagao, K., Prosniak, M., Rice, A. B., Koprowski, H., Schnell, M. J., and Dietzschold, B. (2004). Identification of viral genomic elements responsible for rabies virus neuroinvasiveness. *Proc. Natl. Acad. Sci. USA* **101**(46):16328–16332.

Faber, M., Bette, M., Preuss, M. A., Pulmanausahakul, R., Rehnelt, J., Schnell, M. J., Dietzschold, B., and Weihe, E. (2005a). Overexpression of tumor necrosis factor alpha by a recombinant rabies virus attenuates replication in neurons and prevents lethal infection in mice. *J. Virol.* **79**(24):15405–15416.

Faber, M., Faber, M. L., Papaneri, A., Bette, M., Weihe, E., Dietzschold, B., and Schnell, M. J. (2005b). A single amino acid change in rabies virus glycoprotein increases virus spread and enhances virus pathogenicity. *J. Virol.* **79**(22):14141–14148.

Faber, M., Lamirande, E. W., Roberts, A., Rice, A. B., Koprowski, H., Dietzschold, B., and Schnell, M. J. (2005c). A single immunization with a rhabdovirus-based vector expressing severe acute respiratory syndrome coronavirus (SARS-CoV) S protein results in the production of high levels of SARS-CoV-neutralizing antibodies. *J. Gen. Virol.* **86** (Pt 5):1435–1440.

Faber, M., Li, J., Kean, R. B., Hooper, D. C., Alugupalli, K. R., and Dietzschold, B. (2009). Effective preexposure and postexposure prophylaxis of rabies with a highly attenuated recombinant rabies virus. *Proc. Natl. Acad. Sci. USA* **106**(27):11300–11305.

Faul, E. J., Wanjalla, C. N., McGettigan, J. P., and Schnell, M. J. (2008). Interferon-beta expressed by a rabies virus-based HIV-1 vaccine vector serves as a molecular adjuvant and decreases pathogenicity. *Virology* **382**(2):226–238.

Faul, E., Lyles, D., and Schnell, M. (2009a). Interferon response and viral evasion by members of the family Rhabdoviridae. *Viruses* **1**(3):832–851.

Faul, E. J., Aye, P. P., Papaneri, A. B., Pahar, B., McGettigan, J. P., Schiro, F., Chervoneva, I., Montefiori, D. C., Lackner, A. A., and Schnell, M. J. (2009b). Rabies virus-based vaccines elicit neutralizing antibodies, poly-functional CD8+ T cell, and protect rhesus macaques from AIDS-like disease after SIV(mac251) challenge. *Vaccine* **28**(2):299–308.

Foley, H. D., McGettigan, J. P., Siler, C. A., Dietzschold, B., and Schnell, M. J. (2000). A recombinant rabies virus expressing vesicular stomatitis virus glycoprotein fails to protect against rabies virus infection. *Proc. Natl. Acad. Sci. USA* **97**(26):14680–14685.

Foley, H. D., Otero, M., Orenstein, J. M., Pomerantz, R. J., and Schnell, M. J. (2002). Rhabdo-virus-based vectors with human immunodeficiency virus type 1 (HIV-1) envelopes display HIV-1-like tropism and target human dendritic cells. *J. Virol.* **76**(1):19–31.

Gillet, J. P., Derer, P., and Tsiang, H. (1986). Axonal transport of rabies virus in the central nervous system of the rat. *J. Neuropathol. Exp. Neurol.* **45**(6):619–634.

Gomme, E. A., Faul, E. J., Flomenberg, P., McGettigan, J. P., and Schnell, M. J. (2010). Characterization of a single-cycle rabies virus-based vaccine vector. *J. Virol.* **84** (6):2820–2831.

Graf, W., Gerrits, N., Yatim-Dhiba, N., and Ugolini, G. (2002). Mapping the oculomotor system: The power of transneuronal labelling with rabies virus. *Eur. J. Neurosci.* **15** (9):1557–1562.

Grimm, R. (2002). The history of the eradication of rabies in most European countries. *Hist. Med. Vet.* **27**(1–4):295–301.

Hashimoto, M., Takahara, D., Hirata, Y., Inoue, K., Miyachi, S., Nambu, A., Tanji, J., Takada, M., and Hoshi, E. (2010). Motor and non-motor projections from the cerebellum to rostrocaudally distinct sectors of the dorsal premotor cortex in macaques. *Eur. J. Neurosci.* **31**(8):1402–1413.

Haut, L. H., and Ertl, H. C. (2009). Obstacles to the successful development of an efficacious T cell-inducing HIV-1 vaccine. *J. Leukoc. Biol.* **86**(4):779–793.

Hoshi, E., Tremblay, L., Feger, J., Carras, P. L., and Strick, P. L. (2005). The cerebellum communicates with the basal ganglia. *Nat. Neurosci.* **8**(11):1491–1493.

Huang, Y., Tang, Q., Nadin-Davis, S. A., Zhang, S., Hooper, C. D., Ming, P., Du, J., Tao, X., Hu, R., and Liang, G. (2010). Development of a reverse genetics system for a human rabies virus vaccine strain employed in China. *Virus Res.* **149**(1):28–35.

Inoue, K., Shoji, Y., Kurane, I., Iijima, T., Sakai, T., and Morimoto, K. (2003). An improved method for recovering rabies virus from cloned cDNA. *J. Virol. Methods* **107**(2):229–236.

Ito, N., Takayama, M., Yamada, K., Sugiyama, M., and Minamoto, N. (2001). Rescue of rabies virus from cloned cDNA and identification of the pathogenicity-related gene: Glycoprotein gene is associated with virulence for adult mice. *J. Virol.* **75**(19):9121–9128.

Ito, N., Sugiyama, M., Yamada, K., Shimizu, K., Takayama-Ito, M., Hosokawa, J., and Minamoto, N. (2005). Characterization of M gene-deficient rabies virus with advantages of effective immunization and safety as a vaccine strain. *Microbiol. Immunol.* **49** (11):971–979.

Iwata, K., Miyachi, S., Imanishi, M., Tsuboi, Y., Kitagawa, J., Teramoto, K., Hitomi, S., Shinoda, M., Kondo, M., and Takada, M. (2011). Ascending multisynaptic pathways from the trigeminal ganglion to the anterior cingulate cortex. *Exp. Neurol.* **227**(1):69–78.

Jacotot, E., Cardona, A., Rebouillat, D., Terradillos, O., Marianneau, P., Thoulouze, M. I., Lafon, M., Deubel, V., and Edelman, L. (1999). Combined use of radioimagers and radioactive 3′OH DNA nick end labelling to quantify apoptosis in cell lines and tissue sections: Applications to virus-induced apoptosis. *Apoptosis* **4**(3):169–178.

Karacostas, V., Nagashima, K., Gonda, M. A., and Moss, B. (1989). Human immunodeficiency virus-like particles produced by a vaccinia virus expression vector. *Proc. Natl. Acad. Sci. USA* **86**(22):8964–8967.

Kelly, R. M., and Strick, P. L. (2000). Rabies as a transneuronal tracer of circuits in the central nervous system. *J. Neurosci. Methods* **103**(1):63–71.

Kelly, R. M., and Strick, P. L. (2003). Cerebellar loops with motor cortex and prefrontal cortex of a nonhuman primate. *J. Neurosci.* **23**(23):8432–8444.

Kelly, R. M., and Strick, P. L. (2004). Macro-architecture of basal ganglia loops with the cerebral cortex: Use of rabies virus to reveal multisynaptic circuits. *Prog. Brain Res.* **143**:449–459.

Koff, W. C., Johnson, P. R., Watkins, D. I., Burton, D. R., Lifson, J. D., Hasenkrug, K. J., McDermott, A. B., Schultz, A., Zamb, T. J., Boyle, R., and Desrosiers, R. C. (2006). HIV vaccine design: Insights from live attenuated SIV vaccines. *Nat. Immunol.* **7**(1):19–23.

Koser, M. L., McGettigan, J. P., Tan, G. S., Smith, M. E., Koprowski, H., Dietzschold, B., and Schnell, M. J. (2004). Rabies virus nucleoprotein as a carrier for foreign antigens. *Proc. Natl. Acad. Sci. USA* **101**(25):9405–9410.

Kuang, Y., Lackay, S. N., Zhao, L., and Fu, Z. F. (2009). Role of chemokines in the enhancement of BBB permeability and inflammatory infiltration after rabies virus infection. *Virus Res.* **144**(1–2):18–26.

Kucera, P., Dolivo, M., Coulon, P., and Flamand, A. (1985). Pathways of the early propagation of virulent and avirulent rabies strains from the eye to the brain. *J. Virol.* **55** (1):158–162.

Lafay, F., Coulon, P., Astic, L., Saucier, D., Riche, D., Holley, A., and Flamand, A. (1991). Spread of the CVS strain of rabies virus and of the avirulent mutant AvO1 along the olfactory pathways of the mouse after intranasal inoculation. *Virology* **183**(1):320–330.

Langley, W. A., Bradley, K. C., Li, Z. N., Smith, M. E., Schnell, M. J., and Steinhauer, D. A. (2010). Induction of neutralizing antibody responses to anthrax protective antigen by using influenza virus vectors: Implications for disparate immune system priming pathways. *J. Virol.* **84**(16):8300–8307.

Larsen, D. D., Wickersham, I. R., and Callaway, E. M. (2007). Retrograde tracing with recombinant rabies virus reveals correlations between projection targets and dendritic architecture in layer 5 of mouse barrel cortex. *Front. Neural Circuits* **1**:5.

Le Mercier, P., Jacob, Y., Tanner, K., and Tordo, N. (2002). A novel expression cassette of lyssavirus shows that the distantly related Mokola virus can rescue a defective rabies virus genome. *J. Virol.* **76**(4):2024–2027.

Lentz, T. L., Burrage, T. G., Smith, A. L., and Tignor, G. H. (1983). The acetylcholine receptor as a cellular receptor for rabies virus. *Yale J. Biol. Med.* **56**(4):315–322.

Li, J., McGettigan, J. P., Faber, M., Schnell, M. J., and Dietzschold, B. (2008). Infection of monocytes or immature dendritic cells (DCs) with an attenuated rabies virus results in DC maturation and a strong activation of the NFkappaB signaling pathway. *Vaccine* **26** (3):419–426.

Lois, J. H., Rice, C. D., and Yates, B. J. (2009). Neural circuits controlling diaphragm function in the cat revealed by transneuronal tracing. *J. Appl. Physiol.* **106**(1):138–152.

McAdam, S., Kaleebu, P., Krausa, P., Goulder, P., French, N., Collin, B., Blanchard, T., Whitworth, J., McMichael, A., and Gotch, F. (1998). Cross-clade recognition of p55 by cytotoxic T lymphocytes in HIV-1 infection. *AIDS* **12**(6):571–579.

McGettigan, J. P. (2010). Experimental rabies vaccines for humans. *Expert Rev. Vaccines* **9**(10):1177–1186.

McGettigan, J. P., Foley, H. D., Belyakov, I. M., Berzofsky, J. A., Pomerantz, R. J., and Schnell, M. J. (2001a). Rabies virus-based vectors expressing human immunodeficiency virus type 1 (HIV-1) envelope protein induce a strong, cross-reactive cytotoxic T-lymphocyte response against envelope proteins from different HIV-1 isolates. *J. Virol.* **75**(9):4430–4434.

McGettigan, J. P., Sarma, S., Orenstein, J. M., Pomerantz, R. J., and Schnell, M. J. (2001b). Expression and immunogenicity of human immunodeficiency virus type 1 Gag expressed by a replication-competent rhabdovirus-based vaccine vector. *J. Virol.* **75**(18):8724–8732.

McGettigan, J. P., Naper, K., Orenstein, J., Koser, M., McKenna, P. M., and Schnell, M. J. (2003a). Functional human immunodeficiency virus type 1 (HIV-1) Gag-Pol or HIV-1 Gag-Pol and Env expressed from a single rhabdovirus-based vaccine vector genome. *J. Virol.* **77**(20):10889–10899.

McGettigan, J. P., Pomerantz, R. J., Siler, C. A., McKenna, P. M., Foley, H. D., Dietzschold, B., and Schnell, M. J. (2003b). Second-generation rabies virus-based vaccine vectors expressing human immunodeficiency virus type 1 gag have greatly reduced pathogenicity but are highly immunogenic. *J. Virol.* **77**(1):237–244.

McGettigan, J. P., Koser, M. L., McKenna, P. M., Smith, M. E., Marvin, J. M., Eisenlohr, L. C., Dietzschold, B., and Schnell, M. J. (2006). Enhanced humoral HIV-1-specific immune responses generated from recombinant rhabdoviral-based vaccine vectors co-expressing HIV-1 proteins and IL-2. *Virology* **344**(2):363–377.

McKenna, P. M., Pomerantz, R. J., Dietzschold, B., McGettigan, J. P., and Schnell, M. J. (2003). Covalently linked human immunodeficiency virus type 1 gp120/gp41 is stably anchored in rhabdovirus particles and exposes critical neutralizing epitopes. *J. Virol.* **77**(23):12782–12794.

McKenna, P. M., Aye, P. P., Dietzschold, B., Montefiori, D. C., Martin, L. N., Marx, P. A., Pomerantz, R. J., Lackner, A., and Schnell, M. J. (2004). Immunogenicity study of glycoprotein-deficient rabies virus expressing simian/human immunodeficiency virus SHIV89.6P envelope in a rhesus macaque. *J. Virol.* **78**(24):13455–13459.

McKenna, P. M., Koser, M. L., Carlson, K. R., Montefiori, D. C., Letvin, N. L., Papaneri, A. B., Pomerantz, R. J., Dietzschold, B., Silvera, P., McGettigan, J. P., and Schnell, M. J. (2007). Highly attenuated rabies virus-based vaccine vectors expressing simian–human immunodeficiency virus89.6P Env and simian immunodeficiency virusmac239 Gag are safe in rhesus macaques and protect from an AIDS-like disease. *J. Infect. Dis.* **195**(7):980–988.

Mebatsion, T. (2001). Extensive attenuation of rabies virus by simultaneously modifying the dynein light chain binding site in the P protein and replacing Arg333 in the G protein. *J. Virol.* **75**(23):11496–11502.

Mebatsion, T., and Conzelmann, K. K. (1996). Specific infection of CD4+ target cells by recombinant rabies virus pseudotypes carrying the HIV-1 envelope spike protein. *Proc. Natl. Acad. Sci. USA* **93**(21):11366–11370.

Mebatsion, T., Konig, M., and Conzelmann, K. K. (1996a). Budding of rabies virus particles in the absence of the spike glycoprotein. *Cell* **84**(6):941–951.

Mebatsion, T., Schnell, M. J., Cox, J. H., Finke, S., and Conzelmann, K. K. (1996b). Highly stable expression of a foreign gene from rabies virus vectors. *Proc. Natl. Acad. Sci. USA* **93**(14):7310–7314.

Mebatsion, T., Finke, S., Weiland, F., and Conzelmann, K. K. (1997). A CXCR4/CD4 pseudotype rhabdovirus that selectively infects HIV-1 envelope protein-expressing cells. *Cell* **90**(5):841–847.

Mebatsion, T., Weiland, F., and Conzelmann, K. K. (1999). Matrix protein of rabies virus is responsible for the assembly and budding of bullet-shaped particles and interacts with the transmembrane spike glycoprotein G. *J. Virol.* **73**(1):242–250.

Morcuende, S., Delgado-Garcia, J. M., and Ugolini, G. (2002). Neuronal premotor networks involved in eyelid responses: Retrograde transneuronal tracing with rabies virus from the orbicularis oculi muscle in the rat. *J. Neurosci.* **22**(20):8808–8818.

Morimoto, K., Hooper, D. C., Spitsin, S., Koprowski, H., and Dietzschold, B. (1999). Pathogenicity of different rabies virus variants inversely correlates with apoptosis and rabies virus glycoprotein expression in infected primary neuron cultures. *J. Virol.* **73**(1):510–518.

Morimoto, K., Foley, H. D., McGettigan, J. P., Schnell, M. J., and Dietzschold, B. (2000). Reinvestigation of the role of the rabies virus glycoprotein in viral pathogenesis using a reverse genetics approach. *J. Neurovirol.* **6**(5):373–381.

Morimoto, K., McGettigan, J. P., Foley, H. D., Hooper, D. C., Dietzschold, B., and Schnell, M. J. (2001). Genetic engineering of live rabies vaccines. *Vaccine* **19**(25–26):3543–3551.

Morimoto, K., Shoji, Y., and Inoue, S. (2005). Characterization of P gene-deficient rabies virus: Propagation, pathogenicity and antigenicity. *Virus Res.* **111**(1):61–67.

Nassi, J. J., and Callaway, E. M. (2006). Multiple circuits relaying primate parallel visual pathways to the middle temporal area. *J. Neurosci.* **26**(49):12789–12798.

Ohara, S., Inoue, K., Yamada, M., Yamawaki, T., Koganezawa, N., Tsutsui, K., Witter, M. P., and Iijima, T. (2009). Dual transneuronal tracing in the rat entorhinal-hippocampal circuit by intracerebral injection of recombinant rabies virus vectors. *Front. Neuroanat.* **3**:1.

Ohara, S., Inoue, K., Witter, M. P., and Iijima, T. (2009a). Untangling neural networks with dual retrograde transsynaptic viral infection. *Front. Neurosci.* **3**(3):344–349.

Ohara, S., Inoue, K., Yamada, M., Yamawaki, T., Koganezawa, N., Tsutsui, K., Witter, M. P., and Iijima, T. (2009b). Dual transneuronal tracing in the rat entorhinal-hippocampal circuit by intracerebral injection of recombinant rabies virus vectors. *Front. Neuroanat.* **3**:1.

Orbanz, J., and Finke, S. (2010). Generation of recombinant European bat lyssavirus type 1 and inter-genotypic compatibility of lyssavirus genotype 1 and 5 antigenome promoters. *Arch. Virol.* **155**(10):1631–1641.

Pasteur, L. (1885). Methode pour prevenir la rage apres morsure. *C. R. Acad. Sci.* **101**:765–773.

Peng, B., Wang, L. R., Gomez-Roman, V. R., Davis-Warren, A., Montefiori, D. C., Kalyanaraman, V. S., Venzon, D., Zhao, J., Kan, E., Rowell, T. J., Murthy, K. K., Srivastava, I., *et al.* (2005). Replicating rather than nonreplicating adenovirus-human immunodeficiency virus recombinant vaccines are better at eliciting potent cellular immunity and priming high-titer antibodies. *J. Virol.* **79**(16):10200–10209.

Prevosto, V., Graf, W., and Ugolini, G. (2009). Posterior parietal cortex areas MIP and LIPv receive eye position and velocity inputs via ascending preposito-thalamo-cortical pathways. *Eur. J. Neurosci.* **30**(6):1151–1161.

Publicover, J., Ramsburg, E., and Rose, J. K. (2005). A single-cycle vaccine vector based on vesicular stomatitis virus can induce immune responses comparable to those generated by a replication-competent vector. *J. Virol.* **79**(21):13231–13238.

Pulmanausahakul, R., Faber, M., Morimoto, K., Spitsin, S., Weihe, E., Hooper, D. C., Schnell, M. J., and Dietzschold, B. (2001). Overexpression of cytochrome C by a recombinant rabies virus attenuates pathogenicity and enhances antiviral immunity. *J. Virol.* **75**(22):10800–10807.

Pulmanausahakul, R., Li, J., Schnell, M. J., and Dietzschold, B. (2008). The glycoprotein and the matrix protein of rabies virus affect pathogenicity by regulating viral replication and facilitating cell-to-cell spread. *J. Virol.* **82**(5):2330–2338.

Rathelot, J. A., and Strick, P. L. (2006). Muscle representation in the macaque motor cortex: An anatomical perspective. *Proc. Natl. Acad. Sci. USA* **103**(21):8257–8262.

Rice, C. D., Lois, J. H., Kerman, I. A., and Yates, B. J. (2009). Localization of serotoninergic neurons that participate in regulating diaphragm activity in the cat. *Brain Res.* **1279**:71–81.

Rice, C. D., Weber, S. A., Waggoner, A. L., Jessell, M. E., and Yates, B. J. (2010). Mapping of neural pathways that influence diaphragm activity and project to the lumbar spinal cord in cats. *Exp. Brain Res.* **203**(1):205–211.

Rolland, M., Nickle, D. C., and Mullins, J. I. (2007). HIV-1 group M conserved elements vaccine. *PLoS Pathog.* **3**(11):e157.

Roseveare, C. W., Goolsby, W. D., and Foppa, I. M. (2009). Potential and actual terrestrial rabies exposures in people and domestic animals, upstate South Carolina, 1994–2004: A surveillance study. *BMC Public Health* **9**:65.

Ruigrok, T. J., Pijpers, A., Goedknegt-Sabel, E., and Coulon, P. (2008). Multiple cerebellar zones are involved in the control of individual muscles: A retrograde transneuronal tracing study with rabies virus in the rat. *Eur. J. Neurosci.* **28**(1):181–200.

Russell, N. D., Graham, B. S., Keefer, M. C., McElrath, M. J., Self, S. G., Weinhold, K. J., Montefiori, D. C., Ferrari, G., Horton, H., Tomaras, G. D., Gurunathan, S., Baglyos, L., *et al.* (2007). Phase 2 study of an HIV-1 canarypox vaccine (vCP1452) alone and in combination with rgp120: Negative results fail to trigger a phase 3 correlates trial. *J. Acquir. Immune Defic. Syndr.* **44**(2):203–212.

Schnell, M. J., Mebatsion, T., and Conzelmann, K. K. (1994). Infectious rabies viruses from cloned cDNA. *EMBO J.* **13**(18):4195–4203.

Schnell, M. J., Foley, H. D., Siler, C. A., McGettigan, J. P., Dietzschold, B., and Pomerantz, R. J. (2000). Recombinant rabies virus as potential live-viral vaccines for HIV-1. *Proc. Natl. Acad. Sci. USA* **97**(7):3544–3549.

Schnell, M. J., McGettigan, J. P., Wirblich, C., and Papaneri, A. (2010). The cell biology of rabies virus: Using stealth to reach the brain. *Nat. Rev. Microbiol.* **8**(1):51–61.

Shimizu, K., Ito, N., Mita, T., Yamada, K., Hosokawa-Muto, J., Sugiyama, M., and Minamoto, N. (2007). Involvement of nucleoprotein, phosphoprotein, and matrix protein genes of rabies virus in virulence for adult mice. *Virus Res.* **123**(2):154–160.

Shoji, Y., Inoue, S., Nakamichi, K., Kurane, I., Sakai, T., and Morimoto, K. (2004). Generation and characterization of P gene-deficient rabies virus. *Virology* **318**(1):295–305.

Siler, C. A., McGettigan, J. P., Dietzschold, B., Herrine, S. K., Dubuisson, J., Pomerantz, R. J., and Schnell, M. J. (2002). Live and killed rhabdovirus-based vectors as potential hepatitis C vaccines. *Virology* **292**(1):24–34.

Smart, N. L., and Charlton, K. M. (1992). The distribution of Challenge virus standard rabies virus versus skunk street rabies virus in the brains of experimentally infected rabid skunks. *Acta Neuropathol.* **84**(5):501–508.

Smith, M. E., Koser, M., Xiao, S., Siler, C., McGettigan, J. P., Calkins, C., Pomerantz, R. J., Dietzschold, B., and Schnell, M. J. (2006). Rabies virus glycoprotein as a carrier for anthrax protective antigen. *Virology* **353**(2):344–356.

Stepien, A. E., Tripodi, M., and Arber, S. (2010). Monosynaptic rabies virus reveals premotor network organization and synaptic specificity of cholinergic partition cells. *Neuron* **68**(3):456–472.

Superti, F., Hauttecoeur, B., Morelec, M. J., Goldoni, P., Bizzini, B., and Tsiang, H. (1986). Involvement of gangliosides in rabies virus infection. *J. Gen. Virol.* **67**(Pt 1):47–56.

Taber, K. H., Strick, P. L., and Hurley, R. A. (2005). Rabies and the cerebellum: New methods for tracing circuits in the brain. *J. Neuropsychiatry Clin. Neurosci.* **17**(2):133–139.

Tan, G. S., McKenna, P. M., Koser, M. L., McLinden, R., Kim, J. H., McGettigan, J. P., and Schnell, M. J. (2005). Strong cellular and humoral anti-HIV Env immune responses induced by a heterologous rhabdoviral prime-boost approach. *Virology* **331**(1):82–93.

Tan, G. S., Preuss, M. A., Williams, J. C., and Schnell, M. J. (2007). The dynein light chain 8 binding motif of rabies virus phosphoprotein promotes efficient viral transcription. *Proc. Natl. Acad. Sci. USA* **104**(17):7229–7234.

Tellinghuisen, T. L., Evans, M. J., von Hahn, T., You, S., and Rice, C. M. (2007). Studying hepatitis C virus: Making the best of a bad virus. *J. Virol.* **81**(17):8853–8867.

Thoulouze, M. I., Lafage, M., Schachner, M., Hartmann, U., Cremer, H., and Lafon, M. (1998). The neural cell adhesion molecule is a receptor for rabies virus. *J. Virol.* **72**(9):7181–7190.

Tsiang, H., Derer, M., and Taxi, J. (1983). An *in vivo* and *in vitro* study of rabies virus infection of the rat superior cervical ganglia. *Arch. Virol.* **76**(3):231–243.

Tuffereau, C., Benejean, J., Blondel, D., Kieffer, B., and Flamand, A. (1998). Low-affinity nerve-growth factor receptor (P75NTR) can serve as a receptor for rabies virus. *EMBO J.* **17**(24):7250–7259.

Ugolini, G. (1995). Specificity of rabies virus as a transneuronal tracer of motor networks: Transfer from hypoglossal motoneurons to connected second-order and higher order central nervous system cell groups. *J. Comp. Neurol.* **356**(3):457–480.

Ugolini, G. (2010). Advances in viral transneuronal tracing. *J. Neurosci. Methods* **194**(1):2–20.

Ugolini, G., Klam, F., Doldan Dans, M., Dubayle, D., Brandi, A. M., Buttner-Ennever, J., and Graf, W. (2006). Horizontal eye movement networks in primates as revealed by retrograde transneuronal transfer of rabies virus: Differences in monosynaptic input to "slow" and "fast" abducens motoneurons *J. Comp. Neurol.* **498**(6):762–785.

Viemari, J. C., Bevengut, M., Burnet, H., Coulon, P., Pequignot, J. M., Tiveron, M. C., and Hilaire, G. (2004a). Phox2a gene, A6 neurons, and noradrenaline are essential for development of normal respiratory rhythm in mice. *J. Neurosci.* **24**(4):928–937.

Viemari, J. C., Bevengut, M., Coulon, P., and Hilaire, G. (2004b). Nasal trigeminal inputs release the A5 inhibition received by the respiratory rhythm generator of the mouse neonate. *J. Neurophysiol.* **91**(2):746–758.

von Hahn, T., Yoon, J. C., Alter, H., Rice, C. M., Rehermann, B., Balfe, P., and McKeating, J. A. (2007). Hepatitis C virus continuously escapes from neutralizing antibody and T-cell responses during chronic infection *in vivo*. *Gastroenterology* **132**(2):667–678.

Wall, N. R., Wickersham, I. R., Cetin, A., De La Parra, M., and Callaway, E. M. (2010). Monosynaptic circuit tracing *in vivo* through Cre-dependent targeting and complementation of modified rabies virus. *Proc. Natl. Acad. Sci. USA.* **107**(50):21848–21853.

Wanjalla, C. N., Faul, E. J., Gomme, E. A., and Schnell, M. J. (2010). Dendritic cells infected by recombinant rabies virus vaccine vector expressing HIV-1 Gag are immunogenic even in the presence of vector-specific immunity. *Vaccine* **29**:130–140.

Wen, Y., Wang, H., Wu, H., Yang, F., Tripp, R. A., Hogan, R. J., and Fu, Z. F. (2010). Rabies virus expressing dendritic cell-activating molecules enhances the innate and adaptive immune response to vaccination. *J. Virol* **85**:1634–1644.

Wickersham, I. R., Finke, S., Conzelmann, K. K., and Callaway, E. M. (2007a). Retrograde neuronal tracing with a deletion-mutant rabies virus. *Nat. Methods* **4**(1):47–49.

Wickersham, I. R., Lyon, D. C., Barnard, R. J., Mori, T., Finke, S., Conzelmann, K. K., Young, J. A., and Callaway, E. M. (2007b). Monosynaptic restriction of transsynaptic tracing from single, genetically targeted neurons. *Neuron* **53**(5):639–647.

Wirblich, C., and Schnell, M. J. (2011). Rabies virus glycoprotein expression levels are not critical for pathogenicity of RV. *J. Virol.* **85**:697–704.

Wirblich, C., Tan, G. S., Papaneri, A., Godlewski, P. J., Orenstein, J. M., Harty, R. N., and Schnell, M. J. (2008). PPEY motif within the rabies virus (RV) matrix protein is essential for efficient virion release and RV pathogenicity. *J. Virol.* **82**(19):9730–9738.

Yamada, K., Ito, N., Takayama-Ito, M., Sugiyama, M., and Minamoto, N. (2006). Multigenic relation to the attenuation of rabies virus. *Microbiol. Immunol.* **50**(1):25–32.

Zhao, L., Toriumi, H., Kuang, Y., Chen, H., and Fu, Z. F. (2009). The roles of chemokines in rabies virus infection: Overexpression may not always be beneficial. *J. Virol.* **83**(22):11808–11818.

Zhao, L., Toriumi, H., Wang, H., Kuang, Y., Guo, X., Morimoto, K., and Fu, Z. F. (2010). Expression of MIP-1alpha (CCL3) by a recombinant rabies virus enhances its immunogenicity by inducing innate immunity and recruiting dendritic cells and B cells. *J. Virol.* **84**(18):9642–9648.

CHAPTER **10**

Rabies Virus as a Transneuronal Tracer of Neuronal Connections

Gabriella Ugolini

Contents

Neurobiologie et Développement, UPR3294 CNRS, Institut de Neurobiologie Alfred Fessard (INAF), 1 Avenue de la Terrasse, Bât. 32, 91198 Gif-sur-Yvette, France

Advances in Virus Research, Volume 79
ISSN 0065-3527, DOI: 10.1016/B978-0-12-387040-7.00010-X

Abstract   Powerful transneuronal tracing technologies exploit the ability of some neurotropic viruses to travel across neuronal pathways and to function as self-amplifying markers. Rabies virus is the only viral tracer that is entirely specific, as it propagates exclusively between connected neurons by strictly unidirectional (retrograde) transneuronal transfer, allowing for the stepwise identification of neuronal connections of progressively higher order. Transneuronal tracing studies in primates and rodent models prior to the development of clinical disease have provided valuable information on rabies pathogenesis. We have shown that rabies virus propagation occurs at chemical synapses but not via gap junctions or cell-to-cell spread. Infected neurons remain viable, as they can express their neurotransmitters and cotransport other tracers. Axonal transport occurs at high speed, and all populations of the same synaptic order are infected simultaneously regardless of their neurotransmitters, synaptic strength, and distance, showing that rabies virus receptors are ubiquitously distributed within the CNS. Conversely, in the peripheral nervous system, rabies virus receptors are present only on motor endplates and motor axons, since uptake and transneuronal transmission to the CNS occur exclusively via the motor route, while sensory and autonomic endings are not infected. Infection of sensory and autonomic ganglia requires longer incubation times, as it reflects centrifugal propagation from the CNS to the periphery, via polysynaptic connections from sensory and autonomic neurons to the initially infected motoneurons. Virus is recovered from end organs only after the development of rabies because anterograde spread to end organs is likely mediated by passive diffusion, rather than active transport mechanisms.

I. INTRODUCTION

A landmark event in systems neuroscience has been the development of transneuronal tracers, that is, markers that allow for the identification of the chains of synaptically connected neurons (first-order neurons, second-order, third-order, etc.) that innervate a given organ and mediate a specific behavior (Kuypers and Ugolini, 1990; Morecraft *et al.*, 2009; Ugolini,

1995a, 2010). In order to be effective as transneuronal tracers, such markers should meet several requirements. First, they should propagate *exclusively* by transneuronal transfer between connected neurons (and *not* by cell-to-cell spread among neurons that are not synaptically connected). Second, transneuronal transfer should ideally be unidirectional, to permit unequivocal interpretations. Third, the number of synaptic steps should be easily identifiable. Fourth, the marker should allow for the visualization of *all* groups of neurons that innervate the injection site directly (first-order neurons) and indirectly (second-order neurons, third-order, fourth-order, etc.), in order to permit a comprehensive mapping of the entire connectivity. Fifth, transneuronal labeling should be easily detectable and should not disappear with time. Sixth, the marker should not substantially alter neuronal metabolism, to allow for neurotransmitter and functional studies of the identified neuronal networks.

The first transneuronal tracing methods were based on the use of conventional tracers, and their transfer occurred only when first-order neurons were filled with great quantities of the tracer. Because only a small amount of the tracers crossed synapses, transneuronal labeling was very weak and could be detected, at best, only in some second-order neurons; third-order neurons could not be visualized (Fig. 1A; reviewed by Kuypers and Ugolini, 1990; Morecraft *et al.*, 2009; Ugolini, 1995a, 2010).

Sensitive transneuronal tracing technologies are based on the use of neurotropic viruses as markers (Kuypers and Ugolini, 1990; Loewy, 1995; Ugolini, 1995a, 1996, 2010). They exploit the capacity of some viruses to travel across neuronal pathways, demonstrated by classical studies (e.g., Dietzschold *et al.*, 1985; Dolivo, 1980; Goodpasture and Teague, 1923; Kristensson *et al.*, 1971, 1974, 1982; Kucera *et al.*, 1985; Martin and Dolivo, 1983; Sabin, 1938; Tsiang, 1979). Their superior sensitivity is due to the ability of viruses to function as self-amplifying markers by replicating in recipient neurons, thus overcoming the "dilution" problem of conventional tracers and producing intense transneuronal labeling, as detected immunohistochemically (Kuypers and Ugolini, 1990; Ugolini, 2010; Fig. 1B–D).

There are two main classes of viral transneuronal tracers, derived from alpha-herpesviruses (herpes simplex virus type 1, HSV 1, and pseudorabies, PrV; see Aston-Jones and Card, 2000; Kuypers and Ugolini, 1990; Loewy, 1995; Ugolini, 1995a, 1996, 2010) and a rhabdovirus, that is, rabies virus (the "fixed" CVS-11 strain; Graf *et al.*, 2002; Kelly and Strick, 2000; Morcuende *et al.*, 2002; Prevosto *et al.*, 2009, 2010; Tang *et al.*, 1999; Ugolini, 1995b, 2008, 2010; Ugolini *et al.*, 2006; Figs. 1B, C and 2). These two classes of viral tracers have very different properties (see Section II). Importantly, only rabies virus (Ugolini, 1995b) is completely reliable as transneuronal

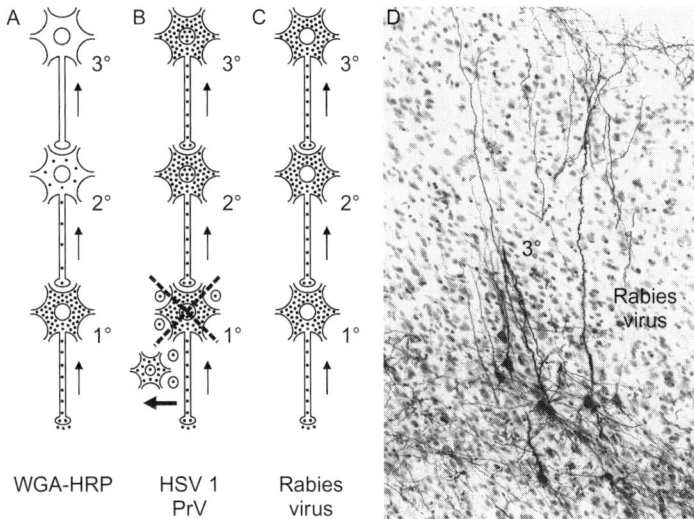

FIGURE 1 Differences in transneuronal labeling obtained with conventional tracers (e.g., wheat germ agglutinin-horseradish peroxidase, WGA-HRP) (A) and neurotropic viruses, that is, alpha-herpesviruses (herpes simplex virus type 1, HSV 1; pseudorabies virus, PrV) (B) and rabies virus (C). With conventional tracers (A), only a small amount of the marker is transferred from first-order neurons (1°) to second-order neurons (2°), resulting in weak transneuronal labeling; third-order neurons (3°) cannot be visualized. Viruses function as self-amplifying markers (B, C): transfer to second-order neurons (2°) is followed by viral replication, resulting in intense transneuronal labeling (2° and 3°; see example in (D)). Alpha-herpesviruses (B) induce neuronal degeneration (X on 1°) and can also propagate nonspecifically, via cell-to-cell spread, to local glial cells and neurons (gray horizontal arrow in (B)); spurious spread of alpha-herpesviruses is dose- and time dependent. In contrast, rabies virus (C) propagates exclusively via retrograde transneuronal transfer, regardless of the dose and postinoculation time. (D) Example of retrograde transneuronal labeling of third-order neurons (3°) with rabies virus (CVS-11 strain) in the cerebral cortex of macaque monkeys. Rabies virus immunohistochemical visualization (immunoperoxidase) is combined with cresyl violet counterstaining of the tissue. Panels (A)–(C) are modified from Ugolini (2010) with permission.

tracer because it propagates *exclusively* by strictly unidirectional (retrograde) transneuronal transfer and allows for the stepwise identification of neuronal networks across a virtually unlimited number of synapses (Fig. 1).

The purpose of this chapter is to highlight the specific properties of rabies virus as a transneuronal tracer, which have been identified by studying viral propagation within the central nervous system (CNS) during the preclinical period in primate and rodent models of known connectivity. The experimental findings have valuable implications for the understanding of rabies pathogenesis, which will be discussed.

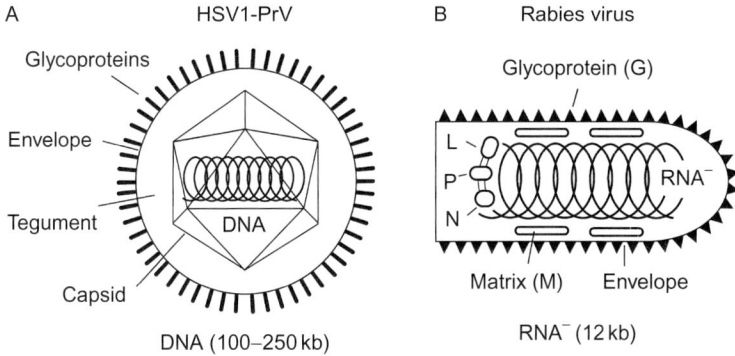

FIGURE 2   Representation of the virion of alpha-herpesviruses (herpes simplex virus type 1, HSV 1, and pseudorabies, PrV) (A) and rabies virus (B). Modified from Ugolini (2010) with permission. (A) The genome of alpha-herpesviruses (linear double-stranded DNA, 100–250 kbp, encoding more than 30 proteins) is enclosed in an icosahedral capsid, overlaid by a tegument and surrounded by a lipid envelope, on which are anchored more than a dozen types of glycoproteins. (B) Rabies virus particles: the virion comprises a central core, containing single-strand, negative sense RNA (less than 12 kb) encapsidated with the nucleoprotein (N), an RNA polymerase (L), and a polymerase cofactor phosphorylated protein (P). The inner core is associated with the matrix protein (M) and is surrounded by a lipid envelope, on which is anchored the glycoprotein (G), which protrudes in trimeric spikes and mediates attachment to cellular receptors.

II. DIFFERENCES IN PROPERTIES OF ALPHA-HERPESVIRUSES AND RABIES VIRUS AS TRANSNEURONAL TRACERS

There are major differences in the properties of alpha-herpesviruses and rabies virus, which make them suitable for different purposes. The first important difference is in their *peripheral uptake*: alpha-herpesviruses can infect *all* categories of neurons that innervate a peripheral site (e.g., a muscle), that is, primary sensory neurons, motoneurons, sympathetic, and parasympathetic neurons (e.g., Goodpasture and Teague, 1923; Kristensson *et al.*, 1982; Kuypers and Ugolini, 1990; Martin and Dolivo, 1983; Sabin, 1938), although not to the same extent. Importantly, alpha-herpesviruses propagate more efficiently in sensory (especially nociceptive) and autonomic pathways than motor pathways (Rotto-Percelay *et al.*, 1992, Ugolini, 1992; Fig. 3). Because of this property, they are especially suitable for studying sensory and autonomic innervation (e.g., Jansen *et al.*, 1995; Standish *et al.*, 1994; Strack and Loewy, 1990) and are the only transneuronal tracers available for these purposes (Loewy, 1995; Ugolini, 1995a, 2010). In contrast, rabies virus, after intramuscular inoculations, is internalized exclusively at motor endplates and propagates to the CNS exclusively from motoneurons (Fig. 4), which makes this virus

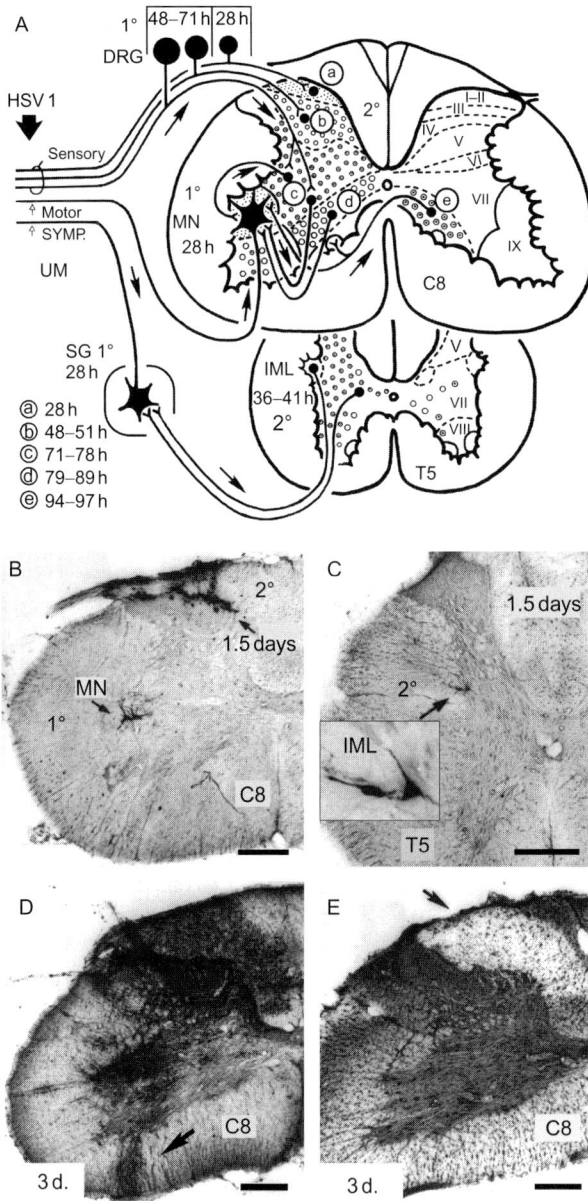

FIGURE 3 (A) Summary of the kinetics of transneuronal transfer of herpes simplex virus type 1 (HSV 1) from mixed limb nerves (ulnar and median, UM) to the spinal cord in rats. Modified from Ugolini (1992) with permission. HSV 1 propagates via the sensory, sympathetic, and motor routes, but not with the same efficiency. Anterograde transneuronal transfer from small (nociceptive) primary sensory afferents to the dorsal horn (2°, a) occurs in less than 1.5 days postinoculation, in synchrony with retrograde transneuronal

the ideal transneuronal tracing tool for studying motor innervation (Graf *et al.*, 2002; Morcuende *et al.*, 2002; Rathelot and Strick, 2006, 2009; Tang *et al.*, 1999; Ugolini, 2010; Ugolini *et al.*, 2006; see Section III.G).

Major pitfalls of alpha-herpesviruses as transneuronal tracers include that they rapidly induce neuronal degeneration and a prominent inflammatory response, leading to focal neurological symptoms and encephalitis (Rinaman *et al.*, 1993; Ugolini, 1992; Ugolini *et al.*, 1987). They can also propagate via cell-to-cell spread between neurons that are not synaptically connected, which is a source of false-positive results when studying connectivity (Loewy, 1995; Ugolini, 1992, 1995a, 2010; Ugolini *et al.*, 1987). Neuronal degeneration and inflammatory response are unavoidable because the replication strategy of alpha-herpesviruses involves host shutoff mechanisms (Laurent *et al.*, 1998; Smith *et al.*, 2005). Moreover, some viral glycoproteins (gB, gD, gH, gL) that are essential for entry and/or transneuronal propagation also play a key role in triggering the innate and adaptive immune response of the host (Morrison, 2004; Reske *et al.*, 2007; Ugolini, 2010). Spurious cell-to-cell spread of alpha-herpesviruses is dependent upon the virus strain, the dose, and the postinoculation time and can be minimized, but not completely abolished, by manipulating these experimental parameters; however, the extent of transneuronal transfer is also reduced (Ugolini, 1995a, 1996, 2010). Typically, the conditions necessary to minimize local spread (use of attenuated strains and injection of low doses, in combination with short time points) do not make it possible to trace further than second-order neurons; higher doses and longer time points, that allow for tracing higher-order neurons, can cause spurious labeling (Loewy, 1995; Ugolini, 1995a, 1996, 2010; Figs. 1B and 3). Another potential difficulty is the bidirectional transfer

---

transfer in autonomic pathways (from the stellate ganglion, SG, 1°, to the intermediolateral cell group; IML, 2°). Anterograde transneuronal transfer from primary sensory afferents of larger caliber, as well as retrograde transneuronal transfer from motoneurons (MN) to the spinal intermediate zone (b, c, d, e), requires longer time points. DRG: dorsal root ganglia. Roman numerals: spinal laminae. (B) HSV 1 immunolabeling in the C8 segment at 1.5 days, showing retrogradely labeled MN (1°) and anterograde transneuronal labeling in superficial sensory laminae of the dorsal horn (2°) and in the dorsal funiculus (glial cells surrounding infected sensory fibers). (C) T5 segment at 1.5 days, showing retrograde transneuronal labeling of sympathetic preganglionic neurons (IML, enlarged in the inset). (D and E) HSV 1 immunolabeling (D) and cresyl violet counterstaining (E) of neighboring sections at C8 at 3 days. Note the loss of Nissl staining of infected glial cells around sensory afferents in the dorsal funiculus (arrow in (E)), and spurious labeling within the ventral roots (arrow in (D)) around the axons of retrogradely infected MN. Spurious spread in the spinal cord at 3 days precedes retrograde transneuronal labeling of supraspinal pathways (that occurs from 3.5 days onward). HSV 1 detection: immunoperoxidase. Bars = 300 μm.

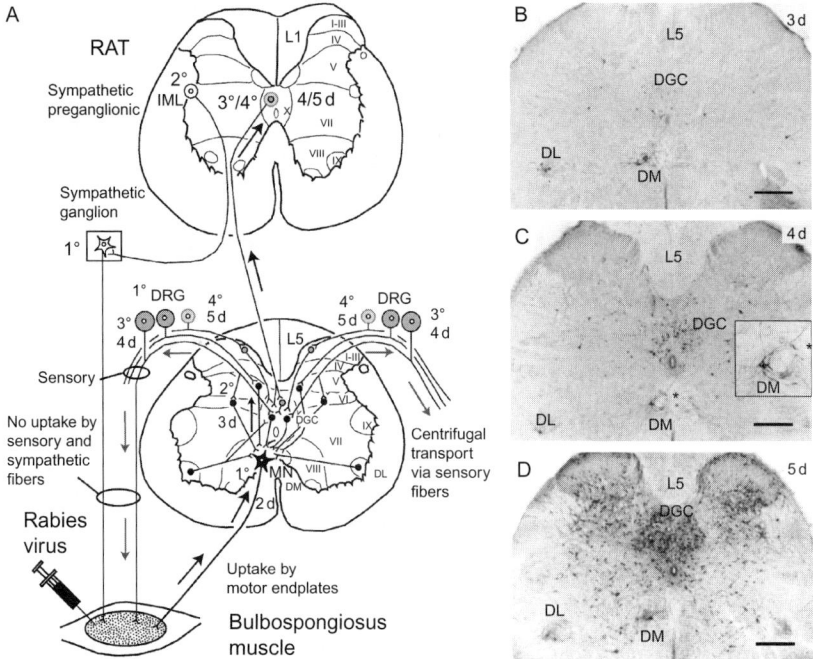

FIGURE 4 (A) Kinetics of propagation of rabies virus (CVS-11 strain) to the spinal cord after inoculation into the left bulbospongiosus (BS) muscle in rats. Modified from Tang *et al.* (1999) and Ugolini (2008) with permission. (B–D) Photomicrograph of rabies virus-immunolabeled neurons (peroxidase antiperoxidase method) in the L5 spinal segment at 3, 4, and 5 days (d) postinoculation (p.i.). Left: ipsilateral side. (A) The BS muscle is innervated by motoneurons (MNs) in the ipsilateral dorsomedian (DM) nucleus, primary sensory neurons in the ipsilateral dorsal root ganglia (DRG) at L5-S1, and neurons in sympathetic ganglia, which receive input from pregaglionic neurons in the intermediolateral cell group (IML) of upper lumbar and lower thoracic spinal segments. Uptake of rabies virus involves only BS MNs (2 days p.i., black). At all time points, infected MNs show normal size and morphology (see inset in (C)). Although they are linked by gap junctions, infected MNs do not become more numerous with time (B–D), showing that rabies virus does not propagate via gap junctions. From BS MNs, rabies virus propagates by retrograde transneuronal transfer at chemical synapses to second-order neurons (see (A), 2°, black; e.g., in dorsal gray commissure, DGC, and dorsolateral nucleus, DL) at 3 days. Higher-order neurons (3°, dark gray; 4°, light gray) are infected at 4 and 5 days p.i., respectively. The bilateral infection of the DRG obtained at 4 and 5 days (A) reflects transneuronal transfer, showing that centrifugal migration to sensory ganglia can already occur during the preclinical period of rabies. Likewise, sympathetic preganglionic populations in the central autonomic area (in lamina X at L1, see (A)), which do not supply the BS muscle, are infected by retrograde transneuronal transfer from BS MNs from 4 days onward. I–X: spinal laminae. Scale bars: 900 μm.

of alpha-herpesviruses (e.g., Aston-Jones and Card, 2000; Ugolini, 1992; see Fig. 3). Only a few strains containing specific mutations have been identified that exhibit unidirectional transfer, mainly in the anterograde direction (the H129 strain of HSV 1) or in the retrograde direction (Bartha PrV and the McIntyre-B HSV 1 strain; see Ugolini, 2010). Finally, due to the restricted host range of alpha-herpesviruses, transneuronal tracing studies can be performed only in a limited number of mammalian species; for example, nonhuman primates are not infected after peripheral inoculations of alpha-herpesviruses (Ugolini, 1995a; 2010).

There are no such drawbacks when using rabies virus as transneuronal tracer because this virus propagates exclusively between connected neurons without inducing spurious spread regardless of the dose and time postinoculation (Figs. 1C, 4, and 5; Clower et al., 2005; Graf et al., 2002; Grantyn et al., 2002; Kelly and Strick, 2003, 2004; Morcuende et al., 2002; Moschovakis et al., 2004; Prevosto et al., 2009, 2010; Tang et al., 1999; Ugolini, 1995b; Ugolini et al., 2006; see Ugolini, 2010). Other major advantages are the fact that axonal transport and transneuronal transfer of rabies virus are strictly unidirectional (retrograde), and neuronal metabolism is not substantially altered for a long time, allowing for the identification of neuronal networks across a virtually unlimited number of synapses (Figs. 1C, 4, and 5; see Section III). Because of the wide host range of rabies virus, transneuronal tracing studies can be performed in all mammals, including primates, after intramuscular and CNS injections (e.g., Grantyn et al., 2002; Kelly and Strick, 2003, 2004; Moschovakis et al., 2004; Prevosto et al., 2009, 2010; Rathelot and Strick, 2006, 2009; Ugolini et al., 2006). Compared with alpha-herpesviruses, another major difference is the long asymptomatic (incubation) period of rabies (usually between 3 weeks and 3 months for human rabies; Jackson, 2002; Plotkin, 2000). With the "fixed" rabies virus strains that are used for transneuronal tracing, depending on the dose and the site of inoculation, the preclinical period is usually 1 week or more, during which the virus can cross at least seven synapses. Because seven synaptic steps are far more than necessary for transneuronal tracing purposes, the absence of any signs of disease for the entire duration of the experiments is a truly important feature of the rabies transneuronal tracing methodology from an ethical viewpoint.

III. RABIES VIRUS

A. Structure of rabies virus

Rabies virus is a single-strand negative RNA virus, from the genus *Lyssavirus* (from *lyssa*, the Greek word for frenzy) of the Rhabdoviruses family (from the Greek *rhabdos*, i.e., "rod" because of its characteristic bullet

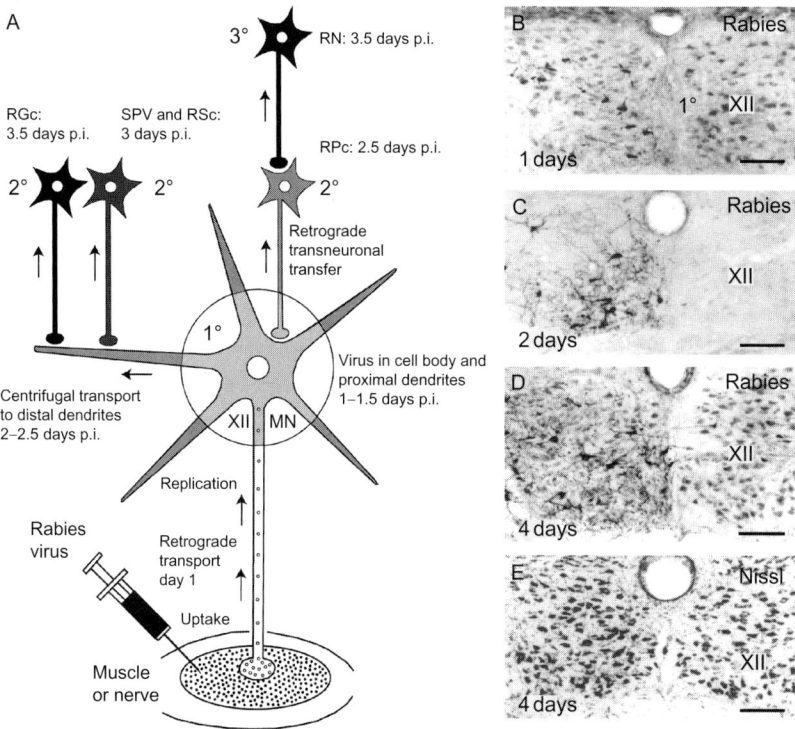

FIGURE 5 Intracellular transport and retrograde transneuronal transfer of rabies virus after inoculation into a muscle or nerve: hypoglossal (XII) model. Modified from Ugolini (2008) (A) and Ugolini (1995b) (B–E) with permission. (A) Uptake at motor endplates or axons is followed by retrograde axonal transport (day 1 postinoculation, p.i.) to first-order neurons (1°, XII motoneurons, MNs), where viral replication occurs. Rabies virus is initially restricted to the cell body and proximal dendrites (light gray, 1–1.5 days p.i.), and is later transported intracellularly to distal dendrites (dark gray, 2–2.5 days p.i.), but not to axons. As a result, transneuronal transfer occurs only in the retrograde direction, that is, from first-order neurons (1°) to presynaptic terminals of second-order neurons (2°). After retrograde axonal transport and replication in 2°, the virus infects third-order neurons (3°). Retrograde transneuronal transfer is time dependent. Different groups of second-order neurons are infected at the same time, regardless of their distance from first-order neurons. The only factor that may sporadically cause asynchronous infection, as illustrated here, is the location of terminals on the neuronal surface: a few neuronal projections targeting exclusively the cell body and proximal dendrites might be infected earlier than projections targeting exclusively distal dendrites. This is due to the fact that viral replication and release from cell bodies precedes centrifugal intracellular transport to distal dendrites. Note, however, that asynchronous visualization of different second-order populations, as illustrated here, has been obtained only when using a rabies virus immunolabeling method that was not very sensitive (see Ugolini, 2010). (B–E) Kinetics of infection of XII MN: at 1 day, labeling is restricted to cell bodies and proximal dendrites (B), and extends to distal dendrites at 2 days (C). Note that even at 4 days, infected MNs show normal size and morphology (D) and normal Nissl staining (E, cresyl violet). Other abbreviations: RGc, nucleus (n.) reticularis gigantocellularis; RPc, n. reticularis parvocellularis; RSc, n. reticularis subcoeruleus; RN, red nucleus; SPV, spinal trigeminal nucleus. Scale bars in (B–E): 150 μm.

shape; Fig. 2B). The viral genome (less than 12 kb) encodes only five proteins: a nucleoprotein (N), an RNA-dependent RNA polymerase (L), a polymerase cofactor phosphorylated protein (the phosphoprotein P), a matrix protein (M), and a single external glycoprotein (G; Dietzschold *et al.*, 2005; Finke and Conzelmann, 2005; Schnell *et al.*, 2010). Rabies virus particles comprise a central core, containing helical RNA and the N, L, and P proteins, that is associated with M protein and surrounded by a lipid envelope, on which is anchored the glycoprotein, which is arranged in trimeric spikes (Fig. 2B; Gaudin *et al.*, 1992; Schnell *et al.*, 2010; Wunner, 2002).

It has been demonstrated that the glycoprotein has a pivotal role in neuroinvasiveness, as its point mutation at position 333 (Coulon *et al.*, 1983; Dietzschold *et al.*, 1983) completely abolishes virulence (Coulon *et al.*, 1989; Dietzschold *et al.*, 1985; Kucera *et al.*, 1985; Lafay *et al.*, 1991) and its gene deletion (Mebatsion *et al.*, 1996a) eliminates transneuronal propagation (Etessami *et al.*, 2000). Moreover, in avirulent strains, neuroinvasiveness is restored by genetic replacement or transcomplementation with the glycoprotein derived from virulent strains (see Dietzschold *et al.*, 2005, 2008; Finke and Conzelmann, 2005). In addition to binding with neuronal receptors, the rabies virus glycoprotein promotes virus and cell membrane fusion (Gaudin, 2000) and confers intracellular transport properties to the internalized virions (see Finke and Conzelmann, 2005; Schnell *et al.*, 2010; Section III.C).

B. Differences among rabies virus strains

There are two types of rabies virus strains: "street" and "fixed" ones. "Street" strains are natural (wild-type) isolates; their properties can be highly variable. "Fixed" strains have been adapted from street strains by repeated passages in mice brains and cell culture, resulting in the selection of strains with stable properties (Wunner and Dietzschold, 1987). Only "fixed" strains are used for transneuronal tracing studies. They are 100–10,000 times less infectious than "street" strains (Dietzschold *et al.*, 2005), in part because they do not replicate in the muscle (Shankar *et al.*, 1991; Ugolini *et al.*, 2006), unlike "street" strains (Charlton and Casey, 1979; Murphy and Bauer, 1974; see also Section III.H). A prototype of fixed strains is the challenge virus standard (CVS) strain (Sacramento *et al.*, 1992). There are several CVS subtypes that differ in their passage history, such as CVS-11, usually grown in baby hamster kidney cells (BHK-21; Seif *et al.*, 1985; Ugolini, 1995b), and the B2c and N2c variants of CVS-24, that were selected by passage in BHK-21 (B2c) or mouse brain and neuroblastoma cells (N2c; Morimoto *et al.*, 1998, 1999).

The properties of rabies virus, reviewed here, refer to the CVS-11 subtype, that is, the "fixed" strain of which the transneuronal propagation has been most thoroughly evaluated (e.g., Akkal *et al.*, 2007; Clower *et al.*, 2005; Graf *et al.*, 2002; Grantyn *et al.*, 2002; Kelly and Strick, 2003, 2004; Morcuende *et al.*, 2002; Moschovakis *et al.*, 2004; Prevosto *et al.*, 2009, 2010; Tang *et al.*, 1999; Ugolini, 1995b; Ugolini *et al.*, 2006). Theoretically, the properties of CVS-11 should not be generalized to all "fixed" strains, as different CVS subtypes, or even variants of the same subtype, can substantially differ in properties (see Morimoto *et al.*, 1998, 1999, for B2c and N2c). Available studies on the transneuronal propagation of the CVS-24 N2c variant suggest unidirectional transport properties as CVS-11 but a higher transfer rate (Hoshi *et al.*, 2005; Kelly and Strick, 2000; but see Rathelot and Strick, 2006, 2009) and also a large variability of the rate of transfer following intramuscular inoculation of different batches of N2c of the same titer (Rathelot and Strick, 2009) that are not observed using CVS-11 (e.g., Moschovakis *et al.*, 2004; Ugolini *et al.*, 2006). To understand whether such differences may be dependent upon intrinsic characteristics of the N2c variant or other experimental parameters, it would be necessary to compare the behavior of N2c and CVS-11 in the same model. The CVS-11 used in our laboratory (Ugolini, 1995b; Ugolini *et al.*, 2006), and other European institutions (e.g., Salin *et al.*, 2008), was originally obtained from P. Atanasiu (Institut Pasteur, FR; Seif *et al.*, 1985). Its glycoprotein sequence (accession no. 1106215A; Seif *et al.*, 1985) shows a difference of 14 AA compared with CVS-11 from the Center for Disease Control and Prevention in Atlanta (accession no. AAC34683; Smith *et al.*, 1973), 11 AA difference with CVS-24 N2c (accession no. AAB97690), and 3 AA with CVS-24 B2c (accession no. AAB97691) from Philadelphia (Morimoto *et al.*, 1998, 1999). Thus, at least with regard to the glycoprotein sequence, the "French" CVS-11 seems closer to CVS-24 B2c than to CVS-24 N2c or to the "American" CVS-11 (see Sacramento *et al.*, 1992, for discrepancies in the recorded lineage of rabies virus strains).

C. Intracellular cycle of rabies virus and unidirectional transport properties

At the site of inoculation, rabies virus is internalized by terminals and transported by fast retrograde axonal transport to the cell bodies of first-order neurons, where a first cycle of transcription and replication begins (Ugolini, 1995b; Fig. 5). Rabies immunolabeling is initially detected only in neuronal cell bodies; later, it extends to dendrites, but not to axons (Ugolini, 1995b; Fig. 5). Because centrifugal intracellular transport is directed exclusively to dendrites, transneuronal transfer occurs *only* in the *retrograde* direction, from neuronal cell bodies and dendrites to presynaptic terminals. From such terminals, virus particles are transported back to the cell body of higher-order neurons, where the next transcription and replication cycle begins (Ugolini, 1995b; Fig. 5). Successive cycles of retrograde axonal transport, transcription, and replication allow for the stepwise retrograde transneuronal infection of synaptically connected neurons of progressively higher order (Fig. 5). The interval required for visualization of each synaptic step mostly depends upon the time devoted to viral replication, as retrograde axonal transport occurs at high speed *in vivo*: different groups of second-order neurons located at various distances from first-order neurons (e.g., 10 μm to 2 cm) are infected at the same time (Graf *et al.*, 2002; Morcuende *et al.*, 2002; Tang *et al.*, 1999; Ugolini, 2008, 2010; Ugolini *et al.*, 2006). *In vitro*, the estimated transport speed is 50–100 mm/day in human dorsal root ganglia (Tsiang *et al.*, 1991), 12–24 mm/day in rat dorsal root ganglia (Lycke and Tsiang, 1987), and slightly more than 8 mm/day in murine neuroblastoma cells (Klingen *et al.*, 2008).

Intracellular transport of rabies virus has also been visualized by live tracking of recombinant virus expressing fluorescent markers in neuroblastoma cells (Klingen *et al.*, 2008); this elegant study showed that retrograde axonal transport of rabies virus involves transport vesicles, in which enveloped virus particles are carried as a cargo; it also confirmed that intracellular anterograde transport is inefficient (Klingen *et al.*, 2008).

Remarkably, *in vivo*, transneuronal transfer of rabies virus is strictly unidirectional also after intracortical injections, despite the fact that such injections provide equal possibilities of axonal transport in the anterograde and retrograde directions (in fact, after such injections, most conventional tracers are transported bidirectionally; Fig. 6). With rabies virus, when retrograde transneuronal transfer has already progressed to third-order neurons providing polysynaptic inputs to the injected cortical area, there is still no evidence of anterograde transneuronal transfer to second-order targets (e.g., recipient regions of the pontine nuclei or basal ganglia; Kelly and Strick, 2003; Prevosto *et al.*, 2009, 2010; see Fig. 6B). The strictly unidirectional transfer of rabies virus is a major advantage, as it enables unequivocal identification of the polysynaptic inputs to the injected CNS or peripheral site of inoculation.

Axonal transport of rabies virus is blocked by colchicine and other substances that disrupt microtubules function (Ceccaldi *et al.*, 1989; Lycke and Tsiang, 1987). Both anterograde and retrograde axonal transport are microtubule dependent but mediated by different molecular motors, that is, kinesins and dynein, respectively (Hirokawa and Takemura, 2005). The exclusively retrograde direction and high speed of intracellular transport of rabies virus can only be explained by active, dynein-dependent mechanisms. The rabies virus glycoprotein is clearly involved, as it confers retrograde axonal transport properties to pseudotyped lentiviruses vectors (Finke and Conzelmann, 2005; Mazarakis *et al.*, 2001). A role in axonal transport has been postulated also for the viral phosphoprotein, because of its strong interactions with the dynein light chain LC8

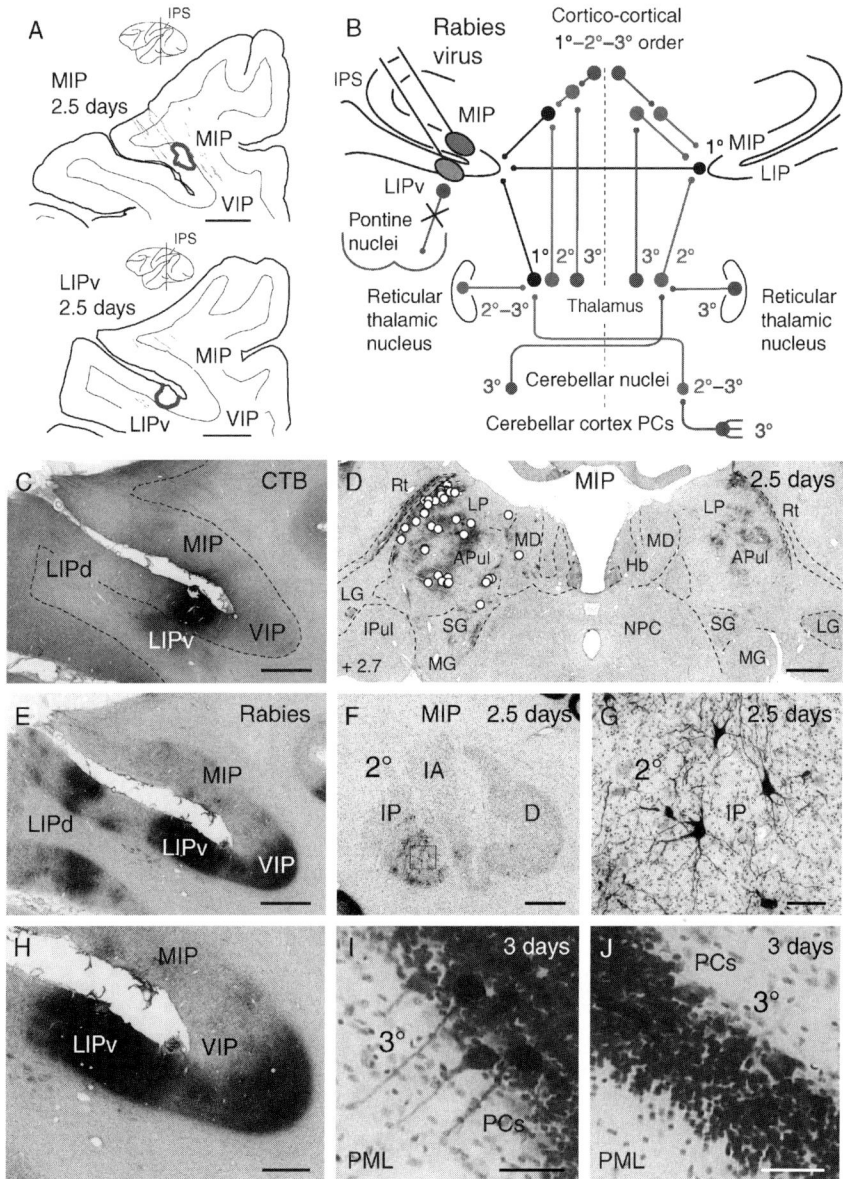

FIGURE 6 Transneuronal transfer of rabies virus after intracortical injections of a mixture of rabies virus and the conventional tracer Cholera Toxin B (CTB) fragment in primates. Modified from Prevosto *et al.* (2010) with permission. (A) Coronal sections showing the center of the injection area (red outlines) into the left medial intraparietal area (MIP) or the ventral lateral intraparietal area (LIPv) of the intraparietal sulcus (IPS), visualized by Cholera toxin B (CTB) immunolabeling at 2.5 days after injection of the rabies virus/CTB mixture. (B) Summary of the pathways of transneuronal transfer of

(Jacob *et al.*, 2000; Raux *et al.*, 2000). However, this would require virus uncoating to occur prior to transport, which has not been demonstrated (Finke and Conzelmann, 2005; Schnell *et al.*, 2010); moreover, deletion of the LC8-binding site in the phosphoprotein does not affect transport of rabies virus (Mebatsion, 2001) but alters its transcription (Tan *et al.*, 2007).

---

rabies virus to the cerebellum after injection of rabies virus/CTB into cortical areas MIP or LIPv: 1° (black), first-order neurons (visualized by the conventional tracer, CTB) in the ipsilateral (left) thalamus (white dots in (D)) and in cortical areas. 2° (blue), second-order neurons infected by retrograde transneuronal transfer of rabies virus at 2.5 days in the contralateral cerebellar nuclei, in the ipsilateral thalamic nuclei and reticular thalamic nucleus, and in the contralateral thalamic nuclei (the latter reflecting projections to IPS areas of the right hemisphere). 3° (red), third-order neurons labeled at 3 days in the contralateral cerebellar cortex (Purkinje cells, PCs) and contralateral reticular thalamic nucleus. Note that anterograde transneuronal transfer (e.g., to the pontine nuclei) did not occur (X, violet). (C, E, H) Photomicrographs of adjoining sections at the LIPv injection site, immunolabeled for CTB (C) and rabies virus (E, H) at 2.5 days postinoculation. The injection area is easily identifiable with CTB (C) but not with rabies virus ((E), enlarged in (H)), because transneuronal transfer of rabies virus produces intense labeling of short-distance projection neurons in neighboring portions of the sulcus (e.g., in dorsal LIP, LIPd, and ventral intraparietal area, VIP). Note (in (E) and (H)) the absence of degeneration at the cortical (LIPv) site of inoculation and the lack of involvement of the white matter. (D) Example of rabies immunolabeling in the caudal thalamus at 2.5 days after injection of the rabies virus/CTB mixture into MIP. Left side is ipsilateral; number on the lower left corner indicates the rostrocaudal distance from the interaural axis. White dots: first-order neurons (CTB) in the thalamus (here in lateralis posterior, LP, anterior pulvinar, APul, and medial dorsal, MD, nuclei; for labeling found at other thalamic levels, see Prevosto *et al.*, 2010). Brown: rabies virus retrograde transneuronal labeling. In this model, labeling in the thalamus provides an internal control for the number of synapses crossed by the rabies virus tracer: note that at this time point (2.5 days), transfer involves second-order neurons (2°: ipsilateral reticular thalamic nucleus, Rt left, and contralateral thalamic nuclei) and not third-order neurons (3°: contralateral Rt); the latter are infected at 3 days (see summary diagram in (B)). Other abbreviations: IPul, inferior pulvinar; LG, lateral geniculate; MG, medial geniculate; NPC, nucleus of the posterior commissure; SG, suprageniculate. (F and G) Examples of rabies immunolabeled second-order neurons (2°) in the contralateral (right) cerebellar nuclei (MIP, 2.5 days): infected cells are found in the dentate nucleus (D) and in the ventrolateral portion of the interpositus posterior nucleus (IP); boxed area in (F) is enlarged in (G). (I–J) Examples of third-order (3°) labeling of PCs in the cerebellar cortex (paramedian lobule, PML) at 3 days (MIP; see also summary figure in (B)). Detection of rabies virus (in (D)–(J)) was based on a sensitive immunoperoxidase protocol and combined with cresyl violet counterstaining of the same section. The results illustrate the power of the rabies transneuronal tracing technology in providing a time-dependent visualization of entire functional neuronal circuits (here, the cerebellar cortical and nuclear modules to MIP implicated in adaptive control of visual and proprioceptive guidance of reaching, arm/ eye/head coordination, and prism adaptation; see Prevosto *et al.*, 2010). Scale bar = C, D, E: 2000 μm; F, H: 1000 μm; G: 100 μm; I, J: 50 μm. (See Page 8 in Color Section at the back of the book.)

D. Rabies virus replication does not cause cell damage

With street rabies virus, cytopathic changes are negligible even at the time of death (see Jackson, 2002; Juntrakul *et al.*, 2005). Similarly, with the virulent "fixed" strains of rabies virus that are used for transneuronal tracing, neurons that have been infected for several days maintain normal size and Nissl staining pattern (Tang *et al.*, 1999; Ugolini, 1995b; Fig. 5B–E). They also remain metabolically viable, as they can still express their neurotransmitters (Fig. 7K and L) and cotransport other tracers (Fig. 6; Graf *et al.*, 2002; Miyachi *et al.*, 2006; Morcuende *et al.*, 2002; Prevosto *et al.*, 2010; Salin *et al.*, 2009; Tang *et al.*, 1999; Ugolini *et al.*, 2006; see Ugolini, 2010 and Section III.E.3). This is due to the fact that rabies virus has developed a multilevel strategy to prevent neuronal impairment. First, its replication does not involve host shutoff mechanisms (Conzelmann, 2005); during the preclinical period, host cell gene expression is downregulated, with a major upregulation occurring only at long time points (6–7 days in mice) and coinciding with the onset of clinical disease (Prosniak *et al.*, 2001, 2003). Second, pathogenicity of rabies virus strains is inversely correlated with their ability to induce apoptosis (programmed cell death) and with the level of glycoprotein expression (Morimoto *et al.*, 1999); virulent strains of rabies virus prevent apoptosis by keeping viral gene expression beyond threshold levels and by interfering with proapoptotic factors (Finke and Conzelmann, 2005; Morimoto *et al.*, 1999; Schnell *et al.*, 2010). Rabies virus has also immunoevasive strategies that involve blocking cellular interferon signaling (Brzózka *et al.*, 2005, 2006; Conzelmann, 2005; Schnell *et al.*, 2010; Vidy *et al.*, 2007) and inactivating "protective" T lymphocytes via overexpression of immunosubversive molecules (Baloul and Lafon, 2003; Baloul *et al.*, 2004; Lafon, 2008).

E. Rabies transneuronal tracing: Methodological aspects

1. Identification of the order of connections and influence of the initial viral load on the speed of transneuronal progression of rabies virus within the CNS

As for the other viral tracers, studying the kinetics of transfer of rabies virus at different time points after the inoculations is of paramount importance for identifying the order of connections. In each model, it is also important to verify the synaptic order based on internal controls (i.e., presence or absence of labeling in known pathways; Ugolini, 2010; see, e.g., Fig. 6B and D). Following peripheral or CNS inoculations, infection of first-order neurons usually requires up to 2 days (because viral uptake is not efficient), whereas each subsequent step of transneuronal transfer to higher-order neurons (second-order, third-order, etc.) occurs much more rapidly, at regular intervals of 12 h or more depending on the initial viral load, the

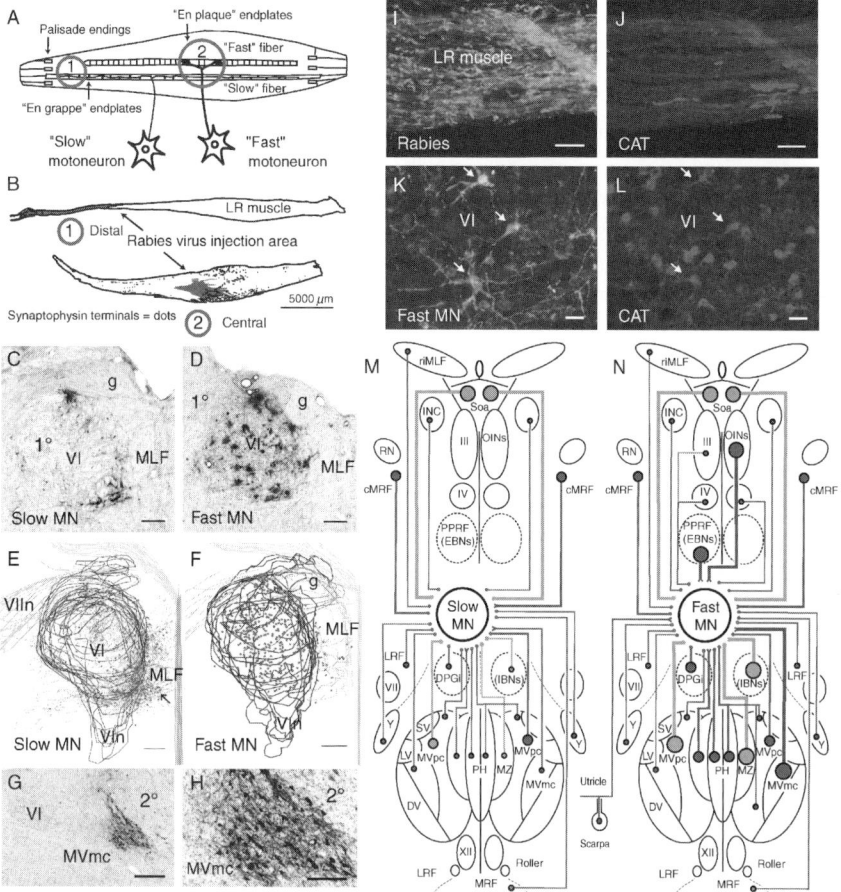

FIGURE 7 Retrograde transneuronal transfer of rabies virus from the left lateral rectus (LR) muscle in primates. Modified from Ugolini *et al.* (2006) with permission. (A and B) Differences in uptake by "slow" and "fast" motoneurons (MNs) after injection of rabies virus into the distal (1) and central (2) parts of the muscle. (A) Distal intramuscular injections (1) involve selectively "en grappe" endplates of "slow" MN, supplying slow muscle fibers. Only injections into the center of the muscle belly (2) involve "en plaque" motor endplates of "fast" MN. (B) Extent of the rabies virus injection site (red) in the muscle, visualized by rabies immunolabeling at 2.5 days (see example in (I)). Note the lack of spread of the infection within the muscle. Black dots: synaptophysin-positive terminals. (C–F) Differences in topography of "slow" (C and E) and "fast" (D and F) MNs (first-order, 1°), illustrated by cross sections (C and D) and three-dimensional reconstructions (E and F) of the abducens (VI) nucleus (dark blue outlines: VI nucleus and emerging roots of the VI nerve). Large red dots: MN cell bodies; small dots in (E): MN dendrites. Light blue outlines on the left in (E) and (F): descending limb of the facial nerve (VIIn). Green outlines in (F): genu (g) and ascending limb of VIIn. Gray vertical lines: midline. Yellow outlines: brainstem dorsal surface. MLF: medial longitudinal fasciculus. (G and H) Examples of second-order neurons (2°) in the contralateral medial vestibular nucleus,

model, and the sensitivity of the rabies immunodetection method (Graf
et al., 2002; Grantyn et al., 2002; Kelly and Strick, 2003, 2004; Morcuende
et al., 2002; Moschovakis et al., 2004; Rathelot and Strick, 2006; Tang et al.,
1999; Ugolini, 1995b; Ugolini et al., 2006; see Ugolini, 2010; Figs. 5–8).

It is important to keep constant the injected amount and concentration
of rabies virus in a series of experiments because the interval required for
visualizing each step of transfer is influenced by the *dose* of the inoculum.
In primates, for example, after inoculation of a constant dose (2 µl intra-
cortically or 110 µl intramuscularly) of CVS-11 at high concentrations (titer
at or above 10^{10} pfu/ml), monosynaptic, disynaptic, and trisynaptic connections to the infected first-order neurons are visualized at 12 h intervals
(at 2.5, 3, and 3.5 days, respectively; Moschovakis et al., 2004; Grantyn et al.,
2002; Prevosto et al., 2009, 2010; Ugolini et al., 2006; see Figs. 6–8). However,

---

magnocellular portion (MVmc) infected at 2.5 days by retrograde transneuronal transfer
of rabies virus from "fast" MNs (injection 2 in (A) and (B)). (I–L) Examples of dual color
immunofluorescence for rabies virus (FITC, green) and choline acetyltransferase (CAT), a
marker for MNs and other cholinergic neurons (Cy3, red) in the LR muscle (I and J) and in
the VI nucleus (K and L). (I) The rabies virus injection area in the muscle can be easily
identified because of viral uptake by fibrocites. (J) Motor endplates (CAT-positive) in the
same section. (K and L) "Fast" MNs (after injection site 2 in (A) and (B)): infected MN (K)
remain viable because they express CAT antigen at normal levels (L, arrows). They are
intermixed with unlabeled MN (CAT-positive but rabies-negative). (M and N) Differences
in the second-order populations that innervate monosynaptically slow (M) and fast (N)
LR MNs (infected by rabies virus at 2.5 days). Marker size: strength of the projections. Red
neuronal markers and forked synapses: excitatory neurons; yellow neuronal markers and
bouton synapses: inhibitory; green neuronal markers and empty bouton synapses: non-
characterized or mixed populations. (M) Slow LR MNs are innervated only by pathways
involved in slow eye movements and gaze holding [supraoculomotor area (Soa), pre-
positus hypoglossi (PH), parvocellular medial vestibular nucleus (MVpc), caudal medullary medial reticular formation (MRF), central mesencephalic reticular formation
(cMRF)]. (J) Pathways to fast LR MNS: retrograde transneuronal transfer of rabies virus
involves *all* known second-order populations of horizontal eye movements pathways,
regardless of the distance and strength of their input to LR MNs [saccade bursters
(excitatory burst neurons, EBNs, in ipsilateral paramedian pontine reticular formation,
PPRF; inhibitory burst neurons, IBNs, in contralateral dorsal paragigantocellular reticular
formation, DPGi), angular vestibulo-ocular reflex (VOR) pathways (excitatory: contralateral magnocellular medial vestibular nucleus, MVmc; inhibitory: ipsilateral parvocellular medial vestibular nucleus, MVpc), linear VOR pathways (ipsilateral Scarpa's
ganglion), pathways involved in coordination of medial rectus (MR)/LR muscles (oculomotor internuclear neurons, OINs), portions of the horizontal velocity-to-position
integrator involved in inhibition of LR MNs during contralateral saccades (contralateral
marginal zone, MZ)]. Rabies virus immunolabeling in (C), (D), (G), and (H) was based on a
sensitive immunoperoxidase protocol and combined with cresyl violet counterstaining
of the same section. Bars = (C)–(F): 400 µm; (G): 600 µm; (H): 200 µm; (I, J): 100 µm; (E, F):
50 µm. For other details, see Ugolini et al. (2006). (See Page 9 in Color Section at the
back of the book.)

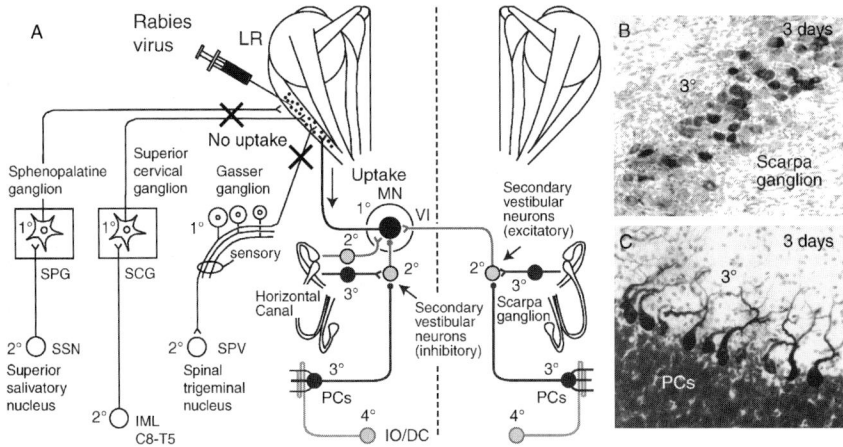

FIGURE 8 Pathways of propagation of rabies virus (CVS strain) after inoculation into the left lateral rectus (LR) muscle in macaque monkeys. Panel (A) is modified from Ugolini (2008) with permission. Uptake and transneuronal propagation of rabies virus occurs exclusively via the motor route (first-order neurons, 1°: LR motoneurons, MNs in the abducens, VI, nucleus), with no propagation in sensory, sympathetic or parasympathetic pathways that innervate the same muscle. [Sensory pathways: first-order neurons (1°), Gasser ganglion; second-order neurons (2°), spinal trigeminal nucleus. Sympathetic pathways: first-order neurons (1°), superior cervical ganglion, SCG; second-order neurons (2°), intermediolateral cell group, IML, of spinal segments C8-T5. Parasympathetic pathways: first-order neurons (1°), sphenopalatine ganglion, SPG; second-order neurons (2°), superior salivatory nucleus, SSN.] Retrograde transneuronal transfer from MNs (first-order, 1°, black) involves sequentially second-order neurons (2°, gray) at 2.5 days, third-order (3°, dark gray) at 3 days, and fourth-order (4°, light gray) at 3.5 days, as exemplified here by a schematic representation of the horizontal vestibulo-ocular reflex (VOR) circuitry to "fast" LR MNs (see also Fig. 7). Retrograde transneuronal transfer of rabies virus involves all known connections, including both excitatory neurons (forked synapses) and inhibitory neurons (bouton synapses). Note that in this model, labeling of the vestibular (Scarpa's) ganglia in the inner ear occurs ipsilaterally at 2.5 days (second-order neurons of linear VOR pathways to "fast" LR MNs; see also Fig. 7N) and bilaterally at 3 days (higher-order neurons of VOR pathways; see example in (B)). (B) Rabies virus-immunolabeled third-order neurons (3°) in Scarpa's ganglion, infected at 3 days by retrograde transneuronal transfer of rabies virus after injection into the LR muscle (see (A)). The infection of Scarpa's ganglion is a striking example of centrifugal spread of rabies virus to sensory ganglia which is mediated by retrograde transneuronal propagation and occurs already during the asymptomatic period. (C) Examples of third-order (3°) labeling of Purkinje cells (PCs) in the cerebellar flocculus at 3 days after injection into the LR muscle (see (A)). In (B) and (C), immunoperoxidase detection of rabies virus was combined with cresyl violet counterstaining of the same section.

the intervals are much longer when using CVS-11 at lower concentrations (10^7 or 10^8 pfu/ml, e.g., Kelly and Strick, 2003, 2004; Miyachi *et al.*, 2005, 2006). Varying the amount or concentration of the inoculum in a series of experiments must be avoided in rabies transneuronal tracing studies, as it can cause variability (e.g., Ruigrok *et al.*, 2008). The virus strain is another important factor, as the N2c strain propagates more rapidly than CVS-11 (Hoshi *et al.*, 2005) and may cause variability of the rate of transfer after intramuscular injection (Rathelot and Strick, 2009), unlike CVS-11 (Ugolini, 2010; Ugolini *et al.*, 2006; see Section III.B). Both the initial viral load and the virus strain may contribute to explain major differences in incubation times in human rabies (Jackson, 2002; Plotkin, 2000).

2. Sensitivity of the rabies immunodetection methods is important

When using the correct experimental parameters (see above), transneuronal tracing with rabies virus allows for a precise identification of the synaptic order because neuronal populations of progressively higher order are visualized sequentially (Ugolini, 2010). Distinction of the synaptic order is facilitated by the fact that transneuronal labeling is not gradual, but occurs stepwise, because replication of rabies virus is necessary for its immunohistochemical detection.

Sensitivity of the rabies immunolabeling protocol is very important: if it is low, modulatory connections that are sparse may not be detected, or may not reach detection threshold until later time points (see Ugolini, 1995b, 2010). For example, we had found in the hypoglossal (XII) model that some second-order cell groups were visualized a little later than other groups of the same synaptic order (Ugolini, 1995b; Fig. 5A). This asynchrony was correlated with the input strength and location of presynaptic terminals: second-order populations providing only weak input and targeting exclusively distal dendrites of XII motoneurons could be visualized a little later than cell groups of the same synaptic order that provide strong input and target motoneuronal cell bodies and proximal dendrites (Ugolini, 1995b; Fig. 5A). This is due to the fact that viral replication in (and transfer from) the cell body precedes centrifugal transport to distal dendrites (Ugolini, 1995b, 2008; Fig. 5A). Moreover, delayed labeling of the last groups of second-order neurons overlapped with the onset of labeling of higher-order neurons (Ugolini, 1995b; Fig. 5A). The asynchrony observed in the XII model was induced by the low sensitivity of the immunolabeling protocol because we have obtained no more evidence of asynchrony once we have started using a rabies virus primary antibody of superior sensitivity (Ugolini, 2010; Ugolini *et al.*, 2006; Figs. 6–8). With the improved rabies immunolabeling protocol, all populations of the same synaptic order are detected simultaneously regardless of the strength and location of the connections, although it is possible to observe differences in labeling intensity between different populations of the same synaptic order (Ugolini, 2010; Ugolini *et al.*, 2006). Thus, labeling that with the old protocol was below detection threshold is now detected, albeit as weaker labeling.

3. Combined visualization of rabies virus and neurotransmitter, cell markers, or other tracers

Because infected neurons remain metabolically viable, rabies immunolabeling can be combined with the identification of other tracers, neurotransmitters or cell markers. In dual immunolabeling protocols, rabies virus transneuronal labeling has been already combined with the visualization of choline acetyltransferase (used as marker for motoneurons and autonomic preganglionic neurons; Graf *et al.*, 2002; Morcuende *et al.*, 2002; Tang *et al.*, 1999; Ugolini *et al.*, 2006; see Fig. 7I–L), oxytocin (Tang *et al.*, 1999), calbindin, parvalbumin, pleiotrophin, and the neuronal form of nitric oxide synthase (Miyachi *et al.*, 2006; Salin *et al.*, 2009).

We have shown that a conventional tracer that is not transferred transneuronally (Cholera toxin B fragment, CTB low salt, List Biological Labs, Campbell, CA; end concentration 0.03%) can be mixed with rabies virus without altering viral uptake (Prevosto *et al.*, 2009, 2010; Ugolini, 2010; Fig. 6A–C, E, and H). Injecting such rabies virus/CTB mixture is a major methodological improvement: first, it allows for the definition of the injection area because CTB immunolabeling reveals the precise extent of the injection site (Fig. 6A and C), which would be difficult using rabies virus alone, because the virus does not induce tissue damage, does not infect glial cells, and does not accumulate at the injection site (Fig. 6E and H; Prevosto *et al.*, 2009, 2010; Ugolini, 2010). Second, the rabies virus/CTB combination makes it possible to identify first-order neurons (CTB) and higher-order neurons (rabies virus) in the same experiment, which is another considerable advantage (Fig. 6; Prevosto *et al.*, 2009, 2010; Ugolini, 2010).

F. Host range and species differences in uptake via different routes of inoculation

Rabies virus can infect all mammals, but not all species are equally susceptible following peripheral routes of inoculation. In mice, CVS-11 propagates efficiently via both the intranasal and the intramuscular routes (Coulon *et al.*, 1989; Lafay *et al.*, 1991), whereas in skunks, the intramuscular route is much less effective (Smart and Charlton, 1992). In rats, guinea pigs, and primates, transneuronal transfer of CVS-11 is very efficient via the intramuscular and intracerebral routes (Graf *et al.*, 2002; Morcuende *et al.*, 2002; Prevosto *et al.*, 2009, 2010; Tang *et al.*, 1999; Ugolini *et al.*, 2006). Once the virus has reached and replicated in first-order neurons, transneuronal transfer progresses at the same rate regardless of the peripheral or intracerebral route of inoculation (Prevosto *et al.*, 2009, 2010; Ugolini *et al.*, 2006). In primates, rats, and guinea pigs, the efficacy of transneuronal transfer and its timing (e.g., the interval required for the infection of second-order neurons) are not influenced by genetic or age differences of the animals, at least in adults. In mice, newborns are more susceptible (Casals, 1940; Morimoto *et al.*, 1998; Nilsson *et al.*, 1968), likely because of immature immune response (Morimoto *et al.*, 1998). Remarkably, after intracerebral inoculation of rabies virus mutants (RV194-2, Av01, SAD-D29) that are significantly less neuroinvasive than the parental strain due to point mutation of the glycoprotein at position 333, adult mice survive and develop neutralizing antibodies at high levels, but newborns die with rabies (Coulon *et al.*, 1983; Dietzschold *et al.*, 1983; Mebatsion, 2001; Seif *et al.*, 1985).

In primates, rats, and guinea pigs, intramuscular injections of CVS-11 result in uptake and propagation to the CNS only via the motor route (see Section III.G). In mice, however, the CVS strain can infect simultaneously motoneurons and primary sensory neurons with equal efficiency via the intramuscular route (Coulon *et al.*, 1989; Jackson, 2002). Moreover, adult mice can develop rabies after oral administration of the "fixed" ERA strain, which is avirulent in monkeys and other mammals via the same route (Lawson *et al.*, 1987). The exceptional susceptibility of mice is presumably due to the fact that CVS and ERA, like other "fixed" strains, were originally mouse adapted (see, e.g., Sacramento *et al.*, 1992). Therefore, studies of the propagation of "fixed" rabies virus strains in mice models are probably less representative of human rabies infection than those performed in other species of rodents and nonhuman primates (Ugolini, 2008, 2010).

G. Entry of rabies virus occurs exclusively via the motor route after peripheral inoculations

In primates, rats, and guinea pigs, we found that CVS-11 enters exclusively via the motor route after *intramuscular* inoculations, that is, sensory and autonomic neurons that innervate the muscle are not infected (Graf *et al.*, 2002; Morcuende *et al.*, 2002; Tang *et al.*, 1999; Ugolini *et al.*, 2006; see also Ugolini, 2008; Figs. 4, 7, and 8). This phenomenon was first documented in rats after inoculation of CVS-11 into the bulbospongiosus muscle (Tang *et al.*, 1999; Fig. 4). This muscle is innervated by motoneurons in the ipsilateral dorsomedial (DM) nucleus at L5-L6, and also primary sensory neurons in the ipsilateral dorsal root ganglia at L5-S1 and sympathetic postganglionic neurons in the lumbar paravertebral sympathetic chain (the latter receiving projections from sympathetic preganglionic neurons that are located in the intermediolateral cell group of lower thoracic and upper lumbar spinal segments; Fig. 4). We found that rabies virus infected only bulbospongiosus motoneurons (first-order), and subsequently progressed, in sequential steps of transfer, to synaptically connected (higher-order) spinal and supraspinal populations of motor pathways (Tang *et al.*, 1999; Fig. 4). Similarly, rabies virus entered only via the motor route after inoculation of CVS-11 into facial muscles (orbicularis oculi) in rats (Morcuende *et al.*, 2002) and into extraocular eye muscles in guinea pigs and primates (Graf *et al.*, 2002; Ugolini *et al.*, 2006; Figs. 7 and 8). The exclusive transneuronal propagation of rabies virus (CVS-11) via the motor route in primates, rats, and guinea pigs is a particularly valuable feature of the rabies transneuronal tracing technology, as it allows for a specific identification of the polysynaptic descending motor pathways involved in the control of single muscles (Graf *et al.*, 2002; Morcuende *et al.*, 2002; Rathelot and Strick, 2006, 2009; Tang *et al.*, 1999; Ugolini, 2010; Ugolini *et al.*, 2006; Figs. 4, 7, and 8). Importantly, this could not be achieved in transneuronal tracing studies with alpha-herpesviruses because they propagate simultaneously in sensory, sympathetic, and motor pathways (see Section II and Fig. 3)

The lack of penetration of rabies virus into peripheral sensory and autonomic endings is not only an exclusive property of the CVS-11 strain, and is not the result of quantitative differences in motor versus sensory and autonomic innervation, because it was also reported after inoculation of the CVS-N2c strain into primates hand muscles, despite their prominent sensory and sympathetic innervation (Rathelot and Strick, 2006). Importantly, we have shown that CVS-11 enters exclusively via the motor route also after inoculations directly into peripheral *nerves* (e.g., the hypoglossal nerve in rats; Ugolini, 1995b), even when the inoculated nerves (e.g., ulnar) contain a great number of sensory and sympathetic axons, in addition to motor axons (Ugolini, unpublished observations). Thus, in the peripheral nervous system, rabies virus "receptors" appear to be present both on motor axons (possibly at the nodes of Ranvier) and on motor endplates, but not on sensory and autonomic axons and terminals.

These experimental findings, obtained by studying the early stages of propagation of "fixed" CVS variants in primates and rodents models, have potential implications for the understanding of the pathophysiology of human rabies. If the penetration of "street" rabies virus similarly prefers the motor route, it would explain why the risk of developing rabies after dog bites is empirically 50 times higher after deep bites into muscles and/or nerves (Hemachudha *et al.*, 2002), allowing for direct contact with motor endplates and motor axons, compared with skin lesions that only permit access to less permissive sensory and sympathetic endings (Ugolini, 2008).

Classic rabies is almost always associated with true rabies virus (genotype 1), usually *canine related*, and can manifest in either the furious or the paralytic forms (Hemachudha *et al.*, 2002, 2006). Clinical diversities are not fully explained by virus variants (since a single dog caused furious rabies to one patient but paralytic rabies to another; Hemachudha *et al.*, 2006) but are related to different neuropathogenetic mechanisms (i.e., peripheral nerve demyelination of autoimmune etiology, which resembles the Guillan–Barré syndrome, in the paralytic form, but not in the furious form; Hemachudha *et al.*, 2005, 2006; Sheikh *et al.*, 2005). Although clinical stages of illness are far too advanced to allow for definite conclusions regarding the early pathways of viral propagation, some clinical, electrophysiological, and neuropathological findings in canine-related human rabies point to a more prominent involvement of motor versus sensory elements (Mitrabhakdi *et al.*, 2005; Sheikh *et al.*, 2005), that could be explained by earlier or preferential infection via the motor route, that is, as observed experimentally for fixed rabies virus (see above). Thus, in *furious* rabies patients, it was shown that sensory and motor nerve conduction studies were normal during the early clinical stages of illness, yet abundant denervation potentials were evident primarily in the bitten limb, that preceded clinical weakness and suggested an acute motor fiber loss, probably at the anterior horn level, in the absence of detectable sensory loss (Mitrabhakdi *et al.*, 2005). Furthermore, in one Chinese *paralytic* rabies patient, Wallerian-like degeneration and inflammatory changes were much more severe in ventral than in dorsal spinal roots (Sheikh *et al.*, 2005), which may be similarly explained by a preferential infection via the motor route.

Bat-related rabies, however, is characterized by nonclassical or atypical clinical features (Hemachudha *et al.*, 2005). Moreover, with bat variants (e.g., silver-haired bat rabies virus), a superficial wound or scratch, that can deliver only negligible amounts of virus, is sufficient to cause infection, despite the fact that the skin contains only sensory and sympathetic endings (Jackson, 2002; Rupprecht and Hemachudha, 2004). The greater neuroinvasiveness of bat variants is likely due to their unique ability to replicate in epidermal cells at lower than normal body temperature (34 °C), that could enable them to amplify at the inoculation site, thereby enhancing the probability of entering nerve endings (Morimoto *et al.*, 1996). Propagation of bat-related strains via sensory and possibly, sympathetic routes, could explain why local neuropathic pain at the bitten area is much more common (70% vs. 30% in dog-related cases; Hemachudha *et al.*, 2002, 2006) as well as objective sensory deficits, Horner's syndrome, and possibly other atypical clinical features of bat-related cases (Hemachudha *et al.*, 2002, 2006).

H. Uptake of rabies virus occurs only within the inoculated portion of the muscle

For transneuronal tracing purposes, it is important to inoculate always the same portion of a muscle in a series of experiments to ensure the same amount of uptake because rabies virus is taken up exclusively by motor endplates in the inoculated portion of the muscle and does not spread within the muscle. We have demonstrated this property of rabies virus in primates, by injecting the CVS-11 strain (110 μl, titer 7.8×10^{10} pfu/ml) into either the distal or central portions of the lateral rectus (LR) muscle, which contain the motor endplates of two different populations of moto-neurons, innervating slow and fast muscle fibers, respectively (Fig. 7; Ugolini *et al.*, 2006). Rabies immunostaining of the muscle at 2.5 days postinoculation showed rabies virus antigen in fibrocytes, and not in myocytes (Ugolini *et al.*, 2006; Fig. 7I). Similarly, even in the case of street rabies virus strains, local replication in the inoculated muscle initially spares myocytes (Charlton and Casey, 1979). In this model, infection of fibrocytes by the CVS-11 strain was probably defective because it did not spread to noninjected portions of the muscle (Fig. 7A and B). In fact, after inoculations into the *distal* portion of the LR muscle, which contains exclusively "en grappe" endplates of "slow" motoneurons, the infection involved only this particular motoneurons population (located at the periphery of the abducens nucleus; Fig. 7C and E; Ugolini *et al.*, 2006). In contrast, "fast" motoneurons (located inside the abducens nucleus; Fig. 7D and F) were infected only after injection into the *central* part of the muscle, that is, the only muscle portion containing "en plaque" motor endplates of these motoneurons (Ugolini *et al.*, 2006; Fig. 7A and B). Retrograde transneuronal transfer of rabies virus from these different groups of motoneurons revealed the existence of major differences in their premotor innervations (Fig. 7G, H, M, and N; Ugolini *et al.*, 2006).

In primate and rodent models, motoneurons were infected in less than 2 days after intramuscular inoculations of CVS-11 at high titer, showing that rabies virus directly infects motor endplates without the need of prior replication within the muscle (Graf *et al.*, 2002; Tang *et al.*, 1999; Ugolini, 1995b; Ugolini *et al.*, 2006). Migration to the CNS without prior replication at the site of inoculation has been documented also following intramus-cular inoculations of the CVS-24 variant in mice (Shankar *et al.*, 1991). These findings stress the importance of complete wound infiltration with rabies immunoglobulins as early as possible, within 2 days after the bite, to prevent the infection. They also explain why postexposure prophylaxis may fail if wound infiltration is either incomplete or undertaken later because rabies virus may have already gained access to motoneurons. Under other conditions, for example, if the titer of the inoculum is low or the inoculation is superficial (or in the case of bat variants, see above), local replication might be necessary before the virus can reach motor endplates, which may explain the particularly long incubation times in some cases of human rabies (e.g., Jackson, 2002; Plotkin, 2000).

I. Ubiquitous propagation of rabies virus at chemical synapses, and lack of transmission via gap junctions or local spread

In all models that have been studied to date, transneuronal transfer of rabies virus has never failed to label known pathways mediated by classical chemical synapses ("wiring transmission"). Propagation is very efficient, as all populations of the same synaptic order are infected simultaneously, regardless of their neurotransmitters, synaptic strength, termination site, or distance (e.g., Graf *et al.*, 2002; Grantyn *et al.*, 2002; Morcuende *et al.*, 2002; Tang *et al.*, 1999; Ugolini, 1995b, 2010; Ugolini *et al.*, 2006; Figs. 6–8).

For example, following inoculation into the LR muscle belly in primates, transfer of rabies virus infected synchronously (at 2.5 days postinoculation) all second-order populations that innervate directly "fast" abducens motoneurons (Figs. 7N and 8A). This included both excitatory populations (e.g., excitatory neurons of angular vestibulo-ocular reflex, VOR, pathways, in the contralateral magnocellular medial vestibular nucleus, MVmc, and excitatory burst neurons, EBNs, of saccade pathways, in the ipsilateral paramedian pontine reticular formation, PPRF) and inhibitory ones (e.g., inhibitory neurons of VOR pathways in the ipsilateral MVmc, inhibitory burst neurons in the contralateral dorsal paragigantocellular reticular formation, DPGi; Fig. 7N; see example of second-order labeling of the contralateral, MVmc in Fig. 7G and H). Similarly, minor pathways to "fast" abducens motoneurons (such as those derived from the ipsilateral Scarpa's ganglion that mediate linear VOR responses) were visualized in synchrony as major ones (e.g., from PPRF, DPGi, MVmc; Ugolini *et al.*, 2006; Fig. 7N). Importantly, short pathways (e.g., from the DPGi) were labeled at the same time as long ones (e.g., from oculomotor internuclear neurons, OINs; Fig. 7N). The same applied to third-order neurons, infected at 3 days in the same model: the infection involved brainstem populations (e.g., saccade-related burst neurons in the superior colliculus; Grantyn *et al.*, 2002) at the same time as layer V cortical neurons in the Frontal Eye Field (Moschovakis *et al.*, 2004), despite major differences in their respective distance from the brainstem oculomotor populations that they innervate.

Similarly, after intracortical inoculations into the posterior parietal cortex in primates, we found that all second-order populations that innervate the injected cortical areas via the thalamus were labeled in synchrony at 2.5 days, despite major differences in neurotransmitters, strength, and type of their terminations (e.g., neurons in the contralateral cerebellar nuclei, which synapse strongly onto single thalamic cells, and in the ipsilateral reticular thalamic nucleus, which issues diffuse terminal projections to the thalamus; Fig. 6B, D, F, and G; Prevosto *et al.*, 2009, 2010).

The only example of poor transneuronal propagation of rabies virus at chemical synapses was the negligible infection of the locus coeruleus (in the XII and bulbospongiosus models; Tang *et al.*, 1999; Ugolini, 1995b). This is a special case because the projections from the locus coeruleus are largely via "volume transmission" (see Fuxe *et al.*, 2007), suggesting that this particular type of synapses might be less conducive to rabies virus (Tang *et al.*, 1999; Ugolini, 1995b, 2010). Interestingly, "volume transmission" pathways are much more extensively infected with alpha-herpesviruses (e.g., XII model; Babic *et al.*, 1993; Ugolini *et al.*, 1987), likely because the spurious (cell-to-cell) spread of alpha-herpesviruses facilitates propagation through this less conducive type of synapses (Ugolini, 2010).

Rabies virus does not propagate at electrical synapses (gap junctions). This was demonstrated in the bulbospongiosus model (Fig. 4): although bulbospongiosus motoneurons are extensively interconnected by gap junctions, the number of infected motoneurons did not increase with time (Fig. 4B–D), showing that gap junctions are not conducive to rabies virus propagation (Tang *et al.*, 1999). In addition to classical electron microscopy findings showing that propagation of rabies virus occurs primarily at synaptic junctions (Charlton and Casey, 1979; Iwasaki and Clark, 1975), it has been unequivocally demonstrated that rabies virus is not transmitted via nonsynaptic (spurious) spread from infected neurons to neighboring, but not synaptically connected cells (Fig. 1C), and is not taken up by fibers of passage even after long standing infection (Tang *et al.*, 1999; Ugolini, 1995b; see Ugolini, 2010).

J. Neuronal receptors for rabies virus

In vivo, rabies virus infects only neurons, even after inoculations directly into the CNS (e.g., Kelly and Strick, 2003; Prevosto *et al.*, 2009, 2010; Fig. 6E and H). The finding that rabies virus propagates at chemical synapses with the same efficiency through all known pathways, regardless of their neurotransmitters and synaptic strength (see Section III.I), indicates that neuronal receptors for rabies virus are ubiquitously distributed within the CNS (e.g., Graf *et al.*, 2002; Grantyn *et al.*, 2002; Morcuende *et al.*, 2002; Tang *et al.*, 1999; Ugolini, 1995b, 2008, 2010; Ugolini *et al.*, 2006).

Molecules that have been proposed to act as rabies virus receptors include the nicotinic acetylcholine receptor (nAChR; Hanham *et al.*, 1993; Lentz *et al.*, 1982), the neuronal cell adhesion molecule (NCAM; Thoulouze *et al.*, 1998), the nerve growth factor receptor (p75; Tuffereau *et al.*, 1998), and perhaps also highly sialylated gangliosides (Superti *et al.*, 1986).

Among these putative receptors for rabies virus, NCAM (Thoulouze *et al.*, 1998) is the most likely candidate in view of its widespread distribution in the adult nervous system, its presynaptic location, and its presence also at the neuromuscular junction (Lafon, 2005). It is possible that additional receptors are utilized as well, since in NCAM-deficient mice, rabies virus propagation is severely impaired, but not completely abolished (Thoulouze *et al.*, 1998). It has been speculated that highly sialylated gangliosides might act in synergy with NCAM, because they are ubiquitously distributed and are important constituents of presynaptic membranes and lipid rafts, to which NCAM is associated (see Lafon, 2005).

Unlike NCAM or gangliosides, the CNS distribution of p75 (Tuffereau *et al.*, 1998) and nAChR (Hanham *et al.*, 1993; Lentz *et al.*, 1982) is not sufficiently ubiquitous in the adult CNS (Lafon, 2005). In fact, p75 is mainly expressed during development, and is not present at the neuromuscular junction (see Lafon, 2005), which is the preferred route of entry of rabies virus (Graf *et al.*, 2002; Tang *et al.*, 1999; Ugolini, 2008, 2010; Ugolini *et al.*, 2006). Expression of p75 in primary sensory neurons is not sufficient for rabies virus binding and infection (Tuffereau *et al.*, 2007). Similarly, neurons in the sympathetic ganglia, which express p75 (Garcia-Suarez *et al.*, 1996), are not infected following peripheral inoculations of rabies virus (Graf *et al.*, 2002; Tang *et al.*, 1999; Ugolini, 2008, 2010; Ugolini *et al.*, 2006). Moreover, rabies infection develops equally well in p75-deficient and normal mice (Jackson and Park, 1999; Tuffereau *et al.*, 2007). Similarly, in the CNS, presence or absence of the nAChR has no appreciable effects, as rabies virus propagates synchronously to cholinergic and noncholinergic populations of the same synaptic order (Ugolini, 2010).

The nAChR, because of its mainly postsynaptic location, cannot directly mediate uptake, but may improve the probability of uptake, by concentrating viral particles in front of the neuromuscular junction (Lafon, 2005; Lentz *et al.*, 1982). Its presence at motor endplates, but not at peripheral sensory and autonomic endings, could explain why in primates, rats, and guinea pigs, peripheral uptake of rabies virus is restricted to motoneurons, while sensory and sympathetic neurons that innervate the same muscle are not infected (Graf *et al.*, 2002; Tang *et al.*, 1999; Ugolini, 2008, 2010; Ugolini *et al.*, 2006; Figs. 4, 7, and 8).

K. Mechanisms mediating centrifugal propagation of rabies virus to end organs

Depending on the site of inoculation, some centrifugal propagation of rabies virus from the CNS to peripheral sensory ganglia can already occur during the preclinical period. It is mediated by retrograde transneuronal transfer, via the polysynaptic connections from sensory ganglia to motoneurons or other initially infected CNS populations (Ugolini, 2008).

We obtained evidence of this phenomenon when studying the kinetics of propagation of CVS-11 following intramuscular inoculations into the bulbospongiosus muscle: rabies virus infected exclusively bulbospongiosus motoneurons (first-order) at 2 days postinoculation. In the spinal cord, subsequent steps of retrograde transneuronal transfer caused the infection of specific populations of second-order spinal interneurons at 3 days, and higher-order neurons at 4 and 5 days postinoculation (Tang *et al.*, 1999) (Fig. 4). In this model, retrograde transneuronal transfer caused the infection of a sympathetic preganglionic population (in the central autonomic area, in lamina X of lumbar segments), which does not innervate the bulbospongiosus muscle (Fig. 4A). Moreover, a great number of primary sensory neurons were infected bilaterally in the dorsal root ganglia starting from 4 days postinoculation (Fig. 4A). Bilateral infection of the dorsal root ganglia in this model cannot be explained by peripheral uptake (which could only cause the infection of ipsilateral dorsal root ganglia; see Fig. 4A). It clearly reflected centrifugal propagation of rabies virus to sensory ganglia via their polysynaptic connections to the infected motoneurons (Fig. 4A).

Examples of centrifugal propagation of rabies virus to peripheral ganglia, occurring already during the preclinical period, were also obtained in other models. Following intramuscular injection into an extraocular muscle (the LR) in primates, retrograde transneuronal transfer of rabies virus from abducens motoneurons caused the infection of the vestibular (Scarpa's) ganglia in the inner ear ipsilaterally at 2.5 days (second-order neurons of linear VOR pathways) and bilaterally at 3 days (higher-order neurons of VOR pathways; Ugolini et al., 2000, 2006; Fig. 8). Similarly, intracortical inoculation into the posterior parietal cortex in primates resulted in the centrifugal propagation of rabies virus to the Scarpa's ganglion already at 3 days postinoculation, which reflected third-order ascending vestibular projections from the labyrinth (via the vestibular nuclei and the thalamus) to the injected cortical area (Prevosto et al., 2006; Ugolini, 2008).

With regard to rabies pathogenesis, the experimental findings show that the motor route is the privileged route of entry of rabies virus into the CNS, whereas sensory ganglia can be infected only secondarily, via transneuronal transfer, which can explain the more prominent involvement of motor versus sensory elements in canine-derived human rabies (Mitrabhakdi et al., 2005; Sheikh et al., 2005; see also Section III.G).

Although some sensory ganglia can be already involved during the preclinical period, rabies virus can be recovered from end organs (salivary gland, skin, hair follicles, muscle fibers) only at late stages of infection, when animals and humans show clinical features of rabies (Jackson, 2002). Thus, centrifugal spread to end organs can only be mediated by transneuronal propagation and must ultimately involve anterograde axonal transport (e.g., from infected sensory ganglia to the skin and hair follicles). This may appear a paradox, in view of the exclusively unidirectional (retrograde) propagation of rabies virus during early stages of infection (see above, Section III.C). However, it is important to consider that the finding that rabies virus can be recovered from end organs only late, when the disease is already declared, is in keeping with the experimental demonstration that anterograde intracellular transport of rabies virus is inefficient (Klingen et al., 2008; see Section III.C). Thus, anterograde axonal spread to end organs is probably mediated by passive diffusion, rather than active transport mechanisms, and likely necessitates a considerable "virus load" of the neurons, explaining why it occurs so late (Ugolini, 2008).

IV. PERSPECTIVES

A. Methodologies: Genetically modified rabies tracers

The development of reverse genetics (Conzelmann, 1996; Mebatsion *et al.*, 1996a,b) has made it possible to manipulate directly the genome of rabies virus, providing outstanding opportunities to improve knowledge of mechanisms involved in viral functions and to design new vaccines (Faul *et al.*, 2009; Finke and Conzelmann, 2005; Schnell *et al.*, 2005).

Preliminary results highlight the potential of reverse genetics approaches also for engineering modified rabies virus tracers that could be tailored for specific purposes (Callaway, 2008; Ugolini, 2010). Research in this direction has two main goals. The first is to develop *defective "single-step" rabies virus vectors* that are not transferred transneuronally, and that could serve to identify direct connections to single neuron or selected cell types. Initial steps in this direction involved engineering a defective (glycoprotein-negative and transcomplemented) rabies virus tracer that labels only first-order neurons that innervate the injection site, like a conventional retrograde tracer (Etessami *et al.*, 2000), and carries a foreign gene as marker (Mebatsion *et al.*, 1996b; Wickersham *et al.*, 2007). Current efforts are aimed at trying to restrict the uptake of such "single-step" rabies tracers to chosen cells (see Callaway, 2008; Ugolini, 2010).

The second major goal is to develop *dual transneuronal tracing methods* based on the use of virulent isogenic rabies virus strains that could serve to identify two different neuronal circuits (controlling two different body sites) in the same experiment. This would be of great importance because only dual transneuronal tracing technologies could clarify unequivocally the extent of convergence and separation of neuronal circuits that control different targets. In the first attempt of this kind (Ohara *et al.*, 2009), isogenic rabies virus recombinants were generated by inserting different reporter genes (β-gal, Venus, or EGFP) into the attenuated HEP-Flury strain of rabies virus, where the glycoprotein gene was replaced with that from CVS in order to restore virulence and mimic the properties of CVS. Tests of dual infection *in vitro* and *in vivo* with these recombinants showed that viral interference for replication was a limiting factor: to achieve efficient double labeling, the two viruses must infect the same neurons within a few hours; otherwise, the efficiency of the second infection decreases exponentially (Ohara *et al.*, 2009). Moreover, the replication and/or propagation speed of the recombinants is modified by the length of the inserted foreign genes (Ohara *et al.*, 2009). While these findings stress the need to adjust the size of the inserted foreign gene and the dose of each virus to achieve optimal dual transneuronal labeling, the successful colocalization of the two isogenic recombinants *in vitro* and *in vivo* (Ohara *et al.*, 2009) clearly illustrates the potential of genetically engineered rabies viruses for dual transneuronal tracing. Since a direct comparison with the propagation properties of CVS has not been carried out yet, it remains to be demonstrated whether such isogenic recombinants are truly as effective as CVS-11 or not, particularly in view of the fact that they still express the matrix protein of the attenuated HEP-Flury strain, and there is evidence that propagation of rabies virus also depends upon the matrix protein (Pulmanausahakul *et al.*, 2008). Thus, isogenic recombinants derived from the CVS background (or carrying the matrix protein gene from CVS) may be preferable. Theoretically, it should be also possible to engineer rabies virus recombinants that would express activity indicators or light-sensitive ion channels, to allow for monitoring or manipulating neuronal activity *in vivo*, which would be a major advance. The capacity of rabies virus to replicate without altering neuronal function, at least during the preclinical period, makes it the most promising viral vector for these purposes.

B. Rabies pathogenesis: Perspectives

While considerable insight has been gained into the mechanisms of propagation of "fixed" strains of rabies virus, neuroanatomical studies of transneuronal transfer of rabies virus during the preclinical period still need to be carried out to elucidate possible differences in the modalities of propagation of "street" rabies virus of canine and bat origin, both in their natural hosts and in suitable rodents and primate models. It is important to consider, for example, that only a few studies are available on the propagation of bat-derived rabies virus variants *in vivo*. Another question to be addressed in neuroanatomical models concerns the mechanisms of neuronal dysfunction, at the level of both single neurons and entire neuronal networks, which are responsible for the behavioral changes ultimately occurring in rabies. In view of their relevance to human rabies, primate models of rabies virus transneuronal propagation would be particularly valuable also for understanding immune evasion mechanisms and testing antiviral strategies, in order to find effective therapies for this deadly disease, which is still one of the most common lethal infections worldwide.

ACKNOWLEDGMENTS

This work was supported by the European Union (QLRT-2001-00151, EUROKINESIS, and BIO4-CT98-0546, TransVirus) and the Centre National de la Recherche Scientifique (CNRS).

REFERENCES

Akkal, D., Dum, R. P., and Strick, P. L. (2007). Supplementary motor area and presupplementary motor area: Targets of basal ganglia and cerebellar output. *J. Neurosci.* **27**:10659–10673.

Aston-Jones, G., and Card, J. P. (2000). Use of pseudorabies virus to delineate multisynaptic circuits in brain: Opportunities and limitations. *J. Neurosci. Methods* **103**:51–61.

Babic, N., Mettenleiter, T. C., Flamand, A., and Ugolini, G. (1993). Role of essential glycoproteins gII and gp50 in transneuronal transfer of pseudorabies virus from the hypoglossal nerves of mice. *J. Virol.* **67**:4421–4426.

Baloul, L., and Lafon, M. (2003). Apoptosis and rabies virus neuroinvasion. *Biochimie* **85**:777–788.

Baloul, L., Camelo, S., and Lafon, M. (2004). Up-regulation of Fas ligand (FasL) in the central nervous system: A mechanism of immune evasion by rabies virus. *J. Neurovirol.* **10**:372–382.

Brzózka, K., Finke, S., and Conzelmann, K. K. (2005). Identification of the rabies virus alpha/beta interferon antagonist: Phosphoprotein P interferes with phosphorylation of interferon regulatory factor 3. *J. Virol.* **79**:7673–7681.

Brzózka, K., Finke, S., and Conzelmann, K. K. (2006). Inhibition of interferon signaling by rabies virus phosphoprotein P: Activation-dependent binding of STAT1 and STAT2. *J. Virol.* **80**:2675–2683.

Callaway, E. M. (2008). Transneuronal circuit tracing with neurotropic viruses. *Curr. Opin. Neurobiol.* **18**:617–623.

Casals, J. (1940). Influence of age factors on susceptibility of mice to rabies virus. *J. Exp. Med.* **72**:445–451.

Ceccaldi, P. E., Gillet, J. P., and Tsiang, H. (1989). Inhibition of the transport of rabies virus in the central nervous system. *J. Neuropathol. Exp. Neurol.* **48**:620–630.

Charlton, K. M., and Casey, G. A. (1979). Experimental rabies in skunks: Immunofluorescence light and electron microscopic studies. *Lab. Invest.* **41**:36–44.

Clower, D. M., Dum, R. P., and Strick, P. L. (2005). Basal ganglia and cerebellar inputs to 'AIP'. *Cereb. Cortex* **15**:913–920.

Conzelmann, K. K. (1996). Genetic manipulation of non-segmented negative-strand RNA viruses. *J. Gen. Virol.* **77**:381–389.

Conzelmann, K. K. (2005). Transcriptional activation of alpha/beta interferon genes: Interference by nonsegmented negative-strand RNA viruses. *J. Virol.* **79**:5241–5248.

Coulon, P., Rollin, P. E., and Flamand, A. (1983). Molecular basis of rabies virus virulence. II. Identification of a site on the CVS glycoprotein associated with virulence. *J. Gen. Virol.* **64**:693–696.

Coulon, P., Derbin, C., Kucera, P., Lafay, F., Prehaud, C., and Flamand, A. (1989). Invasion of the peripheral nervous systems of adult mice by the CVS strain of rabies virus and its avirulent derivative AvO1. *J. Virol.* **63**:3550–3554.

Dietzschold, B., Wunner, W. H., Wiktor, T. J., Lopes, A. D., Lafon, M., Smith, C. L., and Koprowski, H. (1983). Characterization of an antigenic determinant of the glycoprotein that correlates with pathogenicity of rabies virus. *Proc. Natl. Acad. Sci. USA* **80**:70–74.

Dietzschold, B., Wiktor, T. J., Trojanowski, J. Q., Macfarlan, R. I., Wunner, W. H., Torres-Anjel, M. J., and Koprowski, H. (1985). Differences in cell-to-cell spread of pathogenic and apathogenic rabies virus in vivo and in vitro. *J. Virol.* **56**:12–18.

Dietzschold, B., Schnell, M., and Koprowski, H. (2005). Pathogenesis of rabies. *Curr. Top. Microbiol. Immunol.* **292**:45–56.

Dietzschold, B., Li, J., Faber, M., and Schnell, M. (2008). Concepts in the pathogenesis of rabies. *Future Virol.* **3**:481–490.

Dolivo, M. (1980). A neurobiological approach to neurotropic viruses. *Trends Neurosci.* **3**:149–152.

Etessami, R., Conzelmann, K. K., Fadai-Ghotbi, B., Natelson, B., Tsiang, H., and Ceccaldi, P. E. (2000). Spread and pathogenic characteristics of a G-deficient rabies virus recombinant: An in vitro and in vivo study. *J. Gen. Virol.* **81:**147–153.

Faul, E. J., Aye, P. P., Papaneri, A. B., Pahar, B., McGettigan, J. P., Schiro, F., Chervoneva, I., Montefiori, D. C., Lackner, A. A., and Schnell, M. J. (2009). Rabies virus-based vaccines elicit neutralizing antibodies, poly-functional CD8+ T cell, and protect rhesus macaques from AIDS-like disease after SIV(mac251) challenge. *Vaccine* **28:**299–308.

Finke, S., and Conzelmann, K. K. (2005). Replication strategies of rabies virus. *Virus Res.* **111:**120–131.

Fuxe, K., Dahlström, A., Höistad, M., Marcellino, D., Jansson, A., Rivera, A., Diaz-Cabiale, Z., Jacobsen, K., Tinner-Staines, B., Hagman, B., Leo, G., Staines, W., *et al.* (2007). From the Golgi-Cajal mapping to the transmitter-based characterization of the neuronal networks leading to two modes of brain communication: Wiring and volume transmission. *Brain Res. Rev.* **55:**17–54.

Garcia-Suarez, O., Naves, F. J., Del Valle, M. E., Esteban, I., Bronzetti, E., Vazquez, E., and Vega, J. A. (1996). Distribution of p75 and trk-neurotrophin receptor proteins in adult human sympathetic ganglia. *Anat. Embryol. (Berl.)* **193:**577–583.

Gaudin, Y. (2000). Rabies virus-induced membrane fusion pathway. *J. Cell Biol.* **150:**601–612.

Gaudin, Y., Ruigrok, R. W., Tuffereau, C., Knossow, M., and Flamand, A. (1992). Rabies virus glycoprotein is a trimer. *Virology* **187:**627–632.

Goodpasture, E. W., and Teague, O. (1923). Transmission of the virus of herpes febrilis along nerves in experimentally infected rabbits. *J. Exp. Med.* **44:**139–184.

Graf, W., Gerrits, N., Yatim-Dhiba, N., and Ugolini, G. (2002). Mapping the oculomotor system: The power of transneuronal labeling with rabies virus. *Eur. J. Neurosci.* **15:**1557–1562.

Grantyn, A., Brandi, A. M., Dubayle, D., Graf, W., Ugolini, G., Hadjidimitrakis, K., and Moschovakis, A. (2002). Density gradients of trans-synaptically labeled collicular neurons after injection of rabies virus in the lateral rectus muscle of the rhesus monkey. *J. Comp. Neurol.* **451:**346–361.

Hanham, C. A., Zhao, F., and Tignor, G. H. (1993). Evidence from the anti-idiotypic network that the acetylcholine receptor is a rabies virus receptor. *J. Virol.* **67:**530–542.

Hemachudha, T., Laothamatas, J., and Rupprecht, C. E. (2002). Human rabies: A disease of complex neuropathogenetic mechanisms and diagnostic challenges. *Lancet Neurol.* **1:**101–109.

Hemachudha, T., Wacharapluesadee, S., Mitrabhakdi, E., Wilde, H., Morimoto, K., and Lewis, R. A. (2005). Pathophysiology of human paralytic rabies. *J. Neurovirol.* **11:**93–100.

Hemachudha, T., Wacharapluesadee, S., Laothamatas, J., and Wilde, H. (2006). Rabies. *Curr. Neurol. Neurosci. Rep.* **6:**460–468.

Hirokawa, N., and Takemura, R. (2005). Molecular motors and mechanisms of directional transport in neurons. *Nat. Rev. Neurosci.* **6:**201–214.

Hoshi, E., Tremblay, L., Féger, J., Carras, P. L., and Strick, P. L. (2005). The cerebellum communicates with the basal ganglia. *Nat. Neurosci.* **8:**1491–1493.

Iwasaki, Y., and Clark, H. F. (1975). Cell to cell transmission of virus in the central nervous system. II. Experimental rabies in mouse. *Lab. Invest.* **33:**391–399.

Jackson, A. C. (2002). Pathogenesis. *In* "Rabies" (A. C. Jackson and W. H. Wunner, eds.), pp. 245–282. Academic Press, San Diego.

Jackson, A. C., and Park, H. (1999). Experimental rabies virus infection of p75 neurotrophin receptor-deficient mice. *Acta Neuropathol. (Berl.)* **98:**641–644.

Jacob, Y., Badrane, H., Ceccaldi, P. E., and Tordo, N. (2000). Cytoplasmic dynein LC8 interacts with lyssavirus phosphoprotein. *J. Virol.* **74:**10217–10222.

Jansen, A. S., Nguyen, X. V., Karpitskiy, V., Mettenleiter, T. C., and Loewy, A. D. (1995). Central command neurons of the sympathetic nervous system: Basis of the fight-or-flight response. *Science* **270:**644–646.

Juntrakul, S., Ruangvejvorachai, P., Shuangshoti, S., Wacharapluesadee, S., and Hemachudha, T. (2005). Mechanisms of escape phenomenon of spinal cord and brainstem in human rabies. *BMC Infect. Dis.* **5:**104.

Kelly, R. M., and Strick, P. L. (2000). Rabies as a transneuronal tracer of circuits in the central nervous system. *J. Neurosci. Methods* **103:**63–71.

Kelly, R. M., and Strick, P. L. (2003). Cerebellar loops with motor cortex and prefrontal cortex of a nonhuman primate. *J. Neurosci.* **23:**8432–8444.

Kelly, R. M., and Strick, P. L. (2004). Macro-architecture of basal ganglia loops with the cerebral cortex: Use of rabies virus to reveal multisynaptic circuits. *Prog. Brain Res.* **143:**449–459.

Klingen, Y., Conzelmann, K. K., and Finke, S. (2008). Double-labeled rabies virus: Live tracking of enveloped virus transport. *J. Virol.* **82:**237–245.

Kristensson, K., Lycke, E., and Sjöstrand, J. (1971). Spread of herpes simplex virus in peripheral nerves. *Acta Neuropathol.* **17:**44–53.

Kristensson, K., Ghetti, B., and Wiśniewski, H. M. (1974). Study on the propagation of Herpes simplex virus (type 2) into the brain after intraocular injection. *Brain Res.* **69:**189–201.

Kristensson, K., Nennesmo, L., Persson, L., and Lycke, E. (1982). Neuron to neuron transmission of herpes simplex virus. Transport of virus from skin to brainstem nuclei. *J. Neurol. Sci.* **54:**149–156.

Kucera, P., Dolivo, M., Coulon, P., and Flamand, A. (1985). Pathways of the early propagation of virulent and avirulent rabies strains from the eye to the brain. *J. Virol.* **55:**158–162.

Kuypers, H. G. J. M., and Ugolini, G. (1990). Viruses as transneuronal tracers. *Trends Neurosci.* **13:**71–75.

Lafay, F., Coulon, P., Astic, L., Saucier, D., Riche, D., Holley, A., and Flamand, A. (1991). Spread of the CVS strain of rabies virus and of the avirulent mutant AvO1 along the olfactory pathways of the mouse after intranasal inoculation. *Virology* **183:**320–330.

Lafon, M. (2005). Rabies virus receptors. *J. Neurovirol.* **11:**82–87.

Lafon, M. (2008). Immune evasion, a critical strategy for rabies virus. *Dev. Biol. (Basel)* **131:**413–419.

Laurent, A. M., Madjar, J. J., and Greco, A. (1998). Translational control of viral and host protein synthesis during the course of herpes simplex virus type 1 infection: Evidence that initiation of translation is the limiting step. *J. Gen. Virol.* **79:**2765–2775.

Lawson, K. F., Black, J. G., Charlton, K. M., Johnston, D. H., and Rhodes, A. J. (1987). Safety and immunogenicity of a vaccine bait containing ERA strain of attenuated rabies virus. *Can. J. Vet. Res.* **51:**460–464.

Lentz, T. L., Burrage, T. G., Smith, A. L., Crick, J., and Tignor, G. H. (1982). Is the acetylcholine receptor a rabies virus receptor? *Science* **215:**182–184.

Loewy, A. D. (1995). Pseudorabies virus: A transneuronal tracer for neuroanatomical studies. *In* "Viral Vectors: Gene Therapy and Neuroscience Applications" (M. Keplitt and A. D. Loewy, eds.), pp. 349–366. Academic Press, New York.

Lycke, E., and Tsiang, H. (1987). Rabies virus infection of cultured rat sensory neurons. *J. Virol.* **61:**2733–2741.

Martin, X., and Dolivo, M. (1983). Neuronal and transneuronal tracing in the trigeminal system of the rat using the herpes virus suis. *Brain Res.* **273:**253–276.

Mazarakis, N. D., Azzouz, M., Rohll, J. B., Ellard, F. M., Wilkes, F. J., Olsen, A. L., Carter, E. E., Barber, R. D., Baban, D. F., Kingsman, S. M., Kingsman, A. J., O'Malley, K., *et al.* (2001). Rabies virus glycoprotein pseudotyping of lentiviral vectors enables retrograde axonal transport and access to the nervous system after peripheral delivery. *Hum. Mol. Genet.* **10:**2109–2121.

Mebatsion, T. (2001). Extensive attenuation of rabies virus by simultaneously modifying the dynein light chain binding site in the P protein and replacing Arg333 in the G protein. *J. Virol.* **75:**11496–11502.

Mebatsion, T., Konig, M., and Conzelmann, K. K. (1996a). Budding of rabies virus particles in the absence of the spike glycoprotein. *Cell* **84:**941–951.

Mebatsion, T., Schnell, M. J., Cox, J. H., Finke, S., and Conzelmann, K. K. (1996b). Highly stable expression of a foreign gene from rabies virus vectors. *Proc. Natl. Acad. Sci. USA* **93:**7310–7314.

Mitrabhakdi, E., Shuangshoti, S., Wannakrairot, P., Lewis, R. A., Susuki, K., Laothamatas, J., and Hemachudha, T. (2005). Difference in neuropathogenetic mechanisms in human furious and paralytic rabies. *J. Neurol. Sci.* **238:**3–10.

Miyachi, S., Lu, X., Inoue, S., Iwasaki, T., Koike, S., Nambu, A., and Takada, M. (2005). Organization of multisynaptic inputs from prefrontal cortex to primary motor cortex as revealed by retrograde transneuronal transport of rabies virus. *J. Neurosci.* **25:**2547–2556.

Miyachi, S., Lu, X., Imanishi, M., Sawada, K., Nambu, A., and Takada, M. (2006). Somatotopically arranged inputs from putamen and subthalamic nucleus to primary motor cortex. *Neurosci. Res.* **56:**300–308.

Morcuende, S., Delgado-García, J. M., and Ugolini, G. (2002). Neuronal premotor networks involved in eyelid responses: Retrograde transneuronal tracing with rabies virus from the orbicularis oculi muscle in the rat. *J. Neurosci.* **22:**8808–8818.

Morecraft, R. J., Ugolini, G., Lanciego, J. L., Wouterlood, F. G., and Pandya, D. N. (2009). Classic and contemporary neural tract tracing techniques. *In* "Imaging Brain Pathways-Diffusion MRI: From Quantitative Measurement to In-Vivo Neuroanatomy" (H. Johansen-Berg and T. Behrens, eds.), pp. 273–308. Academic Press, Elsevier, Amsterdam.

Morimoto, K., Patel, M., Corisdeo, S., Hooper, D. C., Fu, Z. F., Rupprecht, C. E., Koprowski, H., and Dietzschold, B. (1996). Characterization of a unique variant of bat rabies virus responsible for newly emerging human cases in North America. *Proc. Natl. Acad. Sci. USA* **93:**5653–5658.

Morimoto, K., Hooper, D. C., Carbaugh, H., Fu, Z. F., Koprowski, H., and Dietzschold, B. (1998). Rabies virus quasispecies: Implications for pathogenesis. *Proc. Natl. Acad. Sci. USA* **95:**3152–3156.

Morimoto, K., Hooper, D. C., Spitsin, S., Koprowski, H., and Dietzschold, B. (1999). Pathogenicity of different rabies virus variants inversely correlates with apoptosis and rabies virus glycoprotein expression in infected primary neuron cultures. *J. Virol.* **73:**510–518.

Morrison, L. A. (2004). The Toll of herpes simplex virus infection. *Trends Microbiol.* **12:**353–356.

Moschovakis, A. K., Gregoriou, G. G., Ugolini, G., Doldan, M., Graf, W., Guldin, W., Hadjidimitrakis, K., and Savaki, H. E. (2004). Oculomotor areas of the primate frontal lobes: A transneuronal transfer of rabies virus and [14C]-2-deoxyglucose functional imaging study. *J. Neurosci.* **24:**5726–5740.

Murphy, F. A., and Bauer, S. P. (1974). Early street rabies virus infection in striated muscle and later progression to the central nervous system. *Intervirology* **3:**256–268.

Nilsson, M. R., Sugay, W., Pasqualin, O. L., and Muller, S. B. K. (1968). Rabies diagnosis. Comparative study on susceptibility of adult and sucking mice. *Arq. Inst. Biol. (Sao Paulo)* **35:**43–47.

Ohara, S., Inoue, K., Yamada, M., Yamawaki, T., Koganezawa, N., Tsutsui, K., Witter, M. P., and Iijima, T. (2009). Dual transneuronal tracing in the rat entorhinal-hippocampal circuit by intracerebral injection of recombinant rabies virus vectors. *Front. Neuroanat.* **3:**1.

Plotkin, S. A. (2000). Rabies. *Clin. Infect. Dis.* **30:**4–12.

Prevosto, V., Ugolini, G., Isom, S., and Graf, W. (2006). Differences in ascending vestibular, eye position and somatosensory input to medial (MIP/VIPm) and lateral (VIPl/LIPv) intraparietal areas, revealed by retrograde transneuronal transfer of rabies virus. Program No. 242.18/K12, 2006 Neuroscience Meeting Planner. Atlanta, GA: Society for Neuroscience, 2006. Online.

Prevosto, V., Graf, W., and Ugolini, G. (2009). Posterior parietal cortex areas MIP and LIPv receive eye position and velocity inputs via ascending preposito-thalamo-cortical pathways. *Eur. J. Neurosci.* **30:**1151–1161.

Prevosto, V., Graf, W., and Ugolini, G. (2010). Cerebellar inputs to intraparietal cortex areas LIP and MIP: Functional frameworks for adaptive control of eye movements, reaching, and arm/eye/head movement coordination. *Cereb. Cortex* **20:**214–228.

Prosniak, M., Hooper, D. C., Dietzschold, B., and Koprowski, H. (2001). Effect of rabies virus infection on gene expression in mouse brain. *Proc. Natl. Acad. Sci. USA* **98:**2758–2763.

Prosniak, M., Zborek, A., Scott, G. S., Roy, A., Phares, T. W., Koprowski, H., and Hooper, D. C. (2003). Differential expression of growth factors at the cellular level in virus-infected brain. *Proc. Natl. Acad. Sci. USA* **100:**6765–6770.

Pulmanausahakul, R., Li, J., Schnell, M. J., and Dietzschold, B. (2008). The glycoprotein and the matrix protein of rabies virus affect pathogenicity by regulating viral replication and facilitating cell-to-cell spread. *J. Virol.* **82:**2330–2338.

Rathelot, J. A., and Strick, P. L. (2006). Muscle representation in the macaque motor cortex: An anatomical perspective. *Proc. Natl. Acad. Sci. USA* **103:**8257–8262.

Rathelot, J. A., and Strick, P. L. (2009). Subdivisions of primary motor cortex based on corticomotoneuronal cells. *Proc. Natl. Acad. Sci. USA* **106:**918–923.

Raux, H., Flamand, A., and Blondel, D. (2000). Interaction of the rabies virus P protein with the LC8 dynein light chain. *J. Virol.* **74:**10212–10216.

Reske, A., Pollara, G., Krummenacher, C., Chain, B. M., and Katz, D. R. (2007). Understanding HSV-1 entry glycoproteins. *Rev. Med. Virol.* **17:**205–215.

Rinaman, L., Card, J. P., and Enquist, L. W. (1993). Spatiotemporal responses of astrocytes, ramified microglia, and brain macrophages to central neuronal infection with pseudorabies virus. *J. Neurosci.* **13:**685–702.

Rotto-Percelay, D. M., Wheeler, J. G., Osorio, F. A., Platt, K. B., and Loewy, A. D. (1992). Transneuronal labeling of spinal interneurons and sympathetic preganglionic neurons after pseudorabies virus injections in the rat medial gastrocnemius muscle. *Brain Res.* **574:**291–306.

Ruigrok, T. J., Pijpers, A., Goedknegt-Sabel, E., and Coulon, P. (2008). Multiple cerebellar zones are involved in the control of individual muscles: A retrograde transneuronal tracing study with rabies virus in the rat. *Eur. J. Neurosci.* **28:**181–200.

Rupprecht, C. E., and Hemachudha, T. (2004). Rabies. *In* "Infections of the Central Nervous System" (M. Scheld, R. J. Whitley, and C. Marra, eds.), 3rd edn. pp. 243–259. Lippincott, Williams & Wilkins, Philadelphia.

Sabin, A. B. (1938). Progression of different nasally instilled viruses along different nervous pathways in the same host. *Proc. Soc. Exp. Biol. Med.* **38:**270–275.

Sacramento, D., Badrane, H., Bourhy, H., and Tordo, N. (1992). Molecular epidemiology of rabies virus in France: Comparison with vaccine strains. *J. Gen. Virol.* **73:**1149–1158.

Salin, P., Castle, M., Kachidian, P., Barroso-Chinea, P., López, I. P., Rico, A. J., Kerkerian-Le Goff, L., Coulon, P., and Lanciego, J. L. (2008). High-resolution neuroanatomical tract-tracing for the analysis of striatal microcircuits. *Brain Res.* **1221:**49–58.

Salin, P., López, I. P., Kachidian, P., Barroso-Chinea, P., Rico, A. J., Gómez-Bautista, V., Coulon, P., Kerkerian-Le Goff, L., and Lanciego, J. L. (2009). Changes to interneuron-driven striatal microcircuits in a rat model of Parkinson's disease. *Neurobiol. Dis.* **34:**545–552.

Schnell, M. J., Tan, G. S., and Dietzschold, B. (2005). The application of reverse genetics technology in the study of rabies virus (RV) pathogenesis and for the development of novel RV vaccines. *J. Neurovirol.* **11:**76–81.

Schnell, M. J., McGettigan, J. P., Wirblich, C., and Papaneri, A. (2010). The cell biology of rabies virus: Using stealth to reach the brain. *Nat. Rev. Microbiol.* **8:**51–61.

Seif, I., Coulon, P., Rollin, P. E., and Flamand, A. (1985). Rabies virulence: Effect on pathogenicity and sequence characterization of rabies virus mutations affecting antigenic site III of the glycoprotein. *J. Virol.* **53:**926–934.

Shankar, V., Dietzschold, B., and Koprowski, H. (1991). Direct entry of rabies virus into the central nervous system without prior local replication. *J. Virol.* **65:**2736–2738.

Sheikh, K. A., Ramos-Alvarez, M., Jackson, A. C., Li, C. Y., Asbury, A. K., and Griffin, J. W. (2005). Overlap of pathology in paralytic rabies and axonal Guillain-Barré syndrome. *Ann. Neurol.* **57:**768–772.

Smart, N. L., and Charlton, K. M. (1992). The distribution of challenge virus standard rabies virus versus skunk street rabies virus in the brains of experimentally infected rabid skunks. *Acta Neuropathol.* **84:**501–508.

Smith, J. S., Yager, P. A., and Baer, G. M. (1973). A rapid reproducible test for determining rabies neutralizing antibody. *Bull. World Health Organ.* **48:**535–541.

Smith, R. W., Malik, P., and Clements, J. B. (2005). The herpes simplex virus ICP27 protein: A multifunctional post-transcriptional regulator of gene expression. *Biochem. Soc. Trans.* **33:**499–501.

Standish, A., Enquist, L. W., and Schwaber, J. S. (1994). Innervation of the heart and its central medullary origin defined by viral tracing. *Science* **263:**232–234.

Strack, A. M., and Loewy, A. D. (1990). Pseudorabies virus: A highly specific transneuronal cell body marker in the sympathetic nervous system. *J. Neurosci.* **10:**2139–2147.

Superti, F., Hauttecoeur, B., Morelec, M. J., Goldoni, P., Bizzini, B., and Tsiang, H. (1986). Involvement of gangliosides in rabies virus infection. *J. Gen. Virol.* **67:**47–56.

Tan, G. S., Preuss, M. A., Williams, J. C., and Schnell, M. J. (2007). The dynein light chain 8 binding motif of rabies virus phosphoprotein promotes efficient viral transcription. *Proc. Natl. Acad. Sci. USA* **104:**7229–7234.

Tang, Y., Rampin, O., Giuliano, F., and Ugolini, G. (1999). Spinal and brain circuits to motoneurons of the bulbospongiosus muscle: Retrograde transneuronal tracing with rabies virus. *J. Comp. Neurol.* **414:**167–192.

Thoulouze, M. I., Lafage, M., Schachner, M., Hartmann, U., Cremer, H., and Lafon, M. (1998). The neural cell adhesion molecule is a receptor for rabies virus. *J. Virol.* **72:**7181–7190.

Tsiang, H. (1979). Evidence for an intraaxonal transport of fixed and street rabies virus. *J. Neuropathol. Exp. Neurol.* **38:**286–299.

Tsiang, H., Ceccaldi, P. E., and Lycke, E. (1991). Rabies virus infection and transport in human sensory dorsal root ganglia neurons. *J. Gen. Virol.* **72:**1191–1194.

Tuffereau, C., Bénéjean, J., Blondel, D., Kieffer, B., and Flamand, A. (1998). Low-affinity nerve-growth factor receptor (P75NTR) can serve as a receptor for rabies virus. *EMBO J.* **17:**7250–7259.

Tuffereau, C., Schmidt, K., Langevin, C., Lafay, F., Dechant, G., and Koltzenburg, M. (2007). The rabies virus glycoprotein receptor p75NTR is not essential for rabies virus infection. *J. Virol.* **81:**13622–13630.

Ugolini, G. (1992). Transneuronal transfer of Herpes Simplex virus type 1 (HSV 1) from mixed limb nerves to the CNS. I. Sequence of transfer from sensory, motor and sympathetic nerve fibres to the spinal cord. *J. Comp. Neurol.* **326:**527–548.

Ugolini, G. (1995a). Transneuronal tracing with alpha-herpesviruses: A review of the methodology. *In* "Viral Vectors: Gene Therapy and Neuroscience Applications" (M. Keplitt and A. D. Loewy, eds.), pp. 293–317. Academic Press, New York.

Ugolini, G. (1995b). Specificity of rabies virus as a transneuronal tracer of motor networks: Transfer from hypoglossal motoneurones to connected second order and higher order central nervous system cell groups. *J. Comp. Neurol.* **356:**457–480.

Ugolini, G. (1996). Tracing connected neurons with herpes simplex virus type 1. *In* "Protocols for Gene Transfer in Neuroscience: Towards Gene Therapy of Neurological

Disorders" (P. R. Lowenstein and L. W. Enquist, eds.), pp. 349–364. John Wiley & Sons, Chichester.

Ugolini, G. (2008). Use of rabies virus as a transneuronal tracer of neuronal connections: Implications for the understanding of rabies pathogenesis. *Dev. Biol. (Basel)* **131**:493–506.

Ugolini, G. (2010). Advances in viral transneuronal tracing. *J. Neurosci. Methods* **194**:2–20.

Ugolini, G., Kuypers, H. G. J. M., and Simmons, A. (1987). Retrograde transneuronal transfer of Herpes Simplex Virus type 1 (HSV 1) from motoneurones. *Brain Res.* **422**:242–256.

Ugolini, G., Dubayle, D., Grantyn, A., Brandi, A., Berthoz, A., Büttner-Ennever, J., Moschovakis, A., and Graf, W. (2000). Horizontal eye movement network in primates. II. Polysynaptic input. *Soc. Neurosci. Abstr.* **26**:969(363.6), New Orleans, LA.

Ugolini, G., Klam, F., Doldan Dans, M., Dubayle, D., Brandi, A. M., Büttner-Ennever, J., and Graf, W. (2006). Horizontal eye movement networks in primates as revealed by retrograde transneuronal transfer of rabies virus: Differences in monosynaptic input to 'slow' and 'fast' abducens motoneurons. *J. Comp. Neurol.* **498**:762–785.

Vidy, A., El Bougrini, J., Chelbi-Alix, M. K., and Blondel, D. (2007). The nucleocytoplasmic rabies virus P protein counteracts interferon signaling by inhibiting both nuclear accumulation and DNA binding of STAT1. *J. Virol.* **81**:4255–4263.

Wickersham, I. R., Finke, S., Conzelmann, K. K., and Callaway, E. M. (2007). Retrograde neuronal tracing with a deletion-mutant rabies virus. *Nat. Methods* **4**:47–49.

Wunner, W. H. (2002). Rabies virus. *In* "Rabies" (A. C. Jackson and W. H. Wunner, eds.), pp. 25–77. Academic Press, San Diego.

Wunner, W. H., and Dietzschold, B. (1987). Rabies virus infection: Genetic mutations and the impact on viral pathogenicity and immunity. *Contrib. Microbiol. Immunol.* **8**:103–124.

CHAPTER 11

Molecular Phylogenetics of the Lyssaviruses—Insights from a Coalescent Approach

Susan A. Nadin-Davis* and **Leslie A. Real[†]**

Contents			

Abstract   Technical improvements over the past 2 decades have enormously facilitated the generation of nucleotide sequence data for lyssavirus collections. These databases are amenable to methods of phylogenetic analysis, which attempt to define the taxonomic structure of this genus and predict the evolutionary relationships of current circulating strains. Coupled with a range of mathematical tools to explore the appropriateness of nucleotide substitution models and test for positive selection, the evolutionary process is

* Centre of Expertise for Rabies, Ottawa Laboratory Fallowfield, Canadian Food Inspection Agency, Ottawa, Ontario, Canada
† Department of Biology and Center for Disease Ecology, Emory University, Atlanta, Georgia, USA

Advances in Virus Research, Volume 79
ISSN 0065-3527, DOI: 10.1016/B978-0-12-387040-7.00011-1

being explored in detail. Despite the potential for high viral mutation levels, the operation of purifying selection appears to effectively constrain lyssavirus evolution. The recent development of
coalescent theory has provided additional approaches to data
analysis whereby the time frame of emergence of viral lineages
can be most reliably estimated. Such studies suggest that all currently circulating rabies viruses have emerged within the past
1500 years. Moreover, through the capability of analyzing viral
population dynamics and determining patterns of population size
variation, coalescent approaches can provide insight into the
demographics of viral outbreaks. Whereas human-assisted movement of reservoir host species has clearly facilitated transfer of
rabies between continents, topographical landscape features significantly influence the rate and extent of contiguous disease
spread. Together with empirical studies on virus diversity, the
application of coalescent approaches will help to better understand lyssavirus emergence, evolution, and spread. In particular,
such methods are presently facilitating exploration of the factors
operating to limit the ability of lyssaviruses to establish new persistent virus–host associations and ultimately control the emergence of new species of this genus.

I. INTRODUCTION

The development of the polymerase chain reaction (PCR), which allows
the rapid amplification of virtually any targeted segment of nucleic acid
(Saiki *et al.*, 1988), together with improved methods for generation of
nucleotide sequence data, have revolutionized the field of molecular
epidemiology. Such developments have been of special importance to
the characterization of many classes of viruses including the lyssaviruses,
as the extensive literature on this subject attests (reviewed by Nadin-
Davis, 2007).

More recently, advances in the mathematical approaches to sequence
data analysis have provided the means to discern greater insights into the
processes that generate current viral diversity. Much of the current theory
of phylogenetic reconstruction is based on the "coalescent," first introduced in the 1980s by Kingman (2000). Coalescent theory is a retrospec-
tive mathematical analysis tracing the ancestry of alleles within a given
population back to their most recent common ancestor (MRCA). The
point at which two lineages share a common ancestor is the point at
which these two lineages "coalesce," and the structure of the entire phylogenetic tree is revealed through knowledge of the location and timing of all
coalescent points emanating from a given ancient ancestor. If the accumulation of allelic or molecular variation adheres to a constant rate (the

"molecular clock"), then the time, as well as the state of the MRCA, can be derived. In particular, when the dates of samples are known, then both maximum likelihood (ML) and Bayesian methods can be used to estimate nucleotide substitution rates and to calculate the time to the most recent common ancestor (TMRCA) of clades (Drummond and Rambaut, 2007; Drummond et al., 2002; Rambaut, 2000). Recent theory has facilitated development of genetic analysis software to extend earlier analysis to include relaxed clock (nonconstant rate) estimation of coalescent structure (Drummond et al., 2006). However, many RNA viruses appear to adhere to an almost constant clock-like rate of molecular substitution (Biek et al., 2007), and the use of strict clock coalescent analysis has been very effectively used in a variety of RNA viral diseases (Holmes, 2009).

In addition to predicting time frames of lineage emergence, coalescent methods of phylogenetic analysis can explore the population dynamics of viral outbreaks. A basic tenet of population genetics theory is that the amount of genetic heterogeneity present in a population scales with the effective population size. The larger the effective population, the greater will be the magnitude of extant genetic variation. In an expanding and growing population in which the effective population size is large, it will take more time for any sample of sequences to coalesce into a common ancestor; the smaller the population, the less time to converge to an MRCA. Consequently, knowledge of evolutionary rates and the temporal pattern of coalescent times can be used to estimate changing effective population sizes over time. Such patterns of population size variation are revealed through the construction of the "Skyline Plot" (Drummond et al., 2005) and have been used to analyze the demography of several important viral epidemics both within natural populations (Biek et al., 2007) and within individual patients (Pybus et al., 2001, 2005).

This chapter will focus on the application of such methods to the analysis of the large lyssavirus sequence databases that have been accumulated in efforts to provide greater insights into lyssavirus diversity, spread, evolution, and host adaptation.

II. LYSSAVIRUS PHYLOGENY

As Rhabdoviruses in the order Mononegavirales, members of the *Lyssavirus* genus are, from a phylogenetic standpoint, rather simple viruses. They have a relatively small (12 kb) nonsegmented negative-sense RNA genome that encodes just five genes as illustrated in Fig. 1 (and reviewed by Wunner, 2007). Moreover, observations to date suggest that the *Rhabdoviridae* family does not undergo recombination to any significant degree (Chare et al., 2003). While it has been known for some time that the extent of nucleotide sequence variation between lyssaviruses can vary widely along

G-L
noncoding
region

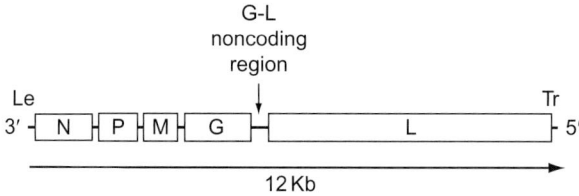

FIGURE 1 *A schematic diagram showing the organization of the 12 kb Pasteur Virus strain of the rabies virus genome (GenBank Accession M13215).* A leader (Le) sequence of 58 nucleotides (nt) at the 3′ terminus is followed by five genes that encode viral proteins thus: N (nucleoprotein), P (phosphoprotein), M (matrix protein), G (glycoprotein), and L (polymerase), The five genes are separated by very short intergenic regions with the exception of the relatively long noncoding region between the G and L genes. A 70 nucleotide trailer (Tr) occurs at the 5′ terminus. Other lyssaviruses exhibit only very minor deviations in size along the length of the genome.

the length of the genome (Delmas *et al.*, 2008; Le Mercier *et al.*, 1997), studies that have compared the utility of different genes for generating phylogenetic trees find that in general similar tree topologies are produced regardless of the genomic region employed (Bourhy *et al.*, 2008; Johnson *et al.*, 2002; Wu *et al.*, 2007). One notable exception was a study examining bat rabies virus (RABV) diversity in which different gene regions predicted rather different tree topologies, perhaps as a result of limitations in representation of certain data sets (Davis *et al.*, 2006). The length of the region targeted will depend in large degree on the purpose of the study. Studies which seek to explore viral variation within sympatric reservoir hosts within a defined spatial area often use partial or complete gene sequence data, usually targeting *N* or *G* genes, to discriminate between closely related viral lineages or strains for surveillance purposes. Studies seeking to classify the entire genus into meaningful groups or to understand more fundamental aspects of virus evolution may use several complete gene sequences if not entire genome sequences.

Both serological and genetic methods of viral characterization have been used to classify the lyssaviruses. On the basis, in particular, of their *N* gene diversity they were, until recently, divided into seven genotypes (see Nadin-Davis, 2007) representing classical RABV as well as six groups of related viruses thus: Lagos Bat virus (LBV), Mokola virus (MOKV), Duvenhage virus (DUVV), European bat lyssaviruses (EBLVs) types 1 and 2, and Australian Bat Lyssavirus (ABLV). All but MOKV were associated with bat species of the Old World or Australia and indeed the role of bats in harboring most present lyssavirus species suggests that the primordial lyssavirus was a bat-associated virus that jumped the species barrier to become associated with terrestrial species during emergence of the RABV lineage (Badrane and Tordo, 2001). These seven genotypes were divided into two phylogroups according to their reported distinct properties of pathogenicity and immunogenicity (Badrane *et al.*, 2001). The more recent discovery of four additional lyssaviruses associated with bats of Eurasia (Kuzmin *et al.*, 2003, 2008a) complicated this taxonomic scheme, making it more difficult to define a threshold of genetic distance that would represent meaningful differences between groups of viruses so as to develop a rational and systematic means of lyssavirus classification. Comparison of the use of all five coding regions for this purpose led to the suggestion that an identity threshold for the complete *N* gene of 82% be considered (Kuzmin *et al.*, 2005, 2008a). Thus viruses having genetic identities across this locus of <82% would be considered to belong to distinct groups. On this basis, the lyssavirus genus is currently divided into 11 distinct species (Table I). However, other studies on collections of the LBV group suggest that, on the basis of these current guidelines, this species should be divided into two distinct species (Delmas *et al.*, 2008; Markotter *et al.*, 2008). Indeed, yet another species has been proposed based on the isolation and sequence characterization of a virus designated Shimoni bat virus (SHIBV; Kuzmin *et al.*, 2010). Again, while this virus, recovered from an insectivorous bat in Kenya, was phylogenetically most similar to the LBV group, it is sufficiently distant genetically to be considered an independent species. Attempts to employ sequence data from other genomic regions yields less convincing patterns since intra- and intergenotypic identity values often overlap. In an alternative approach, the use of concatenated sequence data covering the entire genome may be of some value (Delmas *et al.*, 2008).

One compounding problem with the current classification scheme is that it is based on highly variable numbers of isolates within each species. Thus, of the 11 currently defined species, four (ARAV, KHUV, IRKV, and WCBV) are known by just a single isolate while the other species are represented by anywhere from a few (DUVV) to thousands (RABV) of isolates. It can be anticipated that as additional lyssaviruses are recovered from around the globe, intergroup differences may be further blurred and the current classification scheme may have to be refined so as to best represent the degree of diversity represented by this genus.

III. LYSSAVIRUS PHYLOGEOGRAPHY

It is a principal tenet of lyssavirus biology that although most mammals are susceptible to infection by any lyssavirus, each viral strain is associated with and maintained by a reservoir host. Viral infection of a species that does not normally maintain that virus, referred to as a spillover infection, occurs fairly frequently, but it rarely results in spread of the virus within the new species and thus lyssaviruses are considered to be host adapted at some level (see Section IV). As a result, physical landscape

TABLE I Members of the *Lyssavirus* genus

Lyssavirus species	Abbreviation	Phylogroup	Host reservoir	Range
Rabies virus (prototype)	RABV	1	Mammalian carnivores and bats	Worldwide, except for Australia, Antarctica, and a few island nations[a]
Aravan virus	ARAV	1	Bats	Eurasia
Australian bat lyssavirus	ABLV	1	Pteropid and insectivorous bats	Australia
Duvenhage virus	DUVV	1	Insectivorous bats	Africa
European bat lyssavirus 1	EBLV-1	1	Insectivorous bats	Europe
European bat lyssavirus 2	EBLV-2	1	Insectivorous bats	Europe
Irkut virus	IRKV	1	Bats	Eurasia
Khujand virus	KHUV	1	Bats	Eurasia
Lagos bat virus	LBV	2	Frugivorous bats	Africa
Mokola virus	MOKV	2	Unknown—possibly small mammals	Africa
West Caucasian Bat virus	WCBV	2	Bats	Eurasia
Shimoni bat virus (tentative)	SHIBV	2	Insectivorous bat	Kenya

[a] Several western European countries have recently been declared free of rabies.

features (e.g., large rivers, mountain ranges) that limit spatial spread of a reservoir host or which act to subdivide the host into distinct subpopulations will limit the spread of any virus that it harbors. The only means by which the virus can overcome this limitation is to adapt to a new host. Indeed, for those lyssavirus species for which significant numbers of virus specimens have been genetically characterized, the viruses do exhibit pronounced phylogeographical patterns.

A. Rabies virus

By far the most extensive investigations have been performed on members of the RABV species since this is the virus most frequently encountered both in animals and humans. Using sequence data on several genomic targets (N, G, and P genes and the noncoding G-L region) from hundreds of specimens from around the world, a clear picture of the extent of RABV diversity and phylogeny has emerged (see Badrane and Tordo, 2001; Bourhy et al., 2008; Kissi et al., 1995; Nadin-Davis et al., 2002). An example of such an analysis using selected representative N gene sequences, as summarized in Table II, is illustrated in Fig. 2. RABVs can be grouped into seven major clades designated according to their geographical distribution as follows: "American indigenous," which includes all viruses associated with insectivorous and hematophagous bats of the Americas as well as a small number of viral strains associated with nonflying mammals; "India" including mostly dog viruses from southern India and Sri Lanka; "Asia," comprising dog viruses from China and the countries of southeast Asia, the Philippines, and Indonesia; "Africa 2," canid viruses from western and central Africa; "Africa 3," viruses of the mongoose biotype of southern Africa; "Arctic-related," viruses harbored by red and arctic foxes from circumpolar areas of the northern hemisphere as well as by dogs in several countries of central/western Asia; the "Cosmopolitan" group that is widely distributed across Africa, the Americas, the Middle east, and parts of Europe.

Some early studies employed fairly simplistic approaches to apply time lines to these phylogenies. By applying a single nucleotide substitution rate to all clades, Badrane and Tordo (2001) estimated that carnivore RABVs emerged between 888 and 1459 years ago while TMRCA of the cosmopolitan lineage was dated to 284–504 years ago. In contrast, Holmes et al. (2002) used case surveillance data on the European red fox lineage to estimate rates of synonymous and nonsynonymous mutations for this group and then applied these values to place timescales onto RABV phylogenies; such analyses suggested that the entire diversity of the RABV had occurred within the past 500 years. However, this assumes that the rate of synonymous change does not vary among species.

TABLE II Summary of the sources of sequence data used to construct the phylogenetic tree shown in Fig. 2

Species	Country	Isolate designation	Lineage	Reference or source	GenBank accession no.
RABV	Bosnia (formerly Yugoslavia)	8653.YOU	COSMOPOLITAN	Bourhy et al. (2008)	U42704
RABV	Brazil	DR.BRZ	AMERICAN INDIGENOUS	Nadin-Davis et al. (2010)	AF351847
RABV	Burkina Faso	8636.HAV	AFRICA 2	Kissi et al. (1995)	U22486
RABV	Cambodia	9916.CBG	ASIA	Bourhy et al. (2008)	EU086171
RABV	Cameroon	8801.CAM	AFRICA 2	Kissi et al. (1995)	U22634
RABV	Canada	783T3ON.CAN	ARCTIC	Nadin-Davis et al. (1993)	L20675
RABV	Canada	867SK.CAN	COSMOPOLITAN	Nadin-Davis et al. (1997)	AF344306
RABV	Canada	4055T5.CAN	ARCTIC	Nadin-Davis et al. (1994)	U03770
RABV	Canada	EF31.CAN	AMERICAN INDIGENOUS	Nadin-Davis et al. (2001)	AF351831
RABV	Canada	LAN12.CAN	AMERICAN INDIGENOUS	Nadin-Davis et al. (2001)	AF351840
RABV	Chile	VO13.CH	AMERICAN INDIGENOUS	Nadin-Davis et al. (2001)	AF351850
RABV	China	02046.CHI	ASIA	Bourhy et al. (2008)	EU086182
RABV	China	02045.CHI	ASIA	Bourhy et al. (2008)	EU086181
RABV	Colombia	CO1-04.COL	COSMOPOLITAN	Bourhy et al. (2008)	EU086161
RABV	Estonia	RD9342.EST	COSMOPOLITAN	Bourhy et al. (2008)	U43432
RABV	Ethiopia	8807.ETH	COSMOPOLITAN	Kissi et al. (1995)	U22637
RABV	France	9147.FRA	COSMOPOLITAN	Kissi et al. (1995)	U22474
RABV	French Guiana	9001.GUY	AMERICAN INDIGENOUS	Kissi et al. (1995)	U22478

RABV	Germany	9202.ALL	COSMOPOLITAN	Bourhy et al. (2008)	U42701
RABV	Guinea	9024.GUI	AFRICA 2	Kissi et al. (1995)	U22641
RABV	India	AF374721.IN	INDIA	Jayakumar et al. (2004)	AF374721
RABV	India	RV61.IN	ARCTIC-LIKE	Kuzmin et al. (2004)	AY352493
RABV	Indonesia	03003.IND	ASIA	Bourhy et al. (2008)	EU086192
RABV	Iran	V685.IRN	COSMOPOLITAN	Nadin-Davis et al. (2003)	AY854580
RABV	Iran	V704.IRN	ARCTIC-LIKE	Nadin-Davis et al. (2003)	DQ521212
RABV	Israel	YA6530.ISL	COSMOPOLITAN	David et al. (2007)	DQ837485
RABV	Laboratory strain	PV	COSMOPOLITAN	Tordo et al. (1986)	M13215
RABV	Laboratory strain	SAD-Bern	COSMOPOLITAN	Geue et al. (2008)	EF206708
RABV	Mexico	V587.MEX	AMERICAN INDIGENOUS	Nadin-Davis and Loza-Rubio (2006)	AY854587
RABV	Mexico	V590.MEX	COSMOPOLITAN	Nadin-Davis and Loza-Rubio (2006)	AY854589
RABV	Morocco	9107.MAR	COSMOPOLITAN	Kissi et al. (1995)	U22852
RABV	Mozambique	8631.MOZ	COSMOPOLITAN	Kissi et al. (1995)	U22484
RABV	Myanmar	9909.BIR	ASIA	Bourhy et al. (2008)	EU086164
RABV	Namibia	SN0080.NAM	AFRICA 3	Van Zyl et al. (2010)	FJ392392
RABV	Nepal	9903.NEP	ARCTIC-LIKE	Bourhy et al. (2008)	EU086198
RABV	Nigeria	V461.NIG	AFRICA 2	Nadin-Davis (2007)	AY854600
RABV	Pakistan	196p.PAK	ARCTIC-LIKE	Kuzmin et al. (2004)	AY352495
RABV	Peru	PEHM3230.PR	AMERICAN INDIGENOUS	Warner et al. (1999)	AF045166
RABV	Philippines	94273.PHI	ASIA	Bourhy et al. (2008)	EU086201
RABV	Poland	8618.POL	COSMOPOLITAN	Kissi et al. (1995)	U22840
RABV	Republic S. Africa	32-02.AFS	AFRICA 3	Van Zyl et al. (2010)	FJ392371
RABV	Republic S. Africa	381-06.AFS	AFRICA 3	Van Zyl et al. (2010)	FJ392380

(continued)

TABLE II (*continued*)

Species	Country	Isolate designation	Lineage	Reference or source	GenBank accession no.
RABV	Republic S. Africa	669.90.AFS	AFRICA 3	Van Zyl et al. (2010)	FJ392385
RABV	Republic S. Africa	1500.AFS	AFRICA 3	Kissi et al. (1995)	U22628
RABV	Republic S. Africa	8721.AFS	COSMOPOLITAN	Kissi et al. (1995)	U22633
RABV	Russia	9141.RUS	ARCTIC	Kissi et al. (1995)	U22656
RABV	Saudi Arabia	8706.ARS	COSMOPOLITAN	Kissi et al. (1995)	U22481
RABV	Siberia (Yakutia)	SG19.YAK	ARCTIC	Kuzmin et al. (2008b)	EF611829
RABV	Sri Lanka	1077.SRL	INDIA	Arai et al. (2001)	AB041967
RABV	Tanzania	9221.TAN	COSMOPOLITAN	Kissi et al. (1995)	U22645
RABV	Thailand	8738.THA	ASIA	Kissi et al. (1995)	U22653
RABV	Trinidad	V325DR.TD	AMERICAN INDIGENOUS	Nadin-Davis et al. (2001)	AF351852
RABV	USA, AL	A7007AL.US	ARCTIC	Kuzmin et al. (2008b)	EF611841
RABV	USA, AL	A7033AL.US	ARCTIC	Kuzmin et al. (2008b)	EF611845
RABV	USA, AZ	EF4862AZ.US	AMERICAN INDIGENOUS	Smith et al. Unpublished	AY170397
RABV	USA, CA	LC814CA.US	AMERICAN INDIGENOUS	Smith et al. Unpublished	AF394883
RABV	USA, FL	V125RFL.US	AMERICAN INDIGENOUS	Nadin-Davis et al. (1997)	U27220
RABV	USA, PA	EF136PA.US	AMERICAN INDIGENOUS	Smith et al. Unpublished	AY039226
RABV	USA, TX	CY2204TX.US	COSMOPOLITAN	Velasco-Villa et al. (2008)	FJ228529

RABV	USA, TX	V212SKTX.US	AMERICAN INDIGENOUS	Nadin-Davis et al. Unpublished	EU345003
RABV	USA, TX	TB01TX.US	AMERICAN INDIGENOUS	Nadin-Davis et al. (2001)	AF351849
RABV	USA, WA	MC2847WA.US	AMERICAN INDIGENOUS	Smith et al. Unpublished	AF394872
RABV	Zimbabwe	22107.ZIM	AFRICA 3	Van Zyl et al. (2010)	FJ392391

Nonrabies lyssaviruses

ABLV	Australia	ABLVFF.AUS		Gould et al. (1998)	AF006497
ABLV	Australia	ABLVIB.AUS		Gould et al. (2002)	AF081020
ARAV	Kyrgizstan	ARAV.KYR		Kuzmin et al. (2003)	AY262023
EBLV1	France	EBLV1.FRA		Bourhy et al. (1992)	U22845
EBLV1	Poland	EBLV1.POL		Bourhy et al. (1992)	U22844
EBLV2	Finland	EBLV2.FIN		Bourhy et al. (1992)	U22846
EBLV2	The Netherlands	EBLV2.NTH		Bourhy et al. (1992)	U22847
KHUV	Tajikistan	KHUV.TAJ		Kuzmin et al. (2003)	AY262024
IRKV	Russia	IRKV.RUS		Kuzmin et al. (2005)	AY333112
DUVV	Republic S. Africa	DUVV1.AFS		Bourhy et al. (1993)	U22848
DUVV	Republic S. Africa	DUVV2.AFS		Delmas et al. (2008)	EU293120
LBV	Ethiopia	LBV.ETH		Mebatsion et al. (1993)	AY333110
LBV	Nigeria	LBV.NIG		Bourhy et al. (1993)	U22842
MOKV	Ethiopia	MOKV.ETH		Mebatsion et al. (1993)	AY333111
MOKV	Zimbabwe	MOKV.ZIM		Bourhy et al. (1993)	U22843
SHIBV	Kenya	SHIBV.KYA		Kuzmin et al. (2010)	GU170201
WCBV	Russia	WCBV.RUS		Kuzmin et al. (2005)	AY333113

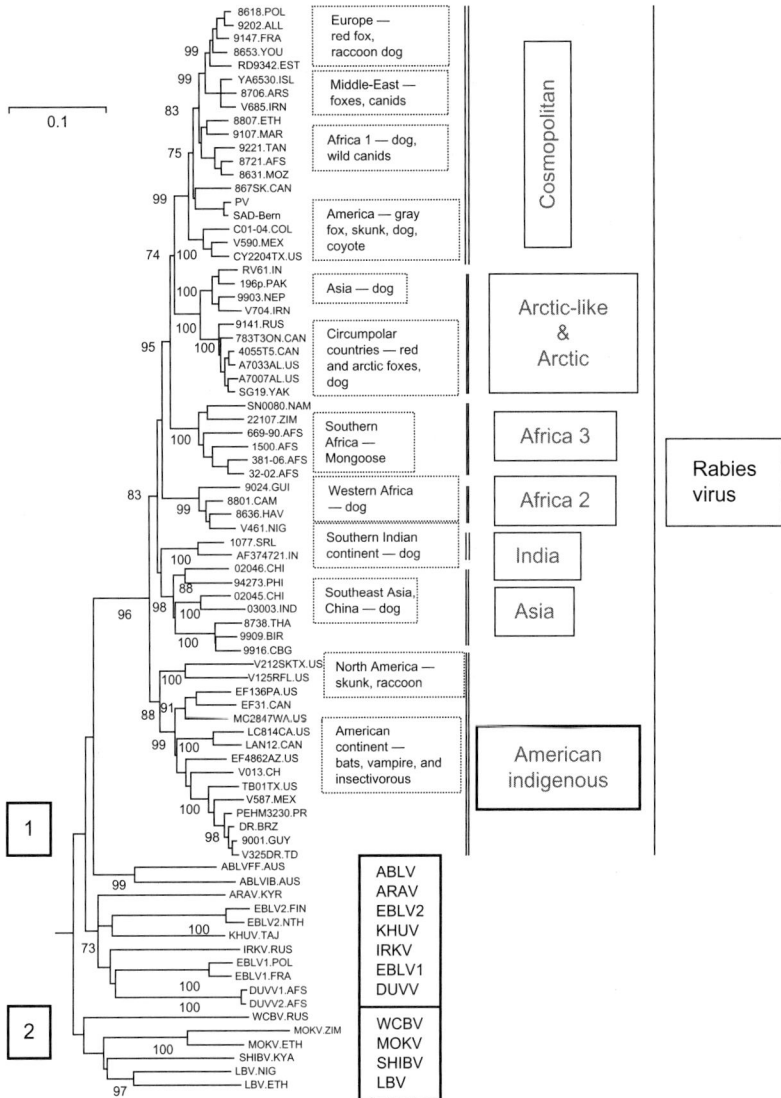

FIGURE 2 *A phylogenetic analysis of 80 viral isolates representative of known lyssavirus diversity.* The phylogenetic tree was generated from an alignment of complete *N* gene coding sequences (1350 bases) produced using the CLUSTALX package (available from http://www.clustal.org/) and analyzed by the neighbor joining method implemented in MEGA version 4 software (available from http://www.megasoftware.net/). The *N* gene sequence of the vesicular stomatitis virus (Indiana subtype) was used as an outgroup (branch not shown). Subdivision of the genus into its two phylogroups is shown in the boxes at bottom left. Species assignments of all clades are shown to the far right of the figure with inclusion of the tentative new species SHIBV. The subdivision of the rabies virus species into seven established viral clades is also indicated thus: Cosmopolitan,

More recently, the application of ML and Bayesian coalescent approaches to analyze lyssavirus nucleotide sequence data provides more robust methods for estimating nucleotide substitution rates and their use for time-line predictions. The substitution rate (number of nucleotide substitutions/site/year) has been reported for a range of strains and genomic targets (Table III). In general, estimates for the substitution rate for RABV-coding regions range from 1×10^{-4} to 4×10^{-4} with no clear variation according to reservoir host or viral gene targeted although some G genes (e.g., the mongoose G gene with a value of 6.875×10^{-4}) did yield rather higher values. Rates for the noncoding G-L region tend to be higher (0.777×10^{-3} to 1.676×10^{-3}) doubtless due to the relaxed constraints on this segment of the genome. Such values are in line with estimates made on other RNA viruses (Belshaw et al., 2008; Drake, 1993). Using these rates of nucleotide substitution, the time of emergence of many lyssavirus lineages has been estimated. Thus, Bourhy et al. (2008) estimated that based on N gene data, TMRCA of all RABVs existed 749 years ago (with a 95% highest posterior density (95% HPD) range of 363–1215 years); an even shorter time period of 583 years ago (95% HPD 222–1116) was estimated using G gene data. Further, again using N gene data, Bourhy et al (2008) estimated that TMRCA for the nonflying mammal-associated viruses circulated 761 years ago (95% HPD of 373–1222 years), a date very close to that calculated for the entire RABV clade. The conclusion was that emergence of the two distinct RABV branches that circulate in American bats and terrestrial hosts occurred at around the same time.

1. Rabies virus lineages

a. India clade   The highly divergent Indian clade (Nanayakkara et al., 2003), which is harbored by dogs, has the most basal position of all RABV lineages associated with nonflying mammals; on this basis, it has been proposed that the ancestor of this clade may have been the progenitor for all RABV lineages except for the American indigenous lineage (Bourhy et al., 2008).

Arctic/Arctic-like, Africa 2, Africa 3, India, Asia, and American indigenous. To the left of each clade name, the countries affected and the main reservoir species are indicated. The scale in the upper left corner depicts the genetic distances represented by all horizontal lines in the tree. Bootstrap values >70%, which strongly support the illustrated branch patterns, are shown either below or to the left of many major branch points. The country of origin of each isolate employed in this analysis is indicated by a two or three letter suffix as indicated in Table II together with additional source information.

TABLE III Estimated nucleotide substitution rates for various lyssaviruses

Species/clade/lineage	Gene target	Nucleotide substitution rate Mean (and 95% HPD range)	Reference
RABV			
All lineages	N	2.3×10^{-4} ($1.1\text{-}3.6 \times 10^{-4}$)	Bourhy et al. (2008)
All lineages	G	3.9×10^{-4} ($1.2\text{-}6.5 \times 10^{-4}$)	Bourhy et al. (2008)
ASIA	G	3.24×10^{-4} ($2.17\text{-}4.36 \times 10^{-4}$)	Gong et al.(2010)
ASIA	G	3.96×10^{-4} ($2.17\text{-}5.99 \times 10^{-4}$)	Ming et al.(2010)
COSMOPOLITAN	N	2.7×10^{-4} ($1.8\text{-}3.7 \times 10^{-4}$)	David et al. (2007)
COSMOPOLITAN (European red fox strain)	N	3.89×10^{-4} ($0.51\text{-}6.70 \times 10^{-4}$)	Kuzmin et al. (2008b)
COSMOPOLITAN (Africa 1)	G-L	16.8×10^{-4} ($6.9\text{-}28.0 \times 10^{-4}$)	Davis et al. (2007)
AFRICA 2	N	3.82×10^{-4} ($2.62\text{-}5.02 \times 10^{-4}$)	Talbi et al. (2009)
AFRICA 2	G	3.25×10^{-4} ($2.22\text{-}4.32 \times 10^{-4}$)	Talbi et al. (2009)
AFRICA 3	N	2.50×10^{-4} ($1.36\text{-}3.76 \times 10^{-4}$)	Van Zyl et al. (2010)
AFRICA 3	G	6.88×10^{-4} ($5.18\text{-}8.51 \times 10^{-4}$)	Van Zyl et al. (2010)
AFRICA 3	G-L	8.26×10^{-4} ($1.49\text{-}15.12 \times 10^{-4}$)	Davis et al. (2007)
ARCTIC-RELATED	N	1.23×10^{-4} ($0.68\text{-}1.83 \times 10^{-4}$)	Kuzmin et al. (2008b)
ARCTIC-RELATED (Ontario fox strain)	G	3.64×10^{-4} ($3.24\text{-}4.04 \times 10^{-4}$)	Real et al. (2005)
AMERICAN INDIGENOUS (Bat strains)	N, P	$2.5\text{-}4.0 \times 10^{-4}$	Davis et al. (2006)
AMERICAN INDIGENOUS (Bat strains)	N	2.32×10^{-4}	Hughes et al. (2005)
AMERICAN INDIGENOUS (Big brown bat strains)	P	1.77×10^{-4}	Nadin-Davis et al. (2010)
AMERICAN INDIGENOUS (Raccoon strain)	G-L	7.77×10^{-4} ($7.69\text{-}7.85 \times 10^{-4}$)	Szanto et al. (2010)
AMERICAN INDIGENOUS (Raccoon strain)	G, N	2.9×10^{-4}	Biek et al. (2007)
EBLV			
EBLV-1	N	0.61×10^{-4} ($0.114\text{-}1.09 \times 10^{-4}$)[a]	Davis et al. (2005)
EBLV-1	G	0.51×10^{-4} ($0.03\text{-}0.92 \times 10^{-4}$)[a]	Davis et al. (2005)
EBLV-1	N	1.1×10^{-4}[b]	Hughes (2008)

[a] Using strict molecular clock.
[b] Using relaxed molecular clock.

b. Asia clade The large heterogeneous Asia clade, estimated variously to have emerged from an MRCA around 1412 (95% HPD 1006–1736; Ming *et al.*, 2010) or around 1654 (95% HPD 1514–1812; Gong *et al.*, 2010), is widely distributed across much of this continent and can be subdivided into a number of regionally localized subgroups (Bourhy *et al.*, 2008; Ito *et al.*, 1999), many of which have been identified in various parts of China (Meng *et al.*, 2007; Zhang *et al.*, 2006, 2009). The dog is the principal reservoir host across the range of this lineage. Phylogenetic studies are consistent with past spread of RABV variants from China to other Asian countries and island nations such as Indonesia and the Philippines during periods of extensive human migration from China (Bourhy *et al.*, 2008; Gong *et al.*, 2010; Nishizono *et al.*, 2002; Susetya *et al.*, 2008). Spatial clustering of viral variants is of course very pronounced in such island nations where human-assisted movements of animals are required for virus spread (Susetya *et al.*, 2008).

c. Cosmopolitan clade The cosmopolitan clade, which includes the group previously referred to as "Africa 1" (Kissi *et al.*, 1995), is believed to have been widely distributed as a result of human-assisted movement of diseased animals from Europe to many parts of the world during colonial activities (Smith *et al.*, 1992; Nadin-Davis and Bingham, 2004). Thus, this clade includes viruses from several parts of the Americas and the Caribbean and large areas of northern, eastern, and southern Africa and those of the Middle East and Europe. In Europe, in recent times, this clade is represented by viruses harbored by the red fox and raccoon dog reservoir species and at least four main clades of viruses associated with these hosts were spatially separated by major rivers and mountain ranges (Bourhy *et al.*, 1999). The emergence of the present European/Middle-eastern variants of this lineage was dated to approximately 1870 (David *et al.*, 2007).

d. Africa 2 clade Examination of the origins of the Africa 2 lineage suggests its introduction into Africa within the past 200 years (TMRCA dated to 1845), a time frame corresponding to a period of extensive colonial activity by Europeans, particularly by the French, in the region (Talbi *et al.*, 2009). This lineage is harbored by canids across western and central Africa. The Sahara desert forms a strong barrier separating this lineage from the Africa 1 lineage that circulates in northern Africa and evidence for an east–west axis of viral spread of the Africa 2 lineage was presented (Talbi *et al.*, 2009). In contrast, another study that explored Bayesian methods for inferring the phylogeographic history of this lineage concluded that the population size of this virus has remained fairly constant over the past 150 years and that it has spread in a continuous manner with little overall directionality, thereby confounding efforts to identify the location of its original introduction into this region of Africa (Lemey *et al.*, 2009).

e. Africa 3 clade   The mongoose lineage of southern Africa (Africa 3) comprises a rather heterogeneous group of viruses that exhibit strong phylogeographical structure with subdivision into five spatially separate subclades (Nel *et al.*, 2005; Van Zyl *et al.*, 2010). Estimates of TMRCA for this lineage range quite widely depending on the gene targeted as well as the data set and assumptions applied. Using sequences of the G-L inter-genic region, Davis *et al.* (2007) estimated TMRCA for this entire lineage at 73 years, 95% HPD 55–181. Van Zyl *et al.* (2010) obtained values varying from 229 years, 95% HPD 135–360 (*N* gene data), to 159 years, 95% HPD 119–202 (*G* gene data). In this study, it was noted that the different ages predicted by these analyses reflect differences in the rates of nucleotide substitution calculated for the three databases; mean values for the rates of nucleotide substitutions were 2.495×10^{-4} (*N* gene), 6.875×10^{-4} (*G* gene), and 0.826×10^{-3} (G-L intergenic region). Thus, the more con-served the genetic region and the lower the nucleotide substitution rate, the greater the age estimate for the lineage, a feature also observed by Bourhy *et al.* (2008) and that will need to be resolved in future studies. Based on a comparative study using G-L sequences of canid RABV in southern Africa, which yielded a mean age for TMRCA of just 30 years, it is clear that the mongoose lineage is the most ancient RABV of the area. Considering anecdotal case records that suggest rabies was present in wildlife of the area in the late 1700s, Van Zyl *et al.* (2010) suggest that the mongoose lineage emerged from a canid RABV that was brought into South Africa during a period of extensive human migration well before the introduction of the cosmopolitan lineage into this region of Africa.

A comparison of the population dynamics of these two distinct RABV variants using a relaxed molecular clock suggested that mongoose RABVs evolve more slowly than those associated with canids (mean evolutionary rates of 0.826 and 1.676×10^{-3}, respectively, for the G-L region). This observation suggests the importance of employing relaxed molecular clocks when examining viruses from multiple host species, whereas when studying viruses within a species, this consideration may be less important. Moreover, this same study revealed that canid RABV popula-tion size has remained fairly constant since being introduced into the area in the 1940s, while the mongoose viral biotype has grown exponentially with a mean epidemic doubling time of about 5 years (Davis *et al.*, 2007). The different population dynamics of these two lineages may be due in part to differences in rabies control efforts in the two hosts; some limited dog rabies control was attempted in the early period of this epizootic while no control was ever instigated for the mongoose reservoir. Differ-ences in host ecology could also of course have impacted viral spread and evolution of the two lineages. The mongoose lives underground in close-knit communities with limited intergroup contact, while dogs and wild canids are less restricted in their movements and contacts (Davis et al., 2007).

f. Arctic-related clade   The existence of a group of distinct viruses that circulated in several countries of northern climes had been known for some time and was referred to as arctic rabies (reviewed by Crandell, 1991), but only relatively recently, with the genetic characterization of several specimens from parts of Asia, including Nepal, India, Pakistan, Korea, and Inner Mongolia as well as the Middle East, was the true extent of this lineage realized (Hyun et al., 2005; Kuzmin et al., 2004; Mansfield et al., 2006; Nadin-Davis et al., 2003; Shao et al., 2011). Given its geographical distribution, it has now come to be referred to more accurately as the arctic-related or arctic-like lineage. Phylogenetic analysis suggested the basal position of samples from India within this clade (Nadin-Davis et al., 2007), thus suggesting that the entire lineage had evolved from Indian dog viruses. Subsequent coalescent studies identified two arctic-like clades from the Middle East and the Indian subcontinent (Arctic-like-1) and eastern Asia (Arctic-like-2) as well as four arctic clades (Arctic-1 to 4) distributed across different ranges of the polar and northern regions (Kuzmin et al., 2008b). The date of TMRCA for the entire lineage was estimated to range between 1255 and 1786, with the Arctic-like-2 clade diverging first followed by the Arctic-like-1 clade; this lineage, in turn, apparently spread northward to spawn the emergence of the true arctic viruses. In North America, this lineage has frequently spread southward in the red fox host into southern populated regions of Canada and such an incursion was well documented in the mid to late 1950s (Tabel et al., 1974). This outbreak entered the province of Ontario, with two distinct waves of infection responsible for populating the eastern and southwestern regions of the province, and caused an epizootic that persisted well into the 1990s until rabies control measures were implemented. Subsequent genetic characterization of viruses collected in the early 1990s identified four main N gene variants across the affected zone (Nadin-Davis et al., 1993) with even further variation identified by G gene analysis (Nadin-Davis et al., 1999). It was speculated that the pattern of variation observed might be due to localized viral drift and/or adaptation as a result of fox host population subdivision by waterways and other landscape features. Later reanalysis of these viral variants showed how their spatial distribution reflected the historical movement of rabies into the area and that the observed patterns of viral variation could be explained by a model based solely on isolation by distance (Real et al., 2005). The MRCA of the Ontario fox strain was estimated to have occurred at around year 1960 in fairly close concordance with the surveillance records.

g. American indigenous clade   This clade, which has often been designated the American bat clade, is more accurately referred to as the
American indigenous clade since it includes not only all bat viruses of
the Americas, but also strains associated with skunks (south central skunk
strain of the southern United States and Mexican skunk strain), raccoons
in eastern North America, and a marmoset species in Brazil (Favoretto
et al., 2001). However, the bat variants form the deepest roots of this clade
suggesting that all of these strains emerged directly or indirectly from a
bat-associated progenitor. Such speculation is supported by the recent
emergence of a new RABV–skunk association following a species jump of
a big brown bat variant to this new host (Leslie *et al.*, 2006). Throughout
the continent, several different viral lineages are associated with particular species of insectivorous bats (de Mattos *et al.*, 2000; Kuzmin and
Rupprecht, 2007; Nadin-Davis *et al.*, 2001; Oliveira *et al.*, 2010; Velasco-
Villa *et al.*, 2006), whereas in Latin America, the viruses associated with
vampire bats (*Desmodus rotundus*) frequently spillover into livestock species and cause large economic losses. In Brazil, the vampire bat strain has
been reported to exhibit strong geographical partitioning according to the
topography of various mountain ranges; this phylogeographic effect was
explained by the limitation that higher ground elevation exerts on vampire bat range (Kobayashi *et al.*, 2008). In Canada, examination of the
distribution of RABV variants associated with the big brown bat found
that several variants were restricted to particular geographical areas with
the Rocky Mountain range in the west forming a significant barrier to both
host and virus dispersal (Nadin-Davis *et al.*, 2010). This study identified
five main viral lineages and demonstrated that recent increases in population size of the lineage were due primarily to the emergence of a
relatively new variant that had spread rapidly across much of the host's
range. TMRCA for these viruses was dated to around 1573 (Fig. 3; Nadin-
Davis *et al.*, 2010), whereas in contrast, a U.S. study dated this progenitor
to the early 1800s and suggested moreover that the diversity of all American bat variants arose from a common progenitor around the mid 1600s
(Hughes *et al.*, 2005). This latter estimate would appear to be inconsistent
with the timescale presented by Bourhy *et al.* (2008) for global RABV
emergence, but the reasons for these discrepancies are unclear.

The raccoon rabies virus (RRABV) strain originally emerged in Florida
with the first reported cases in the 1940s and was subsequently translocated to West Virginia through movement of diseased animals, resulting
in the emergence of the mid-Atlantic strain which was identified in the
early 1970s. Since then it has spread throughout the eastern seaboard of
the United States. Dating of viral phylogenies generated from various
regions of the genome accurately estimated the original emergence of this
lineage in Florida to 1946 (Szanto *et al.*, 2011) and the year of origin of the
mid-Atlantic variant of this strain to 1973 (Biek *et al.*, 2007), dates that

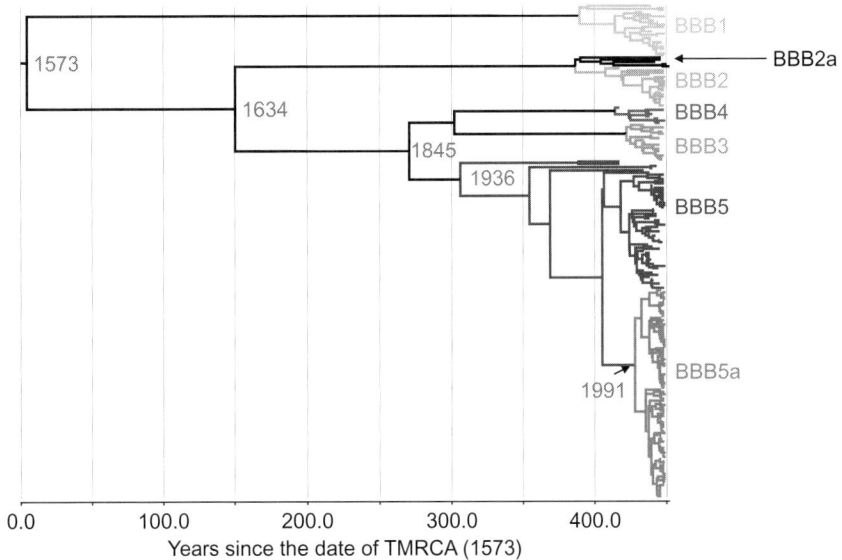

FIGURE 3 *A maximum clade credibility tree generated by partial P gene sequences of the five main viral variants (BBB1 to BBB5) associated with the big brown bat host in Canada.* The tree, slightly modified from that shown in Nadin-Davis *et al.* (2010), was generated by the BEAST software package using a relaxed molecular clock. The estimated mean value for TMRCA is shown to the right of each major branch. Divergence of each lineage occurred in relatively recent times, as illustrated in particular by the BBB5a subgroup that is restricted spatially to Ontario and its provincial borders, and which emerged around the year 1991.

agree well with the surveillance case reports. Moreover, the latter study examined the evolution of the RRABV strain over a 30-year period and demonstrated the validity of using coalescent approaches for exploring viral population history (Biek *et al.*, 2007), a feat that was possible because of the relatively recent emergence of this strain, the availability of extensive epidemiological data for this epizootic, and the fortunate availability of historical viral samples collected from different time points during the course of epidemic expansion that were amenable to nucleotide sequencing. The authors identified seven genetic lineages within the mid-Atlantic strain and showed how each radiated from the first reported cases in West Virginia. Once an area was colonized by a lineage, it persisted within that area. Using sequence data from isolates representing each lineage, it was possible to estimate total numbers of RRABV infections during the course of the epizootic. The data suggested that, rather than a uniform increase, there had been periods of exponential growth followed by periods of population size stasis (Fig. 4). These predictions, as determined by the coalescent approach, matched well with the epidemiological data on the

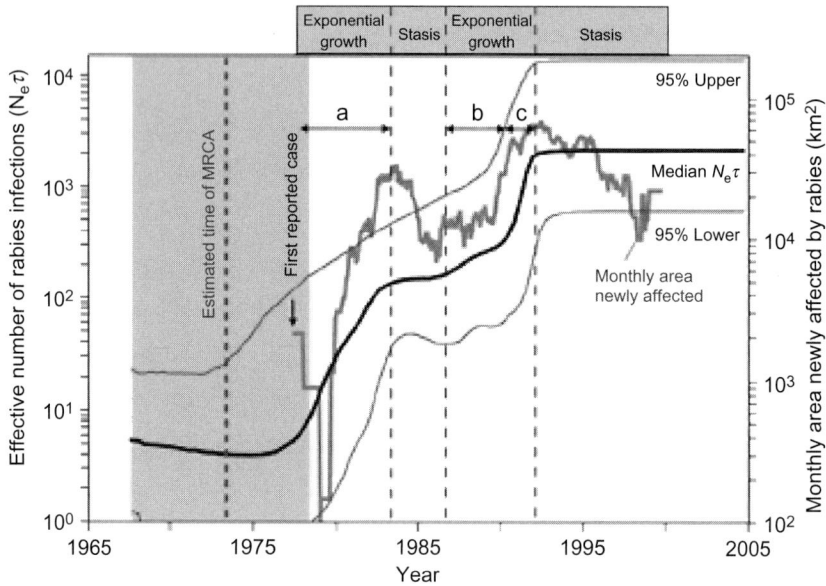

FIGURE 4 *Number of RRABV infections, 1977–2005, estimated from genetic and case data.* Median effective number of RRABV infections (thick black line) was estimated by using a Bayesian skyline plot and represents the product of effective population size (N_e) and generation time (ι) in years. Thin black lines represent 95% highest posterior density (HPD) intervals. Estimated time associated with the most recent common ancestor is indicated by a dashed line with the HPD interval shown as a shaded area. The line identified as "monthly area newly affected" represents the 15-month moving average of the monthly area (in km²) newly affected by RRABV between 1977 and 1999 as an index of the number of rabid raccoons through time.

temporal and spatial expansion of the epizootic with periods of reduced diffusion corresponding to the time at which the wave front of epidemic expansion reached major mountain ranges (i.e., the Allegheny and the Adirondack Mountains). The inference from this study is that the demographic history of a RABV outbreak can be inferred from the genetic signature of its viral variants and that the revealed ecological dynamics can uncover landscape barriers to spread or highlight the effectiveness of spatially specific control strategies, including oral rabies vaccination (ORV) delivery (Biek and Real, 2010). Similar inferences have emerged through study of other RNA viruses (Pybus and Rambaut, 2009).

2. Central role of the dog in spreading RABV

With the exception of the American indigenous clade, it is notable that the dog is the main reservoir host for many RABV clades, including the more basal clades that circulate in India and Asia. While many viral strains are specifically associated with other species of the Canidae and with other carnivore hosts, their lineages are generally interspersed with various dog-associated lineages; this is true for both the arctic-related clade and particularly for the cosmopolitan clade, which includes RABVs that are maintained in a variety of reservoir hosts (foxes, skunks, dogs, mongoose populations of several Caribbean islands, and several other wild canids, possibly including jackals and wolves). This suggests that the emergence of the RABV progenitor was closely associated with dogs, in keeping with the public association of rabies and mad dogs, but that spillover transmissions to other species does, on rare occasions, result in new self-perpetuating virus–host associations. Several regional studies have reported viral phylogenies most consistent with the emergence of RABV strains in wildlife following successful species jumps from dogs. Examples include the emergence of red fox rabies in Europe in the 1930s (Bourhy et al., 1999) and more recently in Turkey (Johnson et al., 2003), the origins of fox rabies in Colombia (Páez et al., 2005) and Brazil (Bernardi et al., 2005; Carnieli et al., 2008), and the emergence in South Africa of distinct rabies lineages in bat-eared foxes (Sabeta et al., 2007) and jackals (Zulu et al., 2009). Despite the many instances of viruses making successful species jumps, the rate of success of this process is relatively low compared to the number of intraspecific virus transmissions. Factors that may limit the success rate of such jumps are addressed in Section IV.

3. Mechanisms of RABV spread

The global study of RABV phylogeny by Bourhy et al. (2008) identified strong population subdivision according to geographical region for most lineages with viral spread occurring mostly across geographically neighboring regions. Two main modes of virus dissemination were discerned: (i) human-assisted migration (e.g., from the Kazakhstan/Russia region to Canada and Greenland, and from China to the Philippines and Indonesia); (ii) viral dispersal by gradual spatial spread of the virus through intraspecific transmission (e.g., canid RABV movements within Africa). Indeed, in many instances, the observed RABV phylogenetic patterns appear to reflect a mixture of human-assisted introduction followed by gradual viral dispersal within its host, with physical landscape features such as mountain ranges, deserts, and large water masses such as rivers and lakes, influencing spread through their effects on reservoir host population structure.

Where surveillance records document the emergence and spread of particular RABV lineages, it has generally been observed that phylogenetic data of current circulating viruses can accurately estimate the time frame of emergence of a specific strain. Undoubtedly as time lines get longer, their 95% confidence range will increase and some inconsistencies have emerged (e.g., American bat lineage). Nevertheless, it is notable that the time frame of emergence of all RABVs currently in circulation appears to stretch over less than a millennium.

B. EBLVs

EBLV-1, which is harbored by the serotine bat, *Eptesicus serotinus*, is the most widespread bat lyssavirus in Europe. It clusters into two phylogenetically distinct subgroups that occupy largely overlapping ranges (Davis *et al.*, 2005). Interestingly, EBLV-1a viruses originating from Germany, the Netherlands, and Denmark showed no geographical clustering, indicating relative ease of movement of host and virus across this region of Europe, whereas French and eastern European samples of this strain were more divergent. The EBLV-1b group, in contrast, exhibited greater genetic diversity and much stronger phylogeographic structure with isolates from specific countries tending to cluster together and those from France forming a basal group. These data suggested a north–south axis of spread of EBLV-1b in western Europe and an east–west axis of spread for EBLV-1a in northern Europe.

With estimated mean values of 5–6×10^{-5} for N and G genes, the EBLV-1 species was reported to exhibit significantly lower substitution rates than RABVs (Davis *et al.*, 2005) and it was argued that the ecology of the reservoir host and the potential existence of nonclinical host carriers might place especially high constraints on these viruses. However, reanalysis of these data using a relaxed molecular clock in place of the strict clock implemented in the original study generated an EBLV-1 substitution rate estimate of 1.1×10^{-4}, a value more in line with that of other lyssaviruses (Hughes, 2008). Since the value of the nucleotide substitution rate directly influences the length of the time line for a group of sequences, optimal estimation of this value through use of the appropriate molecular clock becomes important. TMRCA for the EBLV-1 lineage was estimated to have circulated between 500 and 750 years ago (Davis *et al.*, 2005) or 70 and 300 years ago depending on the substitution rate employed (Hughes, 2008).

Isolates of EBLV-2 have been recovered from two bat species, *Myotis dasycneme* and *Myotis daubentonii*, in several European countries, but more detailed phylogeographic analysis of this virus must await recovery of more specimens.

C. ABLV

Interestingly, the ABLV species is associated with two distinct reservoir hosts, Pteropid bats (flying foxes) of the megachiroptera and insectivorous bats. While viruses of these two biotypes are clearly separate populations that appear to be distributed across the range of their respective hosts, within each host, the viruses exhibit very limited diversity, perhaps an indication that these two lineages have emerged independently, but relatively recently from a common ancestor (Guyatt et al., 2003). Possible candidates include putative bat lyssaviruses of the Philippines, which to date are proposed to exist based solely on serological information (Arguin et al., 2002). Similarly, serological evidence has suggested the circulation of viruses related to ABLV or those from Eurasia in bats on the Asian mainland (Kuzmin et al., 2006; Lumlertdacha et al., 2005; Reynes et al., 2004), but to date no viral specimens have been recovered for genetic analysis.

D. African nonrabies lyssaviruses

Despite relatively limited numbers of isolations of both MOKV and LBV across Africa, it is recognized that different regions of Africa harbor distinct strains of these two viruses (Markotter et al., 2008; Nel et al., 2000). The host reservoir for MOKV is unknown with isolations of this species having been made primarily from shrews and domestic animals, whereas frugivorous bats are believed to harbor LBV. Very few isolates of DUVV, thought to be harbored by insectivorous bats, have been made. These have come mostly from southern Africa where the virus exhibits high levels of genetic identity (Paweska et al., 2006), whereas a single isolate that originated from Kenya was more divergent (Van Thiel et al., 2009). Since it appears that all the RABV lineages currently circulating in Africa (Africa 1, 2, and 3) were all introduced at various times from different European sources, the LBV, MOKV, and DUVV species, together with the proposed SHIBV species, which is currently known by a single isolate from a bat in Kenya (Kuzmin et al., 2010), are probably the only true indigenous lyssaviruses on this continent. However, examination of these species over a wider geographical area will be needed before a detailed understanding of their phylogeographic patterns can be discerned.

E. Eurasian nonrabies lyssaviruses

The Aravan virus (ARAV) was isolated from a lesser mouse-eared bat (*Myotis blythi*) in southern Kyrgyzstan in 1991, whereas Khujand virus (KHUV) was isolated in 2001 from a whiskered bat (*Myotis mystacinus*) in northern Tajikistan; both were recovered during active surveillance of bat populations in central Asia (Kuzmin et al., 2003). Two other viruses were isolated in 2002; Irkut virus (IRKV) was recovered from a greater tube-nosed bat (*Murina leucogaster*) in the town of Irkutsk in the Baikal lake region of Eastern Siberia, whereas the West Caucasian bat virus (WCBV) originated from a common bent-winged bat (*Miniopterus schreibersi*) from the Krasnador region of Western Russia northeast of the Black Sea (Kuzmin *et al.*, 2005). Serological and phylogenetic analysis of all four viruses have demonstrated the distinct nature of each of these viruses and supported their classification as individual lyssavirus species, but since only single isolates of these viruses have been retrieved to date, their natural host reservoirs and spatial distribution are currently unknown.

IV. LYSSAVIRUS ADAPTATION

A. Viral features

Given that particular strains of lyssaviruses are maintained in specific hosts, there is much interest in better understanding the mechanisms that cause this association. While the ecology and behavioral traits of each reservoir species may facilitate specific virus–host associations, it would seem likely that there are certain molecular features of individual viral strains that enable them to adapt to their hosts. Simple alignments of predicted protein sequences have often identified specific amino acid replacements that are associated with variants that circulate in particular hosts; for example, see Oliveira *et al.* (2010) which describes a study on the diversity of insectivorous bat viruses of South America and which identified several amino acid sequences specific to genus-specific clusters of viruses. However, the challenge is to differentiate functionally important changes from neutral mutations that have arisen within a particular lineage purely by chance. Thus, as is the case for many viruses (Holmes and Drummond, 2007), a clear understanding of the factors that operate to influence the success of lyssavirus host species jumps remains elusive. Due to their high mutation rates, large population sizes, and in some species, the ability to reassort and recombine, RNA viruses often comprise genetically highly variable constellations of sequences. These highly variable populations have been termed quasispecies (Domingo *et al.*, 1985; Eigen and Biebricher, 1988; Holland *et al.*, 1992), but the term has recently become quite controversial. The original formulation of the concept required that selection act on the entire constellation of variable sequences rather than on the fitness of individual sequence variants co-occurring within a given population. Selection on the population of sequences can lead to a reduction in the overall average fitness of viral variants but are maintained at this lower fitness level due to the high mutation rate. The evidence for such population-level selection is weak (Holmes, 2010), but under some conditions, especially in the laboratory, such selection may generate true quasispecies (Lauring and Andino, 2010). Given the ambiguity in the evidence and the confusion over the meaning of the term quasispecies, we prefer to use the more accurate and general measure of population sequence heterogeneity to characterize the genetic structure of viral populations.

Many of the lyssaviruses have been characterized by their levels of genetic sequence variation. Benmansour *et al.* (1992) examined a dog strain of RABV by investigating the genetic diversity of the G gene of the viral population and found significant levels of heterogeneity; moreover, when this virus was passaged in cell culture, changes in the distribution of sequence variants occurred suggesting that the virus was able to readily adapt to a new environment. Another study that examined the genetic variation in the mouse-adapted RABV CVS-24 found that, upon passage in BHK cells, a dominant variant (CVS-B2c), distinct from that of the brain-adapted virus (CVS-N2c), was rapidly selected; this transformation was associated with a number of nonsynonymous G gene mutations and a distinct pathogenicity (Morimoto *et al.*, 1998). Both these studies concluded that the variable nature of RABV promoted the emergence of a minor subpopulation of the original virus to be the dominant population when the virus was subjected to environmental change. The ready emergence of viral variants with the greater fitness for the current situation would suggest that RABV might frequently jump over the host species barrier and form new virus–host associations.

As a follow-up to these studies, Kissi *et al.* (1999) studied the dynamics of RABV mutation and genetic population structure during serial passages of a European fox virus in several heterologous hosts, including mice, cell culture, and domestic animals (dogs and cats). Perhaps a little surprisingly, despite confirmation of the highly variable nature of the virus, in most cases, even after multiple passages, the consensus sequence obtained from several regions of the genome (N, a short segment spanning across the N-P intergenic region, a portion of G and the G-L region) remained unchanged; only one exception to this result was observed in the virus that was passaged through adult mice where a single nonsynonymous mutation was observed. The greatest mutation rates were observed in the mouse-passaged virus with nonsynonymous changes predominating in the G gene. The authors explained their findings by proposing two mechanisms of RABV evolution: a slow accumulation of limited numbers of mutations with retention of the original consensus sequence and rarer rapid selective overgrowth of favored variants suggestive of a positive selection process.

In addition to making the connection between population-level variation and response to selection, modern molecular evolutionary techniques can be used to assess if selection is operating (and even identify specific sites under positive selection) through analysis of the pattern of nucleotide substitutions for a group of viruses (Nei and Kumar, 2004). Methods for identifying such selection rely on the estimation of the rates of synonymous (dS) and nonsynonymous (dN) substitutions; the former type of substitution reflects general genetic drift and neutral evolutionary trends while the latter may, if sufficiently pronounced, indicate positive selective forces.

In contrast to the above laboratory constructed populations, when patterns of nucleotide substitution using dN–dS ratios for RABV field specimens are examined, the evidence for positive selection is very limited. By an ML analysis of N and G gene sequences derived entirely from RABV field specimens collected from around the world, Holmes *et al.* (2002) explored these substitution patterns. Both genes were highly constrained and exhibited a fairly constant dS value between 4 and 5.3×10^{-4} indicative of an overall neutral evolutionary process. For both genes, the overall dN was low compared to several other RNA viruses, with the value for the G gene being approximately twice than that for the N gene (5×10^{-5} vs. 2.85×10^{-5}), an observation that might be interpreted as indicating some localized positive selection on the G gene. Comparison of complete lyssavirus genomes revealed decreasing genetic identities for the five proteins in the order $N > L > M > G > P$ (Delmas *et al.*, 2008) with a fourfold difference in the mean dN/dS ratio between the N and P genes reflecting differences in the selective constraints operating on these proteins. Indeed, studies that compare the best fit of RABV sequence data to various models of nucleotide substitution often support the operation of positive selection (Holmes *et al.*, 2002; Szanto *et al.*, 2008). However, in contrast, the majority of studies of RABV field isolates, at both localized and global levels, have concluded that RABV populations exhibit relatively low genetic diversity, with high dS/dN values indicating a high level of constraint operating across the genome and that purifying selection is the predominant evolutionary process (Bourhy *et al.*, 1999, 2008; Kobayashi *et al.*, 2010). Indeed, a broader-based study on several RNA viruses suggested that purifying selection operates generally on these organisms to remove a high proportion of mutations which are deleterious and normally transient in nature, thereby limiting the extent of viral adaptation (Pybus *et al.*, 2007).

Despite this overall evolutionary trend of purifying selection, the possibility remains that a small number of individual amino acids are important for host adaptation by the virus and several efforts to explore this possibility have been documented by identification of specific codons for which the dN/dS value is >1. By this process, the following residues were identified: (i) position 101 of the N gene (Bourhy *et al.*, 1999); (ii) positions 1, 5, and 175 (Bourhy *et al.*, 1999) and residues 183 and 370 (Holmes *et al.*, 2002) of the G gene (the highly variable 183 residue may impact cell tropism since it is next to antigenic site II within a neurotoxin-like region that may be responsible for binding to the nicotinic acetylcholine receptor, one of many putative RABV receptors); and (iii) position 62 of the L gene (Szanto *et al.*, 2008) as identified for the RRABV strain compared to other RABVs. The significance of these findings remain unclear given that other studies failed to identify positive selection at these sites (e.g., Hughes *et al.*, 2005 in a study on N gene variation of American bat rabies variants).

It has been speculated that the life cycle of RABV, which requires the virus to replicate in a variety of cell types (neurons, muscle tissue, salivary glands) may impose particularly high constraints on the evolution of these viruses. Moreover, viral evasion of host immune responses through sequestration of the virus within the CNS may limit the effect of immune selective pressures on evolution of the RABV glycoprotein, unlike the pressures exerted on surface proteins of other RNA viruses (Holmes *et al.*, 2002).

In terms of their ability to adapt to particular hosts, the influenza A viruses are amongst the most studied group of RNA viruses due to their ability to elicit human pandemics. While the receptor-binding capability of its surface hemagglutinin (HA) protein is clearly important with respect to conferring host specificity and virulence, it is now known that other viral proteins, including the products encoding polymerase functions (e.g., PB2), are also important in this regard (Hatta *et al.*, 2001; Matrosovich *et al.*, 2009). Certain amino acids in both the HA and PB2 proteins were shown to be critical for transmission of the H5N1 avian influenza viruses in mammals (Gao *et al.*, 2009), and activity-enhancing mutations of the viral polymerase complex are reported to mediate adaptation to mammalian hosts (Gabriel *et al.*, 2005).

Despite extensive studies on *G* gene variation within the RABV, to date specific residues that are thought to be important for host adaptation have not yet emerged. Moreover, sequence characterization of the *L* gene that encodes the polymerase product has been performed on relatively few lyssavirus isolates although recent interest in whole genome characterization is now focusing more attention on this gene (see Delmas *et al.*, 2008); a search in GenBank (October 5, 2010) yielded 72 complete genome entries. Given the requirement for the *L* gene product to interact with many host cell factors, it is possible that a few critical residues within this protein could significantly impact viral propagation efficiency within specific hosts and thereby contribute substantially to host adaptation. However, until a more extensive lyssavirus *L* gene database is available, its role in this regard will remain unknown.

B. Impact of host behavior and genetics

Two recent studies have explored the effect of genetic divergence of donor and recipient hosts on the emergence of new virus–host associations. Streicker *et al.* (2010) examined the influence of the host on emergence of the American bat RABVs. Since these RABVs have a phylogenetic structure that closely reflects their reservoir host species, clearly most transmissions occur intraspecifically with occasional host shifts that allow emergence of new lineages. Drawing from sequence data on a large collection of bat RABVs originating from across the United

States, it was estimated that cross-species transmissions occur once for approximately every 73 intraspecies transmission events. However, the vast majority of these cross-species events were evolutionary dead-ends for the virus. The role of bat host ecological overlap in affecting rates of cross-species transmission was explored, but it was concluded that similarity of donor and recipient host species in terms of their evolutionary proximity, and hence conservation of cellular and immunological traits, was the primary factor in determining whether infection took place. Secondary effects impacting the likelihood of physical contact of the two bat species (e.g., roosting habits, feeding preferences) also played some role. In other words, geographic overlap of bat hosts is likely to determine the rate of RABV exposure, while the greater the evolutionary distance between the host species, the lower the frequency of RABV infection. In essence, host phylogenetic distance was identified as the principal constraint limiting cross-species events that might result in a successful host jump with emergence of a new successful virus–host association. Sustained transmission of an RABV in a specific host requires optimal balance of intrahost viral replication and viral shedding in salivary glands, achieved through fine-tuning of the virus's association with cell receptors and the cellular machinery that it employs for propagation and spread. It might thus follow that the amount of viral evolution needed to achieve such an optimal state will be lower for a recipient host that is in evolutionary terms close to the donor host, and host species barriers may often prove to be an insurmountable obstacle to RNA virus emergence despite the intrinsic mutability of these pathogens (Streicker *et al.*, 2010).

In a similar type of study generalized to a comparison among all the bat hosts of the lyssaviruses, Rogawski and Real (unpublished data) characterized the influence of genetic and geographic distance between bat hosts as determinants of successful host jumping among all 11 lyssavirus species. Subsequent to the construction of both lyssavirus and bat host phylogenies, host jumps were identified using TreeMap (Bederson *et al.*, 2002), and genetic distance matrices among hosts and virus were computed. Rogawski and Real compared the genetic distances between hosts and overlap of geographic bat ranges for identified host jumps to the same distances for random pairings of hosts. Eight host jumps were identified to explain the current bat host–virus associations. Genetic similarity between donor and recipient hosts does not appear to constrain successful host jumping, and host jumps occurred between both closely related and more distantly related hosts. The genetic distances between hosts of identified jumps were not significantly smaller than those for random pairings of hosts. Conversely, host jumps were more common between hosts with greater overlapping geographic ranges, and hosts involved in jumps generally shared similar foraging and roosting habitats. While genetic similarity may also have an impact, these results suggest that geographic proximity to new hosts and the number and intensity of contacts between species are the driving factors in host jumping events.

It is important to recognize that these two studies on host jumping analyzed two different data sets at two different scales of genetic relatedness. Streicker *et al.* (2010) examined only the RABV among bat hosts for this particular species of lyssavirus, while Rogawski and Real examined host jumping at the level of the *lyssavirus* genus. It may be a general feature of coevolutionary relationships that propensity for genetic relatedness to constrain host switching deteriorates as one moves to higher levels of taxonomic relationship.

V. CONCLUDING REMARKS

Despite the extensive nucleotide sequence information now available for many lyssavirus isolates, a better understanding of the role played by viral variation in host adaptation will emerge only with the characterization of complete viral genomes, since it remains unclear what residues may impact the ability of the virus to propagate optimally in its preferred host. In this regard, more emphasis on *L* gene characterization is needed. Through its ability to apply time frames to phylogenies and examine viral population dynamics, coalescent methodology is becoming a vital tool for studying lyssavirus emergence and spread. By correlating the information obtained by coalescent investigations with accurate disease surveillance records, insights into the effects of landscape features and host habitat on disease spread can be appreciated. Further, we may glean better understanding of host factors that may impact on emergence of new viral–host associations.

One conundrum revealed by recent estimates of the time line of RABV emergence has become evident through such investigations. The clade comprising all terrestrial RABVs is estimated to have emerged in the past millennium, but this appears to be at odds with the interpretation of historical records suggesting the recognition of a rabies-like disease associated with dogs in ancient times of both Western and Eastern civilizations (Baer, 2007; Wu *et al.*, 2009). If indeed current estimates of the evolutionary time line of all RABVs are accurate, this would require that either the disease interpreted as rabies by historical scholars was actually a different disease or alternatively rabies has emerged in this species independently on at least two occasions with die-off of the lineage responsible for cases recorded over 1500 years ago. Given the dynamic nature of virus–host associations, other lyssavirus lineages are likely to emerge in the future; identifying such outbreaks and responding to their threat in a timely manner will be facilitated by genetic characterization (preferably complete viral genome sequencing) coupled with epidemiological data that together should provide essential insights into viral phylodynamics (Holmes and Grenfell, 2009).

REFERENCES

Arai, Y. T., Takahashi, H., Kameoka, Y., Shiino, T., Wimalaratne, O., and Lodmell, D. L. (2001). Characterization of Sri Lanka rabies virus isolates using nucleotide sequence analysis of nucleoprotein gene. *Acta Virol.* **45**:321–333.

Arguin, P. M., Murray-Lillibridge, K., Miranda, M. E. G., Smith, J. S., Calaor, A. B., and Rupprecht, C. E. (2002). Serologic evidence of Lyssavirus infections among bats, the Philippines. *Emerg. Infect. Dis.* **8**:258–262.

Badrane, H., and Tordo, N. (2001). Host switching in *Lyssavirus* history from the Chiroptera to the Carnivora orders. *J. Virol.* **75**:8096–8104.

Badrane, H., Bahloul, C., Perrin, P., and Tordo, N. (2001). Evidence of two *Lyssavirus* phylogroups with distinct pathogenicity and immunogenicity. *J. Virol.* **75**:3268–3276.

Baer, G. M. (2007). The history of rabies. *In* "Rabies" (A. C. Jackson and W. H. Wunner, eds.), 2nd edn. pp. 1–22. Academic Press, London, UK.

Bederson, B. B., Shneiderman, B., and Wattenberg, M. (2002). Ordered and quantum tree-maps: Making effective use of 2D space to display hierarchies. *ACM Trans. Graph.* **21**:833–854.

Belshaw, R., Gardner, A., Rambaut, A., and Pybus, O. G. (2008). Pacing a small cage: Mutation and RNA viruses. *Trends Ecol. Evol.* **23**:188–193.

Benmansour, A., Brahimi, M., Tuffereau, C., Coulon, P., Lafay, F., and Flamand, A. (1992). Rapid sequence evolution of street rabies glycoprotein is related to the highly heterogeneous nature of the viral population. *Virology* **187**:33–45.

Bernardi, F., Nadin-Davis, S. A., Wandeler, A. I., Armstrong, J., Gomes, A. A. B., Lima, F. S., Nogueira, F. R. B., and Ito, F. H. (2005). Antigenic and genetic characterization of rabies viruses isolated from domestic and wild animals of Brazil identifies the hoary fox as a rabies reservoir. *J. Gen. Virol.* **86**:3153–3162.

Biek, R., and Real, L. A. (2010). The landscape genetics of infectious disease emergence and spread. *Mol. Ecol.* **19**:3515–3531.

Biek, R., Henderson, J. C., Waller, L. A., Rupprecht, C. E., and Real, L. A. (2007). A high-resolution genetic signature of demographic and spatial expansion in epizootic rabies virus. *Proc. Natl. Acad. Sci. USA* **104**:7993–7998.

Bourhy, H., Kissi, B., Lafon, M., Sacramento, D., and Tordo, N. (1992). Antigenic and molecular characterization of bat rabies virus in Europe. *J. Clin. Microbiol.* **30**:2419–2426.

Bourhy, H., Kissi, B., and Tordo, N. (1993). Molecular diversity of the *Lyssvirus* genus. *Virology* **194**:70–81.

Bourhy, H., Kissi, B., Audry, L., Smreczak, M., Sadkowska-Todys, M., Kulonen, K., Tordo, N., Zmudzinski, J. F., and Holmes, E. C. (1999). Ecology and evolution of rabies virus in Europe. *J. Gen. Virol.* **80**:2545–2557.

Bourhy, H., Reynes, J.-M., Dunham, E. J., Dacheux, L., Larrous, F., Huong, V. T. Q., Xu, G., Yan, J., Miranda, M. E. G., and Holmes, E. C. (2008). The origin and phylogeography of dog rabies virus. *J. Gen. Virol.* **89**:2673–2681.

Carnieli, P., Jr., de Oliveira Fahl, W., Castilho, J. G., de Novaes Oliveira, R., Macedo, C. I., Durymanova, E., Jorge, R. S. P., Morato, R. G., Spíndola, R. O., Machado, L. M., de Sá, J. E. U., Carrieri, M. L., *et al.* (2008). Characterization of rabies virus isolates from canids and identification of the main wild canid host in Northeastern Brazil. *Virus Res.* **131**:33–46.

Chare, E. R., Gould, E. A., and Holmes, E. C. (2003). Phylogenetic analysis reveals a low rate of homologous recombination in negative-sense RNA viruses. *J. Gen. Virol.* **84:**2691–2703.

Crandell, R. A. (1991). Arctic fox rabies. *In* "The Natural History of Rabies" (G. M. Baer, ed.), 2nd edn. pp. 291–306. CRC Press, Boca Raton.

David, D., Hughes, G. J., Yakobson, B. A., Davidson, I., Un, H., Aylan, O., Kuzmin, I. V., and Rupprecht, C. E. (2007). Identification of novel canine rabies virus clades in the Middle East and North Africa. *J. Gen. Virol.* **88:**967–980.

Davis, P. L., Holmes, E. C., Larrous, F., Van der Poel, W. H. M., Tjørnehøj, K., Alonso, W. J., and Bourhy, H. (2005). Phylogeography, population dynamics, and molecular evolution of European bat lyssaviruses. *J. Virol.* **79:**10487–10497.

Davis, P. L., Bourhy, H., and Holmes, E. C. (2006). The evolutionary history and dynamics of bat rabies virus. *Infect. Genet. Evol.* **6:**464–473.

Davis, P. L., Rambaut, A., Bourhy, H., and Holmes, E. C. (2007). The evolutionary dynamics of canid and mongoose rabies virus in southern Africa. *Arch. Virol.* **152:**1251–1258.

De Mattos, C. A., Favi, M., Yung, V., Pavletic, C., and De Mattos, C. C. (2000). Bat rabies in urban centers in Chile. *J. Wildl. Dis.* **36:**231–240.

Delmas, O., Holmes, E. C., Talbi, C., Larrous, F., Dacheux, L., Bouchier, C., and Bourhy, H. (2008). Genomic diversity and evolution of the Lyssaviruses. *PLoS ONE* 3(4):e2057.

Domingo, E., Martinez-Salas, E., Sobrino, F., de la Torre, J. C., Portela, A., Ortin, J., Lopez-Galindez, C., Pérez-Brena, P., Villanueva, N., Najera, R., Van de Pol, S., Steinhauer, D., *et al.* (1985). The quasispecies (extremely heterogeneous) nature of viral RNA genome populations: Biological relevance—A review. *Gene* **40:**1–8.

Drake, J. W. (1993). Rates of spontaneous mutations among RNA viruses. *Proc. Natl. Acad. Sci. USA* **90:**4171–4175.

Drummond, A. J., and Rambaut, A. (2007). BEAST: Bayesian evolutionary analysis by sampling trees. *BMC Evol. Biol.* **7:**214.

Drummond, A. J., Nicholls, G. K., Rodrigo, A. G., and Solomon, W. (2002). Estimating mutation parameters, population history and genealogy simultaneously from temporally spaced sequence data. *Genetics* **161:**1307–1320.

Drummond, A. J., Rambaut, A., Shapiro, B., and Pybus, O. G. (2005). Bayesian coalescent inference of past population dynamics from molecular sequences. *Mol. Biol. Evol.* **22:**1185–1192.

Drummond, A. J., Ho, S. Y., Phillips, M. J., and Rambaut, A. (2006). Relaxed phylogenies and dating with confidence. *PLoS Biol.* 4(5):e88.

Eigen, M., and Biebricher, C. K. (1988). Sequence space and quasispecies distribution. *In* "RNA Genetics" (E. Domingo, J. J. Holland, and P. Ahlquist, eds.), Vol. III, pp. 211–245. CRC Press, Boca Raton.

Favoretto, S. R., de Mattos, C. C., Morais, N. B., Araújo, F. A. A., and de Mattos, C. A. (2001). Rabies in marmosets (*Callithrix jacchus*), Ceará, Brazil. *Emerg. Infect. Dis.* **7:**1062–1065.

Gabriel, G., Dauber, B., Wolff, T., Planz, O., Klenk, H.-D., and Stech, J. (2005). The viral polymerase mediates adaptation of an avian influenza virus to a mammalian host. *Proc. Natl. Acad. Sci. USA* **102:**18590–18595.

Gao, Y., Zhang, Y., Shinya, K., Deng, G., Jiang, Y., Li, Z., Guan, Y., Tian, G., Li, Y., Shi, J., Liu, L., Zeng, X., *et al.* (2009). Identification of amino acids in HA and PB2 critical for the transmission of H5N1 avian influenza viruses in a mammalian host. *PLoS Pathog.* 5(12):e1000709.

Geue, L., Schares, S., Schnick, C., Kliemt, J., Beckert, A., Freuling, C., Conraths, F. J., Hoffmann, B., Zanoni, R., Marston, D., McElhinney, L., Johnson, N., *et al.* (2008). Genetic characterisation of attenuated SAD rabies virus strains used for oral vaccination of wildlife. *Vaccine* **26:**3227–3235.

Gong, W., Jiang, Y., Za, Y., Zeng, Z., Shao, M., Fan, J., Sun, Y., Xiong, Z., Yu, X., and Tu, C. (2010). Temporal and spatial dynamics of rabies viruses in China and Southeast Asia. *Virus Res.* **150:**111–118.

Gould, A. R., Hyatt, A. D., Lunt, R., Kattenbelt, J. A., Hengstberger, S., and Blacksell, S. D. (1998). Characterisation of a novel lyssavirus isolated from *Pteropid* bats in Australia. *Virus Res.* **54**:165–187.

Gould, A. R., Kattenbelt, J. A., Gumley, S. G., and Lunt, R. A. (2002). Characterisation of an Australian bat lyssavirus variant isolated from an insectivorous bat. *Virus Res.* **89**:1–28.

Guyatt, K. J., Twin, J., Davis, P., Holmes, E. C., Smith, G. A., Smith, I. L., Mackenzie, J. S., and Young, P. L. (2003). A molecular epidemiological study of Australian bat lyssavirus. *J. Gen. Virol.* **84**:485–495.

Hatta, M., Gao, P., Halfmann, P., and Kawaoka, Y. (2001). Molecular basis for high virulence of Hong Kong H5N1 influenza A viruses. *Science* **293**:1840–1842.

Holland, J. J., de la Torre, J. C., and Steinhauer, D. A. (1992). RNA virus populations as quasispecies. *Curr. Top. Microbiol. Immunol.* **176**:1–21.

Holmes, E. C. (2009). RNA virus genomics: A world of possibilities. *J. Clin. Invest.* **119**:2488–2495.

Holmes, E. C. (2010). The RNA virus quasispecies: Fact or fiction? *J. Mol. Biol.* **400**:271–273.

Holmes, E. C., and Drummond, A. J. (2007). The evolutionary genetics of viral emergence. *Curr. Top. Microbiol. Immunol.* **315**:51–66.

Holmes, E. C., and Grenfell, B. T. (2009). Discovering the phylodynamics of RNA viruses. *PLoS Comput. Biol.* **5**(10):e1000505.

Holmes, E. C., Woelk, C. H., Kassis, R., and Bourhy, H. (2002). Genetic constraints and the adaptive evolution of rabies virus in nature. *Virology* **292**:247–257.

Hughes, G. J. (2008). A reassessment of the emergence time of European bat lyssavirus type 1. *Infect. Genet. Evol.* **8**:820–824.

Hughes, G. J., Orciari, L. A., and Rupprecht, C. E. (2005). Evolutionary timescale of rabies virus adaptation to North American bats inferred from the substitution rate of the nucleoprotein gene. *J. Gen. Virol.* **86**:1467–1474.

Hyun, B.-H., Lee, K.-K., Kim, I.-J., Lee, K.-W., Parl, H.-J., Lee, O.-S., An, S.-H., and Lee, J.-B. (2005). Molecular epidemiology of rabies virus isolates from South Korea. *Virus Res.* **114**:113–125.

Ito, N., Sugiyama, M., Oraveerakul, K., Piyaviriyakul, P., Lumlertdacha, B., Arai, Y. T., Tamura, Y., Mori, Y., and Minamoto, N. (1999). Molecular epidemiology of rabies in Thailand. *Microbiol. Immunol.* **43**:551–559.

Jayakumar, R., Tirumurugaan, K. G., Ganga, G., Kumanan, K., and Mahalinga Nainar, A. (2004). Characterization of nucleoprotein gene sequence of an Indian isolate of rabies virus. *Acta Virol.* **48**:47–50.

Johnson, N., McElhinney, L. M., Smith, J., Lowings, P., and Fooks, A. R. (2002). Phylogenetic comparison of the genus *Lyssavirus* using distal coding sequences of the glycoprotein and nucleoprotein genes. *Arch. Virol.* **147**:2111–2123.

Johnson, N., Black, C., Smith, J., Un, H., McElhinney, L. M., Aylan, O., and Fooks, A. R. (2003). Rabies emergence among foxes in Turkey. *J. Wildl. Dis.* **39**:262–270.

Kingman, J. F. C. (2000). Origins of the coalescent: 1974–1982. *Genetics* **156**:1461–1463.

Kissi, B., Tordo, N., and Bourhy, H. (1995). Genetic polymorphism in the rabies virus nucleoprotein. *Virology* **209**:526–537.

Kissi, B., Badrane, H., Audry, L., Lavenu, A., Tordo, N., Brahimi, M., and Bourhy, H. (1999). Dynamics of rabies virus quasispecies during serial passages in heterologous hosts. *J. Gen. Virol.* **80**:2041–2050.

Kobayashi, Y., Sato, G., Mochizuki, N., Hirano, S., Itou, T., Carvalho, A. A. B., Albas, A., Santos, H. P., Ito, F. H., and Sakai, T. (2008). Molecular and geographic analyses of vampire bat-transmitted cattle rabies in central Brazil. *BMC Vet. Res.* **4**:44.

Kobayashi, Y., Suzuki, Y., Itou, T., Carvalho, A. A., Cunha, E. M., Ito, F. H., Gojobori, T., and Sakai, T. (2010). Low genetic diversities of rabies virus populations within different hosts in Brazil. *Infect. Genet. Evol.* **10**:278–283.

Kuzmin, I. V., and Rupprecht, C. E. (2007). Bat rabies. *In* "Rabies" (A. C. Jackson and W. H. Wunner, eds.), 2nd edn. pp. 259–307. Academic Press, London, UK.

Kuzmin, I. V., Orciari, L. A., Arai, Y. T., Smith, J. S., Hanlon, C. A., Kameoka, Y., and Rupprecht, C. E. (2003). Bat lyssaviruses (Aravan and Khujand) from central Asia: Phylogenetic relationships according to N, P and G gene sequences. *Virus Res.* **97:**65–79.

Kuzmin, I. V., Botvinkin, A. D., McElhinney, L. M., Smith, J. S., Orciari, L. A., Hughes, G. J., Fooks, A. R., and Rupprecht, C. E. (2004). Molecular epidemiology of terrestrial rabies in the former Soviet Union. *J. Wildl. Dis.* **40:**617–631.

Kuzmin, I. V., Hughes, G. J., Botvinkin, A. D., Orciari, L. A., and Rupprecht, C. E. (2005). Phylogenetic relationships of Irkut and West Caucasian bat viruses within the *Lyssavirus* genus and suggested quantitative criteria based on the N gene sequence for lyssavirus genotype definition. *Virus Res.* **111:**28–43.

Kuzmin, I. V., Niezgoda, M., Carroll, D. S., Keeler, N., Hossain, M. J., Breiman, R. F., Ksiazek, G., and Rupprecht, C. E. (2006). Lyssavirus surveillance in bats, Bangladesh. *Emerg. Infect. Dis.* **12:**486–488.

Kuzmin, I. V., Wu, X., Tordo, N., and Rupprecht, C. E. (2008a). Complete genomes of Aravan, Khujand, Irkut and West Caucasian bat viruses, with special attention to the polymerase gene and non-coding regions. *Virus Res.* **136:**81–90.

Kuzmin, I. V., Hughes, G. J., Botvinkin, A. D., Gribencha, S. G., and Rupprecht, C. E. (2008b). Arctic and arctic-like rabies viruses: Distribution, phylogeny and evolutionary history. *Epidemiol. Infect.* **136:**509–519.

Kuzmin, I. V., Mayer, A. E., Niezgoda, M., Markotter, W., Agranda, B., Breiman, R. F., and Rupprecht, C. E. (2010). Shimoni bat virus, a new representative of the *Lyssavirus* genus. *Virus Res.* **149:**197–210.

Lauring, A. S., and Andino, R. (2010). Quasispecies theory and the behaviour of RNA viruses. *PLoS Pathog.* **6**(7):e1001005.

Le Mercier, P., Jacob, Y., and Tordo, N. (1997). The complete Mokola virus genome sequence: Structure of the RNA-dependent RNA polymerase. *J. Gen. Virol.* **78:**1571–1576.

Lemey, P., Rambaut, A., Drummond, A. J., and Suchard, M. A. (2009). Bayesian phylogeography finds its roots. *PLoS Comput. Biol.* **5**(9):e1000520.

Leslie, M. J., Messenger, S., Rohde, R. E., Smith, J., Cheshier, R., Hanlon, C., and Rupprecht, C. E. (2006). Bat-associated rabies virus in skunks. *Emerg. Infect. Dis.* **12:**1274–1277.

Lumlertdacha, B., Boongird, K., Wanghongsa, S., Wacharapluesadee, S., Chanhome, L., Khawplod, P., Hemachudha, T., Kuzmin, I., and Rupprecht, C. E. (2005). Survey for bat lyssaviruses, Thailand. *Emerg. Infect. Dis.* **11:**232–236.

Mansfield, K. L., Racloz, V., McElhinney, L. M., Marston, D. A., Johnson, N., Rønsholt, L., Christensen, L. S., Neuvonen, E., Botvinkin, A. D., Rupprecht, C. E., and Fooks, A. R. (2006). Molecular epidemiological study of Arctic rabies virus isolates from Greenland and comparison with isolates from throughout the Arctic and Baltic regions. *Virus Res.* **116:**1–10.

Markotter, W., Kuzmin, I., Rupprecht, C. E., and Nel, L. H. (2008). Phylogeny of Lagos bat virus: Challenges for lyssavirus taxonomy. *Virus Res.* **135:**10–21.

Matrosovich, M., Stech, J., and Klenk, H. D. (2009). Influenza receptors, polymerase and host range. *Rev. Sci. Tech.* **28:**203–217.

Mebatsion, T., Cox, J. H., and Conzelmann, K. K. (1993). Molecular analysis of rabies-related viruses from Ethiopia. *Onderstepoort. J. Vet. Res.* **60:**289–294.

Meng, S.-L., Yan, J.-X., Xu, G.-L., Nadin-Davis, S. A., Ming, P.-G., Liu, S.-Y., Wu, J., Ming, H.-T., Zhu, F.-C., Zhou, D.-J., Xiao, Q.-Y., Dong, G.-M., *et al.* (2007). A molecular epidemiological study targeting the glycoprotein gene of rabies virus isolates from China. *Virus Res.* **124:**125–138.

Ming, P., Yan, J., Rayner, S., Meng, S., Xu, G., Tang, Q., Wu, J., Luo, J., and Yang, X. (2010). A history estimate and evolutionary analysis of rabies virus variants in China. *J. Gen. Virol.* **91:**759–764.

Morimoto, K., Hooper, D. C., Carbaugh, H., Fu, Z. F., Koprowski, H., and Dietzschold, B. (1998). Rabies virus quasispecies: Implications for pathogenesis. *Proc. Natl. Acad. Sci. USA* **95:**3152–3156.

Nadin-Davis, S. A. (2007). Molecular epidemiology. *In* "Rabies" (A. C. Jackson and W. H. Wunner, eds.), 2nd edn. pp. 69–122. Academic Press, London, UK.

Nadin-Davis, S. A., and Bingham, J. (2004). Europe as a source of rabies for the rest of the world. *In* "Historical Perspective of Rabies in Europe and the Mediterranean Basin" (A. A. King, A. R. Fooks, M. Aubert, and A. I. Wandeler, eds.), pp. 259–280. OIE, Paris, France.

Nadin-Davis, S. A., and Loza-Rubio, E. (2006). The molecular epidemiology of rabies associated with chiropteran hosts in Mexico. *Virus Res.* **117:**215–226.

Nadin-Davis, S. A., Casey, G. A., and Wandeler, A. I. (1993). Identification of regional variants of the rabies virus within the Canadian province of Ontario. *J. Gen. Virol.* **74:**829–837.

Nadin-Davis, S. A., Casey, G. A., and Wandeler, A. I. (1994). A molecular epidemiological study of rabies virus in central Ontario and western Quebec. *J. Gen. Virol.* **75:**2575–2583.

Nadin-Davis, S. A., Huang, W., and Wandeler, A. I. (1997). Polymorphism of rabies viruses within the phosphoprotein and matrix protein genes. *Arch. Virol.* **142:**979–992.

Nadin-Davis, S. A., Sampath, M. I., Casey, G. A., Tinline, R. R., and Wandeler, A. I. (1999). Phylogeographic patterns exhibited by Ontario rabies virus variants. *Epidemiol. Infect.* **123:**325–336.

Nadin-Davis, S. A., Huang, W., Armstrong, J., Casey, G. A., Bahloul, C., Tordo, N., and Wandeler, A. I. (2001). Antigenic and genetic divergence of rabies viruses from bat species indigenous to Canada. *Virus Res.* **74:**139–156.

Nadin-Davis, S. A., Abdel-Malik, M., Armstrong, J., and Wandeler, A. I. (2002). Lyssavirus P gene characterisation provides insights into the phylogeny of the genus and identifies structural similarities and diversity within the encoded phosphoprotein. *Virology* **298:**286–305.

Nadin-Davis, S. A., Simani, S., Armstrong, J., Fayaz, A., and Wandeler, A. I. (2003). Molecular and antigenic characterization of rabies viruses from Iran identifies variants with distinct epidemiological origins. *Epidemiol. Infect.* **131:**777–790.

Nadin-Davis, S. A., Turner, G., Paul, J. P. V., Madhusudana, S. N., and Wandeler, A. I. (2007). Emergence of arctic-like rabies lineage in India. *Emerg. Infect. Dis.* **13:**111–116.

Nadin-Davis, S. A., Feng, Y., Mousse, D., Wandeler, A. I., and Aris-Brosou, S. (2010). Spatial and temporal dynamics of rabies virus variants in big brown bat populations across Canada: Footprints of an emerging zoonosis. *Mol. Ecol.* **19:**2120–2136.

Nanayakkara, S., Smith, J. S., and Rupprecht, C. E. (2003). Rabies in Sri Lanka: Splendid isolation. *Emerg. Infect. Dis.* **9:**368–371.

Nei, M., and Kumar, S. (2004). Molecular Evolution and Phylogenetics. Oxford University Press, Oxford, UK.

Nel, L., Jacobs, J., Jaftha, J., von Teichman, B., and Bingham, J. (2000). New cases of Mokola virus infection in South Africa: A genotypic comparison of southern African isolates. *Virus Genes* **20:**103–106.

Nel, L. H., Sabeta, C. T., von Teichman, B., Jaftha, J. B., Rupprecht, C. E., and Bingham, J. (2005). Mongoose rabies in southern Africa: A re-evaluation based on molecular epidemiology. *Virus Res.* **109:**165–173.

Nishizono, A., Mannen, K., Elio-Villa, L. P., Tanaka, S., Li, K., Mifune, K., Arca, B. F., Cabanban, A., Martinez, B., Rodríguez, A., Atienza, V. C., Camba, R., *et al.* (2002). Genetic analysis of rabies virus isolates in the Philippines. *Microbiol. Immunol.* **46:**413–417.

Oliveira, R. N., de Souza, S. P., Lobo, R. S. V., Castilho, J. G., Macedo, C. I., Carnieli, P., Jr., Fahl, W. O., Achkar, S. M., Scheffer, K. C., Kotait, I., Carrieri, M. L., and Brandão, P. E. (2010). Rabies virus in insectivorous bats: Implications of the diversity of the nucleoprotein and glycoprotein genes for molecular epidemiology. *Virology* **405**:352–360.

Páez, A., Saad, C., Núñez, C., and Bóshell, J. (2005). Molecular epidemiology of rabies in northern Colombia 1994–2003. Evidence for human and fox rabies associated with dogs. *Epidemiol. Infect.* **133**:529–536.

Paweska, J. T., Blumberg, L. H., Liebenberg, C., Hewlett, R. H., Grobbelaar, A. A., Leman, P. A., Croft, J. E., Nel, L. H., Nutt, L., and Swanepoel, R. (2006). Fatal human infection with rabies-related Duvenhage virus. *Emerg. Infect. Dis.* **12**:1965–1967.

Pybus, O. G., and Rambaut, A. (2009). Evolutionary analysis of the dynamics of viral infectious disease. *Nat. Rev. Genet.* **10**:540–550.

Pybus, O. G., Charleston, M. A., Gupta, S., Rambaut, A., Holmes, E. C., and Harvey, P. H. (2001). The epidemic behaviour of the hepatitis C virus. *Science* **292**:2323–2325.

Pybus, O. G., Cochrane, A., Holmes, E. C., and Simmonds, P. (2005). The hepatitis C virus epidemic among injecting drug users. *Infect. Genet. Evol.* **24**:845–852.

Pybus, O. G., Rambaut, A., Belshaw, R., Freckleton, R. P., Drummond, A. J., and Holmes, E. C. (2007). Phylogenetic evidence for deleterious mutation load in RNA viruses and its contribution to viral evolution. *Mol. Biol. Evol.* **24**:845–852.

Rambaut, A. (2000). Estimating the rate of molecular evolution: Incorporating non-contemporaneous sequences into maximum likelihood phylogenies. *Bioinformatics* **16**:395–399.

Real, L. A., Henderson, J. C., Biek, R., Snaman, J., Jack, T. L., Childs, J. E., Stahl, E., Waller, L., Tinline, R., and Nadin-Davis, S. (2005). Unifying the spatial population dynamics and molecular evolution of epidemic rabies virus. *Proc. Natl. Acad. Sci. USA* **102**:12107–12111.

Reynes, J.-M., Molia, S., Audry, L., Hout, S., Ngin, S., Walston, J., and Bourhy, H. (2004). Serologic evidence of lyssavirus infection in bats, Cambodia. *Emerg. Infect. Dis.* **10**:2231–2234.

Sabeta, C. T., Mansfield, K. L., McElhinney, L. M., Fooks, A. R., and Nel, L. H. (2007). Molecular epidemiology of rabies in bat-eared foxes (*Otocyon megalotis*) in South Africa. *Virus Res.* **129**:1–10.

Saiki, R. K., Gelfand, D. H., Stoffel, S., Scharf, S. J., Higuchi, R., Horn, G. T., Mullis, K. B., and Erlich, H. A. (1988). Primer-directed enzymatic amplification of DNA with a thermostable DNA polymerase. *Science* **239**:487–491.

Shao, X. Q., Yan, X. J., Luo, G. L., Zhang, H. L., Chai, X. L., Wang, F. X., Wang, J. K., Zhao, J. J., Wu, W., Cheng, S. P., Yang, F. H., Qin, X. C., *et al.* (2011). Genetic evidence for domestic raccoon dog rabies caused by arctic-like rabies virus in Inner Mongolia, China. *Epidemiol. Infect.* **139**:629–635.

Smith, J. S., Orciari, L. A., Yager, P. A., Seidel, H. D., and Warner, C. K. (1992). Epidemiologic and historical relationships among 87 rabies virus isolates as determined by limited sequence analysis. *J. Infect. Dis.* **166**:296–307.

Streicker, D. G., Turmelle, A. S., Vonhof, M. J., Kuzmin, I. V., McCracken, G. F., and Rupprecht, C. E. (2010). Host phylogeny constrains cross-species emergence and establishment of rabies virus in bats. *Science* **329**:676–679.

Susetya, H., Sugiyama, M., Inagaki, A., Ito, N., Mudiarto, G., and Minamoto, N. (2008). Molecular epidemiology of rabies in Indonesia. *Virus Res.* **135**:144–149.

Szanto, A. G., Nadin-Davis, S. A., and White, B. N. (2008). Complete genome sequence of a raccoon rabies virus isolate. *Virus Res.* **136**:130–139.

Szanto, A. G., Nadin-Davis, S. A., Rosatte, R. C., and White, B. N. (2011). Genetic tracking of the raccoon variant of rabies virus in eastern North America. *Epidemics.* in press, doi:10.1016/j.epidem.2011.02.002.

Tabel, H., Corner, A. H., Webster, W. A., and Casey, G. A. (1974). History and epizootiology of rabies in Canada. *Can. Vet. J.* **15**:271–281.

Talbi, C., Holmes, E. C., de Benedictis, P., Faye, O., Nakouné, E., Gamatié, D., Diarra, A., Elmamy, B. O., Sow, A., Adjogoua, E. V., Sangare, O., Dundon, W. G., et al. (2009). Evolutionary history and dynamics of dog rabies virus in western and central Africa. J. Gen. Virol. **90:**783–791.

Tordo, N., Poch, O., Ermine, A., Keith, G., and Rougeon, F. (1986). Walking along the rabies genome: Is the large G-L intergenic region a remnant gene. Proc. Natl. Acad. Sci. USA **83:**3914–3918.

Van Thiel, P.-P., de Bie, R. M., Eftimov, F., Tepaske, R., Zaaijer, H. L., van Doornum, G. J., Schutten, M., Osterhaus, A. D., Majoie, C. B., Aronica, E., Fehlner-Gardiner, C., Wandeler, A. I., et al. (2009). Fatal human rabies due to Duvenhage virus from a bat in Kenya: Failure of treatment with coma-induction, ketamine, and antiviral drugs. PLOS Negl. Trop. Dis. **3**(7):e428.

Van Zyl, N., Markotter, W., and Nel, L. H. (2010). Evolutionary history of African mongoose rabies. Virus Res. **150:**93–102.

Velasco-Villa, A., Orciari, L. A., Juárez-Islas, V., Gómez-Sierra, M., Padilla-Medina, I., Flisser, A., Souza, V., Castillo, A., Franka, R., Escalante-Mañe, M., Sauri-González, I., and Rupprecht, C. E. (2006). Molecular diversity of rabies viruses associated with bats in Mexico and other countries of the Americas. J. Clin. Microbiol. **44:**1697–1710.

Velasco-Villa, A., Reeder, S. A., Orciari, L. A., Yager, P. A., Franka, R., Blanton, J. D., Zuckero, L., Hunt, P., Oertli, E. H., Robinson, L. E., and Rupprecht, C. E. (2008). Enzootic rabies elimination from dogs and re-emergence in wild terrestrial carnivores, United States. Emerg. Infect. Dis. **14:**1849–1854.

Warner, C. K., Zaki, S. R., Shieh, W. J., Whitfield, S. G., Smith, J. S., Orciari, L. A., Shaddock, J. H., Niezgoda, M., Wright, C. W., Goldsmith, C., and Rupprecht, C. E. (1999). Laboratory investigation of human deaths from vampire bat rabies in Peru. Am. J. Trop. Med. Hyg. **60:**502–507.

Wu, X., Franka, R., Velasco-Villa, A., and Rupprecht, C. E. (2007). Are all lyssavirus genes equal for phylogenetic analyses? Virus Res. **129:**91–103.

Wu, X., Hu, R., Zhang, Y., Ding, G., and Rupprecht, C. E. (2009). Reemerging rabies and lack of systemic surveillance in People's Republic of China. Emerg. Infect. Dis. **15:**1159–1164.

Wunner, W. H. (2007). Rabies virus. In "Rabies" (A. C. Jackson and W. H. Wunner, eds.), pp. 23–68. Academic Press, London, UK.

Zhang, Y.-Z., Xiong, C.-L., Zou, Y., Wang, D.-M., Jiang, R.-J., Xiao, Q.-Y., Hao, Z.-Y., Zhang, L.-Z., Yu, Y.-X., and Fu, Z. F. (2006). Molecular characterization of rabies virus isolates in China during 2004. Virus Res. **121:**179–188.

Zhang, Y.-Z., Xiong, C.-L., Lin, X.-D., Zhou, D.-J., Jiang, R.-J., Xiao, Q.-Y., Xie, X.-Y., Yu, X.-X., Tan, Y.-J., Li, M. H., Ai, Q.-S., Zhang, L.-J., et al. (2009). Genetic diversity of Chinese rabies viruses: Evidence for the presence of two distinct clades in China. Infect. Genet. Evol. **9:**87–96.

Zulu, G. C., Sabeta, C. T., and Nel, L. H. (2009). Molecular epidemiology of rabies: Focus on domestic dogs (Canis familiaris) and black-backed jackals (Canis mesomelas) from northern South Africa. Virus Res. **140:**71–78.

CHAPTER 12

Bats and Lyssaviruses

Ashley C. Banyard,* David Hayman,*,†,‡
Nicholas Johnson,* Lorraine McElhinney,*,§ and
Anthony R. Fooks*,§

Contents

* Rabies and Wildlife Zoonoses Group, Department of Virology, Veterinary Laboratories Agency, Weybridge, New Haw, Addlestone, Surrey, United Kingdom
† Cambridge Infectious Diseases Consortium, Department of Veterinary Medicine, Cambridge, United Kingdom
‡ Institute of Zoology, Regent's Park, London, United Kingdom
§ National Centre for Zoonosis Research, University of Liverpool, Leahurst, Neston, Wirral, United Kingdom

Advances in Virus Research, Volume 79
ISSN 0065-3527, DOI: 10.1016/B978-0-12-387040-7.00012-3

Abstract   Numerous bat species have been identified as important reservoirs of zoonotic viral pathogens. Rabies and rabies-related viruses constitute one of the most important viral zoonoses and pose a significant threat to public health across the globe. Whereas rabies virus (RABV) appears to be restricted to bats of the New World, related lyssavirus species have not been detected in the Americas and have only been detected in bat populations across Africa, Eurasia, and Australia. Currently, 11 distinct species of lyssavirus have been identified, 10 of which have been isolated from bat species and all of which appear to be able to cause encephalitis consistent with that seen with RABV infection of humans. In contrast, whereas lyssaviruses are apparently able to cause clinical disease in bats, it appears that these lyssaviruses may also be able to circulate within bat populations in the absence of clinical disease. This feature of these highly encephalitic viruses, alongside many other aspects of lyssavirus infection in bats, is poorly understood. Here, we review what is known of the complex relationship between bats and lyssaviruses, detailing both natural and experimental infections of these viruses in both chiropteran and nonchiropteran models. We also discuss potential mechanisms of virus excretion, transmission both to conspecifics and spill-over of virus into nonvolant species, and mechanisms of maintenance within bat populations. Importantly, we review the significance of neutralizing antibodies reported within bat populations and discuss the potential mechanisms by which highly neurovirulent viruses such as the lyssaviruses are able to infect bat species in the absence of clinical disease.

I. INTRODUCTION

The most significant zoonotic pathogen of bat origin is rabies virus (RABV). This virus and other members of the genus to which it belongs, the lyssaviruses, cause fatal encephalitis for which there is no effective treatment. Approximately, 20% of mammalian species are bats with more than 1100 species being recognized worldwide (Teeling *et al.*, 2005). They have many characteristics that differentiate them from other mammalian species, and at the same time, they exhibit an enormous degree of intraspecies diversity. Bats are hypothesized to have evolved between 50 and 70 million years ago and have undergone a rapid diversification during this period (Simmons *et al.*, 2008, Teeling *et al.*, 2005). All bat species belong to the Order Chiroptera that is subdivided into two suborders, *Yangochiroptera* and *Yinpterochiroptera*, the latter including the superfamily Pteropodidae, the old world fruit bats, and Rhinolophoidea (Giannini and Simmons, 2003). Scientific interest in bats has increased substantially following the identification of bats as important reservoirs of pathogens of both zoonotic and veterinary importance (Calisher *et al.*, 2006; Dominguez *et al.*, 2007; Field, 2009; Towner *et al.*, 2009; Wang and Eaton, 2007).

Lyssavirus infection of bats occurs across much of the globe, although different virus species are present in different regions and tend to infect particular bat species (Streicker *et al.*, 2010). In the Americas, only RABV is associated with bats, whereas across Europe, Africa, Asia, and Australia, the remaining lyssaviruses predominate in the complete absence of bat-associated RABV. The reasons for this geographical separation of viruses in bat populations remain the subject of much speculation, and the evolution of bat lyssaviruses remains an enigma (Vos *et al.*, 2007). The current global distribution of bat lyssaviruses is illustrated in Fig. 1. The exception to this geographical partitioning is RABV (species 1; Anonymous, 2009), which is endemic worldwide in carnivores with the exception of a number of regions where the disease has been controlled or excluded (Australia and Great Britain) or eliminated through vaccination campaigns (Western Europe). Well-established RABV reservoir hosts are present in North America (e.g., skunks, foxes, and raccoons), Africa (e.g., mongoose, bat-eared foxes, and jackals), and Eurasia (e.g., foxes and raccoon dogs). Terrestrial wildlife reservoirs are apparently absent in South America and Australasia. RABV variants have been reported to undergo genetic adaptation to particular hosts, sometimes leading to a diversity of clades or biotypes with infection of wild terrestrial carnivore reservoirs varying according to species present within the local fauna. For example, in South Africa, RABV circulates in dogs and jackals in the northern region, dogs in the eastern region, bat-eared foxes in the western region, and mongooses (*Herpestidae*) (a different biotype) in the interior (Nel and Rupprecht, 2007).

Phylogenetic analyses and virus–host relationships suggest that all lyssaviruses, including RABV, likely originated in bats. With the exception of Mokola virus (MOKV), all lyssaviruses have been isolated from bats (Badrane and Tordo, 2001; Nel and Rupprecht, 2007). Thus, it remains of great importance to study bat lyssaviruses to understand both virus and chiropteran host ecology and to determine the potential for spill-over transmission into both humans and nonvolant mammal populations. The current taxonomic classification of the lyssaviruses is

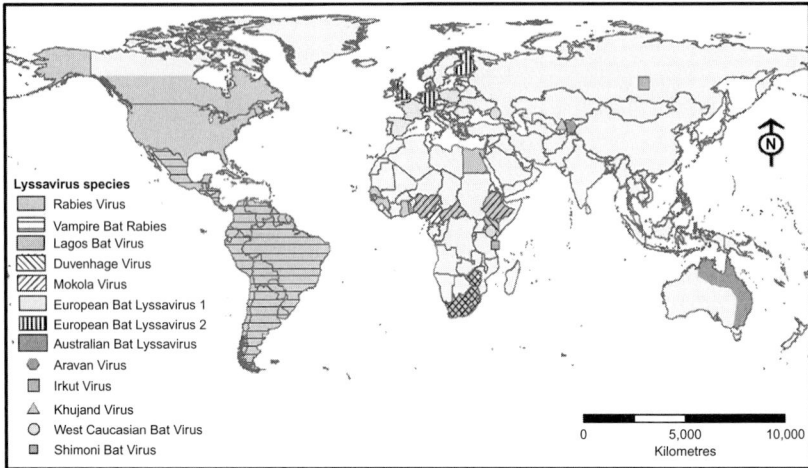

FIGURE 1   Geographical distribution of bat lyssavirus isolates across the globe. Countries are shaded according to the detection of different lyssavirus species in bats. Where only single isolates have been detected, viruses are denoted by symbols. Lyssavirus species are colored according to the key. (See Page 9 in Color Section at the back of the book.)

based on genetic analyses of the viral genome (Kuzmin *et al.*, 2005, 2010) and differentiates viruses into 11 genetically divergent species: (1) *Rabies virus* (RABV), (2) *Lagos bat virus* (LBV), (3) *Mokola virus* (MOKV), (4) *Duvenhage virus* (DUVV), (5) *European bat lyssavirus type 1* (EBLV-1), (6) *European bat lyssavirus type 2* (EBLV-2), (7) *Australian bat lyssavirus* (ABLV), (8) *Irkut virus* (IRKV), (9) *Aravan virus* (ARAV), (10) *Khujand virus* (KHUV), and (11) *West Caucasian Bat Virus* (WCBV) (Anonymous, 2009). A 12th genetically related virus, *Shimoni bat virus* (SHIV), is yet to be classified but is believed to represent a further lyssavirus species, given that it has 80% nucleotide identity with other lyssaviruses (Kuzmin *et al.*, 2010).

Representative isolates from all lyssaviruses have been sequenced and all are approximately 12 kb in length (Gould *et al.*, 2002; Kuzmin *et al.*, 2003, 2005, 2008a, 2010; Marston *et al.*, 2007). A phylogenetic analysis of the lyssaviruses and representative mammalian species that they have each been found to infect is shown in Fig. 2. The arrangement of the five gene-coding regions (nucleoprotein (N)-phosphoprotein (P)-matrix protein (M)-glycoprotein (G)-polymerase protein (L)) is conserved across the genus (Tordo *et al.*, 1988). Each gene is flanked by intergenic regions that have a high degree of divergence both inter- and intragenotypically (Marston *et al.*, 2007). Variation at intergenic regions is typically seen in the form of sequence divergence or the presence of short insertions

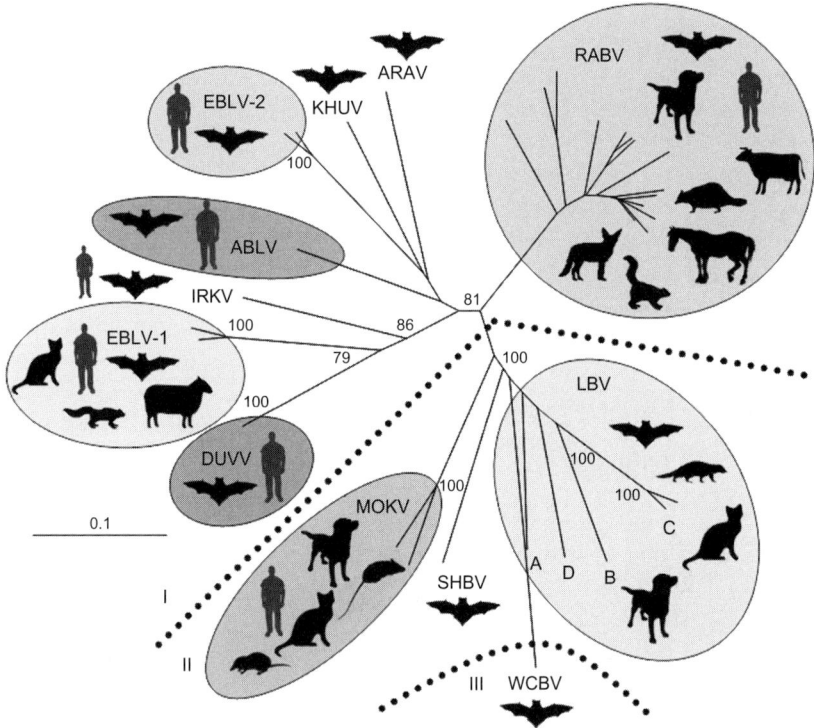

FIGURE 2   Phylogenetic analysis of characterized lyssavirus isolates based on 405 nucleotides of the nucleoprotein. Sequences were aligned using the ClustalW, and the tree was visualized using Treeview (Version 3.2). Bootstrap values at significant nodes are shown. For each lyssavirus species, animals found naturally infected are silhouetted at branch termini. Differentiation into phylogroups according to antigenicity is labeled and separated by dashed lines.

(Johnson *et al.*, 2007; Marston *et al.*, 2007), as well as in some isolates, the presence of a long uncharacterized genetic element present between the G- and L-coding regions (Ravkov *et al.*, 1995; Tordo *et al.*, 1986). The cause of variation within genomes is not clear but could be related to polymerase errors during replication (Assenberg *et al.*, 2010).

The lyssavirus species can also be grouped into phylogroups (Badrane *et al.*, 2001) (Fig. 2). Within the lyssavirus genus, phylogroup I includes all species apart from LBV, MOKV, WCBV, and SHIV. LBV, MOKV, and the recently isolated SHIV are each distributed in Africa and are members of phylogroup II (Badrane *et al.*, 2001; Horton *et al.*, 2010; Kuzmin *et al.*, 2005, 2010). The phylogroup II viruses have greater divergence at the amino acid level on the glycoprotein ectodomain and were initially reported to be less pathogenic than phylogroup I lyssaviruses. However, this property of phylogroup II viruses has been challenged by more complete pathogenicity studies (Markotter *et al.*, 2009). In addition, the sporadic spill-over infections of these viruses to a number of host species argue that they share the pathogenic characteristics of other phylogroups (Fig. 2). WCBV could be categorized in a new phylogroup, phylogroup III. However, only a single isolation of this virus has been made, and clarification through detection of further WCBV isolates must occur before a novel phylogroup distinction can be officially accepted (Kuzmin *et al.*, 2005). The division of lyssaviruses into phylogroups is partly due to antigenic divergence, and vaccines derived from classical RABV strains have been shown to confer little or no protection against members of phylogroups II and III in experimental studies (Badrane *et al.*, 2001; Hanlon *et al.*, 2001, 2005; Weyer *et al.*, 2010). However, as for WCBV, few isolates are available for a number of the lyssaviruses and early studies were limited to mouse models, so the influence of genetic and antigenic variation to biological differences between species requires further study. Recently, phylogenetic analysis has suggested greater genetic diversity within the LBV isolates than observed for other species, with four lineages suggested (Kuzmin *et al.*, 2010). Currently, it is thought that all four LBV phylogroups are present in Africa, with serological evidence of WCBV having been reported in African bat populations (Kuzmin *et al.*, 2008c; Wright *et al.*, 2010). The greater genetic diversity and serological cross-reactivity of African lyssaviruses have led to the hypothesis that lyssaviruses originated from Africa (Badrane and Tordo, 2001; Badrane *et al.*, 2001; Nel and Rupprecht, 2007).

II. BAT LYSSAVIRUSES: EURASIA AND AUSTRALASIA

There are currently seven distinct lyssaviruses associated with bats in Europe, Asia, and Australia. Of these, four have been associated with human fatalities, and a clinical presentation consistent with rabies has been observed (Table I; Allworth *et al.*, 1996; Belikov *et al.*, 2009; Fooks *et al.*, 2003; Selimov *et al.*, 1989). Available data suggest that, like RABV, bat lyssaviruses are neurotropic viruses with similar pathogenesis, that is, retrograde axonal transport of virus through the peripheral nervous system with ascension within the spinal cord followed by extensive replication in the brain (Fig. 3A; Johnson *et al.*, 2006a). However, these viruses show clear epidemiological differences with RABV in their restricted geographical distribution and their association with particular bat species. This may represent reduced virulence when compared to RABV or coevolution with a particular reservoir species. As well as infection in humans, there have been rare reports of nonrabies lyssaviruses present in nonvolant mammals (Dacheux *et al.*, 2009; Muller

TABLE I Bat-associated human cases of lyssaviruses of Europe, Asia, and Australia

Virus	Distribution	Bat species	Latin name	Incidence in humans	Reference
EBLV-1	Continental Europe	Serotine bat	*Eptesicus serotinus*	3[a]	Roine et al. (1988), Selimov et al. (1989), Botvinkin et al. (2005)
EBLV-2	The Netherlands, Switzerland, Finland, United Kingdom, Germany	Daubenton's bat	*Myotis daubentonii*	2	Lumio et al. (1986), Fooks et al. (2003)
ABLV	Australia	Pteropid and insectivorous bat species	ND	2	Allworth et al. (1996), Hanna et al. (2000)
ARAV	Kyrgyzstan	Lesser mouse-eared bat	*Myotis blythi*	None	n/a
IRKV	Russia	Greater tube-nosed bat	*Murina leucogaster*	1	Belikov et al. (2009)
KHUV	Tajikistan	Whiskered bat	*Myotis mystacinus*	None	n/a
WCBV	Russia	Common bent-winged bat	*Miniopterus schreibersii*	None	n/a

n/a, not applicable; ND, not determined.

[a] Two further reports of human deaths have been reported following encounters with bats in Europe, although neither has been confirmed as EBLV-1.

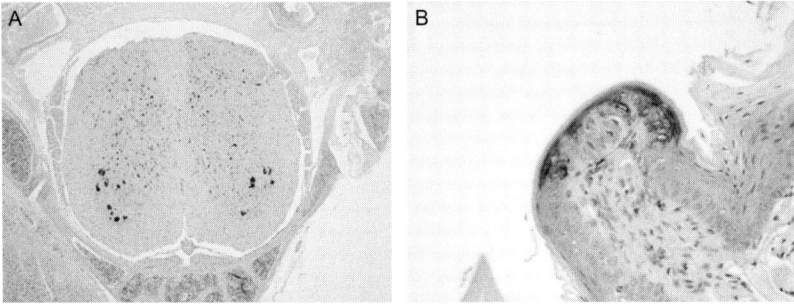

FIGURE 3 (A) Detection of lyssavirus nucleoprotein (brown staining) in a cross section of the spine of a Daubenton's bat naturally infected with EBLV-2 (5×). Neurons show staining in the gray matter of the spinal cord and particularly involve ventral horn cells. (B) Detection of lyssavirus antigen (brown staining) in a taste bud within the tongue of a serotine bat experimentally infected with EBLV-1 (40×). More than 50% of the taste buds observed showed immunolabeling for antigen. Images courtesy of Dr. Alex Nunez, Department of Histopathology, Veterinary Laboratories Agency. (See Page 10 in Color Section at the back of the book.)

et al., 2004; Tjornehoj *et al.*, 2006). Below we discuss the particular features of each of the Eurasian and Australian lyssaviruses with emphasis on the pathogenesis studies undertaken on each to assess virulence and transmission within the reservoir host.

A. European bat lyssavirus type 1

The first report of a rabid bat in Europe was made from observations in 1954 (Mohr, 1957). Only with the advent of antigenic typing using monoclonal antibodies (Schneider and Cox, 1994) could the virus isolated in European bats be distinguished from RABV present in both European fox populations and North American bats. Genomic sequencing has enabled further characterization and has led to an estimation of between 500 and 750 years for EBLV-1 divergence from the other lyssavirus species (Davis *et al.*, 2005, 2006). EBLV-1 has only been reported in Europe, although some authors have speculated that it may be present in North Africa due to shared bat populations north and south of the Mediterranean Sea (Freuling *et al.*, 2009a). Two lineages of EBLV-1 have been defined (Amengual *et al.*, 1997). EBLV-1a is detected throughout northern Europe with most isolations reported from France, the Netherlands, Germany, and Poland. Surveillance in Germany for EBLV-1 has reported most cases from the northern regions of the country that are at lower elevations and where the highest density of serotine bats (*Eptesicus serotinus*) is suspected (Muller *et al.*, 2007). In contrast, EBLV-1b has been reported from southern Germany, France, and Spain. However, bat surveillance is variable in

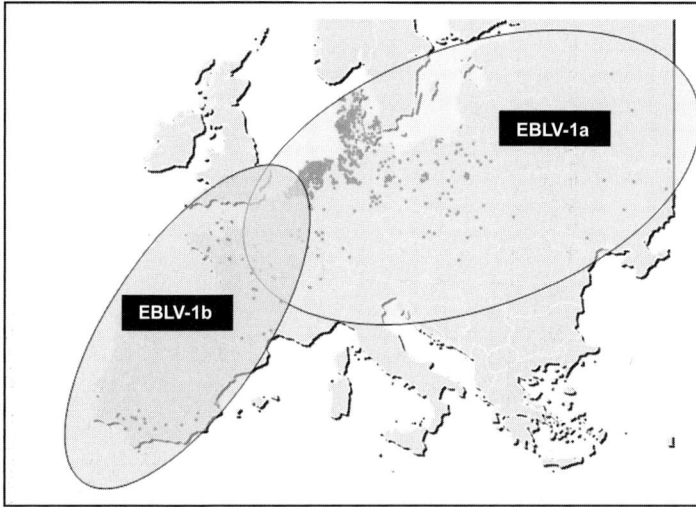

FIGURE 4   Distribution of EBLV-1a and 1b cases across Europe. Individual cases are marked, whereas the approximate ranges of each of the EBLV 1a and 1b subtypes are shaded.

Europe, and a recent report demonstrated an EBLV-1b isolate in central Poland (Smreczak *et al.*, 2008), suggesting that the distribution of this lineage is more widespread in Europe than previously considered (Fig. 4). Despite the presence of serotine bats in southern England and long-term active and passive surveillance for lyssaviruses in the native bat population, EBLV-1 virus has never been isolated. However, specific antibodies have been detected in a single serotine bat, suggesting that the virus may also be present in UK bat populations (Harris *et al.*, 2009).

   Both EBLV-1 lineages are mainly associated with the serotine bat with 99% of cases being associated with this species. The exception to this appears to be in Spain where EBLV-1 has been reported from a range of species including the greater mouse-eared bat (*Myotis myotis*), the Natterer's bat (*Myotis nattereri*), the greater horseshoe bat (*Rhinolophus ferrumequinum*), and the common bent-winged bat (*Miniopterus schreibersii*; Amengual *et al.*, 2007; Serra-Cobo *et al.*, 2002). However, caution should be exercised when identifying a reservoir species, and the species most frequently reported may prove misleading. For example, the species most likely to be submitted for diagnosis may also be those with an anthropophilic habitat, those that are not experiencing a decline in population size or those that succumb to clinical infections. The distribution of *E. serotinus* is widespread across Western Europe (including southern regions of the United Kingdom), north to Denmark and southern Sweden, south to North Africa, eastward to the Himalayas, and north to Korea and is possibly expanding its range in Europe. This species is not commonly migratory, but movements of up to 330 km (200 miles) have been recorded from Eastern Europe. It appears that most bats survive infection, as evidenced by the repeat captures of individual seropositive bats over a number of years during both active and passive serological surveillance initiatives across Europe (Brookes *et al.*, 2005; Echevarria *et al.*, 2001; Harris *et al.*, 2009; Serra-Cobo *et al.*, 2002). Indeed, Amengual *et al.* (2007) provided evidence for subclinical infection with EBLV-1 in a longitudinal study of naturally infected greater mouse-eared bats (*M. myotis*) in maternal colonies in Spain; however, the finding of lyssavirus antigen in blood clots remains a controversial observation. This study used capture–mark–recapture (CMR) techniques to understand EBLV-1 infection within the colonies (range 120–804 bats/colony) over a 12-year period. The study generated data on both survival rate and population size of *M. myotis* and provided evidence of fluctuating antibody titers, with 20 of 37 seropositive recaptured bats losing detectable immunity during this period (Amengual *et al.*, 2007).

Where clinical disease is seen, bats are often weak and unable to fly and display abnormal behavior, including uncoordinated movements, spasms, and occasionally paralysis. Serotine bats usually inhabit relatively small roosts, although nursery colonies may include up to 300 animals. This species is also known to cohabit roosts with other insectivorous bat species, although nursery colonies are usually species specific. Incidents of spill-over infections of EBLV-1 into a stone marten (Muller *et al.*, 2004), sheep (Tjornehoj *et al.*, 2006), and domestic cats (Dacheux *et al.*, 2009) have occurred but are rare and none have led to the establishment of a terrestrial reservoir for the virus as seen in North America with spill-over of rabies from bats to both skunks and foxes (Daoust *et al.*, 1996; Leslie *et al.*, 2006).

Experimentally, EBLV-1 causes disease in bats indistinguishable from that observed with RABV infection of North American bats. Direct inoculation of EBLV-1 into the brain of Egyptian flying foxes (*Rousettus aegyptiacus*) caused neurological disease and death in five of eight (63%) inoculated animals, although surprisingly not all (Van der Poel *et al.*, 2000). Bats surviving in this instance must be considered to have had an aborted infection, although such observations are rare and further explanations for such unusual outcomes cannot preclude inoculation failure or error. This was also observed in one of two experimental studies of EBLV-1 in the North American big brown bat (*Eptesicus fuscus*) (Franka *et al.*, 2008). In the *E. fuscus* study, inoculation by the intramuscular route led to the development of disease in 50% of challenged animals. In a further study by the same authors, using the proposed EBLV-1 reservoir host, the serotine bat, 100% induction of rabies by intracranial inoculation was demonstrated (Freuling *et al.*, 2009b). Intramuscular inoculation was less successful in causing productive infection with only one of seven bats developing disease. By contrast, subdermal inoculation caused the development of disease in three of seven bats with concomitant shedding of virus in saliva immediately before the development of disease. Further, clear evidence for virus infection of taste buds was observed (Fig. 3B), which has been reported previously in human rabies (Jackson *et al.*, 1999), although it remains unclear if infection of taste buds could result in viral excretion. The principal experimental observations of bat studies with EBLVs are summarized in Table II.

B. European bat lyssavirus type 2

EBLV-2 was originally isolated from a Pond bat (*Myotis dasycneme*) in the Netherlands (Nieuwenhuijs, 1987). Since then the virus has been isolated sporadically across a number of countries of Northern Europe but has only been associated with *Myotis daubentonii*, the Daubenton's bat. Virus detection has also occurred in Switzerland (Amengual *et al.*, 1997), the United Kingdom (Banyard *et al.*, 2009), Germany (Freuling *et al.*, 2008), and Finland (Jakava-Viljanen *et al.*, 2010). Two cases of human infection have been reported (Fooks *et al.*, 2003; Lumio *et al.*, 1986) and, as with spill-over in humans with EBLV-1, the clinical presentation was similar to that observed for infection with RABV. EBLV-2 infection in bats also results in disease indistinguishable from rabies. Typically, the infected animal is grounded, agitated, and aggressive. When approached, infected bats have made repeated attempts to bite the handler or objects that are placed in front of them (Johnson *et al.*, 2003). In diseased bats, EBLV-2 was always detected in the brain and to a lesser extent in other organs, including the tongue and salivary glands (Johnson *et al.*, 2006b). In comparative studies in a variety of species, EBLV-2 appears less virulent than EBLV-1 (Brookes *et al.*, 2007; Cliquet *et al.*, 2009; Vos *et al.*, 2004).

Little is understood about the persistence of EBLV-2 in its natural host. In the United Kingdom, the virus is endemic within the Daubenton's bat population with isolation of virus being reported on at least one occasion each year (Banyard *et al.*, 2010). Seroprevalence studies also suggest a low-level persistence in the bat population (Harris *et al.*, 2009) with a prevalence estimate between 1% and 4%, but when, where, and how transmission occurs in the natural environment are still unclear. Infection studies with Daubenton's bats have demonstrated that direct intracranial inoculation leads to rapid development of disease. However, inoculation via peripheral routes, such as intramuscular and intranasal, did not lead to infection or seroconversion of the animals challenged. One of seven bats inoculated by the subdermal route developed disease (Table II). This implies that the most effective route of transmission is through biting, because virus was detected in oral swabs of the infected bat

TABLE II Experimental studies on Eurasian lyssaviruses in bats

Virus	Bat species	Latin name	Inoculation routes	Mortality (%)	Incubation period (days)	Salivary excretion	Reference
EBLV-1	Egyptian fruit bat	*Rousettus aegyptiacus*	IC	62.5	11–34	NM	Van der Poel *et al.* (2000)
ABLV	Gray-headed flying fox	*Pteropus poliocephalus*	IM	33	15–24	Y	McColl *et al.* (2002)
ARAV	Big brown bat	*Eptesicus fuscus*	IM	75	16–22	N	Hughes *et al.* (2006)
KHUV				60	14–20	Y	
IRKV				54.5	7–16	Y	
EBLV-1	Big brown bat	*Eptesicus fuscus*	IM	44	12–58	Y	Franka *et al.* (2008)
			SD	0	–	N	
			PO	0	–	N	
			IN	0	–	N	
EBLV-2	Daubenton's bat	*Myotis daubentonii*	IC	100	12–14	N	Johnson *et al.* (2008a)
			IM	0	–	N	
			IN	0	–	N	
			SD	14	33	Y	
EBLV-1	Serotine bat	*Eptesicus serotinus*	IC	100	7–13	N	Freuling *et al.* (2009b)
			IM	14	26	N	
			IN	0	–	N	
			SD	43	17–20	Y	

IC, intracranially; IM, intramuscular; SD, subdermal; PO, oral (per os); IN, intranasal; Y, yes; N, no; NM, not measured.

(Johnson *et al.*, 2008a). Scratches or bites might explain the infection of two bat biologists with histories of encounters with Daubenton's bats (Fooks *et al.*, 2003). However, in a number of *in vivo* studies, there have been no reports of an infected bat biting another bat and that bat developing disease. The potential for infection via low transmissibility (basic reproduction number, R0) rates may confer an evolutionary advantage to these viruses. Indeed, if transmissibility rates are high, disease may occur and individuals succumb, reducing the potential for further spread. The dissemination of EBLV-2 within experimentally infected bats is identical to that reported in bats infected with RABV, and neuroinvasion activates the same innate immune responses (Johnson *et al.*, 2006a), both suggesting a similar pathology. However, the limited geographical distribution and host range imply that EBLV-2 is different than RABV. Whether this constraint is virological or ecological is yet to be defined (Vos *et al.*, 2007).

C. Australian bat lyssavirus

Australia was reported to be free of rabies within its wildlife population with only occasional cases of imported human rabies being observed (Johnson *et al.*, 2008b; McCall *et al.*, 2000). However, in 1996, investigation of a female black flying fox (*Pteropus alecto*) that was unable to fly resulted in the isolation of a lyssavirus (Crerar *et al.*, 1996; Fraser *et al.*, 1996). Surveillance initiatives also confirmed the presence of lyssavirus in both Pteropid (Gould *et al.*, 1998) and insectivorous bats (Gould *et al.*, 2002; Hooper *et al.*, 1997), and later, human infections were reported following encounters with both fruit and insectivorous bats (Allworth *et al.*, 1996; Hanna *et al.*, 2000; Warrilow, 2005; Warrilow *et al.*, 2002). Indeed, ABLV has now been isolated from five different bat species, all four species of *Pteropodidae* in Australia and from an insectivorous bat species, the yellow-bellied sheath-tailed bat (*Saccolaimus flaviventris*), with two distinct lineages apparently circulating in insectivorous and frugivorous bats (Fraser *et al.*, 1996; Gould *et al.*, 1998, 2002; Guyatt *et al.*, 2003). Phylogenetically and serologically, ABLV isolates appear to be more closely related to RABV than any of the other Old World lyssaviruses (Fig. 2). Although the black flying fox is a native fruit bat to Australia and is present on islands to the north, ABLV has only been isolated in Australia. However, serosurveillance of bat populations in the Philippines has suggested that lyssavirus infection of bats might be more widespread than previously thought (Arguin *et al.*, 2002).

Experimental infections with ABLV have been undertaken in one of the native fruit bat species, the gray-headed flying fox (*Pteropus poliocephalus*). Intramuscular inoculation resulted in 3 of 10 animals developing clinical signs of disease (Table II), including muscle weakness, trembling, and limb paralysis (McColl *et al.*, 2002). ABLV was detected in the brain of each animal. The remaining animals all survived to the end of the study with evidence of neutralizing antibodies against ABLV. Further ABLV inoculation experiments have been conducted to assess the susceptibility of companion animals to infection (McColl *et al.*, 2007). Although a number of subjects, both dogs and cats, showed occasional neurologic signs, these did not develop further and all survived to the end of the experimentation. All animals seroconverted, and no ABLV antigen or viral genome was detectable in tissue samples investigated following necropsy.

D. Eurasian lyssaviruses

Four Eurasian lyssaviruses have been identified from diverse locations throughout Eurasia (Table I). ARAV and KHUV viruses were isolated from bats trapped in Kyrgyzstan and Tajikistan, respectively (Botvinkin *et al.*, 2003; Kuzmin *et al.*, 1992, 2003). IRKV was isolated from a bat trapped in Eastern Siberia, whereas WCBV was isolated from a bat in southern Russia near the border with Georgia (Botvinkin *et al.*, 2003). All have been fully sequenced and fit into the phylogeny of the lyssavirus genus (Kuzmin *et al.*, 2003, 2005).

Little is known about the epidemiology of these lyssaviruses because only single isolations from bats have been made. Serosurveys of bats in Asia and Africa have identified cross-reactivity with existing lyssaviruses with bat serum samples taken during surveys demonstrating neutralization with: ARAV, KHUV, IRKV, and ABLV in Thailand (Lumlertdacha, 2005); ARAV and KHUV in Bangladesh (Kuzmin *et al.*, 2006); and WCBV in Kenya (Kuzmin *et al.*, 2008a). These studies suggest that these viruses may be more widespread, but such studies have not been supported by isolations of virus in any of the bat species collected. A recent report has suggested that a human case of rabies has occurred due to infection with an Irkut-like virus (Belikov *et al.*, 2009) in East Siberia. It seems likely that more lyssaviruses will be isolated in bat species, particularly in Asia. Interestingly, there have been anecdotal reports of RABVs being detected across Asia with evidence being found in fruit bats in Thailand (Smith *et al.*, 1967), India (Pal *et al.*, 1980), and China, where a bat bite was suspected in relation to a human infection. Postmortem analysis was not, however, attempted in the human case, and so it cannot be verified as RABV or a related lyssavirus (Tang *et al.*, 2005).

Experimental infections in bat models have been conducted with all of the Eurasian bat lyssaviruses (Hughes *et al.*, 2006; Kuzmin *et al.*, 1994, 2008d). In each, a number of experimental subjects developed rabies-like clinical signs following inoculation, although some survived to the end of the experimental period (Table II). Analysis of virus tissue distribution revealed the brain as the most highly infected tissue confirming the neurotropism of these viruses. Further, virus excretion in saliva was demonstrated shortly before the development of clinical signs. In these experiments, uninoculated bats were held in the same cage as those that developed an infection, and no evidence for horizontal transmission was identified (Hughes *et al.*, 2006).

WCBV has only been isolated from a single *M. schreibersi* in southeastern Europe (Botvinkin *et al.*, 2003), although WCBV seropositive bats have been detected in Kenya (Kuzmin *et al.*, 2008c), suggesting a large geographical distribution. WCBV is the most divergent member of the lyssavirus genus, and has long genetic distances and lacks serological cross-reactivity to other lyssaviruses (Horton *et al.*, 2010; Kuzmin *et al.*, 2005, 2008a; Wright *et al.*, 2010). Pathogenicity of lyssavirus isolates for different species is of scientific interest, especially following reports of highly variable pathogenicity between phylogroups I and II lyssaviruses in mice. Interestingly, infection of ferrets with IRKV caused substantial clinical disease and death, whereas experimental infection in ferrets with ARAV and KHUV suggested little or no pathogenicity (Hanlon *et al.*, 2005).

Experimental infection of 21 North American big brown bats with WCBV led to three of eight animals inoculated intramuscularly in neck muscles succumbing to rabies between 10 and 18 days postinoculation (Kuzmin *et al.*, 2008d). Of the surviving animals inoculated in the masseter ($n = 7$) and neck muscles (5 of 8), or orally ($n = 6$), all survived to 6 months with no antigen detectable in those tissues tested. Four surviving bats inoculated in the masseter muscles seroconverted with WCBV neutralizing antibodies detectable until the end of the experiment 6 months later (Kuzmin *et al.*, 2008d). Interpretation of these observations is complicated, however, not only because these studies were undertaken in bats of North American origin but also because of the fact that the animals were either of wild origin (and therefore of unknown immunological status against RABV, which circulates among North American bats) or were survivors of a previously undertaken IRKV challenge study. In those bats previously infected with IRKV, IRKV-neutralizing antibodies were detected to the end of observation. This was despite being 12 months after the IRKV challenge and included those not boosted by WCBV inoculation. This *in vivo* bat study, as with those involving other members of the lyssavirus genus (detailed below), has only just begun to attempt to address some of the questions regarding lyssavirus pathogenesis and host immune response to infection in bats.

III. BAT LYSSAVIRUSES: AFRICA

Given the diversity of lyssaviruses detected in Africa and with most nonrabies lyssaviruses being isolated from bats, there is substantial circumstantial evidence to support the hypothesis that lyssaviruses originated and evolved in African bats (Badrane and Tordo, 2001; Nel and Rupprecht, 2007). The ecology of MOKV has not been investigated and is poorly understood. Bats were first suggested as the hosts in which lyssaviruses evolved in the 1980s, when authors suggested that plant and arthropod rhabdoviruses had adapted to mammalian hosts (Shope, 1982). Subsequently, authors have suggested that the close genetic relationship between EBLV-1 and DUVV may provide evidence of viruses from Africa entering Europe (Amengual *et al.*, 1997; Serra-Cobo *et al.*, 2002; Schneider and Cox, 1994). In contrast, the isolation of WCBV from the West Caucuses and detection of antibodies against WCBV in Africa provides the first evidence of a bat lyssavirus infection throughout the Old World (Botvinkin *et al.*, 2003; Kuzmin *et al.*, 2008c). The geographical distribution of the African lyssaviruses, including the serological detection of WCBV neutralising antibodies, is detailed in Fig. 5. Below, we describe what is currently understood regarding host tropism, pathogenicity, and phylogenetic relationships between each of the viruses currently characterized.

A. Lagos bat virus

There have been more isolations of LBV than any of the other African bat lyssaviruses recognized, with the virus apparently circulating among bats in sub-Saharan Africa. Several bat species have been associated with LBV infection, including Wahlberg's epauletted fruit bat (*Epomorphorus wahlbergi*), the straw-colored fruit bat (*Eidolon helvum*) (Fig. 6), the Egyptian fruit bat (*R. aegyptiacus*), and an insectivorous bat, the Gambian slit-faced bat (*Nycteris gambiensis*). Spill-over events of LBV from bats into other mammals have been reported, albeit infrequently (Markotter *et al.*, 2006a, b) with infection of humans never having been demonstrated (Markotter *et al.*, 2008a). It is of note that whereas LBV has not been implicated in human fatalities, rabies cases are grossly under-diagnosed in Africa (Mallewa *et al.*, 2007) and testing of tissues at postmortem, where undertaken, typically uses nonspecific tests that may allow fatal LBV infections to be categorized as RABV infections.

LBV was first isolated from pooled *E. helvum* brain material in Nigeria in 1956 (Boulger and Porterfield, 1958). Initially, lack of Negri body formation in experimentally infected mice and an inability of the virus to be neutralized by rabies immune serum led researchers to disregard its relationship to RABV (Boulger and Porterfield, 1958). However, in 1970,

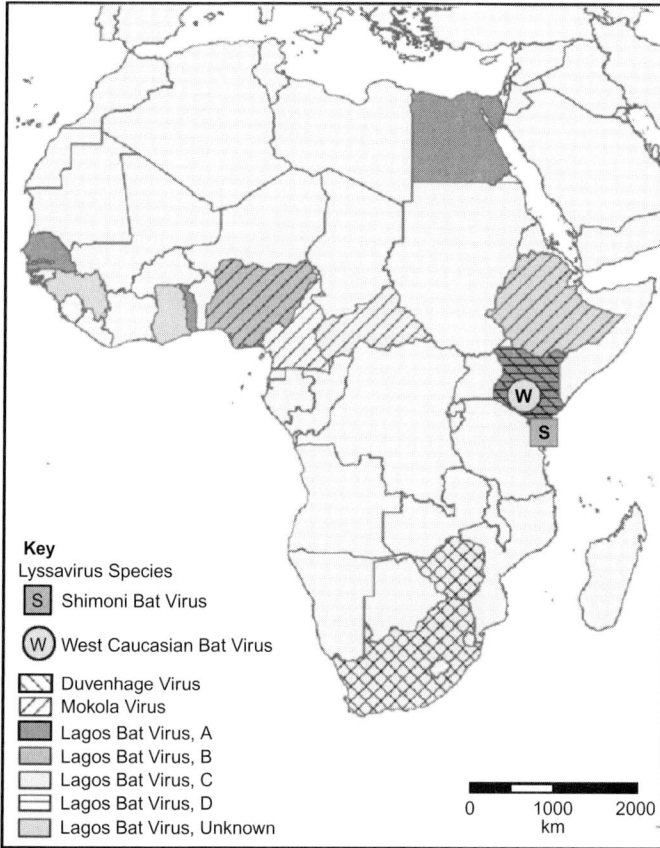

FIGURE 5 Geographical distribution of both bat-associated lyssavirus isolates and detection of WCBV neutralising antibodies across Africa. Isolates are colored as shown in the key. (See Page 10 in Color Section at the back of the book.)

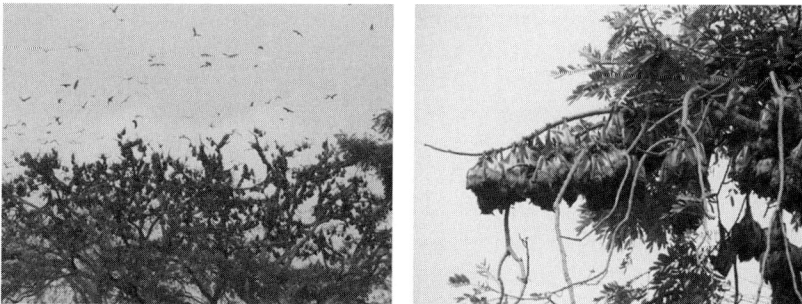

FIGURE 6 Colonies of *E. helvum* roosting in trees in Accra, Ghana. Images courtesy of David Hayman.

reactivity in complement fixation and virus neutralization tests established a link with RABV (Shope *et al.*, 1970). Since 1956, there have been numerous isolations of LBV (Table III).

More recent studies have revealed a high seroprevalence of antibodies against LBV in two colonial fruit bat species, *E. helvum* and *R. aegyptiacus* (Dzikwi, *et al.*, 2010; Hayman *et al.*, 2008; Kuzmin *et al.*, 2008b). Seroprevalence ranged from 14% to 67% in *E. helvum* and 29% to 46% in *R. aegyptiacus*, with adult *R. aegyptiacus* having a higher seroprevalence (60%) than subadults (31%). As previously reported, a substantial proportion (38%) of sera that neutralized LBV also neutralized MOKV (Badrane *et al.*, 2001; Hanlon *et al.*, 2005; Kuzmin *et al.*, 2008b; Wright *et al.*, 2010). Studies by Kuzmin *et al.* (2008b) have reported an absence of detectable LBV from 931 oral swabs from healthy bats by nested RT-PCR but generated sequences from brain material of one dead bat from which LBV was isolated (Kuzmin *et al.*, 2008b). Other studies have also demonstrated seropositivity in both *E. helvum* and the Gambian epauletted fruit bat (*Epomorphorus gambianus*) in Nigeria (Dzikwi *et al.*, 2010; Hayman *et al.*, 2008).

The discovery of further LBV isolates and their genome analysis have suggested that LBV phylogeny is more complex than originally thought (Kuzmin *et al.*, 2008b, 2010; Nadin-Davis *et al.*, 2002). A Senegalese (1985), a Kenyan (2007), and a French isolate (either Togolese or Egyptian origin, 1999) are highly similar (>99% nucleotide identity across the *N* gene) and constitute lineage A. The original isolate (Nigeria, 1956) is genetically distant from lineage A isolates and constitutes lineage B, whereas a third lineage (C) is made up of isolates from the Central African Republic, Zimbabwe, and South Africa (Markotter *et al.*, 2006a). Most recently, a fourth lineage (D) has been characterized in Kenya from an Egyptian fruit bat having only 79.5–80.9% similarity to lineages A–C (Kuzmin *et al.*, 2010) (Fig. 2; Table III). These four distinct groups are geographically clustered with the eight isolates from South Africa showing very little sequence variation, despite isolations occurring over a 25-year period (Markotter *et al.*, 2008a). Divergence between lineages is high with lineage A sharing <80% identity with the other lineages across a fragment of the *N* gene, a percentage cutoff value previously suggested as suitable for lyssavirus genotype division (Bourhy *et al.*, 1993; Kissi *et al.*, 1995). However, differentiation criteria must be scrutinized, as phylogeny on alternative regions of the genome shows less divergence between lineages. Virus classification (ICTV) does not recognize "genotypes," accepting only "species." Differentiation using *N* gene sequences is sufficient to characterize a virus to a particular "genotype," but sequence identity alone is not sufficient for acceptance as a species. Characteristics such as antigenic properties, geographical distribution, and host range must also be taken into consideration. Consequently, whereas the LBV isolates

TABLE III Detection/isolation and genetic characterization of LBV

Bat species	Latin name	Year	Location	Detection method	Clinical disease/comments	Lineage	Reference
Straw-colored fruit bat	*Eidolon helvum*	1956	Nigeria	VI	Unknown/isolation from a pool of eight brains	B	Boulger and Porterfield (1958)
		1985	Senegal	VI	Unknown	A	Swanepoel (1994)
		2007	Ghana	S	Healthy	ND	Hayman *et al.* (2008)
		2007	Kenya	VI	Dead	A	Kuzmin *et al.* (2008b, 2010)
		2006–2007	Kenya	S	Healthy	ND	Kuzmin *et al.* (2008b)
		2008	Nigeria	S	Healthy	ND	Dzikwi *et al.* (2010)
Dwarf epaulet fruit bats	*Micropteropus pussilus*	1974	Central African Republic	VI	Unknown	C	Sureau *et al.* (1977)
Wahlberg's epauletted fruit bat	*Epomophorus wahlbergi*	1980	South Africa	VI	Clinical rabies[a]	C	King and Crick (1988)
		1990	South Africa	VI	Dead	ND	Swanepoel (1994)
		2003–2004	South Africa	VI	Dead	C	Markotter *et al.* (2006b)
		2005	South Africa	VI	Clinically rabid, then died	C	Markotter *et al.* (2006b)
Egyptian fruit bat	*Rousettus aegypticus*	1999	France (ex-Togo or Egypt)	VI	Clinical rabies	A	Aubert (1999)
		2008	Kenya	VI	Healthy	D	Kuzmin *et al.* (2010)

(continued)

TABLE III (continued)

Bat species	Latin name	Year	Location	Detection method	Clinical disease/ comments	Lineage	Reference
Gambian epauletted fruit bat	*Epomophorus gambianus*	2007	Ghana	S	Healthy	ND	Hayman *et al.* (2008)
Buettikofer's epauletted fruit bat	*Epomops buettikoferi*	2007	Ghana	S	Healthy	ND	Hayman *et al.* (2008)
Gambian slit-faced bat	*Nycteris gambiensis*	1985	Guinea	VI	Unknown	ND	Swanepoel (1994)
Domestic cat	*Felis catus*	1982	South Africa	VI	Clinical rabies	ND	King and Crick (1988)
		1986	Zimbabwe	VI	Clinical rabies	C	King and Crick (1988)
Domestic dog	*Canis familiaris*	1989–1990	Ethiopia	VI	Dead	ND	Mebatsion *et al.* (1992)
		2003	South Africa	VI	Clinical rabies	ND	Markotter *et al.* (2008b)
Water mongoose	*Atilax paludinosus*	2004	South Africa	VI	Clinical rabies	C	Markotter *et al.* (2006a)

Animal previously vaccinated against rabies. S, serological detection; VI, virus isolation; lineage A, light gray; lineage B, dark gray with black text; lineage C, dark gray with white text; lineage D, black with white text; ND, not determined.

[a] Ten further LBV cases were reported but not isolated; where genetic characterization has been possible, lineage differentiations are shaded.

studied could be differentiated into four separate lineages (Table III), they are proposed as a single species (Kuzmin *et al.*, 2010). This phylogenetic relationship is depicted in Fig. 2.

Experimental infection *in vivo* with LBV has been examined to determine the relative pathogenicity of the virus in different species. Early studies suggested that LBV was not able to cause disease in guinea pigs ($n = 2$, intramuscular inoculation), rabbits ($n = 2$, one intramuscular and one intracerebral inoculation), or an individual *Cercocebus torquatus* monkey (subcutaneous inoculation; Boulger and Porterfield, 1958). Such experimental studies and others (Badrane *et al.*, 2001) led to suggestions that the phylogroup II viruses characterized at the time, LBV and MOKV, had a reduced pathogenicity, when compared with studies with RABV isolates, with inoculation by the peripheral route. In contrast, both LBV and MOKV caused death when inoculated intracranially into dogs and monkeys (Tignor *et al.*, 1973). These limited studies were, however, undertaken using only a single representative of each lyssavirus species (Badrane *et al.*, 2001). Genetic differences including the amino acid substitution at position 333 of the viral glycoprotein were suggested to play a key role in the reduced pathogenicity, as had been reported for some fixed (laboratory-adapted) RABV isolates (Coulon *et al.*, 1998; Dietzschold *et al.*, 1983; Seif *et al.*, 1985). The correlates of pathogenicity, however, remain poorly understood for the lyssaviruses, and both host-driven restrictions and tissue culture-derived mutations may affect the pathogenicity of any one virus isolate. Evidence for such restrictions is provided by spill-over events, which have caused rabies in a range of species (Crick *et al.*, 1982; King and Crick, 1988; Markotter *et al.*, 2006a,b; Mebatsion *et al.*, 1992). One recent experimental study compared LBV isolates to RABV and MOKV isolates in the murine model via different routes of inoculation (Markotter *et al.*, 2009). Intracranial inoculation of mice with each lyssavirus produced 100% mortality, whereas intramuscular inoculation caused comparative mortality between LBV and RABV and survivorship following infection with MOKV remained higher than with LBV and RABV (Markotter *et al.*, 2009). Therefore, despite the early reports of low pathogenicity of LBV in the laboratory (Badrane *et al.*, 2001; Boulger and Porterfield, 1958), subsequent investigation has shown that there is substantial variation in pathogenicity between LBV isolates (Markotter *et al.*, 2009). Unfortunately, no original unpassaged virus exists for the primary Nigerian LBV isolate and, hence, analysis of its pathogenic potential cannot currently be undertaken. However, molecular tools may be used to generate this virus in future from full genome sequence data derived from original material and establish growth characteristics *in vitro* and pathogenicity *in vivo*.

B. Mokola virus

Whereas MOKV has not been isolated from bats, isolates are available from other species and the host reservoir(s) remain unknown (Meredith *et al.*, 1996; Sabeta *et al.*, 2007). MOKV clearly has an African distribution and is closely related genetically to the other lyssaviruses. MOKV was first isolated from shrews (*Crocidura* sp.) in Nigeria in 1968 (Kemp *et al.*, 1972) and since then has also been isolated from domestic cats in South Africa in 1970 and 1995–1998 (Nel *et al.*, 2000; Schneider *et al.*, 1985), shrews (*Crocidura* sp.) in Cameroon in 1974 (Le Gonidec *et al.*, 1978; Swanepoel, 1994), domestic cats and a dog in Zimbabwe in 1981 and 1982 (Foggin, 1982), the rusty-bellied brush-furred rat (*Lophuromys sikapusi*) from the Central Africa Republic in 1983 (Swanepoel, 1994), and between 1989 and 1990 in domestic cats in Ethiopia (Mebatsion *et al.*, 1992). Two human infections have also been reported in Nigeria in 1969 and 1971, although only one of these was fatal (Familusi *et al.*, 1972) whereas the other isolation may have been a laboratory contaminant (Familusi and Moore, 1972). Cross-neutralization shown by LBV seropositive bat sera (Dzikwi *et al.*, 2010; Kuzmin *et al.*, 2008b) suggests that bats cannot yet be ruled out as reservoirs; however, the lack of sampling of rodents, shrews, and other potential reservoirs in Africa is notable.

C. Duvenhage virus

DUVV was first isolated in South Africa in 1970 from a human who died following a bat bite (Meredith *et al.*, 1971). Further isolations from insectivorous bats occurred from *M. schreibersii* in South Africa in 1981 and *Nycteris thebaica* in Zimbabwe in 1986 (King and Crick, 1988; Paweska *et al.*, 2006). Interestingly, the *N. thebaica* was trapped in a survey, with no clinical signs of rabies reported (Foggin, 1988). Two further cases of DUVV in humans have been reported, one from South Africa (Paweska *et al.*, 2006) and the other from the Netherlands, the virus being of Kenyan origin (van Thiel *et al.*, 2008).

D. West Caucasian bat virus

As detailed in Section II, WCBV appears to have a wide geographical range, including both Eurasia and at least parts of Africa. A recent study reported neutralizing antibodies against WCBV in *Miniopterus* bats collected in Kenya with prevalence ranging from 17% to 26% in sampled bats (Kuzmin *et al.*, 2008c). WCBV seropositive bats were detected in four of five locations sampled across Kenya. This report provides evidence that WCBV, originally isolated in Europe, may emerge in other continents.

Further isolations of WCBV or serological detection are required to understand its epidemiology and relationships with the other lyssaviruses.

E. Shimoni bat virus

Isolated in 2009, SHBV represents the most recently detected bat lyssavirus, potentially a new species, isolated from the brain of a dead Commerson's leaf-nosed bat (*Hipposideros commersoni*) in Kenya. The virus lies antigenically within phylogroup II, being classified phylogenetically between MOKV and WCBV (Kuzmin *et al.*, 2010). The *Hipposideros* subfamily has a broad distribution in the Old World from tropical Africa to China. Therefore, further sampling of these genera will be interesting to determine if this is another virus that may have crossed from Africa to Eurasia, as appears to have been the case from the limited data available from WCBV (Kuzmin *et al.*, 2010).

Interestingly, *M. schreibersii*, a species from which EBLV-1, DUVV, and WCBV have been isolated or RNA detected, has a distribution from the Middle East and Caucasus, across southern Europe and down through Africa. This species may, therefore, act as a host to facilitate the cross-continental transmission and emergence of lyssaviruses from Africa, along with species from the *Hipposideros* subfamily.

IV. BAT RABIES AND THE AMERICAS

The Americas are geographically divided into three major regions encompassing a total of 48 defined countries, island nations, and territories: North America including the United States, Mexico, and Canada; Central America, including all the mainland countries as well as the island nations of the Caribbean; and South America, including some of the most densely populated countries of the Americas. Whereas terrestrial rabies in domestic animals is reported to have been eliminated from North America (Belotto *et al.*, 2005), other sylvatic terrestrial reservoirs remain. These reservoirs appear to maintain RABV variants within populations that can spill-over into domestic animals and occasionally into humans. Bat-associated rabies is also reported frequently and now constitutes a recognized public health threat in North America. Domestic- and bat-associated rabies also continues to be an important economic and public health concern in Latin America. As in North America, concerted mass vaccination campaigns targeting domestic cats and dogs have led to a dramatic decrease in urban rabies. However, RABV transmitted by hematophagous bats is currently an increasing problem across Latin America, and vampire bat rabies is now considered the most significant threat to livestock health as well as posing considerable risk to humans

(Ruiz and Chavez, 2010; Schneider *et al.*, 2005). Indeed, RABV occurs in both hematophagous and nonhematophagous bats across the New World and, despite widespread surveillance, only RABV has been isolated, without documentation of detection of the other recognized lyssavirus species. Here, we document what is currently understood regarding diversity, transmission, and virus–host dynamics within bat populations in the Americas.

A. Vampire bat rabies

The human population across Central America and vast regions of South America remains at risk of RABV transmission from bats, in particular, hematophagous or vampire bats. There are only three species of hematophagous bat that consume blood exclusively as their diet: the common vampire bat (*Desmodus rotundus*), the white-winged vampire bat (*Diaemus youngi*), and the hairy-legged vampire bat (*Diphylla ecaudata*). The common vampire bat is present across much of Latin America. It has been postulated that the introduction of domesticated livestock to the Americas has increased vampire bat densities considerably over the past 300 years through an increase in available prey species such as cattle, horses, goat, and sheep (Altringham, 1996; Constantine, 1988). Its current distribution is considered to be increasing as a result of alterations in climatic conditions. It has been suggested that an increase in temperature over the next few decades could result in a substantial expansion of its current habitat along the east and west coasts of Mexico and into Southern states of the United States, potentially including Texas, Florida, and Arizona. (Shahroukh and Moreno-Valdez, 2009). Alongside this, both deforestation and the introduction of prey species such as livestock into new areas provide a food source that will help increase populations of vampire bats. The white-winged vampire bat is found from Mexico to southern Argentina and is also present on the islands of Trinidad and Isla Margarita. In Trinidad, white-winged vampire bats have been found cohabiting roosts in caves with *D. rotundus* as well as insectivorous bats such as the great sac-winged bat (*Saccopteryx bilineata*). The hairy-legged vampire is subdivided into two subspecies with *D. ecaudata centralis* being present from Western Panama to Mexico whereas *D. ecaudata ecaudata* is found from Brazil and eastern Peru to eastern Panama (Greenhall and Schmidt, 1988; Nowak, 1999).

The hematophagous nature of these bats provides a unique mechanism of transmission for RABV. Interestingly, there appears to be some preference in prey species utilized for feeding in that the common vampire bat appears to prefer predation on bovids; the hairy-legged bat is most commonly associated with feeding on bovids and equids, whereas the white-winged vampire bat favors avian species (Greenhall, 1961).

Transmission events from hematophagous bats to livestock species were first documented in Central and South America at the beginning of the past century (Carini, 1911; Hurst and Pawan, 1931) with attacks on live-stock species causing rabies outbreaks in cattle in the 1920s (Haupt and Rehaag, 1921). Indeed, the RABV lineage associated with vampire bats is postulated to be phylogenetically the most ancient among American bat isolates (Hughes *et al.*, 2005), although the actual origin of the virus remains unknown (Davis *et al.*, 2006).

Mechanisms of transmission between vampire bats within roosts remain speculative, but their roost structure and behavioral adaptation to feed on blood suggest several obvious mechanisms for spread of infection within the roost. Vampire bats not only have a unique adaptation in their requirement for blood but are also known to regurgitate ingested blood for mutual feeding purposes. This may serve as a mechanism of transmission alongside potential delivery of virus through allogrooming, biting, licking, or inhalation of aerosolized virus. Experimental studies to attempt to elucidate mechanisms of transmission of virus between bats have addressed the possibility of excretion from vampire bats. Whereas salivary excretion has been documented in swabs from bats just before the onset of clinical disease, excretion from healthy animals has not generally been detected (Moreno and Baer, 1980) apart from in exceptionally rare cases where human error could not be ruled out (Franka *et al.*, 2008). A recent study looked at the effect of dose on survivorship within vampire bats (Almeida *et al.*, 2005). This study corroborated earlier observations that are of general interest. First, the detection of early clinical signs was not possible merely through observation, and it was not until animals were separated and forced to move around that disease signs were evident. This suggests that bats that have become separated from a roost with clear clinical disease may be in a late stage of infection, although it remains unknown how clinical disease progression correlates with virus excretion. This may have significant consequences for contact and transmission rates within bat species. Second, as reported previously (Aguilar-Setien *et al.*, 1998; Pawan, 1936; Rodrigues and Tamayo, 2000), not all animals that succumbed to infection displayed observable clinical disease. These findings, however, may not be surprising, given that checks were performed daily, and it is likely that diagnosing signs of disease in wild animals may be difficult. This is especially true if during the prodromal phase animals display nonspecific clinical signs and/or if progression to death is rapid. Those that may have had clinical illness did not necessarily display the aggressive behavior reported in other studies either (Pawan, 1936). Another similar study by Aguilar-Setien *et al.* (2005) sought to assess virus excretion in the vampire bat model using a large dose (10^6 MICLD$_{50}$) of a vampire bat rabies virus isolate. As previously reported, a decrease in feeding was observed following the onset of clinical disease in those that succumbed leading to dehydration and reduced salivation. Infected bats were swabbed prior to and following the onset of clinical disease. No viral material was detected in swabs from clinical animals; however, virus isolation in tissue culture was successful from three bats that survived infection after 6 ($n = 2$) or 21 ($n = 1$) days postinoculation. All three bats remained healthy and had rabies neutralizing antibodies by the end of the experimentation (Aguilar-Setien *et al.*, 2005). Clearly, mechanisms by which virus is maintained, excreted, or cleared remain poorly understood, and future experimentation is needed to confirm these findings. However, design of future experimentation must rationalize dose administration because a very high viral dose may cause an "unnatural infection" with neurological disease and death occurring before virus is shed in salivary glands.

Vampire bat rabies infections of humans and herbivores appear to be increasing in Central and South America (Ruiz and Chavez, 2010) with *D. rotundus* being the main reservoir across Mexico, Brazil, Argentina, and Chile (Cisterna *et al.*, 2005; Mayen, 2003; Nadin-Davis and Loza-Rubio, 2006; Yung *et al.*, 2002). Often, high human population densities are associated with people living in conditions of extreme poverty in these regions (Castilho *et al.*, 2010). Such areas have been associated with high incidences of vampire bat rabies transmission to both humans and herbivores and have identified the circulation of specific virus lineages within localized geographical locations. It is hypothesized that topological features such as dense jungle may restrict vampire bat movement and that this results in the generation of viral sublineages circulating within distinct regions (Castilho *et al.*, 2010; Kobayashi *et al.*, 2007, 2008; Paez *et al.*, 2007; Velasco-Villa *et al.*, 2006).

B. Insectivorous bat-associated rabies

Initial detection of RABV in insectivorous and frugivorous bats was made during surveys into hematophagous bat populations and rabies transmission in South America (Carini, 1911; Pawan, 1936). It was not until the first detection of rabies in an insectivorous bat in the early 1950s that insectivorous bats were also found to harbor the virus in North America (Baer and Smith, 1991; Brass, 1994; Sulkin and Greve, 1954). A recent study in Brazil documented that 41 species of bat have historically been associated with transmission of bat rabies, including 25 genera and three bat families: the *Phyllostomidae*, the *Vespertilionidae*, and the *Molossidae* (Sodre *et al.*, 2010). Across the Americas, 16% of wildlife-associated rabies cases were reported from bat species, mostly nonhematophagous bats, between 1993 and 2002 (Belotto *et al.*, 2005). With the elimination of terrestrial RABV in companion animals across North America, the transmission of RABV to humans from bats has become of increasing importance as a public health risk (Messenger *et al.*, 2002). Both increased surveillance and general scientific interest in RABV as a viral pathogen and the ecology and biology of bat species has seen a dramatic surge in the number of bat rabies cases being reported in the United States (Blanton *et al.*, 2010). Despite the large number of different bat species associated with RABV transmission in Central and Southern America, association of RABV infection in North America has highlighted a key role in infection of certain bat species. The big brown bat (*E. fuscus*), the little brown bat (*Myotis lucifigus*), and the Brazilian (Mexican) free-tailed bat (*Tadaria brasiliensis*) are most commonly submitted for rabies testing, although only a fraction of those submitted are found to be positive for RABV infection (Blanton *et al.*, 2010). Interestingly, the species that are most frequently associated with transmission to humans are silver-haired bats (n=6) (*Lasionycteris noctivagans*), eastern pipistrelle bats (n=4) (*Perimyotis subflavus*) and Brazilian (Mexican) free-tailed bats (n=5) (*T. brasiliensis*) in the United States between 2000 and 2009 (Blanton *et al.*, 2010; Brass, 2009). Recent studies have also highlighted an apparent host restriction seen within circulating bat RABV variants in North America with a suggestion that phylogenetic barriers exist to cross-species trans-mission at the level of both initial infection and sustained transmission within the newly infected species (Streicker *et al.*, 2010). Current genetic data depicting the phylogenetic relationship between different bat rabies isolates from species across the Americas are shown in Fig. 7 and Table IV. As with lyssavirus infections seen across Europe, a skewed geographical distribution exists for the detection of RABV following human encounters due to disproportionate density of human populations alongside the acknowledgment of preferred roost habitats for different bat species (Streicker *et al.*, 2010).

Numerous experimental studies have been undertaken with nonhe-matophagous bat rabies variants *in vivo* both in chiropteran and in terres-trial animal models. A series of experiments in the late 1950s highlighted potential mechanisms for virus persistence by virtue of body temperature as well as suggesting a possible role for the adipose tissue of hibernating bats in the maintenance of RABV (Sulkin, 1962; Sulkin *et al.*, 1957, 1960), although later studies were unsuccessful in corroborating an involvement of brown fat in virus maintenance through periods of torpor (Kuzmin *et al.*, 1994). Throughout the 1960s, extensive studies were undertaken in caves where naturally infected insectivorous bats were present to attempt to elucidate potential transmission mechanisms. Caged coyotes and foxes were positioned under large roosts and monitored, and the caged animals invariably developed clinical rabies (Constantine, 1962, 1967) highlight-ing the potential for aerosol transmission of RABV (Constantine, 1966). However, it is not clear that biting can be ruled out as a potential trans-mission mechanism in this study. Whereas natural exposure via the

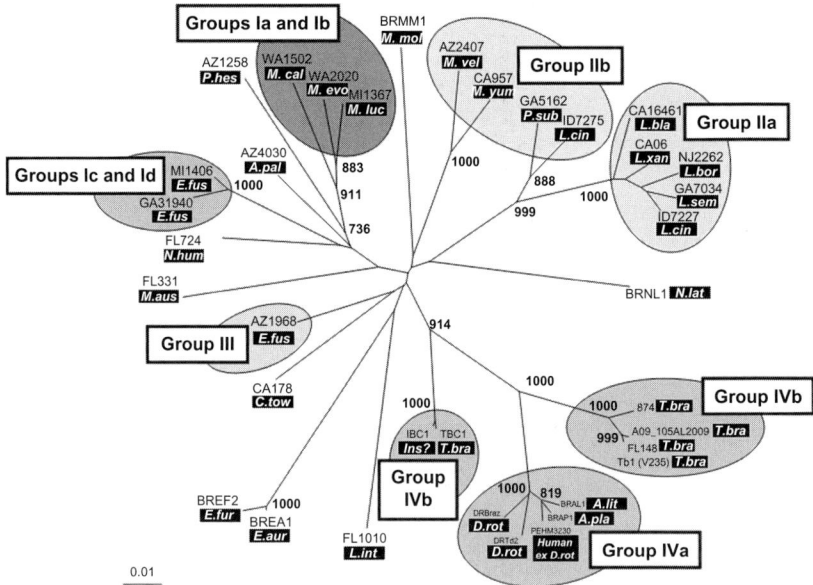

FIGURE 7 Maximum likelihood phylogenetic tree of 36 partial *N* gene sequences (590 nucleotides) of RABV isolated from at least 27 different bat species from across the Americas. Previously identified bat RABV lineages are shown (Nadin-Davis *et al.*, 2001). Significant bootstrap values ($>70\%$, 1000 replicates) are indicated. Latin names of bats are detailed in black boxes (white text) with sample identification codes corresponding to Table IV.

aerosol route has been reported (Winkler, 1968; Winkler *et al.*, 1973), more recent experimental attempts to infect mice by this route have had success with RABVs but not with other lyssaviruses (Johnson *et al.*, 2006c). In other experiments with bats, rabid animals have been observed biting cage mates, although disease did not develop in these animals (Shankar *et al.*, 2004). Most recently, the effect of multiple exposures to virus has been addressed in *E. fuscus* with a RABV isolate (Turmelle *et al.*, 2010). Following initial exposure, mortality reached almost 40% with only 35% developing neutralizing antibodies. Of the 17 bats (39%) that succumbed following the first inoculation, only one bat had developed neutralizing antibody titers, and then only on the day of euthanasia. Those that survived the first inoculation were kept for a total of 175 days between inoculations and prior to the second inoculation, the number of seropositive bats had decreased to 12%. This suggests that antibody titers wane to levels that are not detectable using the current tests. A similar factor was hypothesized previously when vampire bats selected for experimental inoculation were seronegative prior to inoculation but developed a strong antibody response following RABV inoculation (Aguilar-Setien *et al.*,

TABLE IV   Details of samples used to generate Fig. 7

Species of bat	Abbreviated name	Year of isolation	Location	Accession number
Antrozous pallidus	*A. pal*	2005	USA, Arizona	GU644641
Artibeus lituratus	*A. lit*	1998	Brazil	AB117969
Artibeus planirostris	*A. pla*	1998	Brazil	AB117972
Corynorhinus townsendii	*C. tow*	2003	USA, California	GU644759
Desmodus rotundus	*D. rot*	1986	Brazil	AF351847
Desmodus rotundus	*D. rot*	1995	Trinidad	AF351852
Eptesicus furinalis	*E. fur*	2001	Brazil	AB201812
Eptesicus fuscus	*E. fus*	2004	USA, Georgia	GU644652
Eptesicus fuscus	*E. fus*	2004	Arizona	GU644642
Eptesicus fuscus	*E. fus*	2003	USA, Michigan	GU644659
Eumops auripendulus	*E. aur*	1998	Brazil	AB201809
Human ex vampire bat	*Hu ex D. rot*	1996	Peru	AF045166
Insectivorous bat (?)	*Ins*	1988	Chile	AF351850
Lasionycteris noctivagans	*L. Noc*	2005	USA, Idaho	GU644923
Lasiurus blossevillii	*L. blo*	2002	USA, California	GU644696
Lasiurus borealis	*L. bor*	2005	USA, New Jersey	GU644702
Lasiurus cinereus	*L. cin*	2005	USA, Idaho	GU644715
Lasiurus intermedius	*L. int*	2002	USA, Florida	GU644914
Lasiurus seminolus	*L. sem*	2003	USA, Georgia	GU644732
Lasiurus xanthinus	*L. xan*	2004	USA, California	GU644740
Molossus molossus	*M. mol*	1999	Brazil	AB201815
Myotis austroriparius	*M. aus*	2001	USA, Florida	GU644742
Myotis californicus	*M. cal*	2004	USA, Washington	GU644745
Myotis evotis	*M. evo*	2005	USA, Washington	GU644747
Myotis lucifugus	*M. luc*	2005	USA, Michigan	GU644749
Myotis velifer	*M .vel*	2004	USA, Arizona	GU644960
Myotis yumanensis	*M. yum*	2004	USA, California	GU644753
Nycticeius humeralis	*N. hum*	2003	USA, Florida	GU644969
Nyctinomops laticaudatus	*N. lat*	1998	Brazil	AB201806
Parastrellus hesperus	*P. hes*	2004	USA, Arizona	GU644755
Perimyotis subflavus	*P. sub*	2005	USA, Georgia	GU644975
Tadarida brasiliensis	*T. bra*	2004	USA, Florida	GU644777
Tadarida brasiliensis	*T. bra*	1988	USA, Florida	AF394876
Tadarida brasiliensis	*T. bra*	?	USA, Texas	AF351849
Tadarida brasiliensis	*T. bra*	1987	Chile	AF070450
Tadarida brasiliensis	*T. bra*	2009	Mexico	GU991832

2005). These observations may suggest that bats had undetectable levels of antibody prior to inoculation through natural exposure and support the use of techniques that measure binding antibodies (e.g., ELISA) rather than relying solely on methods that detect neutralizing antibodies (e.g., RFFIT, FAVN) for prescreening of sera. In the repeat exposure study, mortality following the second inoculation was not significantly lower than that observed following primary inoculation (36%) and only 60% seroconverted (including three of the nine that succumbed). A tertiary inoculation was also performed and one further animal succumbed. Following tertiary exposure, 17% of bats seroconverted (Turmelle *et al.*, 2010). Clearly, the role of antibody development following infection differs between individuals, and ultimately, other immunological components such as cell-mediated mechanisms play an important role in host response to infection.

Other studies have addressed the susceptibility of different bat species to infection and again there appears to be a virus–host dependence on the outcome of infection. Numerous observations suggest that both hematophagous and nonhematophagous bats that form highly social roosts appear to be less susceptible to disease with indigenous RABV isolates. Where infection occurs, clinical disease is observed as a nonaggressive, paralytic form of rabies. In direct contrast, less social bats appear to have a heightened susceptibility to RABV variants and appear more likely to develop a furious form of the disease following infection (reviewed in Kuzmin and Rupprecht, 2007). Further studies have analyzed serological responses to both natural and experimental infection with lyssaviruses with some demonstrating fluctuation through time in antibody responses within some species (Constantine, 1967; O'Shea *et al.*, 2003; Shankar *et al.*, 2004; Steece and Altenbach, 1989; Turmelle *et al.*, 2010). Despite these studies, the development, role, and significance of seropositivity within a bat population remain poorly understood.

C. Bat rabies and host switching

Successful species-to-species transmission of viral pathogens is an important factor in the emergence and evolution of microorganisms. For viruses, such transmission can lead to host switching whereby a virus can spill-over into a novel host and theoretically alter its genome to enable efficient replication and maintenance within the recipient species. This fact is of particular importance for zoonotic pathogens where host switching may lead to establishment of novel human pathogens with altered virulence. Host switching has been proposed as the evolutionary mechanism by which lyssaviruses have evolved through spill-over from bats to infect terrestrial mammals (Badrane and Tordo, 2001). The mutability of lyssaviruses to enable such transmission and adaptation is thought to be a result of the error prone nature of the virally encoded RNA-dependent RNA polymerase enzyme that facilitates both transcription and replication of the viral genome (Assenberg *et al.*, 2010).

In the majority of cases, spill-over events are dead-end infections. However, if productive infection is established in the new host and excretion occurs, then further transmission within the new species may occur. This is the mechanism by which lyssaviruses successfully switch hosts and establish further cycles of infection. Genetic analysis of glycoprotein sequences from viruses circulating in both bat and terrestrial carnivore species suggests that host switching of lyssaviruses from bats to other mammals has occurred repeatedly and successfully in history (Badrane and Tordo, 2001).

The rabies situation in wildlife across the Americas is complicated due to the presence of different terrestrial and bat vector species. Among domestic animals, cats and dogs are the most important animal reservoirs for spill-over cases of RABV to humans, whereas within wildlife species, foxes, raccoons, and skunks constitute the greatest threat to spill over into both humans and domestic animals. Despite the complexity of the situation, these terrestrial species may be limited in their distribution: with raccoons (*Procyon lotor*) being present across much of the eastern United States; the gray fox (*Urocyon cinereoargenteus*) in Arizona and Texas; and both red (*Vulpes vulpes*) and arctic (*Alopex lagopus*) foxes in Alaska and parts of Canada; although precise species distributions have not been defined. Oral vaccination programs have, however, successfully reduced the number of rabies cases in foxes reported in some regions (MacInnes *et al.*, 2001; Sidwa *et al.*, 2005). Terrestrial rabies associated with both raccoons and skunks, particularly the striped skunk (*Mephitis mephitis*) and the eastern spotted skunk (*Spilogale putorius*), covers much of the north central and south central United States with a combined total of 3930 cases, 64% of the total cases reported from wild terrestrial species, being reported in 2009 (Blanton *et al.*, 2010).

Whereas RABV infection attributed to specific species is clearly defined, spill-over into other wildlife species occurs, but only rarely initiates a new cycle of maintenance of virus within the new host. Transmission between animals of the same species maintains the levels of infected individuals and at the regional level may lead to continued circulation of a virus variant within a local population for decades (Blanton *et al.*, 2010; Childs *et al.*, 2001). Whereas it is apparently rare, two case reports provide evidence for maintenance of virus in a terrestrial species following presumed transmission from a bat species. In 1993, a small outbreak of rabies cases occurred in foxes on Prince Edward Island, Canada. The genetic detection of a bat RABV variant within this fox population was confirmed, and from the detection of low levels of virus in salivary gland material, it was assumed that some degree of intraspecific transmission among the foxes had occurred (Daoust *et al.*, 1996). A second report from Arizona, USA in 2001, highlighted the infection of a number of skunks with a bat RABV variant. This virus was phylogenetically most similar to that known to be present in *Eptesicus* and *Myotis* sp. populations from the same region (Leslie *et al.*, 2006). Sustained intraspecies transmission of this bat variant of RABV in the skunk population was the most likely explanation as the skunk cases occurred over a period of only 7 months (Leslie *et al.*, 2006).

V. DISCUSSION

The role that bats play in the maintenance, transmission, and evolution of lyssaviruses is complex and generally poorly understood. The protected nature of numerous bat species across the developed world has made experimental studies with lyssaviruses, in what are considered to be the reservoir host species, problematic. The zoonotic potential of these viruses coupled with the lack of protection afforded by standard rabies vaccines against some of these pathogens has further complicated the issue through the need for experimentation to be undertaken in high containment with stringent biosecurity. There is currently a lack of knowledge at both the pathogen and the host level, and further studies are necessary to bridge this gap in knowledge. Below we attempt to address the current thinking regarding bat exposure and infection with lyssaviruses and highlight questions that need to be answered if we are to gain further insight into lyssavirus infection of bats.

A. Receptor usage and virus replication upon exposure

It is widely recognized that lyssaviruses are neurotropic. However, the receptors utilized by different lyssavirus isolates, and under what circumstances, are not known. It is clear, however, that for bats to transmit virus either within roosts or to terrestrial mammals, there has to be a mechanism for virus cell entry. At the molecular level, this interaction is determined primarily by receptor availability and usage. Currently, three receptors are proposed to act as key molecules by which RABVs gain entry into cells. These include the nicotinic acetylcholine receptor (nAchR), responsible for interneuronal communication within the central nervous system and the peripheral nerve network; neural cell adhesion molecule (NCAM), present at the nerve termini and deep within the neuromuscular junctions at the postsynaptic membranes; and the neurotrophin receptor (p75NTR), which plays a role in cellular death, synaptic transmission, and axonal elongation (Dechant and Barde, 2002; Lafon, 2005). However, recent studies have suggested that the p75NTR molecule is probably not important for RABV entry (Tuffereau *et al.*, 2007). When observed in bats, clinical manifestations of disease include neurological signs, indicating that bat virus variants are also highly neurotropic. These receptor molecules, however, have primarily been implicated in cell entry using murine and canine *in vitro* and *in vivo* systems, and the presence of viable receptors in bat and other species tissues has received little attention. Again, despite partial characterization of these molecules as receptors for RABV, it is currently unknown to what extent each of these proposed receptors is utilized by lyssaviruses. Replication of lyssaviruses in other cell lines has suggested that there may be a ubiquitous receptor molecule utilized by different isolates, although the replication of wild-type isolates in nonneuronal cell lines other than baby hamster kidney (BHK) cells has not been studied in detail. Novel species-specific bat cell lines that have recently been developed (Crameri *et al.*, 2009) may further elucidate mechanisms by which lyssaviruses enter cells and help determine whether or not they can be maintained in nonneuronal cells *in vitro*.

Such studies may also elucidate restrictions that appear to be in place for infection of different species. Certainly, infection with EBLV-1 and -2 appears in the main to be restricted to *E. serotinus* and *M. daubentonii*, respectively. European bat species have been suggested to mix at both swarming sites and within roosts, potentially enabling a mechanism of cross-species transmission. However, the inaccessibility of underground roosts and caves means that our understanding of bat ecology across Europe remains poor (Rivers *et al.*, 2006). Whether or not the species restriction of EBLVs is real or whether, like some bat variants of RABVs, virus can be maintained in numerous bat reservoirs requires further analysis (Streicker *et al.*, 2010). In addition, further receptor analysis is required for lyssaviruses, such as LBV, that appear to be promiscuous and infect several bat species across several genera. How lyssaviruses compare with regard to their receptor usage may give important insights into host restriction mechanisms and is an area for future study. In the absence of extensive *in vivo* research, novel *in vitro* methodologies may provide answers to such questions.

B. Bat population structures, sizes, and ecology

Our current understanding of bat ecology and epidemiology is not sufficient to explain maintenance and transmission of lyssaviruses within bat populations. It is clear that lyssaviruses are able to infect a wide range of bat species across the globe. However, bat species have an incredibly wide range of habitats, life cycles, and population sizes. The movement of bats between roosts in widely dispersed locations may also influence virus maintenance. Some bat species have relatively localized movements, for example, insectivorous bats such as *M. daubentonii*, whereas larger migratory bat species (e.g., *E. helvum*) fly great distances between roosts for as yet undefined purposes. Indeed, in such large migratory species, telemetry has been used to track individual bats moving over 370 km in a single night and traveling over 2500 km during migration, although tracking individuals often proves difficult (Richter and Cumming, 2008). Whereas it is clear that some bats move to locations that are known to be roost sites, bats also "disappear" for considerable lengths of time occasionally returning to known roosts. This includes both insectivorous species where maternal roosts are unknown and migratory species such as *E. helvum* where 100,000s of bats migrate annually (Thomas, 1983). Knowledge of the size and structure of such metapopulations, and the degree of connectivity between them where they exist across continents, would greatly enhance our understanding of the potential for virus maintenance and transmission within them. Numerous studies have reported virus-specific neutralizing antibodies within healthy individuals of such bat species. However, isolation of live virus is rare, and mechanisms of maintenance remain unknown. In addition, the aging of wild animals is difficult and precludes a detailed analysis of age-specific seroprevalence, in turn reducing the information available from serological surveys.

C. Bat immunobiology and the carrier state hypothesis

The basic immunobiological status of bats, particularly with respect to exposure to lyssaviruses, is poorly understood. With the recent detection of numerous zoonotic pathogens in bats, considerable studies are now being focused on both bat ecology and pathogen interactions (Calisher *et al.*, 2006; Cui *et al.*, 2007; Dominguez *et al.*, 2007; Field, 2009; Towner *et al.*, 2009; Wang and Eaton, 2007; Wibbelt *et al.*, 2007). Early findings in this novel area of host–pathogen interactions have looked at bat genomics for indicators of immune regulators and have made comparisons with established findings in more extensively studied experimental animal models (Allen *et al.*, 2009; Mayer and Brunner, 2007; Omatsu *et al.*, 2008). The concept of the existence of an RABV carrier state in bats has been postulated for many years. This hypothesizes that bats are somehow able to support virus infection in an as yet undefined tissue type but remain free of clinical disease for long periods and being able to transmit virus to conspecifics within roosts. However, there is little empirical evidence to support this hypothesis. Further, it is plausible that bats may eventually succumb to disease during periods of reduced immunocompetence, with the protracted incubation times of lyssaviruses perhaps providing a more heterogeneous immunological landscape over time for lyssaviruses than for other classical acute RNA viral infections. Clearly, both baseline immunological characteristics of bats and the immunological response following infection are poorly understood. For many species, the bat life cycle is intrinsically linked to numerous ecological factors that determine key stages of bat biology such as periods of hibernation and/or torpor, the necessity to migrate, and the timing of mating and resultant birth of offspring. The role of the environment, including temperature, humidity, food availability, parasite load, and infection with other bat pathogens may also all play a role in the outcome of exposure to lyssaviruses. The effect of torpor, for example, was experimentally demonstrated to prolong mean incubation period by the duration of torpor itself (Sulkin, 1962; Sulkin et al., 1960). The biological diversity within bat species means that these factors and requirements are particularly varied across different species, and as such, potential carrier status and/or reactivation of virus from a latent stage may be plausible but without any evidence to support it. However, there is scant knowledge on the driving forces behind a number of these factors, and so mechanisms of virus maintenance within healthy bats remain unknown. It is interesting to postulate that alterations to environmental conditions may affect the potential for bats to resist, transmit, or even expose other mammalian populations to virus through spill-over events. Long incubation periods have been described for dead-end hosts such as humans (Johnson et al., 2008b) and also in instances in which captive bats have been apparently healthy upon capture and have developed disease while in captivity (Aguilar-Setien et al., 2005; Almeida et al., 2005; Turmelle et al., 2010), occasionally following long periods (Pajamo et al., 2008). This may reflect the variable incubation period or possibly a delicate host–pathogen relationship in which the immune status may be essential for resisting active viral replication; however, ultimately, these reports may be related to the route of exposure, viral dose received, primary site of replication, and other unknown factors. Continued research into basic bat immunobiology is essential, therefore, to gain a better understanding of the host–pathogen relationship in these unique mammals.

D. Bat lyssavirus serology: Infection or exposure?

The continued serological assessment of different bat species for exposure to lyssaviruses, as well as other viral pathogens of interest to the scientific community, has established that bat populations across the globe are frequently exposed to lyssaviruses. Numerous serosurveillance initiatives have reported serological positivity for virus exposure for several representatives of lyssavirus species (Harris et al., 2009, 2006; Hayman et al., 2008; Kuzmin et al., 2006, 2008b,c; Lumlertdacha 2005; Pal et al., 1980; Smith et al., 1967; Wright et al., 2010). Indeed, the presence of virus-neutralizing antibodies in healthy bats remains an interesting aspect of lyssavirus biology (Arguin *et al.*, 2002; Serra-Cobo *et al.*, 2002; Turmelle *et al.*, 2010). In nonchiropteran hosts, infection with lyssaviruses generally leads to the development of disease, and ultimately death, with seroconversion either occurring late during the symptomatic phase or not at all. Few studies have reported circulation of virus in terrestrial species with rare seropositivity within terrestrial carnivore populations being suggested (East *et al.*, 2001; Lembo *et al.*, 2007). In bat species, so-called abortive infection, that is, the development of a neutralizing antibody response in the absence of disease, appears to be relatively common. Indeed, what constitutes an exposure that is able to prime an immune response in the absence of development of disease remains an enigma.

Studies with lyssaviruses in a wide spectrum of animal models have shown that both the route of exposure and viral dose play important roles in the outcome of infection. Experimental studies in insectivorous bats have attempted to explain the importance of route of inoculation in the natural host, but a clear trend with regard to how virus is transmitted between bats in the roost has not yet been fully defined. Most reliably as an experimental route of inoculation, direct inoculation of viable virus intracranially invariably leads to infection, neurological disease, and death. In limited studies, intranasal inoculation does not appear to be a successful route of exposure if clinical disease is sought (Franka *et al.*, 2008; Freuling *et al.*, 2009b; Johnson *et al.*, 2008a), perhaps reflecting the scarcity of reports on natural infection via this mechanism (Winkler, 1968). Lack of clinical disease following attempted infection via this route may be through a lack of exposure to aerosols containing high enough concentrations of virus for initiation of a productive infection. Studies with *T. brasiliensis*, however, did report intranasal infection to be a viable infection route, resulting in extreme aggression in the inoculated bat (Baer and Bales, 1967). It has also been postulated that aerosolized RABV, possibly encountered at roosting sites, is sufficient to lead to seroconversion (Davis *et al.*, 2007), although not necessarily clinical disease. Certainly in species that roost at high density in caves, this mechanism could lead to exposures. However, for other species such as the Daubenton's bat in the United Kingdom, where comparatively small colonies form, and tree roosting species such as *E. helvum*, even where high roosting densities are seen, such a mechanism seems unlikely.

Experimental inoculation at intramuscular or subdermal locations has also proved to be of limited success in different animal models. However, where different peripheral routes have been assessed, there are often differences in virus origin, tissue culture passage history prior to inoculation, and inoculated viral dose. With little or no standardization of sample preparation seen between different reports, comparison between studies becomes difficult. However, it seems likely that for peripheral inoculation, the degree of innervation at the inoculation site plays a significant role in experimental outcome, although as discussed earlier, receptor usage is also of great importance and remains largely unknown although clearly wild-type viruses will have evolved to exploit natural entry routes.

In no study has a bat been observed to survive following development of clinical disease, and there is little evidence for subclinical infection, although in natural infections, the presence of antibodies supports this observation. Interestingly, however, excretion of virus in the absence of disease development has been reported twice (Aguilar-Setien *et al.*, 2005; Franka *et al.*, 2008) although these findings need to be confirmed by additional studies. Generally, most studies indicate that transmission between bats is likely to be through bites from an infected animal to a conspecific and not by aerosolization of virus within bat roosts. In support of this means of transmission, salivary excretion of virus has been observed immediately before the development of disease in a number of studies (Freuling *et al.*, 2009b; Hughes *et al.*, 2006; Johnson *et al.*, 2008a). However, this is at low levels, usually requiring molecular tools to detect viral genome or repeated passage in tissue culture to detect live virus. There is also some evidence from experimental studies with EBLV-1 that dose may influence the period between exposure to virus and development of disease (Franka *et al.*, 2008). This has been demonstrated for RABV within experimental models (Niezgoda *et al.*, 1997) and combined with the low levels of virus being excreted by bats suggest that the incubation period for naturally infected bats is measured in months, particularly in adults. This may explain why conspecific infection in experimental studies has not been observed as most have been terminated after 3 months. There has been one example of a Daubenton's bat developing disease after 9 months in isolated captivity, and in this instance, an unknown mechanism of latency and virus reactivation may have occurred (Pajamo *et al.*, 2008). Potential mechanisms for a delay in the establishment of a productive infection are unknown but may be similar across all species where reports of variable incubation periods have been made. Long incubation periods would be beneficial to the virus in bats from temperate climates enabling persistence during extended winter hibernation and emergence during the following spring when temperate insectivorous bats become active. Long incubation periods may also allow persistence in migratory populations and species when contact rates in colonies change from high to low, such as during mating or seasonal movements. These factors are hypothesized to select for long incubation periods to allow persistence within metapopulations by increasing chances of an infected individual being introduced into a colony (Boots and Sasaki, 1999; Boots *et al.*, 2004; Ewald, 1993; Keeling and Grenfell, 1999). The same factors are, however, also expected to select for reduced pathogenicity and prolonged infectious periods so as not to reduce the probability of infection transmission between individuals by removing infected individuals from the population (Boots and Sasaki, 1999).

Long-term studies in the greater mouse-eared bat suggest that sero-prevalence can reach high levels and fluctuate within colonies over time (Amengual *et al.*, 2007). To attempt to explain this observation, at least two possible hypotheses should be considered: (1) the bat has been infected, although replication in the peripheral and/or central nervous system may not have occurred, and survived infection; (2) the bat has been exposed to virus, possibly repeatedly, at levels that are sufficient to trigger an immune response but not to cause neuronal infection. These two hypotheses are not mutually exclusive. These hypotheses challenge our current understanding of lyssavirus biology, and whereas the second may be possible, there are currently no biological tools available with which to address these issues. Where repeat infection has been attempted, myriad serological outcomes have been encountered. Further experimental data from studies with bats have only increased uncertainty regarding the role of the antibody response with some experiments showing seroconversion in response to inoculation of high titers of virus (Franka *et al.*, 2008; McColl *et al.*, 2002), whereas other studies using similar titers have failed to find any evidence of seroconversion (Freuling *et al.*, 2009b; Johnson *et al.*, 2008a) despite administration of significant inocula. A recent study looking at the effect of multiple exposures to RABV infection in the North American big brown bat highlighted significant differences between seroconversion probabilities of those that survived and those that succumbed to infection. Interestingly, whereas high seroconversion rates following primary inoculation generally led to survival following repeat exposure, seropositivity did not necessarily preclude survivorship as some bats did not seroconvert but still survived repeat exposure (Turmelle *et al.*, 2010). This factor may be a consequence of limited sensitivity of current neutralization tests to assess serologic status and, indeed, bats chosen for experimental studies may have been naturally exposed to RABV previously but have been seronegative prior to experimental inoculation by neutralization tests. Again, interpretation of serologic status may need revision especially if relying solely on the detection of neutralizing antibodies. Seroprevalence studies continue to be used as a useful means of studying virus epidemiology in protected bat species. However, the significance and interpretation of results with respect to host–virus interaction are unclear.

E. Virus transmission between bats

Fundamentally, it appears that bats are able to transmit lyssaviruses between conspecifics within roosts. The mechanisms by which these viruses can be passed between animals in the absence of clinical disease remain unknown. Whereas clinical disease in bats appears to be rare, there have been unusual reports of large numbers of animals succumbing to RABV infection (Baer and Smith, 1991). A number of lyssavirus species have only been detected as a result of a bat exhibiting clinical disease, and when possible, such occasions have resulted in the isolation of live virus from samples, generally brain material, of the infected animal (Banyard *et al.*, 2009). Where bats are seen to exhibit clinical disease, the potential transmission rates to conspecifics is also completely unknown, although if a bat is acting aggressively and potentially shedding virus within a roost then it would be logical to assume that transmission would occur through biting and scratching. However, as yet the rate of transmission from one rabid bat within a population to conspecifics remains unknown. Further, the potential for a bat exhibiting clinical disease to be actively excreting virus is not defined. Experimental studies have suggested that bats may shed virus during a prodromal stage (Aguilar-Setien *et al.*, 2005), whereas others have detected virus excretion in saliva immediately preceding or during clinical disease (Franka *et al.*, 2008; Freuling *et al.*, 2009b; Hughes *et al.*, 2005; Johnson *et al.*, 2008a; McColl *et al.*, 2002; Turmelle *et al.*, 2010). The restricted use of bats for large-scale pathogenesis studies and difficulties of observational field studies has prevented evaluation of the timing and role of excretion following infection and the onset of clinical disease.

F. Vaccine protection and the bat lyssaviruses

Of importance to public health is the efficacy of current rabies vaccines against infection with other lyssaviruses. Rabies vaccines are all based on a number of classical RABV strains, and a fundamental question is whether they provide sufficient cross-reactivity for African and Eurasian lyssaviruses. Vaccination and challenge studies in animal models suggest that there is protection provided by rabies vaccines against both the EBLVs and ABLV (Brookes *et al.*, 2006) and some of the recently identified Asian lyssaviruses (Hanlon *et al.*, 2005). LBV infection in rabies-vaccinated companion animals has highlighted the lack of protection against nonrabies lyssaviruses following vaccination (King and Crick, 1988; Markotter *et al.*, 2008b). Further, pre- and postexposure vaccination failed to prevent disease and death in an animal model of WCBV infection (Hanlon *et al.*, 2005). These factors suggest that more cross-reactive vaccine formulations may be necessary in areas where a threat to the human population comes from nonrabies lyssaviruses. Recent advances in the antigenic characterization of different lyssaviruses may also aid future cross-reactive vaccine design (Horton *et al.*, 2010).

G. Concluding remarks

Clearly, a number of important factors remain to be addressed to enable a better understanding of bat lyssavirus infections. It is worth considering what is most advantageous for these viruses both at the "within-host" and the "within-population" levels. Novel *in vitro* cell culture systems may improve our understanding of host-specific receptor usage as well as the potential requirement of different viruses for host cell proteins to enable efficient replication. At the population level, evolutionary theory predicts that virulence at the host level should be subject to selection for an optimal level, which is determined by trade-offs between transmission and/or recovery with immunity (O'Keefe, 2005). Highly virulent pathogens kill their hosts rapidly but are classically associated with higher transmission rates; however, these diminish once virulence increases to a level that individuals are killed too rapidly and therefore equilibrate where intermediate mortality and transmission rates occur. Whereas some analyses with spatially structure populations and long-lived immunity in the hosts have shown that viruses can increase pathogen virulence even in directly transmitted viruses (Boots *et al.*, 2004), bat lyssaviruses may be a special case worth further analysis, if the case-fatality rate is the same as canine rabies. Hampson *et al.* (2009) demonstrated that the basic reproductive rate for rabies in dogs across the globe did not vary in a density-dependent way. Therefore, given the different life histories of bats across the world, this genus of viruses may be a useful model to test theories regarding pathogen virulence and infection maintenance within populations. In summary, through as yet undefined mechanisms, it appears that lyssaviruses have evolved to enable their perpetuation within this unique group of flying mammals, bats.

ACKNOWLEDGMENTS

This study was supported by The UK Department for Environment, Food and Rural Affairs (Defra grants SEV3500 and SEO421).

REFERENCES

Aguilar-Setien, A., Brochier, B., Tordo, N., De Paz, O., Desmettre, P., Peharpre, D., and Pastoret, P. P. (1998). Experimental rabies infection and oral vaccination in vampire bats (*Desmodus rotundus*). *Vaccine* **16**:1122–1126.
Aguilar-Setien, A., Loza-Rubio, E., Salas-Rojas, M., Brisseau, N., Cliquet, F., Pastoret, P. P., Rojas-Dotor, S., Tesoro, E., and Kretschmer, R. (2005). Salivary excretion of rabies virus by healthy vampire bats. *Epidemiol. Infect.* **133**:517–522.
Allen, L. C., Turmelle, A. S., Mendonca, M. T., Navara, K. J., Kunz, T. H., and McCracken, G. F. (2009). Roosting ecology and variation in adaptive and innate immune system function in the Brazilian free-tailed bat (*Tadarida brasiliensis*). *J. Comp. Physiol. B Biochem. Syst. Environ. Physiol.* **179**:315–323.
Allworth, A., Murray, K., and Morgan, J. (1996). A human case of encephalitis due to a lyssavirus recently identified in fruit bats. *Commun. Dis. Intell.* **20**:504.

Almeida, M. F., Martorelli, L. F., Aires, C. C., Sallum, P. C., Durigon, E. L., and Massad, E. (2005). Experimental rabies infection in haematophagous bats *Desmodus rotundus*. *Epidemiol. Infect.* **133**:523–527.

Altringham, A. J. D. (1996). Bats, Biology and Behaviour. Oxford University Press, Oxford.

Amengual, B., Whitby, J. E., King, A., Serra-Cobo, J., and Bourhy, H. (1997). Evolution of European bat lyssaviruses. *J. Gen. Virol.* **78**(Pt. 9):2319–2328.

Amengual, B., Bourhy, H., Lopez-Roig, M., and Serra-Cobo, J. (2007). Temporal dynamics of European bat lyssavirus type 1 and survival of *Myotis myotis* bats in natural colonies. *PLoS ONE* **2**:e566.

Anonymous (2009). *ICTV Official Taxonomy* updates since the 8th report, 2009.

Arguin, P. M., Murray-Lillibridge, K., Miranda, M. E., Smith, J. S., Calaor, A. B., and Rupprecht, C. E. (2002). Serologic evidence of lyssavirus infections among bats, the Philippines. *Emerg. Infect. Dis.* **8**:258–262.

Assenberg, R., Delmas, O., Morin, B., Graham, S. C., De Lamballerie, X., Laubert, C., Coutard, B., Grimes, J. M., Neyts, J., Owens, R. J., Brandt, B. W., Gorbalenya, A., *et al.* (2010). Genomics and structure/function studies of Rhabdoviridae proteins involved in replication and transcription. *Antiviral Res.* **87**:149–161.

Aubert, M. F. (1999). Rabies in individual countries, France. *Rabies Bull. Europe* **23**:6.

Badrane, H., and Tordo, N. (2001). Host switching in Lyssavirus history from the Chiroptera to the Carnivora orders. *J. Virol.* **75**:8096–8104.

Badrane, H., Bahloul, C., Perrin, P., and Tordo, N. (2001). Evidence of two Lyssavirus phylogroups with distinct pathogenicity and immunogenicity. *J. Virol.* **75**:3268–3276.

Baer, G. M., and Bales, G. L. (1967). Experimental rabies infection in the Mexican freetail bat. *J. Infect. Dis.* **117**:82–90.

Baer, G. M., and Smith, J. S. (1991). Rabies in nonhematophagous bats. *In* "The Natural History of Rabies", (G. M. Baer, ed.), pp. 341–366. CRC Press, Boca Raton, FL, USA.

Banyard, A. C., Johnson, N., Voller, K., Hicks, D., Nunez, A., Hartley, M., and Fooks, A. R. (2009). Repeated detection of European bat lyssavirus type 2 in dead bats found at a single roost site in the UK. *Arch. Virol.* **154**:1847–1850.

Banyard, A. C., Hartley, M., and Fooks, A. R. (2010). Reassessing the risk from rabies: A continuing threat to the UK? *Virus Res.* **152**:79–84.

Belikov, S. I., Leonova, G. N., Kondratov, I. G., Romanova, E. V., and Pavlenko, E. V. (2009). Isolation and genetic characterisation of a new lyssavirus strain in the Primorskiy kray. *East Siberian J. Infect. Pathol.* **16**:68–69.

Belotto, A., Leanes, L. F., Schneider, M. C., Tamayo, H., and Correa, E. (2005). Overview of rabies in the Americas. *Virus Res.* **111**:5–12.

Blanton, J. D., Palmer, D., and Rupprecht, C. E. (2010). Rabies surveillance in the United States during 2009. *J. Am. Vet. Med. Assoc.* **237**:646–657.

Boots, M., and Sasaki, A. (1999). 'Small worlds' and the evolution of virulence: Infection occurs locally and at a distance. *Proc. R. Soc. Lond. B Biol. Sci.* **266**:1933–1938.

Boots, M., Hudson, P. J., and Sasaki, A. (2004). Large shifts in pathogen virulence relate to host population structure. *Science* **303**:842–844.

Botvinkin, A. D., Poleschuk, E. M., Kuzmin, I. V., Borisova, T. I., Gazaryan, S. V., Yager, P., and Rupprecht, C. E. (2003). Novel lyssaviruses isolated from bats in Russia. *Emerg. Infect. Dis.* **9**:1623–1625.

Botvinkin, A., Selnikova, O. P., Anotonova, L. A., Moiseeva, A. B., and Nesterenko, E. Y. (2005). Human rabies case caused from a bat bite in Ukraine. *Rabies Bull. Europe* **29**:5–7.

Boulger, L. R., and Porterfield, J. S. (1958). Isolation of a virus from Nigerian fruit bats. *Trans. R. Soc. Trop. Med. Hyg.* **52**:421–424.

Bourhy, H., Kissi, B., and Tordo, N. (1993). Molecular diversity of the Lyssavirus genus. *Virology* **194**:70–81.

Brass, D. A. (1994). Rabies in Bats: Natural History and Public Health Implications. Livia Press, Ridgefield, CN.

Brass, D. A. (2009). Rabies vaccine strategies: Concepts of rabies prophylaxis for the caving community. *PRS* **109:**6–16.

Brookes, S. M., Aegerter, J. N., Smith, G. C., Healy, D. M., Jolliffe, T. A., Swift, S. M., Mackie, I. J., Pritchard, J. S., Racey, P. A., Moore, N. P., and Fooks, A. R. (2005). European bat lyssavirus in Scottish bats. *Emerg. Infect. Dis.* **11:**572–578.

Brookes, S. M., Healy, D. M., and Fooks, A. R. (2006). Ability of rabies vaccine strains to elicit cross-neutralising antibodies. *Dev. Biol. (Basel)* **125:**185–193.

Brookes, S. M., Klopfleisch, R., Muller, T., Healy, D. M., Teifke, J. P., Lange, E., Kliemt, J., Johnson, N., Johnson, L., Kaden, V., Vos, A., and Fooks, A. R. (2007). Susceptibility of sheep to European bat lyssavirus type-1 and -2 infection: A clinical pathogenesis study. *Vet. Microbiol.* **125:**210–223.

Calisher, C. H., Childs, J. E., Field, H. E., Holmes, K. V., and Schountz, T. (2006). Bats: Important reservoir hosts of emerging viruses. *Clin. Microbiol. Rev.* **19:**531–545.

Carini, A. (1911). About one large epizootie of rabies. *Ann. Inst. Pasteur (Paris)* **25:**843–846.

Castilho, J. G., Carnieli, P., Jr., Durymanova, E. A., Fahl Wde, O., Oliveira Rde, N., Macedo, C. I., Travassos da Rosa, E. S., Mantilla, A., Carrieri, M. L., and Kotait, I. (2010). Human rabies transmitted by vampire bats: Antigenic and genetic characterization of rabies virus isolates from the Amazon region (Brazil and Ecuador). *Virus Res.* **153:**100–105.

Childs, J. E., Curns, A. T., Dey, M. E., Real, A. L., Rupprecht, C. E., and Krebs, J. W. (2001). Rabies epizootics among raccoons vary along a North-South gradient in the Eastern United States. *Vector Borne Zoonotic Dis.* **1:**253–267.

Cisterna, D., Bonaventura, R., Caillou, S., Pozo, O., Andreau, M. L., Fontana, L. D., Echegoyen, C., de Mattos, C., Russo, S., Novaro, L., Elberger, D., and Freire, M. C. (2005). Antigenic and molecular characterization of rabies virus in Argentina. *Virus Res.* **109:**139–147.

Cliquet, F., Picard-Meyer, E., Barrat, J., Brookes, S. M., Healy, D. M., Wasniewski, M., Litaize, E., Biarnais, M., Johnson, L., and Fooks, A. R. (2009). Experimental infection of foxes with European Bat Lyssaviruses type-1 and 2. *BMC Vet. Res.* **5:**19.

Constantine, D. G. (1962). Rabies transmission by nonbite route. *Public Health Rep.* **77:**287–289.

Constantine, D. G. (1966). Transmission experiments with bat rabies isolates: Responses of certain Carnivora to rabies virus isolated from animals infected by nonbite route. *Am. J. Vet. Res.* **27:**13–15.

Constantine, D. G. (1967). Rabies Transmission by Air in Bat Caves. Public Health service Publication, Washington DC.

Constantine, D. G. (1988). Transmission of pathogenic microorganisms by vampire bats. *In* "Natural History of Vampire Bats", (A. M. Greenhall and U. Schmidt, eds.), pp. 167–189. CRC Press, Boca Raton.

Coulon, P., Ternaux, J. P., Flamand, A., and Tuffereau, C. (1998). An avirulent mutant of rabies virus is unable to infect motoneurons *in vivo* and *in vitro*. *J. Virol.* **72:**273–278.

Crameri, G., Todd, S., Grimley, S., McEachern, J. A., Marsh, G. A., Smith, C., Tachedjian, M., De Jong, C., Virtue, E. R., Yu, M., Bulach, D., Liu, J. P., *et al.* (2009). Establishment, immortalisation and characterisation of pteropid bat cell lines. *PLoS ONE* **4:**e8266.

Crerar, S., Longbottom, H., Rooney, J., and Thornber, P. (1996). Human health aspects of a possible lyssavirus in a flying fox. *Commun. Dis. Intell.* **20:**325.

Crick, J., Tignor, G. H., and Moreno, K. (1982). A new isolate of Lagos bat virus from the Republic of South Africa. *Trans. R. Soc. Trop. Med. Hyg.* **76:**211–213.

Cui, J., Han, N., Streicker, D., Li, G., Tang, X., Shi, Z., Hu, Z., Zhao, G., Fontanet, A., Guan, Y., Wang, L., Jones, G., *et al.* (2007). Evolutionary relationships between bat coronaviruses and their hosts. *Emerg. Infect. Dis.* **13:**1526–1532.

Dacheux, L., Larrous, F., Mailles, A., Boisseleau, D., Delmas, O., Biron, C., Bouchier, C., Capek, I., Muller, M., Ilari, F., Lefranc, T., Raffi, F., *et al.* (2009). European bat lyssavirus transmission among cats, Europe. *Emerg. Infect. Dis.* **15:**280–284.

Daoust, P. Y., Wandeler, A. I., and Casey, G. A. (1996). Cluster of rabies cases of probable bat origin among red foxes in Prince Edward Island, Canada. *J. Wildl. Dis.* **32:**403–406.

Davis, P. L., Holmes, E. C., Larrous, F., Van der Poel, W. H., Tjornehoj, K., Alonso, W. J., and Bourhy, H. (2005). Phylogeography, population dynamics, and molecular evolution of European bat lyssaviruses. *J. Virol.* **79:**10487–10497.

Davis, P. L., Bourhy, H., and Holmes, E. C. (2006). The evolutionary history and dynamics of bat rabies virus. *Infect. Genet. Evol.* **6:**464–473.

Davis, A. D., Rudd, R. J., and Bowen, R. A. (2007). Effects of aerosolized rabies virus exposure on bats and mice. *J. Infect. Dis.* **195:**1144–1150.

Dechant, G., and Barde, Y. A. (2002). The neurotrophin receptor p75(NTR): Novel functions and implications for diseases of the nervous system. *Nat. Neurosci.* **5:**1131–1136.

Dietzschold, B., Wunner, W. H., Wiktor, T. J., Lopes, A. D., Lafon, M., Smith, C. L., and Koprowski, H. (1983). Characterization of an antigenic determinant of the glycoprotein that correlates with pathogenicity of rabies virus. *Proc. Natl. Acad. Sci. USA* **80:**70–74.

Dominguez, S. R., O'Shea, T. J., Oko, L. M., and Holmes, K. V. (2007). Detection of group 1 coronaviruses in bats in North America. *Emerg. Infect. Dis.* **13:**1295–1300.

Dzikwi, A. A., Kuzmin, I. I., Umoh, J. U., Kwaga, J. K., Ahmad, A. A., and Rupprecht, C. E. (2010). Evidence of Lagos bat virus circulation among Nigerian fruit bats. *J. Wildl. Dis.* **46:**267–271.

East, M. L., Hofer, H., Cox, J. H., Wulle, U., Wiik, H., and Pitra, C. (2001). Regular exposure to rabies virus and lack of symptomatic disease in Serengeti spotted hyenas. *Proc. Natl. Acad. Sci. USA* **98:**15026–15031.

Echevarria, J. E., Avellon, A., Juste, J., Vera, M., and Ibanez, C. (2001). Screening of active lyssavirus infection in wild bat populations by viral RNA detection on oropharyngeal swabs. *J. Clin. Microbiol.* **39:**3678–3683.

Ewald, P. W. (1993). The evolution of virulence. *Sci. Am.* **268:**86–93.

Familusi, J. B., and Moore, D. L. (1972). Isolation of a rabies related virus from the cerebro-spinal fluid of a child with 'aseptic meningitis'. *Afr. J. Med. Sci.* **3:**93–96.

Familusi, J. B., Osunkoya, B. O., Moore, D. L., Kemp, G. E., and Fabiyi, A. (1972). A fatal human infection with Mokola virus. *Am. J. Trop. Med. Hyg.* **21:**959–963.

Field, H. E. (2009). Bats and emerging zoonoses: Henipaviruses and SARS. *Zoonoses Public Health* **56:**278–284.

Foggin, C. M. (1982). Atypical rabies virus in cats and a dog in Zimbabwe. *Vet. Rec.* **110:**338.

Foggin, C. M. (1988). Rabies and Rabies Related Viruses in Zimbabwe: Historical, Virological and Ecological Aspects. University of Zimbabwe, Harare.

Fooks, A. R., McElhinney, L. M., Pounder, D. J., Finnegan, C. J., Mansfield, K., Johnson, N., Brookes, S. M., Parsons, G., White, K., McIntyre, P. G., and Nathwani, D. (2003). Case report: Isolation of a European bat lyssavirus type 2a from a fatal human case of rabies encephalitis. *J. Med. Virol.* **71:**281–289.

Franka, R., Johnson, N., Muller, T., Vos, A., Neubert, L., Freuling, C., Rupprecht, C. E., and Fooks, A. R. (2008). Susceptibility of North American big brown bats (*Eptesicus fuscus*) to infection with European bat lyssavirus type 1. *J. Gen. Virol.* **89:**1998–2010.

Fraser, G. C., Hooper, P. T., Lunt, R. A., Gould, A. R., Gleeson, L. J., Hyatt, A. D., Russell, G. M., and Kattenbelt, J. A. (1996). Encephalitis caused by a lyssavirus in fruit bats in Australia. *Emerg. Infect. Dis.* **2:**327–331.

Freuling, C., Grossmann, E., Conraths, F. J., Schameitat, A., Kliemt, J., Auer, E., Greiser-Wilke, I., and Muller, T. (2008). First isolation of EBLV-2 in Germany. *Vet. Microbiol.* **131**:26–34.

Freuling, C., Vos, A., Johnson, N., Fooks, A. R., and Muller, T. (2009a). Bat rabies—A Gordian knot? *Berl. Munch. Tierarztl. Wochenschr.* **122**:425–433.

Freuling, C., Vos, A., Johnson, N., Kaipf, I., Denzinger, A., Neubert, L., Mansfield, K., Hicks, D., Nunez, A., Tordo, N., Rupprecht, C. E., Fooks, A. R., *et al.* (2009b). Experimental infection of serotine bats (*Eptesicus serotinus*) with European bat lyssavirus type 1a. *J. Gen. Virol.* **90**:2493–2502.

Giannini, N. P., and Simmons, N. B. (2003). A phylogeny of megachiropteran bats (Mammalia: Chiroptera: Pteropodidae) based on direct optimization analysis of one nuclear and four mitochondrial genes. *Cladistics* **19**:496–511.

Gould, A. R., Hyatt, A. D., Lunt, R., Kattenbelt, J. A., Hengstberger, S., and Blacksell, S. D. (1998). Characterisation of a novel lyssavirus isolated from Pteropid bats in Australia. *Virus Res.* **54**:165–187.

Gould, A. R., Kattenbelt, J. A., Gumley, S. G., and Lunt, R. A. (2002). Characterisation of an Australian bat lyssavirus variant isolated from an insectivorous bat. *Virus Res.* **89**:1–28.

Greenhall, A. M. (1961). Bats in Agriculture. A Ministry of Agriculture Publication, Trinidad and Tobago.

Greenhall, A. M., and Schmidt, U. (1988). Natural History of Vampire Bats. CRC Press, Boca Raton, FL.

Guyatt, K. J., Twin, J., Davis, P., Holmes, E. C., Smith, G. A., Smith, I. L., Mackenzie, J. S., and Young, P. L. (2003). A molecular epidemiological study of Australian bat lyssavirus. *J. Gen. Virol.* **84**:485–496.

Hampson, K., Dushoff, J., Cleaveland, S., Haydon, D. T., Kaare, M., Packer, C., and Dobson, A. (2009). Transmission dynamics and prospects for the elimination of canine rabies. *PLoS Biol.* **7**:e1000053.

Hanlon, C. A., DeMattos, C. A., DeMattos, C. C., Niezgoda, M., Hooper, D. C., Koprowski, H., Notkins, A., and Rupprecht, C. E. (2001). Experimental utility of rabies virus-neutralizing human monoclonal antibodies in post-exposure prophylaxis. *Vaccine* **19**:3834–3842.

Hanlon, C. A., Kuzmin, I. V., Blanton, J. D., Weldon, W. C., Manangan, J. S., and Rupprecht, C. E. (2005). Efficacy of rabies biologics against new lyssaviruses from Eurasia. *Virus Res.* **111**:44–54.

Hanna, J. N., Carney, I. K., Smith, G. A., Tannenberg, A. E., Deverill, J. E., Botha, J. A., Serafin, I. L., Harrower, B. J., Fitzpatrick, P. F., and Searle, J. W. (2000). Australian bat lyssavirus infection: A second human case, with a long incubation period. *Med. J. Aust.* **172**:597–599.

Harris, S. L., Brookes, S. M., Jones, G., Hutson, A. M., and Fooks, A. R. (2006). Passive surveillance (1987 to 2004) of United Kingdom bats for European bat lyssaviruses. *Vet. Rec.* **159**:439–446.

Harris, S. L., Aegerter, J. N., Brookes, S. M., McElhinney, L. M., Jones, G., Smith, G. C., and Fooks, A. R. (2009). Targeted surveillance for European bat lyssaviruses in English bats (2003–06). *J. Wildl. Dis.* **45**:1030–1041.

Haupt, H., and Rehaag, H. (1921). Epizootic rabies in a herd from Santa Carina (south-east Brazil) transmitted by bats. *Zeitschr. Infektions Hyg. Haustiere* **76–90**(XXII):104–107.

Hayman, D. T., Fooks, A. R., Horton, D., Suu-Ire, R., Breed, A. C., Cunningham, A. A., and Wood, J. L. (2008). Antibodies against Lagos bat virus in megachiroptera from West Africa. *Emerg. Infect. Dis.* **14**:926–928.

Hooper, P. T., Lunt, R. A., Gould, A. R., Samaratunga, H., Hyatt, A. D., Gleeson, L. J., Rodwell, B. J., Rupprecht, C. E., Smith, J. S., and Murray, P. K. (1997). A new lyssavirus—The first endemic rabies related virus recognised in Australia. *Bull. Inst. Pasteur* **94**:209–218.

Horton, D. L., McElhinney, L. M., Marston, D. A., Wood, J. L., Russell, C. A., Lewis, N., Kuzmin, I. V., Fouchier, R. A., Osterhaus, A. D., Fooks, A. R., and Smith, D. J. (2010). Quantifying antigenic relationships among the Lyssaviruses. *J. Virol.* **84**:11841–11848.

Hughes, G. J., Orciari, L. A., and Rupprecht, C. E. (2005). Evolutionary timescale of rabies virus adaptation to North American bats inferred from the substitution rate of the nucleoprotein gene. *J. Gen. Virol.* **86**:1467–1474.

Hughes, G. J., Kuzmin, I. V., Schmitz, A., Blanton, J., Manangan, J., Murphy, S., and Rupprecht, C. E. (2006). Experimental infection of big brown bats (*Eptesicus fuscus*) with Eurasian bat lyssaviruses Aravan, Khujand, and Irkut virus. *Arch. Virol.* **151**:2021–2035.

Hurst, E. W., and Pawan, J. L. (1931). An outbreak of rabies in Trinidad. *Lancet Infect. Dis.* **2**:622–628.

Jackson, A. C., Ye, H., Phelan, C. C., Ridaura-Sanz, C., Zheng, Q., Li, Z., Wan, X., and Lopez-Corella, E. (1999). Extraneural organ involvement in human rabies. *Lab. Invest.* **79**:945–951.

Jakava-Viljanen, M., Lilley, T., Kyheroinen, E. M., and Huovilainen, A. (2010). First encounter of European bat lyssavirus type 2 (EBLV-2) in a bat in Finland. *Epidemiol. Infect.* **138**:1581–1585.

Johnson, N., Selden, D., Parsons, G., Healy, D., Brookes, S. M., McElhinney, L. M., Hutson, A. M., and Fooks, A. R. (2003). Isolation of a European bat lyssavirus type 2 from a Daubenton's bat in the United Kingdom. *Vet. Rec.* **152**:383–387.

Johnson, N., McKimmie, C. S., Mansfield, K. L., Wakeley, P. R., Brookes, S. M., Fazakerley, J. K., and Fooks, A. R. (2006a). Lyssavirus infection activates interferon gene expression in the brain. *J. Gen. Virol.* **87**:2663–2667.

Johnson, N., Phillpotts, R., and Fooks, A. R. (2006b). Airborne transmission of lyssaviruses. *J. Med. Microbiol.* **55**:785–790.

Johnson, N., Wakeley, P. R., Brookes, S. M., and Fooks, A. R. (2006c). European bat lyssavirus type 2 RNA in *Myotis daubentonii*. *Emerg. Infect. Dis.* **12**:1142–1144.

Johnson, N., Freuling, C., Marston, D. A., Tordo, N., Fooks, A. R., and Muller, T. (2007). Identification of European bat lyssavirus isolates with short genomic insertions. *Virus Res.* **128**:140–143.

Johnson, N., Fooks, A., and McColl, K. (2008a). Human rabies case with long incubation, Australia. *Emerg. Infect. Dis.* **14**:1950–1951.

Johnson, N., Vos, A., Neubert, L., Freuling, C., Mansfield, K. L., Kaipf, I., Denzinger, A., Hicks, D., Nunez, A., Franka, R., Rupprecht, C. E., Muller, T., *et al.* (2008b). Experimental study of European bat lyssavirus type-2 infection in Daubenton's bats (*Myotis daubentonii*). *J. Gen. Virol.* **89**:2662–2672.

Keeling, M., and Grenfell, B. (1999). Stochastic dynamics and a power law for measles variability. *Philos. Trans. R. Soc. Lond. B Biol. Sci.* **354**:769–776.

Kemp, G. E., Causey, O. R., Moore, D. L., Odelola, A., and Fabiyi, A. (1972). Mokola virus. Further studies on IbAn 27377, a new rabies-related etiologic agent of zoonosis in Nigeria. *Am. J. Trop. Med. Hyg.* **21**:356–359.

King, A., and Crick, J. (1988). Rabies-related viruses. *In* "Rabies", (K. M. Charlton and J. B. Campbell, eds.), pp. 177–200. Kluwer Academic Publishers, Boston.

Kissi, B., Tordo, N., and Bourhy, H. (1995). Genetic polymorphism in the rabies virus nucleoprotein gene. *Virology* **209**:526–537.

Kobayashi, Y., Sato, G., Kato, M., Itou, T., Cunha, E. M., Silva, M. V., Mota, C. S., Ito, F. H., and Sakai, T. (2007). Genetic diversity of bat rabies viruses in Brazil. *Arch. Virol.* **152**:1995–2004.

Kobayashi, Y., Sato, G., Mochizuki, N., Hirano, S., Itou, T., Carvalho, A. A., Albas, A., Santos, H. P., Ito, F. H., and Sakai, T. (2008). Molecular and geographic analyses of vampire bat-transmitted cattle rabies in central Brazil. *BMC Vet. Res.* **4:**44.

Kuzmin, I. V., and Rupprecht, C. E. (2007). Bat rabies. *In* "Rabies", (A. Jackson and W. Wunner, eds.), pp. 276–277. Academic Press, San Diego, London, Amsterdam.

Kuzmin, I. V., Botvinkin, A. D., Rybin, S. N., and Baialiev, A. B. (1992). A lyssavirus with an unusual antigenic structure isolated from a bat in southern Kyrgyzstan. *Vopr. Virusol.* **37:**256–259.

Kuzmin, I. V., Botvinkin, A. D., and Shaimardanov, R. T. (1994). Experimental lyssavirus infection in chiropters. *Vopr. Virusol.* **39:**17–21.

Kuzmin, I. V., Orciari, L. A., Arai, Y. T., Smith, J. S., Hanlon, C. A., Kameoka, Y., and Rupprecht, C. E. (2003). Bat lyssaviruses (Aravan and Khujand) from Central Asia: Phylogenetic relationships according to N, P and G gene sequences. *Virus Res.* **97:**65–79.

Kuzmin, I. V., Hughes, G. J., Botvinkin, A. D., Orciari, L. A., and Rupprecht, C. E. (2005). Phylogenetic relationships of Irkut and West Caucasian bat viruses within the Lyssavirus genus and suggested quantitative criteria based on the N gene sequence for lyssavirus genotype definition. *Virus Res.* **111:**28–43.

Kuzmin, I. V., Niezgoda, M., Carroll, D. S., Keeler, N., Hossain, M. J., Breiman, R. F., Ksiazek, T. G., and Rupprecht, C. E. (2006). Lyssavirus surveillance in bats, Bangladesh. *Emerg. Infect. Dis.* **12:**486–488.

Kuzmin, I. V., Franka, R., and Rupprecht, C. E. (2008a). Experimental infection of big brown bats (*Eptesicus fuscus*) with West Caucasian bat virus (WCBV). *Dev. Biol. (Basel)* **131:**327–337.

Kuzmin, I. V., Niezgoda, M., Franka, R., Agwanda, B., Markotter, W., Beagley, J. C., Urazova, O. Y., Breiman, R. F., and Rupprecht, C. E. (2008b). Lagos bat virus in Kenya. *J. Clin. Microbiol.* **46:**1451–1461.

Kuzmin, I. V., Niezgoda, M., Franka, R., Agwanda, B., Markotter, W., Beagley, J. C., Urazova, O. Y., Breiman, R. F., and Rupprecht, C. E. (2008c). Possible emergence of West Caucasian bat virus in Africa. *Emerg. Infect. Dis.* **14:**1887–1889.

Kuzmin, I. V., Wu, X., Tordo, N., and Rupprecht, C. E. (2008d). Complete genomes of Aravan, Khujand, Irkut and West Caucasian bat viruses, with special attention to the polymerase gene and non-coding regions. *Virus Res.* **136:**81–90.

Kuzmin, I. V., Mayer, A. E., Niezgoda, M., Markotter, W., Agwanda, B., Breiman, R. F., and Rupprecht, C. E. (2010). Shimoni bat virus, a new representative of the Lyssavirus genus. *Virus Res.* **149:**197–210.

Lafon, M. (2005). Rabies virus receptors. *J. Neurovirol.* **11:**82–87.

Le Gonidec, G., Rickenbach, A., Robin, Y., and Heme, G. (1978). Isolation of a strain of Mokola virus in Cameroon. *Ann. Microbiol. A* **129:**245–249.

Lembo, T., Haydon, D. T., Velasco-Villa, A., Rupprecht, C. E., Packer, C., Brandao, P. E., Kuzmin, I. V., Fooks, A. R., Barrat, J., and Cleaveland, S. (2007). Molecular epidemiology identifies only a single rabies virus variant circulating in complex carnivore communities of the Serengeti. *Proc. R. Soc. Lond. B Biol. Sci.* **274:**2123–2130.

Leslie, M. J., Messenger, S., Rohde, R. E., Smith, J., Cheshier, R., Hanlon, C., and Rupprecht, C. E. (2006). Bat-associated rabies virus in skunks. *Emerg. Infect. Dis.* **12:**1274–1277.

Lumio, J., Hillbom, M., Roine, R., Ketonen, L., Haltia, M., Valle, M., Neuvonen, E., and Lahdevirta, J. (1986). Human rabies of bat origin in Europe. *Lancet* **1:**378.

Lumlertdacha, B. (2005). Laboratory techniques for rabies diagnosis in animals at QSMI. *J. Med. Assoc. Thai.* **88:**550–553.

MacInnes, C. D., Smith, S. M., Tinline, R. R., Ayers, N. R., Bachmann, P., Ball, D. G., Calder, L. A., Crosgrey, S. J., Fielding, C., Hauschildt, P., Honig, J. M., Johnston, D. H., *et al.* (2001). Elimination of rabies from red foxes in eastern Ontario. *J. Wildl. Dis.* **37:**119–132.

Mallewa, M., Fooks, A. R., Banda, D., Chikungwa, P., Mankhambo, L., Molyneux, E., Molyneux, M. E., and Solomon, T. (2007). Rabies encephalitis in malaria-endemic area, Malawi, Africa. *Emerg. Infect. Dis.* **13**:136–139.

Markotter, W., Kuzmin, I., Rupprecht, C. E., Randles, J., Sabeta, C. T., Wandeler, A. I., and Nel, L. H. (2006a). Isolation of Lagos bat virus from water mongoose. *Emerg. Infect. Dis.* **12**:1913–1918.

Markotter, W., Randles, J., Rupprecht, C. E., Sabeta, C. T., Taylor, P. J., Wandeler, A. I., and Nel, L. H. (2006b). Lagos bat virus, South Africa. *Emerg. Infect. Dis.* **12**:504–506.

Markotter, W., Kuzmin, I., Rupprecht, C. E., and Nel, L. H. (2008a). Phylogeny of Lagos bat virus: Challenges for lyssavirus taxonomy. *Virus Res.* **135**:10–21.

Markotter, W., Van Eeden, C., Kuzmin, I. V., Rupprecht, C. E., Paweska, J. T., Swanepoel, R., Fooks, A. R., Sabeta, C. T., Cliquet, F., and Nel, L. H. (2008b). Epidemiology and pathogenicity of African bat lyssaviruses. *Dev. Biol. (Basel)* **131**:317–325.

Markotter, W., Kuzmin, I. V., Rupprecht, C. E., and Nel, L. H. (2009). Lagos bat virus virulence in mice inoculated by the peripheral route. *Epidemiol. Infect.* **137**:1155–1162.

Marston, D. A., McElhinney, L. M., Johnson, N., Muller, T., Conzelmann, K. K., Tordo, N., and Fooks, A. R. (2007). Comparative analysis of the full genome sequence of European bat lyssavirus type 1 and type 2 with other lyssaviruses and evidence for a conserved transcription termination and polyadenylation motif in the G-L 3′ non-translated region. *J. Gen. Virol.* **88**:1302–1314.

Mayen, F. (2003). Haematophagous bats in Brazil, their role in rabies transmission, impact on public health, livestock industry and alternatives to an indiscriminate reduction of bat population. *J. Vet. Med. B Infect. Dis. Vet. Public Health* **50**:469–472.

Mayer, F., and Brunner, A. (2007). Non-neutral evolution of the major histocompatibility complex class II gene DRB1 in the sac-winged bat *Saccopteryx bilineata*. *Heredity* **99**:257–264.

McCall, B. J., Epstein, J. H., Neill, A. S., Heel, K., Field, H., Barrett, J., Smith, G. A., Selvey, L. A., Rodwell, B., and Lunt, R. (2000). Potential exposure to Australian bat lyssavirus, Queensland, 1996–1999. *Emerg. Infect. Dis.* **6**:259–264.

McColl, K. A., Chamberlain, T., Lunt, R. A., Newberry, K. M., Middleton, D., and Westbury, H. A. (2002). Pathogenesis studies with Australian bat lyssavirus in grey-headed flying foxes (*Pteropus poliocephalus*). *Aust. Vet. J.* **80**:636–641.

McColl, K. A., Chamberlain, T., Lunt, R. A., Newberry, K. M., and Westbury, H. A. (2007). Susceptibility of domestic dogs and cats to Australian bat lyssavirus (ABLV). *Vet. Microbiol.* **123**:15–25.

Mebatsion, T., Cox, J. H., and Frost, J. W. (1992). Isolation and characterization of 115 street rabies virus isolates from Ethiopia by using monoclonal antibodies: Identification of 2 isolates as Mokola and Lagos bat viruses. *J. Infect. Dis.* **166**:972–977.

Meredith, C. D., Prossouw, A. P., and Koch, H. P. (1971). An unusual case of human rabies thought to be of chiropteran origin. *S. Afr. Med. J.* **45**:767–769.

Meredith, C. D., Nel, L. H., and von Teichman, B. F. (1996). Further isolation of Mokola virus in South Africa. *Vet. Rec.* **138**:119–120.

Messenger, S. L., Smith, J. S., and Rupprecht, C. E. (2002). Emerging epidemiology of bat-associated cryptic cases of rabies in humans in the United States. *Clin. Infect. Dis.* **35**:738–747.

Mohr, W. (1957). Die Tollwut. *Med. Klin.* **52**:1057–1060.

Moreno, J. A., and Baer, G. M. (1980). Experimental rabies in the vampire bat. *Am. J. Trop. Med. Hyg.* **29**:254–259.

Muller, T., Cox, J., Peter, W., Schafer, R., Johnson, N., McElhinney, L. M., Geue, J. L., Tjornehoj, K., and Fooks, A. R. (2004). Spill-over of European bat lyssavirus type 1 into a stone marten (*Martes foina*) in Germany. *J. Vet. Med. B Infect. Dis. Vet. Public Health* **51**:49–54.

Muller, T., Johnson, N., Freuling, C. M., Fooks, A. R., Selhorst, T., and Vos, A. (2007). Epidemiology of bat rabies in Germany. *Arch. Virol.* **152:**273–288.

Nadin-Davis, S. A., Huang, W., Armstrong, J., Casey, G. A., Bahloul, C., Tordo, N., and Wandeler, A. I. (2001). Antigenic and genetic divergence of rabies viruses from bat species indigenous to Canada. *Virus Research* **74:**139–156.

Nadin-Davis, S. A., and Loza-Rubio, E. (2006). The molecular epidemiology of rabies associated with chiropteran hosts in Mexico. *Virus Res.* **117:**215–226.

Nadin-Davis, S. A., Abdel-Malik, M., Armstrong, J., and Wandeler, A. I. (2002). Lyssavirus P gene characterisation provides insights into the phylogeny of the genus and identifies structural similarities and diversity within the encoded phosphoprotein. *Virology* **298:**286–305.

Nel, L. H., and Rupprecht, C. E. (2007). Emergence of lyssaviruses in the Old World: The case of Africa. *Curr. Top. Microbiol. Immunol.* **315:**161–193.

Nel, L., Jacobs, J., Jaftha, J., von Teichman, B., Bingham, J., and Olivier, M. (2000). New cases of Mokola virus infection in South Africa: A genotypic comparison of Southern African virus isolates. *Virus Genes* **20:**103–106.

Nieuwenhuijs, J. H. (1987). Veterinary Chief Inspection for Public Health. Rabies in Bats. *Tijdschr. Diergeneeskd* **112:**1193–1197.

Niezgoda, M., Briggs, D. J., Shaddock, J., Dreesen, D. W., and Rupprecht, C. E. (1997). Pathogenesis of experimentally induced rabies in domestic ferrets. *Am. J. Vet. Res.* **58:**1327–1331.

Nowak, R. M. (1999). Walker's Mammals of the World. 6th edn. Johns Hopkins University Press, Baltimore.

O'Keefe, K. J. (2005). The evolution of virulence in pathogens with frequency-dependent transmission. *J. Theor. Biol.* **233:**55–64.

Omatsu, T., Bak, E. J., Ishii, Y., Kyuwa, S., Tohya, Y., Akashi, H., and Yoshikawa, Y. (2008). Induction and sequencing of Rousette bat interferon alpha and beta genes. *Vet. Immunol. Immunopathol.* **124:**169–176.

O'Shea, T. J., Shankar, V., Bowen, R. A., Rupprecht, C. E., and Wimsatt, J. H. (2003). Do bats acquire immunity to rabies? Evidence from the field *Bat Res. News* **44:**161.

Paez, A., Velasco-Villa, A., Rey, G., and Rupprecht, C. E. (2007). Molecular epidemiology of rabies in Colombia 1994–2005 based on partial nucleoprotein gene sequences. *Virus Res.* **130:**172–181.

Pajamo, K., Harkess, G., Goddard, T., Marston, D., McElhinney, L., Johnson, N., and Fooks, A. R. (2008). Isolation of European bat lyssavirus type 2 (EBLV-2) in a Daubenton's bat in the UK with a minimum incubation period of 9 months. *Rabies Bull. Europe* **32:**6–7.

Pal, S. R., Arora, B., Chhuttani, P. N., Broor, S., Choudhury, S., Joshi, R. M., and Ray, S. D. (1980). Rabies virus infection of a flying fox bat, *Pteropus policephalus* in Chandigarh, Northern India. *Trop. Geogr. Med.* **32:**265–267.

Pawan, J. L. (1936). Rabies in the vampire bat of Trinidad, with special reference to the clinical course and the latency of infection. *Ann. Trop. Med. Parasitol.* **30:**410–422.

Paweska, J. T., Blumberg, L. H., Liebenberg, C., Hewlett, R. H., Grobbelaar, A. A., Leman, P. A., Croft, J. E., Nel, L. H., Nutt, L., and Swanepoel, R. (2006). Fatal human infection with rabies-related Duvenhage virus, South Africa. *Emerg. Infect. Dis.* **12:**1965–1967.

Ravkov, E. V., Smith, J. S., and Nichol, S. T. (1995). Rabies virus glycoprotein gene contains a long 3′ noncoding region which lacks pseudogene properties. *Virology* **206:**718–723.

Richter, H. V., and Cumming, G. S. (2008). First application of satellite telemetry to track African straw-coloured fruit bat migration. *J. Zool.* **275:**172–176.

Rivers, N. M., Butlin, R. K., and Altringham, J. D. (2006). Autumn swarming behaviour of Natterer's bats in the UK: Population size, catchment area and dispersal. *Biol. Conserv.* **127:**215–226.

Rodrigues, Y. J. L., and Tamayo, J. G. (2000). Pathology of experimental infection with the rabies virus in hematophagous bat (*Desmodus rotundus*). *Rev. Fac. Cs. Vets.* **41:**71–72.

Roine, R. O., Hillbom, M., Valle, M., Haltia, M., Ketonen, L., Neuvonen, E., Lumio, J., and Lahdevirta, J. (1988). Fatal encephalitis caused by a bat-borne rabies-related virus. Clinical findings. *Brain* **111:**1505–1516.

Ruiz, M., and Chavez, C. B. (2010). Rabies in Latin America. *Neurol. Res.* **32:**272–277.

Sabeta, C. T., Markotter, W., Mohale, D. K., Shumba, W., Wandeler, A. I., and Nel, L. H. (2007). Mokola virus in domestic mammals, South Africa. *Emerg. Infect. Dis.* **13:**1371–1373.

Schneider, L. G., and Cox, J. H. (1994). Bat lyssaviruses in Europe. *Curr. Top. Microbiol. Immunol.* **187:**207–218.

Schneider, L. G., Barnard, B. J. H., and Schneider, H. P. (1985). Application of monoclonal antibodies for epidemiological investigations and oral vaccination studies: I—African viruses. In "Rabies in the Tropics", (C. M. E. Kuwert, H. Koprowski, and K. Bogel, eds.), pp. 49–53. Springer-Verlag, Berlin.

Schneider, M. C., Belotto, A., Ade, M. P., Leanes, L. F., Correa, E., Tamayo, H., Medina, G., and Rodrigues, M. J. (2005). Epidemiologic situation of human rabies in Latin America in 2004. *Epidemiol. Bull.* **26:**2–4.

Seif, I., Coulon, P., Rollin, P. E., and Flamand, A. (1985). Rabies virulence: Effect on pathogenicity and sequence characterization of rabies virus mutations affecting antigenic site III of the glycoprotein. *J. Virol.* **53:**926–934.

Selimov, M. A., Tatarov, A. G., Botvinkin, A. D., Klueva, E. V., Kulikova, L. G., and Khismatullina, N. A. (1989). Rabies-related Yuli virus; identification with a panel of monoclonal antibodies. *Acta Virol.* **33:**542–546.

Serra-Cobo, J., Amengual, B., Abellan, C., and Bourhy, H. (2002). European bat lyssavirus infection in Spanish bat populations. *Emerg. Infect. Dis.* **8:**413–420.

Shahroukh, M., and Moreno-Valdez, A. (2009). Climate change, vampire bats, and rabies: Modeling range shifts on the US-Mexico border. 94th ESA Annual Meeting, Alburquerque Conference Center, Alburquerque, Mexico.

Shankar, V., Bowen, R. A., Davis, A. D., Rupprecht, C. E., and O'Shea, T. J. (2004). Rabies in a captive colony of Big Brown bats (Eptesicus fuscus). *J. Wildl. Dis.* **40:**403–413.

Shope, R. E. (1982). Rabies-related viruses. *Yale J. Biol. Med.* **55:**271–275.

Shope, R. E., Murphy, F. A., Harrison, A. K., Causey, O. R., Kemp, G. E., Simpson, D. I., and Moore, D. L. (1970). Two African viruses serologically and morphologically related to rabies virus. *J. Virol.* **6:**690–692.

Sidwa, T. J., Wilson, P. J., Moore, G. M., Oertli, E. H., Hicks, B. N., Rohde, R. E., and Johnston, D. H. (2005). Evaluation of oral rabies vaccination programs for control of rabies epizootics in coyotes and gray foxes: 1995–2003. *J. Am. Vet. Med. Assoc.* **227:**785–792.

Simmons, N. B., Seymour, K. L., Habersetzer, J., and Gunnell, G. F. (2008). Primitive early Eocene bat from Wyoming and the evolution of flight and echolocation. *Nature* **451:**818–821.

Smith, P. C., Lawhaswasdi, K., Vick, W. E., and Stanton, J. S. (1967). Isolation of rabies virus from fruit bats in Thailand. *Nature* **216:**384.

Smreczak, M., Trebas, P., Orlowska, A., and mudzinski,, J. F. (2008). Rabies surveillance in Poland (1992–2006). *Dev. Biol. (Basel)* **131:**249–256.

Sodre, M. M., da Gama, A. R., and de Almeida, M. F. (2010). Updated list of bat species positive for rabies in Brazil. *Rev. Inst. Med. Trop. São Paulo* **52:**75–81.

Steece, R., and Altenbach, J. S. (1989). Prevalence of rabies specific antibodies in the Mexican free-tailed bat (*Tadarida brasiliensis mexicana*) at Lava Cave, New Mexico. *J. Wildl. Dis.* **25:**490–496.

Streicker, D. G., Turmelle, A. S., Vonhof, M. J., Kuzmin, I. V., McCracken, G. F., and Rupprecht, C. E. (2010). Host phylogeny constrains cross-species emergence and establishment of rabies virus in bats. *Science* **329:**676–679.

Sulkin, S. E. (1962). Bat rabies: Experimental demonstration of the "reservoiring mechanism" *Am. J. Public Health* **52:**489–498.

Sulkin, S. E., and Greve, M. J. (1954). Human rabies caused by bat bite. *Tex. State J. Med.* **50:**620–621.

Sulkin, S. E., Krutzsch, P. H., Wallis, C., and Allen, R. (1957). Role of brown fat in pathogenesis of rabies in insectivorous bats (*Tadaria b. mexicana*). *Proc. Soc. Exp. Biol. Med.* **96:**461–464.

Sulkin, S. E., Allen, R., Sims, R., Krutzsch, P. H., and Kim, C. H. (1960). Studies on the pathogenesis of rabies in insectivorous bats II. Influence of environmental temperature. *J. Exp. Med.* **112:**595–617.

Sureau, P., Germain, M., Herve, J. P., Geoffroy, B., Cornet, J. P., Heme, G., and Robin, Y. (1977). Isolation of the Lagos-bat virus in the Central African Republic. *Bull. Soc. Pathol. Exot. Filiales* **70:**467–470.

Swanepoel, R. (1994). Rabies. *In* "Infectious Diseases of Livestock with Special Reference to Southern Africa", (J. A. W. Coetzer, G. R. Thompson, and R. C. Tustin, eds.), pp. 493–553. Oxford University Press/NECC, Cape Town.

Tang, X., Luo, M., Zhang, S., Fooks, A. R., Hu, R., and Tu, C. (2005). Pivotal role of dogs in rabies transmission, China. *Emerg. Infect. Dis.* **11:**1970–1972.

Teeling, E. C., Springer, M. S., Madsen, O., Bates, P., O'Brien, S. J., and Murphy, W. J. (2005). A molecular phylogeny for bats illuminates biogeography and the fossil record. *Science* **307:**580–584.

Thomas, D. W. (1983). The annual migrations of three species of West African fruit bats (Chiroptera: Pteropodidae). *Can. J. Zool.* **61:**2266–2272.

Tignor, G. H., Shope, R. E., Bhatt, P. N., and Percy, D. H. (1973). Experimental infection of dogs and monkeys with two rabies serogroup viruses, Lagos bat and Mokola (IbAn 27377): Clinical, serologic, virologic, and fluorescent-antibody studies. *J. Infect. Dis.* **128:**471–478.

Tjornehoj, K., Fooks, A. R., Agerholm, J. S., and Ronsholt, L. (2006). Natural and experimental infection of sheep with European bat lyssavirus type-1 of Danish bat origin. *J. Comp. Pathol.* **134:**190–201.

Tordo, N., Poch, O., Ermine, A., Keith, G., and Rougeon, F. (1986). Walking along the rabies genome: Is the large G-L intergenic region a remnant gene? *Proc. Natl. Acad. Sci. USA* **83:**3914–3918.

Tordo, N., Poch, O., Ermine, A., Keith, G., and Rougeon, F. (1988). Completion of the rabies virus genome sequence determination: Highly conserved domains among the L (polymerase) proteins of unsegmented negative-strand RNA viruses. *Virology* **165:**565–576.

Towner, J. S., Amman, B. R., Sealy, T. K., Carroll, S. A., Comer, J. A., Kemp, A., Swanepoel, R., Paddock, C. D., Balinandi, S., Khristova, M. L., Formenty, P. B., Albarino, C. G., *et al.* (2009). Isolation of genetically diverse Marburg viruses from Egyptian fruit bats. *PLoS Pathog.* **5:**e1000536.

Tuffereau, C., Schmidt, K., Langevin, C., Lafay, F., Dechant, G., and Koltzenburg, M. (2007). The rabies virus glycoprotein receptor p75NTR is not essential for rabies virus infection. *J. Virol.* **81:**13622–13630.

Turmelle, A. S., Jackson, F. R., Green, D., McCracken, G. F., and Rupprecht, C. E. (2010). Host immunity to repeated rabies virus infection in big brown bats. *J. Gen. Virol.* **91:**2360–2366.

Van der Poel, W. H., Van der Heide, R., Van Amerongen, G., Van Keulen, L. J., Wellenberg, G. J., Bourhy, H., Schaftenaar, W., Groen, J., and Osterhaus, A. D. (2000). Characterisation of a recently isolated lyssavirus in frugivorous zoo bats. *Arch. Virol.* **145:**1919–1931.

van Thiel, P. P., van den Hoek, J. A., Eftimov, F., Tepaske, R., Zaaijer, H. J., Spanjaard, L., de Boer, H. E., van Doornum, G. J., Schutten, M., Osterhaus, A., and Kager, P. A. (2008). Fatal case of human rabies (Duvenhage virus) from a bat in Kenya: The Netherlands, December 2007. *Euro Surveill.* **13:**8007.

Velasco-Villa, A., Orciari, L. A., Juarez-Islas, V., Gomez-Sierra, M., Padilla-Medina, I., Flisser, A., Souza, V., Castillo, A., Franka, R., Escalante-Mane, M., Sauri-Gonzalez, I., and Rupprecht, C. E. (2006). Molecular diversity of rabies viruses associated with bats in Mexico and other countries of the Americas. *J. Clin. Microbiol.* **44:**1697–1710.

Vos, A., Muller, T., Cox, J., Neubert, L., and Fooks, A. R. (2004). Susceptibility of ferrets (*Mustela putorius furo*) to experimentally induced rabies with European bat lyssaviruses (EBLV). *J. Vet. Med. B Infect. Dis. Vet. Public Health* **51:**55–60.

Vos, A., Kaipf, I., Denzinger, A., Fooks, A. R., Johnson, N., and Muller, T. (2007). European bat lyssaviruses: An ecological enigma. *Acta Chiropterologica* **9:**283–296.

Wang, L. F., and Eaton, B. T. (2007). Bats, civets and the emergence of SARS. *Curr. Top. Microbiol. Immunol.* **315:**325–344.

Warrilow, D. (2005). Australian bat lyssavirus: A recently discovered new rhabdovirus. *Curr. Top. Microbiol. Immunol.* **292:**25–44.

Warrilow, D., Smith, I. L., Harrower, B., and Smith, G. A. (2002). Sequence analysis of an isolate from a fatal human infection of Australian bat lyssavirus. *Virology* **297:**109–119.

Weyer, J., Kuzmin, I. V., Rupprecht, C. E., and Nel, L. H. (2008). Cross-protective and cross-reactive immune responses to recombinant vaccinia viruses expressing full-length lyssavirus glycoprotein genes. *Epidemiol. Infect.* **136:**670–678.

Wibbelt, G., Kurth, A., Yasmum, N., Bannert, M., Nagel, S., Nitsche, A., and Ehlers, B. (2007). Discovery of herpesviruses in bats. *J. Gen. Virol.* **88:**2651–2655.

Winkler, W. G. (1968). Airborne rabies virus isolation. *Wildl. Dis.* **4:**37–40.

Winkler, W. G., Fashinell, T. R., Leffingwell, L., Howard, P., and Conomy, P. (1973). Airborne rabies transmission in a laboratory worker. *J. Am. Med. Assoc.* **226:**1219–1221.

Wright, E., Hayman, D. T., Vaughan, A., Temperton, N. J., Wood, J. L., Cunningham, A. A., Suu-Ire, R., Weiss, R. A., and Fooks, A. R. (2010). Virus neutralising activity of African fruit bat (Eidolon helvum) sera against emerging lyssaviruses. *Virology* **408:**183–189.

Yung, V., Favi, M., and Fernandez, J. (2002). Genetic and antigenic typing of rabies virus in Chile. *Arch. Virol.* **147:**2197–2205.

CHAPTER 13

Postexposure Prophylaxis for Rabies in Resource-Limited/ Poor Countries

Prapimporn Shantavasinkul* and **Henry Wilde**[†]

Contents		

Abstract

Human rabies is essentially a fatal disease once clinical signs develop. Rabies postexposure prophylaxis (PEP) consists of thorough wound care in combination with administration of rabies immunoglobulin and rabies vaccine. This is highly effective in rabies prevention if carried out diligently. Preexposure rabies prophylaxis simplifies PEP in the event of an exposure by eliminating the need for immunoglobulin. Shortened and more convenient and economical PEP regimens are being developed with promising results. They reduce the cost of PEP as well as travel expenses for the often very poor patients. The intradermal PEP regimen can now reduce the

* Queen Saovabha Memorial Institute, The Thai Red Cross Society (World Health Organization Collaborating Center for Research on Rabies Pathogenesis and Prevention), Bangkok, Thailand
† WHO-CC for Research and Training on Viral Zoonoses and Infectious Disease Division, Faculty of Medicine, Chulalongkorn University, Bangkok, Thailand

Advances in Virus Research, Volume 79
ISSN 0065-3527, DOI: 10.1016/B978-0-12-387040-7.00013-5

vaccine cost by ~60–70%. Although PEP in humans can prevent death, controlling the canine vector by sustained vaccination remains the mainstay of rabies elimination.

I. INTRODUCTION

Rabies is an acute progressive fatal encephalitis, caused by RNA viruses from the family *Rhabdoviridae*, genus *Lyssavirus*, which includes seven genotypes (Rupprecht *et al.*, 2002). Although a number of carnivore and bat species serve as natural reservoirs, worldwide rabies in dogs is the source of 99% of human infections and poses a threat to >3.3 billion people (Knobel *et al.*, 2005). There are an estimated 60,000 human rabies-related deaths worldwide each year. Most cases occur in Asia and Africa (Warrell *et al.*, 2007).

In humans, rabies is almost invariably fatal once clinical symptoms develop. However, rabies deaths are virtually always preventable, provided postexposure prophylaxis (PEP) is implemented promptly and competently after an exposure. It has been estimated that >15 million people receive PEP yearly (Anonymous, 2010). PEP, for people bitten by rabid mammals, consists of a combination of aggressive wound cleansing, passive immunization with rabies immunoglobulin (RIG), and active immunization with tissue culture rabies vaccine. This has proven highly effective in preventing infections and deaths (Anonymous, 2005, 2007).

II. LOCAL WOUND CARE

After a potential rabies exposure, rabies PEP should be initiated as soon as possible. Rabies PEP consists of thorough local wound care and adminis-tration of both rabies vaccine and RIG. The importance of wound care with soap and an antiseptic agent was documented decades ago (Dean *et al.*, 1963), but it is often completely neglected in rabies-endemic countries. First aid treatment of rabies-exposed victims requires immedi-ate vigorous wound cleansing with flowing water and soap or detergent, preferably under pressure, of all bite wounds or scratches (for at least 15 min, depending on the number of injuries). Washing with water may decrease the size of the viral inoculums (Anonymous, 1997). Soap and antiseptic agents denature the virus and may prevent invasion. All wounds must be irrigated with either iodine-containing or similar viru-cidal agents before going to the nearest health-care center for risk evalua-tion and consideration of vaccination and RIG injection. Wound suturing should be postponed to reduce the risk of infection, and definite wound closure is best done several days later. During this time, wound inspection and daily dressing of wounds should be done. Antitetanus vaccination and antibiotics should be administered as indicated. If it is necessary to approximate a severely lacerated or large bleeding wound by suturing on the first day, then intensive wound cleansing, antiseptic application, and RIG injection should first be carried out. Suturing the wound should be as minimal as possible and should follow waiting for a period of one or more hours after RIG injection in order to allow neutralization of virus.

III. EVALUATION OF RISK OF RABIES EXPOSURE

Factors that should be considered to determine whether PEP is initiated include (1) extent of exposure and the type of contact (Table I), (2) species of and the behavior of the suspect animal, and (3) availability and

TABLE I Postexposure rabies prophylaxis

Category	Type of contact with the suspected animal[a]	Treatment
I	Touching or feeding of animals Licks on intact skin	None. May be opportunity to provide preexposure for certain subjects at future risk
II	Nibbling of uncovered skin Minor scratches or abrasions without bleeding	Start vaccine immediately[b] and stop treatment if FAT negative or dog/cat remains well after 10 days[c]
III	Single or multiple transdermal bites or scratches, licks on broken skin Contamination of mucous membrane with saliva (i.e., licks) Exposures to bats[d]	Inject RIG into and around bite sites. Remainder of volume (if any) IM, followed by vaccine series immmediately[b]. Stop vaccine if FAT negative or dog/cat remains healthy after 10 days[c]

[a] Exposure to rodents, rabbits, and hares in rabies-endemic area may require rabies PEP, but expert opinion should be obtained where available.

[b] In a low rabies-endemic or rabies-free region, observing a biting dog for 10 days before starting rabies prophylaxis may be an option after expert consultation. However, doing this in a canine rabies-endemic country could place patients at grave risk.

[c] Observation prior to PEP applies only to dogs and cats; other domestic and wild animals suspected as rabid should be humanely killed and their brains examined for the presence of rabies antigen using appropriate laboratory techniques.

[d] Postexposure prophylaxis should be considered when contact between a human and a bat has occurred unless the exposed person can rule out a bite or scratch, or exposure to a mucous membrane. Bat bites can be virtually painless.

reliability of laboratory testing of the responsible animal. The World Health Organization (WHO) classified risk of exposures into three categories and their guidelines depend on the severity of the exposure (Anonymous, 2010).

Category I.   Touching or feeding of animals. Licks on intact skin. These are not exposures, and they require no treatment. There may be an opportunity for preexposure prophylaxis (PREP) if patient remains at risk.

Category II.   Nibbling of uncovered skin, minor scratches, or abrasions without bleeding. These are potential exposures and they require rabies vaccination without RIG.

Category III.   Single or multiple transdermal bites or scratches, contamination of mucous membrane with saliva, licks on broken skin, any exposure to bats. They are the most severe form and require immediate RIG injection into and around the wounds and rabies vaccination. Bat bite exposures may be trivial resulting in undetectable wounds that are often painless. They are also listed as category III exposures because of the unique ability of this virus to replicate in the epidermis and dermis.

The next step issue before initiation of PEP is to evaluate the species and history of the responsible animal and whether it is likely to carry rabies in the environment where the bite occurred. Rabies virus can infect any mammal, but dogs and cats are the most important vectors for transmission to humans. Rabies is most commonly transmitted by bites or scratches. However, the virus can be transmitted through aerosol in cave explorers and in laboratory accidents (Johnson et al., 2006; Rupprecht et al., 2002). Human-to-human transmission can occur by transplantation of infected tissues (Anonymous, 1981; Baer et al., 1982; Bronnert et al., 2007; Houff et al., 1979). Regions with unsupervised dog populations present the greatest risk to humans. Canines that live in close proximity to humans are the principal vectors worldwide. Raccoons, skunks, foxes, wolves, bats, and other wild carnivores are threats in some parts of the world but account only for a relatively small portion of the large number of human rabies deaths. Monkeys, cats, rats, and other domestic and agricultural mammals are all potential accidental vectors as they live in close proximity to dogs and bats. Proven reports of rabies in rats and other rodents are extremely rare (Kamoltham et al., 2002; Smith et al., 1968; Wimalaratne, 1997), although rat bites are common in many countries. Documentation of rabies in rats has occurred in Bandicota rats (B. bengalensis, indica, or savilei) but not in marsupial bandicoots of Australia. Rats are quite numerous in many Asian cities and are able to survive an attack by a rabid dog or cat. It is virtually impossible for a nurse or physician to distinguish a large Norwegian or Brown rat from a *Bandicota*. Rat bites are, therefore, being treated in the same manner as dog or cat bites in several Asian countries.

The history of symptoms and signs of rabies in offending dogs is not always reliable. Provoked or unprovoked bites do not predict the risk of rabies in dogs (Siwasontiwat *et al.*, 1992). A history of prior rabies vaccination in dogs cannot guarantee that the animal will not be infected. A significant number of dogs that had been immunized with rabies vaccine were found rabid in a Thai study (Tepsumethanon and Mitmoonpitak, 2010). Some Asian countries (notably Indonesia) manufacture their own canine vaccines and they may have very low potency. The immune response to rabies vaccine is influenced by many factors such as the route of immunization (intramuscular or subcutaneous), the number of vaccinations, the age of the dog when vaccinated, the quality of vaccine, and the frequency of repeat vaccinations (Cliquet *et al.*, 2003; Mansfield *et al.*, 2004; Sage *et al.*, 1993; Tepsumethanon *et al.*, 1991). Even in the United States, rabies has been found in previously vaccinated dogs and cats (Murray *et al.*, 2009).

In well-developed countries, which have a low incidence of rabies, it is usually decided to observe a suspected dog or cat or to euthanize and examine it by a competent laboratory. However, in the developing world, with a large stray dog population, the animal is often unavailable for observation and laboratory examination. Moreover, there are few local animal quarantine facilities and reliable diagnostic laboratories. The risk of rabies virus infection in such an endemic area is much higher, and the threshold for PEP should be very low. It is best to initiate PEP unless immediate competent necropsy and laboratory examination of the responsible animal exclude rabies. Delays in starting PEP during animal observation should be avoided in order to prevent PEP failures due to delay.

PEP may be discontinued if (1) the suspected animal is proven to be free of rabies by a reliable laboratory using direct fluorescent antibody testing of animal brain by an experienced staff (Tepsumethanon *et al.*, 1997), and (2) the responsible animal is a domestic dog or cat that remains well after 10 days observation counting from the day of exposure (Tepsumethanon *et al.*, 2004).

IV. POSTEXPOSURE PROPHYLAXIS OF PREVIOUSLY UNVACCINATED PATIENTS

A. Rabies vaccines

In unvaccinated rabies-exposed patients, after local wound care, RIG and vaccine administration must be started as soon as possible. If there has been delay, PEP should be initiated regardless of the time interval between exposure and initiation of PEP. The incubation period may be as short as a few days or as long as several years. This depends on the site of the bite (distance to the CNS and presence of many peripheral nerve endings), the size of the inoculum, and unknown host factors (Hemachudha and Rupprecht, 2004).

Purified cell-culture and embryonated egg-based rabies vaccines have been proved to be safe and effective in preventing rabies. Vaccines can be used for pre- and postexposure rabies prevention. PEP has been safely administered to millions of people worldwide. WHO recommends that all cell-culture vaccines should have a minimum potency of 2.5 IU per single intramuscular dose from 0.5 or 1.0 mL volumes after reconstitution of the lyophilized ampoule. This depends on the type of vaccines, which are supplied with either 0.5 or 1.0 mL diluents (Anonymous, 2010). WHO also recommends that the volume injected using an intradermal schedule should always be 0.1 mL, whether it comes from a 0.5 or 1.0 mL ampoule. Following reconstitution with the accompanying sterile volume of diluent, the vaccines should be used within 6–8 h if kept at +2 to +8 °C. Despite the availability of cell-culture vaccines on the international market, Pakistan is still producing and using nerve-tissue-derived vaccine (Semple type), which can induce severe adverse reactions and which is of questionable immunogenicity. This vaccine should be avoided and WHO has long recommended that manufacture of nerve-tissue-derived vaccines should be discontinued.

Active immunization with rabies vaccine stimulates the host immune response, and rabies-neutralizing antibodies (RNAb) appear in the circulation ~7–10 days after start of vaccination. RNAb reach a peak on day 14–30 (Khawplod et al., 2002a,b; Shantavasinkul et al., 2010a,b,c) at a level of at least 0.5 IU/mL (Anonymous, 2010), which is maintained until day 28 or 30 (Anonymous, 2007) and for at least one year. This is generally considered adequate to prevent human rabies. Therefore, there is a window period for up to 7–10 days before a protective natural antibody level from vaccine has been reached. This is the rationale for injecting RIG into and around wounds in order to neutralize the virus and prevent its entry into peripheral nerves, where it would be in an immune-protected environment allowing transit to the central nervous system.

Currently, the rabies expert committee of WHO has recognized three rabies PEP schedule of which only the first is also approved by the US CDC:

1. The Essen intramuscular regimen

This gold standard regimen consists of one IM injection of cell-culture vaccine in the deltoid or anterolateral thigh area on days 0, 3, 7, 14, and 28. It consumes five ampoules of vaccine (0.5 or 1 mL volume depending on the type of vaccine) and requires five clinic visits over 1 month. Recently, the

American Advisory Committee on Immunization Practice (ACIP) has revised the PEP treatment guideline (Rupprecht et al., 2010). The new recommendation reduced the number of vaccinations from 5 to 4 doses on days 0, 3, 7, and 14. Accumulated evidence indicates that four vaccinations in combination with RIG, when indicated, elicit an adequate immune response. The fifth injection on day 28 does not contribute to more favorable outcomes in immunocompetent individuals. Nevertheless, immunocompromised persons such as those that are currently taking corticosteroids, antimalarial drugs, and other immunosuppressive agents, or have HIV infection, should receive the original 5-dose IM vaccine regimen. The WHO approved the 4-dose IM regimen, initially as an alternative regimen for healthy and immunocompetent individuals (Anonymous, 2010).

Rabies vaccine should be administered IM at the deltoid area of the arm. For small children, vaccine can be injected at the anterolateral thigh area. The gluteal area is not a reliable site for injection due to the presence of fat, which may retard an adequate RNAb response and may result in PEP failures (Fishbein et al., 1988; Shill et al., 1987).

2. The Zagreb or 2-1-1 regimen

This regimen requires two intramuscular injections at two different sites on day 0 and at one each on days 7 and 21. It consumes four full ampoules of vaccine and requires three clinic visits over 3 weeks. The disadvantage of this regimen is that the physician cannot assess early signs of infection of the bite wound on day 3, which often become manifest by that time.

3. The two-site ID regimen (TRC-ID regimen)

Rabies ID vaccination is capable of achieving a comparable immune response to the intramuscular route, yet using a lower vaccine dose (Chutivongse et al., 1990), and reduces vaccine cost by ~60–70% compared to the standard IM regimen (Wilde et al., 1999). Further, previous studies showed that ID rabies vaccination results in detectable cell-mediated immunoreactivity by day 7, which is earlier than with the "gold standard" Essen intramuscular regimen (day 14; Phanuphak et al., 1987; Ratanavongsiri et al., 1985). This faster reactivity can be attributed to repeated intradermal injections at different lymphatic drainage sites. Intradermal injections are more immunogenic than equivalent single intramuscular ones due to the presence of dendritic cells in skin (Nicolas and Guy, 2008). Recently, it has been shown that the ID route induces a predominant Th2 response, as compared to the predominant Th1 response induced by IM injections of rabies vaccine (Saraya et al., 2010). This presumably enhances the transport of antigen to receptors.

Originally, the TRC-ID regimen consisted of two injections of 0.1 mL of any WHO recognized tissue culture vaccine at two different lymphatic drainage sites on days 0, 3, 7, and one injection on days 28 and 90.

It consumed 0.8 mL of vaccine and required five clinic visits over 3 months. Many patients did not return for the day 90 injection and there were no known treatment failures among this group in Thailand. It was then simplified to two injections on days 0, 3, 7, and 28 and the original day 90 visit was omitted (Khawplod *et al.*, 2006). This schedule has been approved by WHO and replaces the original version (Anonymous, 2010; Table II).

The eight-site intradermal (Oxford) regimen consisted of one injection of vaccine at eight different body sites on day 0, at four sites on day 7, and at one site on days 28 and 90 (Warrell *et al.*, 1985). In order to simplify and facilitate the use of intradermal PEP, the consultation of WHO experts recommended deleting the rarely used eight-site ID regimen from the list of WHO-approved postexposure rabies regimens (Anonymous, 2010).

Recent research from Queen Saovabha Memorial Institute, Bangkok, Thailand, indicated that it might be possible to develop a 1-week ID PEP that would reduce travel time and costs as well as noncompliance. The 1-week ID PEP consists of four-site ID injections over both deltoids and thighs on days 0, 3, and 7 with or without RIG. RNAb were found to be present after vaccinations for at least 1 year. The new regimen could induce significantly higher RNAb on days 14 and 28 over the standard two-site ID PEP (Shantavasinkul *et al.*, 2010a,b,c). The study looks promising and is now being reassessed in additional Phase III studies at three other Asian centers.

TABLE II   WHO-approved rabies vaccination schedules

Schedules	Details
ESSEN regimen (IM)	One full dose of cell-cultured vaccine injected intramuscularly into deltoid or anterolateral thigh on days 0, 3, 7, 14, and 28. The days 14 and 28 dose of the vaccine can be omitted if the animal is known to have remained healthy
Zagreb regimen (IM)	Two full vaccines doses injected intramuscularly at different sites on day 0 and one dose on days 7 and 21. The day 21 dose of the vaccine can be omitted if the animal is known to have remained healthy
Thai Red Cross Intradermal regimen (ID)	Two intradermal injections of 0.1 mL at both deltoids on days 0, 3, 7, and 28. The day 28 dose of the vaccine can be omitted if the animal is known to have remained healthy

Modified from WHO, US CDC, and Thai Red Cross Society recommendations (Anonymous, 2010; Rupprecht *et al.*, 2010).

Rabies is a fatal disease once clinical signs develop and there is no contraindication for rabies PEP. PEP has been shown to be safe in 202 pregnant mothers and their infants (Chutivongse *et al.*, 1995). The infants were followed for 1 postpartum year, and complications were comparable to the matched control group.

Immunocompromised individuals or subjects who are on immuno-suppressive agents, antimalarial drugs, or chloroquine may not produce an adequate RNAb response from rabies vaccinations. AIDS patients with very low CD4 counts may not mount an adequate RNAb response to rabies vaccines (Jaijaroensup *et al.*, 1999). Thorough wound cleansing, followed by RIG injection and a full PEP series, is nevertheless of utmost importance in such cases. Providing preexposure vaccination (PREP) for HIV infected children in canine endemic regions while they are still immunocompetent has been recommended (Thisyakorn *et al.*, 2000, 2001). In immunocompetent persons, no routine antibody screening is recommended following PREP or PEP. Patients with immune-compromising medications or conditions should have evaluation of RNAb 14–28 days after vaccination in order to consider additional vacci-nation and possible changes in lifestyle. Consultation with a rabies expert or infectious diseases specialist is indicated after a rabies exposure of an immunocompromised individual.

B. Rabies immunoglobulins

RIG is indicated only once in previously unvaccinated persons to provide passive immunity and neutralize rabies virus until endogenous antibody production commences. A protective endogenous level of RNAb cannot be expected before days 7–10. During this window period, passive immu-nity by using RIG must be provided as soon as possible after exposure. RIG must be administered in combination with rabies vaccine on day 0 or as soon as possible after exposure in all category III patients and also in immunocompromised patients with category II exposures (Anonymous, 2010). RIG can be safely administered up to 7 days after the first vaccine dose (Khawplod *et al.*, 1996a,b). RIG is not indicated after day 7 when natural antibody has been generated, which may then be neutralized by the delayed RIG injection. None of the vaccine regimens can substitute for the use of RIG. Although some regimens can induce higher RNAb titers, none can elicit a protective antibody level before day 7 (Wilde *et al.*, 2002). RIG must therefore be used as indicated to reduce the risk of PEP failure.

There are two types of RIG. Human rabies immunoglobulin (HRIG) is preferable when it is available. If it is not, equine rabies immunoglobulin (ERIG) is also effective to neutralize virus. The dose of HRIG is 20 IU/kg of body weight. For ERIG, the dose is 40 IU/kg because ERIG has a shorter half-life. RIG should not be administered in the same syringe or at the same body site as vaccine since RIG may inactivate the vaccine. No more than the recommended dose should be administered in order to avoid immune suppression. Skin testing for sensitivity to equine serum products is virtually useless (Tantawichien et al., 1995). There is no standardization of the skin testing method or of the interpretation of skin test results. Skin testing does not predict serum sickness. Anaphylaxis with modern purified ERIG is extremely rare. Of the patients who received ERIG at the Thai Red Cross Society, Bangkok, Thailand and who developed serum sickness, all had negative skin tests. We have encountered only two cases in more than 150,000 subjects that had received ERIG. Both patients had negative skin tests and fully recovery after treatment using adrenaline and diphenhydramine. Corticosteroids were not used in serum sickness or anaphylaxis because they might suppress the antibody response from rabies vaccination (Suwansrinon et al., 2007).

RIG administration should be done after aggressive wound cleansing. It must be infiltrated into and around all bite wounds slowly. All of the calculated RIG dose, or as much as anatomically possible, should be infiltrated into the wound. The remaining RIG should be injected intramuscularly at a distant site from the area of vaccine injection (usually at the lateral thigh and avoiding the gluteal area). Fingers or toes, where there is little space for expansion, are often the sites of canine or cat bites. These areas are associated with a high risk of rabies virus infection since there are many nerve endings. Many physicians try to avoid RIG injection of fingers and toes because it is painful and they fear a compartment syndrome. Actually, it is a safe procedure if carried out with care by experienced staff (Suwansrinon et al., 2006). RIG injection is performed using number 26 or 28 needles through one or two skin puncture-sites or directly into the open bite wounds. Some pressure can be exerted, but injection is stopped when blanching or excessive swelling of the digit becomes apparent. In a prospective study of 100 such injections of digits at our clinic, neither have we encountered a compartment syndrome nor can we recall any past cases over the past two decades. We are aware of the fact that several other clinics use local anesthetics to block the RIG injection site. It has, however, been our experience that this can be as painful or more painful than primary RIG injection into and around the bite wound (Suwansrinon et al., 2006). Almost 50% of animal bites and rabies cases worldwide are in children. This is because they are small and often bitten in high risk areas such as face, head, neck, or hands. With a child's low body weight, the calculated volume of RIG may not be enough to infiltrate all wounds. RIG can be diluted to a sufficient volume for all wounds to be effectively and safely infiltrated. RIG injection into some, but not all, bite wounds may be a cause of PEP failures (Wilde, 2007). All bite wounds are contaminated by animal saliva and many patients come to the clinic with delay. The bite wounds often show evidence of infection at presentation. We have shown in a prospective study that an infected wound can be injected safely with RIG as long as it is properly cleansed and antibiotics are administered (Wilde *et al.*, 1992).

V. POSTEXPOSURE PROPHYLAXIS IN PREVIOUSLY VACCINATED PATIENTS

Previously vaccinated patients are those who have received a complete course of PREP or PEP with cell-cultured vaccine. Such subjects require no routine booster vaccination unless an exposure occurs. It has been shown that cell-cultured vaccines establish long lasting immunity that results in an accelerated antibody response if booster injections are administered. Persons who had received a prior PREP or PEP with a cell-culture vaccine up to 21 years earlier, all developed good anamnestic responses after booster injections (Suwansrinon *et al.*, 2006).

Patients with a history of prior nerve-tissue-derived (Semple or suckling mouse brain) vaccine in the past are treated as if they have never been rabies vaccinated (vaccine plus RIG when indicated). The reason for this is that nerve-tissue-derived vaccines do not always provide a reliable immune response. In one study, some recipients had high anamnestic responses to new vaccination and others had no detectable titers prior to revaccination and did not show an accelerated immune response to PEP (Khawplod *et al.*, 1996a,b). This was presumably due to absent or low potency of some batches of the nerve-tissue vaccine used (Semple or suckling mouse brain products in this study).

When a rabies exposure occurs in a previous recipient of PREP or PEP, local wound care is still an important part of rabies PEP and booster vaccination should be administered immediately. However, RIG is contraindicated because it may actually interfere with the antibody response. Currently recommended booster vaccination consists of only two vaccine doses with cell-culture vaccine. The first dose is administered immediately and the second dose 3 days later at the deltoid or lateral thigh. The US CDC (Manning *et al.*, 2008; Rupprecht *et al.*, 2010) recommends only intramuscular booster administration. However, it has been proven that two booster vaccinations using the intradermal method are as effective as the IM route (Kositprapa *et al.*, 1997; Suwansrinon *et al.*, 2006). The currently recommended booster regimens require two clinic visits and are inconvenient for many rural residents in developing countries where they usually have to travel considerable distances and thereby lose working time and incur transportation expenses that they can ill afford. Moreover, tourists may have to change travel schedules in order to receive the second dose on day 3 (Table III).

TABLE III   Rabies postexposure prophylaxis

Vaccination status	Treatment	Regimen
Previously unvaccinated	Wound care	Immediate thorough wound cleansing with water and soap. If available, use a virucidal agent (hypochloride—Dakin's solution[a] or povidone-iodine) to irrigate the wounds
	Rabies immunoglobulin	Administer HRIG 20 IU/kg body weight or ERIG 40 IU/kg. Skin test is not recommended by WHO before ERIG administration
	Vaccine	Full series of rabies vaccine as per Table II
Previously vaccinated with Semple or suckling mouse brain vaccine[b]	Wound care	Immediate thorough wound cleansing with water and soap. If available, use a virucidal agent (hypochloride—Dakin's solution[a] or povidone-iodine) to irrigate the wounds. Administer complete course of PEP as per Table II
	Rabies immunoglobulin	If Category III exposure
	Vaccine	Full series of rabies vaccine as per Table II

Modified from WHO, US CDC, and Thai Red Cross Society recommendations (Anonymous, 2010; Rupprecht et al., 2010).
[a] Dakin's solution is made by boiling four cups of water, adding ¼ teaspoon baking soda, and adding one tablespoon of Clorax® (sodium hypochloride solution 5.25%).
[b] Any person with a history of complete course of preexposure rabies prophylaxis or at least three doses of PEP with cell-cultured vaccine and those who have been documented to have adequate rabies-neutralizing antibody response of at least 0.5 IU/mL.

An alternative regimen was approved by the WHO in 2010. This regimen consists of 0.1 mL of cell-cultured vaccine administered as one dose each in both deltoids and thighs. It can be done in one visit and has been demonstrated to actually result in higher and earlier RNAb than the recommended 2-IM or ID (Tantawichien *et al.*, 1999, 2001). The four-site ID booster was also shown to induce an anamnestic response in previously vaccinated patients when used with purified vero-cell rabies vaccine (PVRV), purified chick embryo cell vaccine (PCECV; Khawplod *et al.*, 2002a,b; Tantawichien *et al.*, 2001) and human diploid cell vaccine (HDCV; Khawplod *et al.*, 2002a,b). It has been used safely and effectively in over 5000 previously immunized patients at the Queen Saovabha Memorial Institute, Bangkok, Thailand since 1998 without any cases of PEP failure (Shantavasinkul *et al.*, 2010a,b,c).

VI. POSTEXPOSURE PROPHYLAXIS FAILURES

Although PEP is very effective, failure cases have been reported. Most reported PEP failures were associated with deviations from current guidelines. The most commonly encountered causes of such PEP management failures are (1) RIG is not used at all (Devriendt *et al.*, 1982; Gacouin *et al.*, 1999; Sriaroon *et al.*, 2003), it is injected only intramuscularly and not into wounds or not all bite wounds have been injected (Wilde *et al.*, 1996); (2) vaccine or RIG is of low potency or incorrectly administered (Anonymous, 1988; Shill *et al.*, 1987; Wilde *et al.*, 1989); (3) wound care was not done or inadequately performed; (4) there was delay in starting treatment; and (5) the wound was sutured before RIG administration. Nevertheless, there have been rare case reports of human rabies deaths in which PEP had been carried out fully according to WHO guidelines (Hemachudha *et al.*, 1999; Shantavasinkul *et al.*, 2010a,b,c; Wilde, 2007). Such probable true prophylaxis failures are exceedingly rare, and the cases reported represent a very small number compared to the millions of PEPs that are administered worldwide every year. It is noteworthy that the apparently true failures reported had wounds in highly innervated regions such as hands and face. Nevertheless, every such failure case is a tragedy and analyzing and reporting it should be mandatory. To our knowledge, no human deaths from rabies have been reported among patients who received booster vaccination after a prior PREP series of rabies vaccination. Controlling the canine and feline rabies vector in endemic areas of rabies and preexposure rabies administration of high risk groups remains an essential goal for rabies elimination.

REFERENCES

Anonymous (1981). Human-to-human transmission of rabies via corneal transplant—Thailand. *MMWR Morb. Mortal. Wkly. Rep.* **30:**473–474.

Anonymous (1988). Leads from the MMWR. Human rabies despite treatment with rabies immune globulin and human diploid cell rabies vaccine—Thailand . *JAMA* **259:**25–26.

Anonymous (1997). WHO recommendations on rabies post-exposure treatment and the correct technique of intradermal immunization against rabies. WHO publication WHO/EMC/ZOO/96.6, p. 1–24.

Anonymous (2005). WHO Expert Consultation on rabies . *World Health Organ. Tech. Rep. Ser.* **931:**1–88.

Anonymous (2007). WHO Expert Committee on biological standardization. World Health Organ Tech Rep Ser1-340, back cover.

Anonymous (2010). Rabies vaccines: WHO position paper. *Wkly. Epidemiol. Rec.* **85:**309–320.

Baer, G. M., Shaddock, J. H., Houff, S. A., Harrison, A. K., and Gardner, J. J. (1982). Human rabies transmitted by corneal transplant. *Arch. Neurol.* **39:**103–107.

Bronnert, J., Wilde, H., Tepsumethanon, V., Lumlertdacha, B., and Hemachudha, T. (2007). Organ transplantations and rabies transmission. *J. Travel Med.* **14:**177–180.

Chutivongse, S., Wilde, H., Supich, C., Baer, G. M., and Fishbein, D. B. (1990). Postexposure prophylaxis for rabies with antiserum and intradermal vaccination. *Lancet* **335:**896–898.

Chutivongse, S., Wilde, H., Benjavongkulchai, M., Chomchey, P., and Punthawong, S. (1995). Postexposure rabies vaccination during pregnancy: Effect on 202 women and their infants. *Clin. Infect. Dis.* **20:**818–820.

Cliquet, F., Verdier, Y., Sagne, L., Aubert, M., Schereffer, J. L., Selve, M., Wasniewski, M., and Servat, A. (2003). Neutralising antibody titration in 25, 000 sera of dogs and cats vaccinated against rabies in France, in the framework of the new regulations that offer an alternative to quarantine. *Rev. Sci. Tech.* **22:**857–866.

Dean, D. J., Baer, G. M., and Thompson, W. R. (1963). Studies on the local treatment of rabies-infected wounds. *Bull. World Health Organ.* **28:**477–486.

Devriendt, J., Staroukine, M., Costy, F., and Vanderhaeghen, J. J. (1982). Fatal encephalitis apparently due to rabies. Occurrence after treatment with human diploid cell vaccine but not rabies immune globulin. *JAMA* **248:**2304–2306.

Fishbein, D. B., Sawyer, L. A., Reid-Sanden, F. L., and Weir, E. H. (1988). Administration of human diploid-cell rabies vaccine in the gluteal area. *N. Engl. J. Med.* **318:**124–125.

Gacouin, A., Bourhy, H., Renaud, J. C., Camus, C., Suprin, E., and Thomas, R. (1999). Human rabies despite postexposure vaccination. *Eur. J. Clin. Microbiol. Infect. Dis.* **18:**233–235.

Hemachudha, T., and Rupprecht, C. E. (2004). Rabies. *In* "Principle of Neurologic Infectious Disease" (M. Karen, M. Karen, and L. Roos, eds.), pp. 151–174. McGraw-Hill, New York.

Hemachudha, T., Mitrabhakdi, E., Wilde, H., Vejabhuti, A., Siripataravanit, S., and Kingnate, D. (1999). Additional reports of failure to respond to treatment after rabies exposure in Thailand. *Clin. Infect. Dis.* **28:**143–144.

Houff, S. A., Burton, R. C., Wilson, R. W., Henson, T. E., London, W. T., Baer, G. M., Anderson, L. J., Winkler, W. G., Madden, D. L., and Sever, J. L. (1979). Human-to-human transmission of rabies virus by corneal transplant. *N. Engl. J. Med.* **300:**603–604.

Jaijaroensup, W., Tantawichien, T., Khawplod, P., Tepsumethanon, S., and Wilde, H. (1999). Postexposure rabies vaccination in patients infected with human immunodeficiency virus. *Clin. Infect. Dis.* **28:**913–914.

Johnson, N., Phillpotts, R., and Fooks, A. R. (2006). Airborne transmission of lyssaviruses. *J. Med. Microbiol.* **55:**785–790.

Kamoltham, T., Tepsumethanon, V., and Wilde, H. (2002). Rat rabies in Phetchabun Province, Thailand. *J. Travel Med.* **9:**106–107.

Khawplod, P., Wilde, H., Chomchey, P., Benjavongkulchai, M., Yenmuang, W., Chaiyabutr, N., and Sitprija, V. (1996a). What is an acceptable delay in rabies immune globulin administration when vaccine alone had been given previously? *Vaccine* **14:**389–391.

Khawplod, P., Wilde, H., Yenmuang, W., Benjavongkulchai, M., and Chomchey, P. (1996b). Immune response to tissue culture rabies vaccine in subjects who had previous postexposure treatment with Semple or suckling mouse brain vaccine. *Vaccine* **14:**1549–1552.

Khawplod, P., Benjavongkulchai, M., Limusanno, S., Chareonwai, S., Kaewchompoo, W., Tantawichien, T., and Wilde, H. (2002a). Four-site intradermal postexposure boosters in previously rabies vaccinated subjects. *J. Travel Med.* **9:**153–155.

Khawplod, P., Wilde, H., Tepsumethanon, S., Limusanno, S., Tantawichien, T., Chomchey, P., Ayuthaya, A. B., and Wangroonsarb, Y. (2002b). Prospective immunogenicity study of multiple intradermal injections of rabies vaccine in an effort to obtain an early immune response without the use of immunoglobulin. *Clin. Infect. Dis.* **35:**1562–1565.

Khawplod, P., Wilde, H., Sirikwin, S., Benjawongkulchai, M., Limusanno, S., Jaijaroensab, W., Chiraguna, N., Supich, C., Wangroongsarb, Y., and Sitprija, V. (2006). Revision of the Thai Red Cross intradermal rabies post-exposure regimen by eliminating the 90-day booster injection. *Vaccine* **24:**3084–3086.

Knobel, D. L., Cleaveland, S., Coleman, P. G., Fevre, E. M., Meltzer, M. I., Miranda, M. E., Shaw, A., Zinsstag, J., and Meslin, F. X. (2005). Re-evaluating the burden of rabies in Africa and Asia. *Bull. World Health Organ.* **83:**360–368.

Kositprapa, C., Limsuwun, K., Wilde, H., Jaijaroensup, W., Saikasem, A., Khawplod, P., Kriaksorn, U., and Supich, C. (1997). Immune response to simulated postexposure rabies booster vaccinations in volunteers who received preexposure vaccinations. *Clin. Infect. Dis.* **25:**614–616.

Manning, S. E., Rupprecht, C. E., Fishbein, D., Hanlon, C. A., Lumlertdacha, B., Guerra, M., Meltzer, M. I., Dhankhar, P., Vaidya, S. A., Jenkins, S. R., Sun, B., and Hull, H. F. (2008). Human rabies prevention—United States, 2008: Recommendations of the Advisory Committee on Immunization Practices. *MMWR Recomm. Rep.* **57:**1–28.

Mansfield, K. L., Burr, P. D., Snodgrass, D. R., Sayers, R., and Fooks, A. R. (2004). Factors affecting the serological response of dogs and cats to rabies vaccination. *Vet. Rec.* **154:**423–426.

Murray, K. O., Holmes, K. C., and Hanlon, C. A. (2009). Rabies in vaccinated dogs and cats in the United States, 1997–2001. *J. Am. Vet. Med. Assoc.* **235:**691–695.

Nicolas, J. F., and Guy, B. (2008). Intradermal, epidermal and transcutaneous vaccination: From immunology to clinical practice. *Expert Rev. Vaccines* **7:**1201–1214.

Phanuphak, P., Khawplod, P., Sirivichayakul, S., Siriprasomsub, W., Ubol, S., and Thaweepathomwat, M. (1987). Humoral and cell-mediated immune responses to various economical regimens of purified Vero cell rabies vaccine. *Asian Pac. J. Allergy Immunol.* **5:**33–37.

Ratanavongsiri, J., Sriwanthana, B., Ubol, S., and Phanuphak, P. (1985). Cell-mediated immune response following intracutaneous immunisation with human diploid cell rabies vaccine. *Asian Pac. J. Allergy Immunol.* **3:**187–190.

Rupprecht, C. E., Hanlon, C. A., and Hemachudha, T. (2002). Rabies re-examined. *Lancet Infect. Dis.* **2:**327–343.

Rupprecht, C. E., Briggs, D., Brown, C. M., Franka, R., Katz, S. L., Kerr, H. D., Lett, S. M., Levis, R., Meltzer, M. I., Schaffner, W., and Cieslak, P. R. (2010). Use of a reduced (4-dose) vaccine schedule for postexposure prophylaxis to prevent human rabies: Recommendations of the advisory committee on immunization practices. *MMWR Recomm. Rep.* **59:**1–9.

Sage, G., Khawplod, P., Wilde, H., Lobaugh, C., Hemachudha, T., Tepsumethanon, W., and Lumlertdaecha, B. (1993). Immune response to rabies vaccine in Alaskan dogs: Failure to achieve a consistently protective antibody response. *Trans. R. Soc. Trop. Med. Hyg.* **87:**593–595.

Saraya, A., Wacharapluesadee, S., Khawplod, P., Tepsumethanon, S., Briggs, D., Asawavichienjinda, T., and Hemachudha, T. (2010). A preliminary study of chemo- and cytokine responses in rabies vaccine recipients of intradermal and intramuscular regimens. *Vaccine* **28:**4553–4557.

Shantavasinkul, P., Tantawichien, T., Jaijaroensup, W., Lertjarutorn, S., Banjongkasaena, A., Wilde, H., and Sitprija, V. (2010a). A 4-site, single-visit intradermal postexposure pro- phylaxis regimen for previously vaccinated patients: Experiences with >5000 patients. *Clin. Infect. Dis.* **51:**1070–1072.

Shantavasinkul, P., Tantawichien, T., Wacharapluesadee, S., Jeamanukoolkit, A., Udomchaisakul, P., Chattranukulchai, P., Wongsaroj, P., Khawplod, P., Wilde, H., and Hemachudha, T. (2010b). Failure of rabies postexposure prophylaxis in patients present- ing with unusual manifestations. *Clin. Infect. Dis.* **50:**77–79.

Shantavasinkul, P., Tantawichien, T., Wilde, H., Sawangvaree, A., Kumchat, A., Ruksaket, N., Lohsoonthorn, V., and Khawplod, P. (2010c). Postexposure rabies prophy- laxis completed in 1 week: Preliminary study. *Clin. Infect. Dis.* **50:**56–60.

Shill, M., Baynes, R. D., and Miller, S. D. (1987). Fatal rabies encephalitis despite appropriate post-exposure prophylaxis. A case report. *N. Engl. J. Med.* **316:**1257–1258.

Siwasontiwat, D., Lumlertdacha, B., Polsuwan, C., Hemachudha, T., Chutvongse, S., and Wilde, H. (1992). Rabies: Is provocation of the biting dog relevant for risk assessment? *Trans. R. Soc. Trop. Med. Hyg.* **86:**443.

Smith, P. C., Lawhaswasdi, K., Vick, W. E., and Stanton, J. S. (1968). Enzootic rabies in rodents in Thailand. *Nature* **217:**954–955.

Sriaroon, C., Daviratanasilpa, S., Sansomranjai, P., Khawplod, P., Hemachudha, T., Khamoltham, T., and Wilde, H. (2003). Rabies in a Thai child treated with the eight-site post-exposure regimen without rabies immune globulin. *Vaccine* **21:**3525–3526.

Suwansrinon, K., Jaijaroensup, W., Wilde, H., and Sitprija, V. (2006). Is injecting a finger with rabies immunoglobulin dangerous? *Am. J. Trop. Med. Hyg.* **75:**363–364.

Suwansrinon, K., Jaijareonsup, W., Wilde, H., Benjavongkulchai, M., Sriaroon, C., and Sitprija, V. (2007). Sex- and age-related differences in rabies immunoglobulin hypersen- sitivity. *Trans. R. Soc. Trop. Med. Hyg.* **101:**206–208.

Tantawichien, T., Benjavongkulchai, M., Wilde, H., Jaijaroensup, W., Siakasem, A., Chareonwai, S., Yountong, C., and Sitprija, V. (1995). Value of skin testing for predicting reactions to equine rabies immune globulin. *Clin. Infect. Dis.* **21:**660–662.

Tantawichien, T., Benjavongkulchai, M., Limsuwan, K., Khawplod, P., Kaewchompoo, W., Chomchey, P., and Sitprija, V. (1999). Antibody response after a four-site intradermal booster vaccination with cell-culture rabies vaccine. *Clin. Infect. Dis.* **28:**1100–1103.

Tantawichien, T., Supit, C., Khawplod, P., and Sitprija, V. (2001). Three-year experience with 4-site intradermal booster vaccination with rabies vaccine for postexposure prophylaxis. *Clin. Infect. Dis.* **33:**2085–2087.

Tepsumethanon, V. L. B., and Mitmoonpitak, C. (2010). Does history-taking help predict rabies diagnosis in dogs? Brief communication (original). *Asian Biomed.* **4:**811–815.

Tepsumethanon, W., Polsuwan, C., Lumlertdaecha, B., Khawplod, P., Hemachudha, T., Chutivongse, S., Wilde, H., Chiewbamrungkiat, M., and Phanuphak, P. (1991). Immune response to rabies vaccine in Thai dogs: A preliminary report. *Vaccine* **9:**627–630.

Tepsumethanon, V., Lumlertdacha, B., Mitmoonpitak, C., Fagen, R., and Wilde, H. (1997). Fluorescent antibody test for rabies: Prospective study of 8,987 brains. *Clin. Infect. Dis.* **25:**1459–1461.

Tepsumethanon, V., Lumlertdacha, B., Mitmoonpitak, C., Sitprija, V., Meslin, F. X., and Wilde, H. (2004). Survival of naturally infected rabid dogs and cats. *Clin. Infect. Dis.* **39:**278–280.

Thisyakorn, U., Pancharoen, C., Ruxrungtham, K., Ubolyam, S., Khawplod, P., Tantawichien, T., Phanuphak, P., and Wilde, H. (2000). Safety and immunogenicity of preexposure rabies vaccination in children infected with human immunodeficiency virus type 1. *Clin. Infect. Dis.* **30:**218.

Thisyakorn, U., Pancharoen, C., and Wilde, H. (2001). Immunologic and virologic evaluation of HIV-1-infected children after rabies vaccination. *Vaccine* **19:**1534–1537.

Warrell, M. J., Nicholson, K. G., Warrell, D. A., Suntharasamai, P., Chanthavanich, P., Viravan, C., Sinhaseni, A., Chiewbambroongkiat, M. K., Pouradier-Duteil, X., Xueref, C., *et al.* (1985). Economical multiple-site intradermal immunisation with human diploid-cell-strain vaccine is effective for post-exposure rabies prophylaxis. *Lancet* **1:**1059–1062.

Warrell, D. A., and Gutiérrez, J. M. (2007). World Health Organization. Rabies and envenomings: A neglected public health issue: Report of a consultative meeting, World Health Organization, Geneva, 10 January 2007. World Health Organization, Geneva.

Wilde, H. (2007). Failures of post-exposure rabies prophylaxis. *Vaccine* **25:**7605–7609.

Wilde, H., Choomkasien, P., Hemachudha, T., Supich, C., and Chutivongse, S. (1989). Failure of rabies postexposure treatment in Thailand. *Vaccine* **7:**49–52.

Wilde, H., Bhanganada, K., Chutivongse, S., Siakasem, A., Boonchai, W., and Supich, C. (1992). Is injection of contaminated animal bite wounds with rabies immune globulin a safe practice? *Trans. R. Soc. Trop. Med. Hyg.* **86:**86–88.

Wilde, H., Sirikawin, S., Sabcharoen, A., Kingnate, D., Tantawichien, T., Harischandra, P. A., Chaiyabutr, N., de Silva, D. G., Fernando, L., Liyanage, J. B., and Sitprija, V. (1996). Failure of postexposure treatment of rabies in children. *Clin. Infect. Dis.* **22:**228–232.

Wilde, H., Tipkong, P., and Khawplod, P. (1999). Economic issues in postexposure rabies treatment. *J. Travel Med.* **6:**238–242.

Wilde, H., Khawplod, P., Hemachudha, T., and Sitprija, V. (2002). Postexposure treatment of rabies infection: Can it be done without immunoglobulin? *Clin. Infect. Dis.* **34:**477–480.

Wimalaratne, O. (1997). Is it necessary to give rabies post-exposure treatment after rodent (rats, mice, squirrels and bandicoots) bites? *Ceylon Med. J.* **42:**144.

CHAPTER **14**

Neuroimaging in Rabies

Jiraporn Laothamatas,* Witaya Sungkarat,* and Thiravat Hemachudha†

Contents

Abstract

Rabies remains a virtually incurable disease once symptoms develop. Neuroimaging studies demonstrate lesions in the different parts of the neuroaxis, even before brain symptoms are evident. These abnormalities have been detailed in both rabies virus-infected humans and dogs with magnetic resonance imaging (MRI). MRI disturbances were similar in both forms (furious or paralytic) in human rabies; however, they were more pronounced in paralytic than in furious rabies virus-infected dogs in which examination was done early in the disease course. Abnormalities were not confined only to neuronal structures of hippocampus, hypothalamus, basal ganglia, and brain stem but also extended to

* Advanced Diagnostic Imaging and Image-Guided Minimal Invasive Therapy Center (AIMC) and Department of Radiology, Ramathibodi Hospital, Faculty of Medicine, Mahidol University, Bangkok, Thailand
† Department of Medicine (Neurology) and WHO Collaborating Center in Research and Training on Viral Zoonoses, Faculty of Medicine, Chulalongkorn University, Bangkok, Thailand

Advances in Virus Research, Volume 79
ISSN 0065-3527, DOI: 10.1016/B978-0-12-387040-7.00014-7

white matter. The blood–brain barrier (BBB) has been clearly shown to be intact during the time rabies virus-infected patients and dogs remained conscious, whereas leakage was demonstrated as soon as they became comatose. Although the location of MRI abnormalities can help diagnosing rabies, the intensities of signals are usually not very distinct and sometimes not recognizable. Newer techniques and protocols have been developed and utilized, such as diffusion-weighted imaging and diffusion tensor imaging, and the latter provides both qualitative and quantitative data. These techniques have been applied to normal and rabies virus-infected dogs to construct fractional anisotropy and mean diffusivity maps. Results showed clear-cut evidence of BBB intactness with absence of vasogenic brain edema and preservation of most neuronal structures and tracts except at the level of brainstem in paralytic rabies-infected dogs. Neuroimaging is one of the most useful tools for the *in vivo* study of central nervous system infections.

I. INTRODUCTION

Rabies is acute and invariably fatal encephalitis in humans. Dog variant of genotype 1 in the genus *Lyssavirus* is responsible for the vast majority of human rabies deaths worldwide, whereas bat variant (from hematophagous and nonhematophagous bats) has been associated with sporadic cases and outbreaks in the Americas. After successful introduction of virus into the wound, the virus gains entry to the central nervous system (CNS) by fast axonal transport along the nerves (Dirk *et al.*, 2001; Hemachudha and Phuapradit, 1997; Hemachudha *et al.*, 2002, 2005). Various degrees of inflammation of the peripheral nerves, dorsal root ganglia, and spinal cord, especially at the level of bite site, have been observed at postmortem examination. They are in accord with the findings of electrophysiological and neuroimaging studies (Laothamatas *et al.*, 2003; Mitrabhakdi *et al.*, 2005). Myelinopathy or axonopathy underlies motor weakness in the case of human paralytic rabies (Mitrabhakdi *et al.*, 2005; Sheikh *et al.*, 2005). CNS innate immunity, inversely correlated with viral load in the brain, may be responsible for variable results in magnetic resonance imaging (MRI) of the brains in furious and paralytic dogs (Laothamatas *et al.*, 2008). Despite differences in MR signal intensities in the rabies virus-infected dog brains with furious and paralysis, the abnormalities are localized in similar brain regions in both clinical forms. Presence of abnormal, albeit trivial, brain MR signals during the presymptomatic phase and the lack of correlation between clinical limbic involvement and MR localization suggest functional and/or microstructural damage at vulnerable sites. This requires alternative strategies that can focus on the integrity of neurons and tracts interconnecting different brain regions. The status of the blood–brain barrier (BBB) and nature of edematous processes (cytotoxic and vasogenic types) should also be monitored in parallel.

II. NEUROIMAGING TECHNIQUES

Neuroimaging techniques are composed of structural imaging, including computerized tomography (CT) and MRI as well as advanced imaging that can demonstrate functions and molecular and chemical metabolites in the CNS. Upon viewing the images of the CNS in encephalitis, it must be noted that they result from the process of infection itself and the host reaction, which can be variable from necrosis to apoptosis or other type of neuronal cell death process. This may be further complicated by insult(s) from accompanied systemic (such as prolonged hypoxia, shock, bleeding disorder) or metabolic (e.g., electrolyte imbalance or renal insufficiency) derangements. Preferential sites of involvement as shown by neuroimaging can be used as signatures for encephalitis caused by particular pathogens. This is particularly useful when combined with information about the clinical stage of disease (e.g., level of consciousness, cardiopulmonary status), presence of comorbidity of other organ systems, presence of single or multiple sites of involvement along the neuroaxis (brain alone vs. combination of brain, brainstem, spinal cord, and nerve roots), symmetrical or asymmetrical involvement, and status of the BBB. Iodinated contrast enhancement in CT or gadolinium enhancement in MRI depends on the breakdown of the BBB caused by the pathology. In early rabies encephalitis, BBB permeability remains preserved (Hemachudha *et al.*, 2003), and therefore, no parenchymal enhancement is detected. However, in the late or comatose phase of the disease, there is BBB breakdown along the midline structures of the brain and spinal cord associated with gadolinium-enhancing lesions (Laothamatas *et al.*, 2003).

A. CT images

CT scan is one of the structural image techniques based on density information technology (Goldman, 2007). The gray scale levels of the images indicate density of the structures, such as air and bone shown as dark and white, respectively. The gray matter has a higher gray level than the white matter. Water and fluid have levels of gray according to their contents. In edematous brain, a slightly decreased CT density is shown as compared to the normal brain parenchyma. In the diffuse or localized brain infections, such as caused by neurotropic viruses, mild mass effect causing effacement of the sulci and gyri and slightly decreased density of adjacent structures are expected findings. In certain circumstances, there may be associated focal or multiple foci of hemorrhages demonstrated as high-density signals with mass effect such as in the case of Japanese encephalitis and herpes simplex encephalitis (Kalita *et al.*, 2003). CT scan of the brain is not useful in diagnosing human rabies, which is due to very subtle changes in brain structure. Very late cases may suffer from hypoxia and show mild diffuse brain swelling, hyperdensity of bilateral basal ganglia, or cerebral hemorrhage (Awasthi *et al.*, 2001). Cerebral blood flow or perfusion studies have no clinical value in the diagnosis of human rabies. Claims of the clinical significance of cerebral arterial vasospasm as the result of deficiency of neural metabolites in human rabies have led to potentially harmful administration of vasodilators (Willoughby *et al.*, 2008). There has been no clinical or radiological evidence of vascular territory ischemia or infarction in any case of rabies patients during life. This is also true in postmortem examination (Hemachudha and Wilde, 2009).

B. MR techniques

MR is the imaging technique of choice when confronted with patients with encephalopathy/encephalitis because of its high sensitivity in detecting brain parenchymal abnormalities (Jacobs *et al.*, 2007; Kastrup *et al.*, 2005, 2008). Differentiation between fat, blood products, and pathological tissue with high-proteinaceous content is also accurate. In addition, there are several advanced MR techniques to demonstrate functional and molecular and metabolites in the CNS (Chavhan *et al.*, 2009; Poustchi-Amin *et al.*, 2001). These are functional MRI, perfusion MRI, diffusion MRI, diffusion tensor imaging (DTI), tractography (Lee *et al.*, 2005), and MR spectroscopy.

1. MR pulse sequences

There are multiple MR pulse sequences to demonstrate the structures and changes in CNS structures. These include T1-weighted images for anatomy evaluation, T2-weighted images for tissue abnormality detection, and T2-fluid attenuation inversion recovery (FLAIR) images (Simonson *et al.*, 1996), which are T2-weighted images with subtraction of the high water signal intensity enabling better detection of the abnormality along the sulci and periventricular areas. Gradient pulse sequence and susceptibility images are sensitive for paramagnetic effects such as blood products and calcification (Haacke *et al.*, 2009; Mittal *et al.*, 2009; Rauscher *et al.*, 2005; Tong *et al.*, 2008), which are particularly helpful in detecting minute hemorrhages.

2. Diffusion-weighted images and DTI

Diffusion-weighted images (DWI) demonstrate the degree of Brownian movement of the water (H_2O) molecules in tissues (Hagmann *et al.*, 2006; Thomas *et al.*, 2006). In biologic tissues, the interaction between the cellular structures and water molecules determines the degree of diffusion of H_2O molecules, representing the tissue structure at the microscopic level, so-called molecular imaging. When there is neuronal cell swelling or cytotoxic edema, causing narrowing of the interstitial spaces, H_2O molecules then move slower or become trapped causing bright signal on DWI and decreased or hyposignal on apparent diffusion coefficient (ADC) images, indicating restriction in diffusion of the H_2O molecules. In the case of vasogenic edema or gliosis, which results in wider interstitial spaces, the H_2O molecules are likely to move freely. Therefore, this results in increased water diffusion demonstrated as hyposignal in DWI and increased or hypersignal on ADC images. In the early encephalitis phase, with only mild neuronal swelling and no apparent breakdown of cell membranes or leakage of the BBB, no or only subtle changes are evident on T2-weighted or FLAIR images. DWI has been reported to be a sensitive technique at this stage of the disease (Kiroğlu *et al.*, 2006; Prakash *et al.*, 2004).

DTI measures both the direction and magnitude of the H_2O molecules movement designated as fractional anisotropy (FA). Quantification units of diffusion are mean diffusivity (MD) measured in mm^2/s. In CNS tissues, due to the presence of white matter tracts, the diffusion of the H_2O molecules is not equal in all directions but preferentially moves along white matter tracts. Such movement is limited across the white matter tracts, which is the so-called anisotropic phenomenon. This phenomenon can be used to assess the integrity of the white matter tract, such as in demyelinating processes, in which there are decreased FA values. Quantification of FA values between the diseased brain and normal brain can aid the early detection of demyelination (Assaf and Pasternak, 2008).

3. Proton MR spectroscopy

Proton MR spectroscopy is an advanced MR technique using chemical shift phenomenon of hydrogen atoms in different tissues shown as spectra of different metabolites in the brain with definite locations of each metabolite in part per million (ppm) regardless of magnet field strength (Barker, 2009; Barker and Lin, 2006; Dirk *et al.*, 2001; Jansen *et al.*, 2006; Mark, 2006; Yael and Robert, 2007). Examples are N-acetyl aspartase (NAA) peak, a neuronal marker, at 2.0 ppm; choline (Cho) peak, a cell membrane metabolite, at 3.2 ppm; creatine (Cr) peak, a mitochondrial energy metabolism marker, at 3.0 ppm; myo-inositol (mI) peak, a glial/astrocyte-specific marker, at 3.5 ppm; Lactate (Lac) peak, anaerobic respiratory marker, at 1.3–1.5 ppm; Glutamine/Glutamate (Glx) peak, neuronal transmitter marker, at 2.1–2.4 and 3.6–3.8 ppm; and the lipid peak, tissue necrosis marker, at 0.9–1.2 ppm. In the case of encephalitis with neuronal cell damage and inflammatory change/gliosis, proton MR spectroscopy demonstrates decreased NAA peak indicating neuronal cell damage, increased Cho peak due to cell membrane breakdown, and mildly increased mI peak due to glial cell damage (Gillard, 2009). Proton MR spectroscopy has been applied in the study of rabies in dogs (Laothamatas, unpublished data) (Fig. 1).

III. NEUROIMAGING IN RABIES

There have been several reported neuroimaging studies of human rabies associated with dog- and bat variants and organ transplantation (Burton *et al.*, 2005; Desai *et al.*, 2002; Hemachudha *et al.*, 2002; Laothamatas *et al.*, 2003; Pleasure and Fischbein, 2000). The imaging findings of these cases were similar although some aspects varied, such as the extent of involvement and degree of signal intensity and presence of contrast enhanced lesions. These findings might be dependent on the time after clinical onset when the examination was done, the status of immune responses in the brain, and the nature of virus variants. An intense reaction and widespread brain involvement were noted in the cases of rabies associated with organ transplantation in which immunosuppressive agents were withdrawn. This might reflect an immune reconstitution inflammatory-like syndrome (Johnson and Nath, 2009). Preferential sites in human rabies, as demonstrated in MR images, are spinal cord, brain stem, thalami, limbic structures, and white matter with hypersignal T2 changes, but with a very mild degree of mass effect. Some degree of progression involving basal ganglia and cortical gray matter can subsequently develop during the disease course, probably due to virus-induced neuronal injury as well as superimposed hypoxic insult (Awasthi *et al.*, 2001; Burton *et al.*, 2005; Desai *et al.*, 2002; Laothamatas *et al.*, 2003). Owing to the lack of specific patterns in differentiating between furious and paralytic rabies in humans, which might be due to the delay in the timing of examinations, MR studies in early stages of dog rabies were performed (Fig. 2; Laothamatas *et al.*, 2008).

In theory, all main imaging techniques, both basic and advanced MR, should be employed due to its high sensitivity in detecting tissue abnormalities at all levels of peripheral nerves, brachial plexus, spinal cord, and the brain, especially the brain stem and thalami. Quantitative imaging techniques such as MD and FA maps can be used for early detection, prior

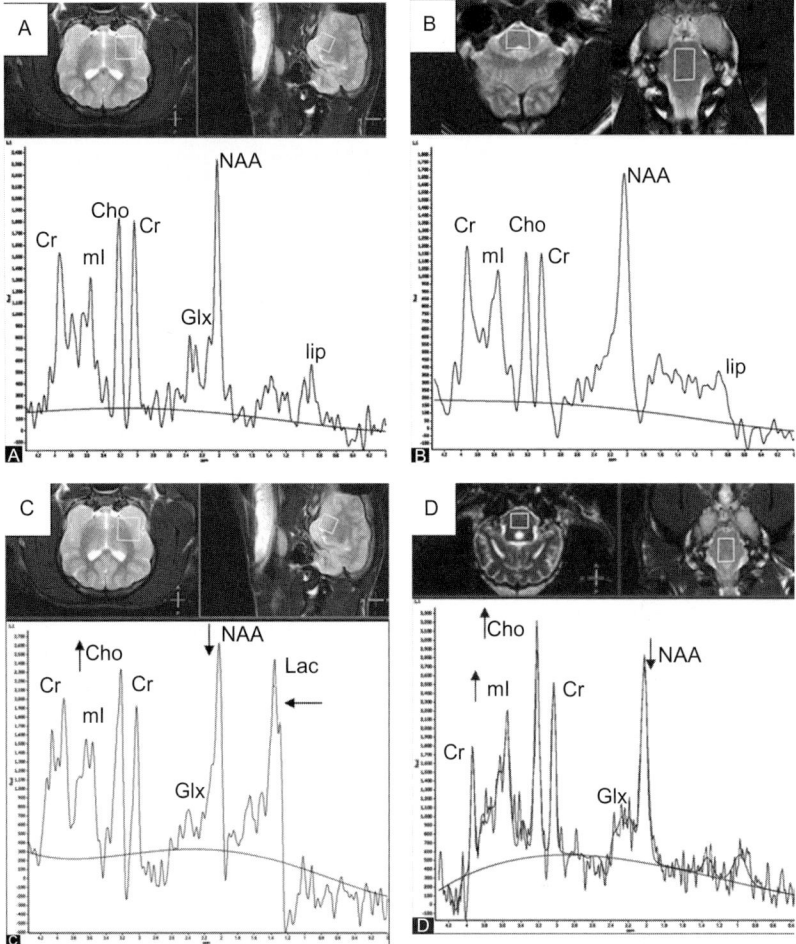

FIGURE 1 Single voxel proton MR spectroscopy with short TE. (A and B) MR spectroscopy of the normal dog brain at the temporal lobe (A) and brain stem (B). (C and D) MR spectroscopy of a dog with furious rabies at the temporal lobe (C) and the brain stem (D) demonstrating decreased NAA peak at 2.0 ppm, indicating neuronal loss, mild increased Cho peak at 3.2 ppm, indicating cell membrane destruction either from neuronal damage or a demyelinating process. Also seen is increased mI peak at 3.56 ppm, indicating glial cells/astrocyte damage, and the presence of a Lac peak is observed at 1.3 ppm, indicating anaerobic respiratory cycle of the rabid dog compared to the normal dog spectra.

to stages of disease with obvious structural damage. Nevertheless, MD or FA map is neither presently available nor reliable without the normative values of healthy controls. Brain metabolite abnormalities can assist in diagnosis and follow-up for the progression of the disease.

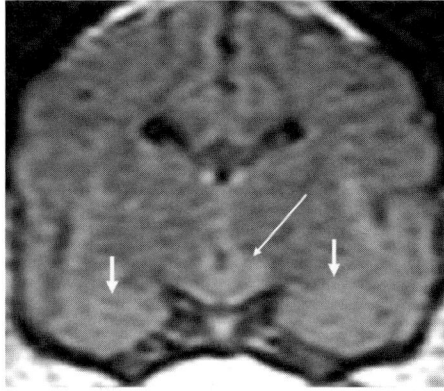

FIGURE 2   Coronal fluid attenuated inversion recovery (FLAIR) T2-weighted MR image of the early paralytic rabies-infected dog demonstrating ill-defined moderate hyper-signal T2 changes involving the bilateral temporal lobes (short white arrows) and hypothalamus (long thin white arrow) that spares the bilateral frontal cortices.

A. MRI in human rabies during different stages

1. Prodromal phase

It is difficult to diagnose rabies at this stage based on clinical grounds alone unless local neuropathic pain involving the bitten limb is experienced. Although there is no clinical evidence of brain or spinal cord involvement, there has been a report (Laothamatas *et al.*, 2003) of MR abnormalities in a furious rabies patient demonstrated as enhancing hypersignal T2 changes along the brachial plexus and associated spinal nerve roots at the corresponding levels of the bitten extremity (Fig. 3). Also demonstrated are nonenhancing ill-defined mild hypersignal T2 intensity changes of the spinal cord and temporal lobe cortices and the hippocampal gyri as well as the cerebral white matter (Fig. 4) (Laothamatas *et al.*, 2003). Electrophysiologic studies of the nerves and muscles, done at the same time, showed sensory neuronopathy and evidence of subclinical anterior horn cell dysfunction (Mitrabhakdi *et al.*, 2005).

2. Acute neurological phase

MRI in both clinical forms is indistinguishable regardless of virus variants (dog or bat). A similar pattern, as previously described, in the prodromal phase, is still seen but with slight progression in space and in degree of signal intensity along the spinal cord, thalami, hypothalami, white matter, and temporal lobes. BBB remains intact as long as the patient remains rousable (Fig. 5). Prominent diffuse hypersignal T2 changes of the cerebral white matter were noted in a furious rabies patient who had received

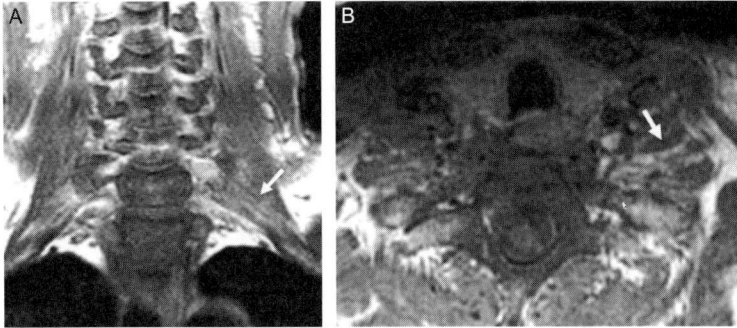

FIGURE 3   MR images of the brachial plexus of a 50-year-old male with furious rabies encephalitis during the prodromal phase. Coronal (A) and axial (B) postgadolinium T1-weighted MR images with fat suppression demonstrating enhancing left brachial plexus located between the anterior scalene and middle/posterior scalene muscles (white arrows in A and B). A is reproduced with permission from Laothamatas *et al.* (2003).

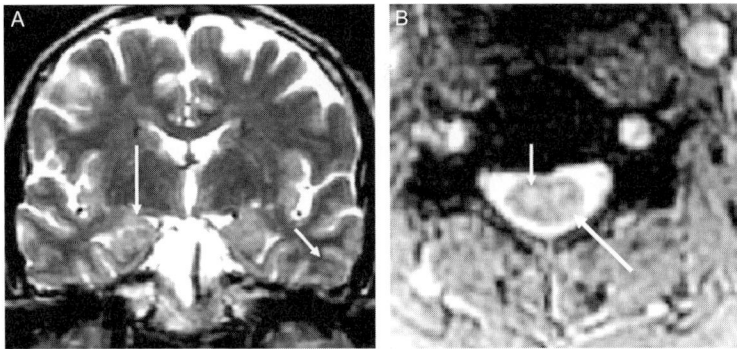

FIGURE 4   MR images of a 50-year-old male with furious rabies during the prodromal phase. (A) coronal fast spin echo T2-weighted images of the brain demonstrating ill-defined nonenhancing mild to moderate hypersignal T2 change at the amygdala and hippocampi (long white arrow) and adjacent temporal cortical gray matter (short white arrow). (B) axial gradient T2-weighted image of the cervical cord at the C4 level demonstrating ill-defined moderate hypersignal T2 changes of the cervical cord involving both central gray and left posterolateral white matter column (short and long white arrows).

very high dose of intravenous human rabies immune globulin (HRIG; Hemachudha *et al.*, 2003). An immune-mediated process may have also contributed to such white matter changes in this case. Prominent cerebral white matter changes can also be seen in patients with acute disseminated encephalomyelitis following rabies postexposure prophylaxis with brain tissue-derived vaccine (Desai *et al.*, 2002).

3. Comatose phase

Superimposed insults, such as hypoxia and ischemia, complicate the imaging findings (Burton *et al.*, 2005; Desai *et al.*, 2002). However, the striking change is BBB leakage that is noted as moderate enhancement along the hypothalamus, mammillary bodies, thalami, substantia nigra, tectal plates, brain stem, spinal cord, deep gray nuclei, cranial nerve nuclei, and optic tracts, and mild enhancement of the cisternal fifth and sixth cranial nerves (Figs. 6 and 7). Vivid enhancement of the intrathecal

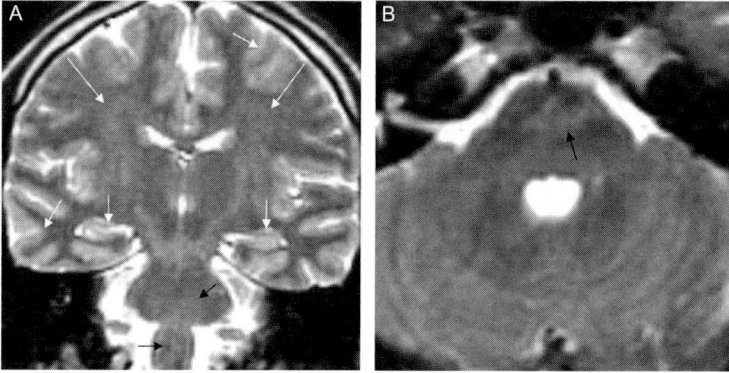

FIGURE 5   MR images of a patient with furious rabies in an acute neurological phase receiving high-dose intravenous human rabies immune globulin. Coronal (A) and axial (B) fast spin echo T2-weighted MR images of the frontal and temporal lobes and brain stem demonstrating extensive moderate ill-defined nonenhancing hypersignal T2 change involving bilateral hippocampi, temporal lobes, and frontal cortices (short white arrows in A); frontal subcortical and deep white matter (long thin white arrows in A); and the brainstem (small black arrows in A and B).

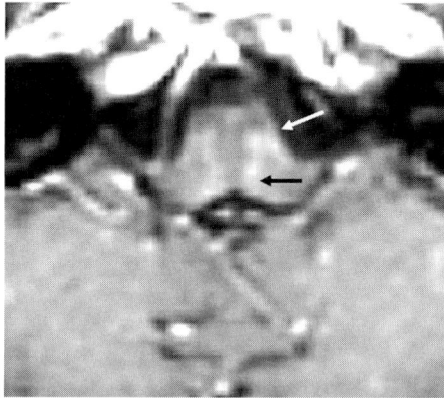

FIGURE 6   MR images of a 72-year-old comatose patient with paralytic rabies. Post-gadolinium axial T1-weighted image of the medulla demonstrating moderate enhancing olivary nuclei (white arrow) and hypoglossal nerve nuclei (black arrow).

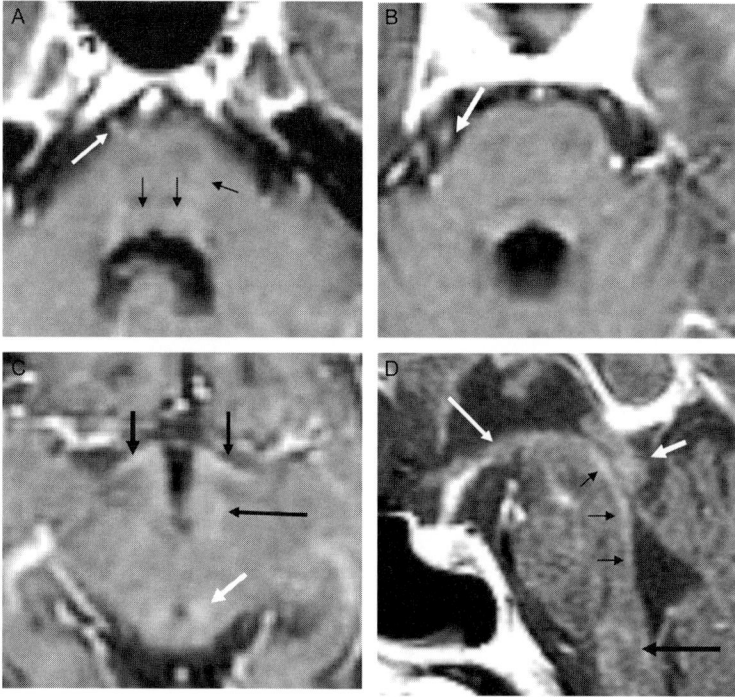

FIGURE 7 Postgadolinium axial T1-weighted images of a comatose patient with paralytic rabies at the brain stem (A, B), midbrain and hypothalamus (C), and mid sagittal view
(D) demonstrating mild enhancement of the right sixth and fifth cranial nerves (white
arrows in A and B) and the optic tracts (small black arrows in C). Moderate enhancement
of the facial colliculi and nuclei of the sixth and seventh, cranial nerves and their tracts
(small black arrows in A), the tectal plates and third cranial nerve nuclei (white arrows in
C and D) and enhancement along the floor of the aqueduct of Sylvius and fourth
ventricle (small black arrows in D) and the medulla (long black arrow in D). Moderate
enhancement of the hypothalamus including the mamillary bodies (long white arrows in
C and D). D is reproduced with permission from Laothamatas *et al.* (2003).

ventral and dorsal nerve roots could also be demonstrated (Fig. 8; Burton
et al., 2005; Hemachudha *et al.*, 2002; Laothamatas *et al.*, 2003; Pleasure and
Fischbein, 2000).

It should be emphasized that MR images were similar in rabies
patients associated with dog or bat variants in terms of location and
pattern of abnormal signal intensity (Pleasure and Fischbein, 2000;
van Thiel, 2009). Features of MR images in rabies are summarized in
Table I.

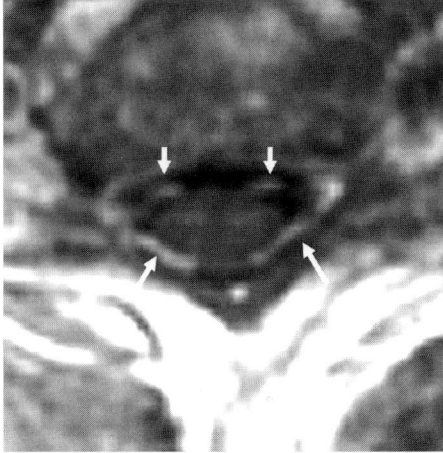

FIGURE 8 Axial T1-weighted postgadolinium MR images at the C7 level of a 70-year-old comatose patient with paralytic rabies demonstrating vivid enhancement of bilateral intrathecal dorsal and ventral nerve roots (white arrows).

B. Dog rabies as a model in studying furious and paralytic presentations

Sites of lesions in dog rabies at early stages remain similar in furious and paralytic clinical forms and are not different to those found in humans. However, diffuse ill-defined hyperintense T2 abnormalities are seen more frequently in furious dogs than in dogs with paralytic disease. More pronounced hyperintense T2 signals are noted more frequently in paralytic rabies (Laothamatas *et al.*, 2008). These are in accord with the findings of viral load in the brain and degree of CNS innate immune response as determined by cytokine mRNA transcripts. A greater viral load and less CNS immunity are demonstrated in furious rabies (Laothamatas *et al.*, 2008). There is correlation between the degree of hypersignal T2 abnormality and that of CNS immunity as seen in dogs with paralytic rabies (Fig. 2).

IV. NEWER NEUROIMAGING TECHNIQUES IN RABIES

Advanced MRI technology for early detection of abnormalities at the molecular level, DWI and DTI, has greater sensitivity than basic MR in demonstrating micro- and macrostructural damages (Nucifora *et al.*, 2007; Thomas *et al.*, 2006). They can be quantifiable and constructed as MD and FA maps of the brain. When compared with the normal map, these maps can demonstrate areas of abnormality at the level of statistical significance

TABLE I Summary of magnetic resonance imaging findings in human rabies[a]

Area of examination	Furious rabies			Paralytic rabies		
	Prodromal to early acute neurological phase[b]	Acute neurological to lethargic phase[c]	Comatose phase	Prodromal to early acute neurological phase	Acute neurological to lethargic phase	Comatose phase
Brachial plexus at bitten limb	++[d]	N/A[e]	N/A	N/A	N/A	N/A
Spinal cord	++	N/A	++	++	N/A	++
Spinal nerve	+	N/A	N/A	N/A	N/A	+++
Brain stem	++	++	+++	+++	N/A	+++
Hypothalamus	+	++	+++	++	N/A	++
Basal ganglia	+	++	+++	+	N/A	+++
Thalamus	+	++	+++	+	N/A	++
Temporal lobe and hippocampus	+	++	+++	++	N/A	++
Frontal lobe	+	++	++	−	N/A	++
Parietal lobe	+	++	++	−	N/A	++

(continued)

TABLE I (continued)

	Furious rabies			Paralytic rabies		
Cerebral WM[f]	+	++	++	N/A	+	++
Cranial nerves	N/A	+	+	N/A	N/A	+
BBB[g] breakdown	No	Yes	Yes	N/A	No	Yes

[a] See details in text and figures for the MR studies. Data summarized from reports elsewhere (Awasthi et al., 2001; Desai et al., 2002; Hemachudha et al., 2002; Laothamatas et al., 2003, 2008; Mitrabhakdi et al., 2005).

[b] Prodromal to early acute neurological phase: at this stage, the patients do not exhibit an altered sensorium and they are fully alert and rational. The patients studied with magnetic resonance imaging included one with brain-free symptoms who presented with only local neuropathic pain at the bitten limb and patients who had phobic spasms but remained fully conscious.

[c] Acute neurological to lethargic phase: the patients exhibit alteration of consciousness between lucid calm and restlessness, which progresses to severe agitation and depressed sensorium, and they remain rousable.

[d] + = degree of abnormalities in terms of signal intensity and/or enhancement.

[e] N/A = not applicable.

[f] WM (white matter) represents subcortical and deep white matter.

[g] BBB = Blood–brain barrier, gadolinium-enhanced lesion represents area with BBB breakdown.

(Fig. 9). The status of BBB can also be assessed by DWI and DTI. BBB is intact with no evidence of gadolinium enhancement and this is also confirmed by a finding of decreased MD, indicating neuronal cells

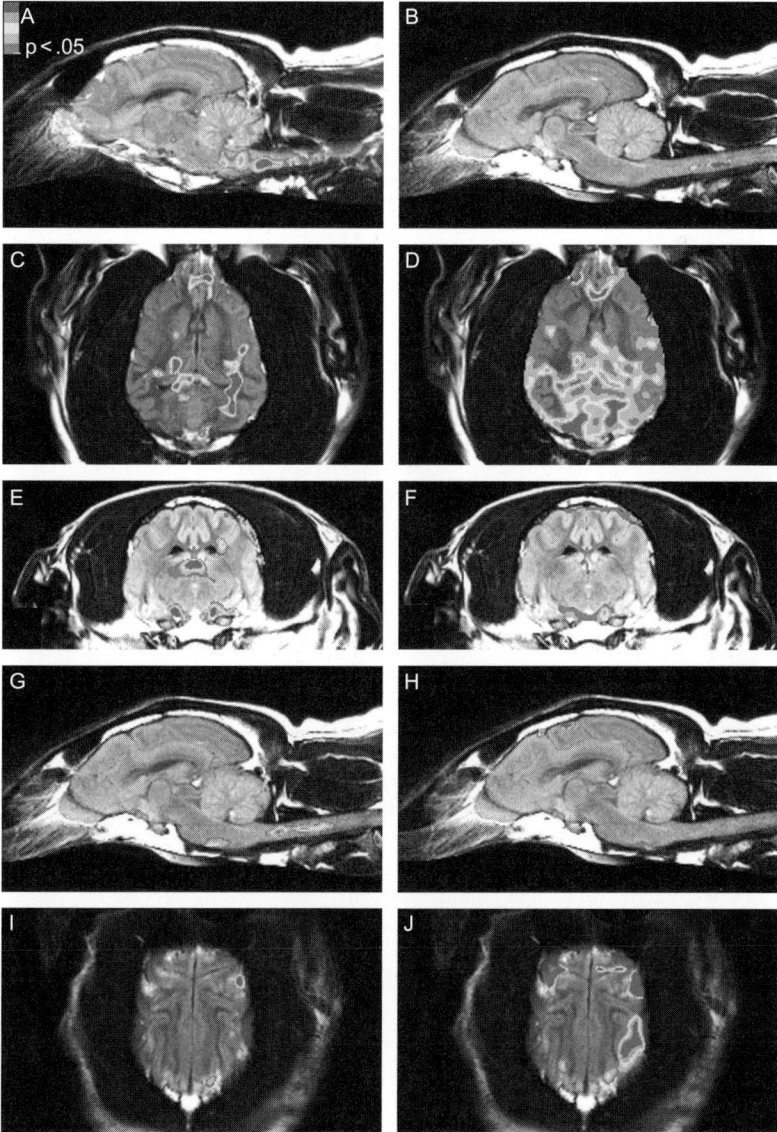

FIGURE 9 *In vivo* MR imaging of the rabies-infected dogs using quantified voxel-based group analyses of normal (*n* = 8) and paralytic (*n* = 4) and furious (*n* = 2) dogs at *p* < 0.05 (scale from blue to red: blue = lower passing threshold, red = highest passing

swelling and limited interstitial spaces. MR spectroscopy also demonstrates the spectra of neuronal damage, glial cell injury, and cell membrane breakdown (Mark, 2006) as shown in a dog with furious rabies
compared to a normal dog (Fig. 1). They can also be used to follow up the
disease condition and progression by comparing between the quantified
MD and FA values and MR spectral ratio.

In the future, molecular imaging of the brain with tissue- or pathogen-
specific labeling such as "rabies virus antibody tagged MR contrast" or
"iron tagged rabies viruses" may help in the study of viral pathogenesis
at an early phase and during the course of the disease and also help in the
design of therapeutic strategies (de Backer *et al.*, 2010; Hoehn *et al.*, 2008;
Long and Bulte, 2009).

V. CONCLUSIONS

Neuroimaging using both basic and advanced MR techniques has been
described in rabies virus-infected humans and dogs and presently should
be considered as important tools not only in rabies but also in other
encephalitides. Preferential sites of CNS involvement are similar in both
clinical forms of human and dog victims. Virus variants, dog or bat, may
not have impact upon the pattern of MR abnormalities. Advanced MR
techniques may offer opportunities to monitor the sites and degree of
micro- and macrostructural changes in the CNS as well as to *in vivo*
tracking of viral spread and of host immune cells from the circulation
into the CNS parenchyma.

---

threshold). (A and C) FA voxel-based group analysis map of the paralytic dogs; (B and D)
FA voxel-based group analysis map of the furious dogs; (E) Mean diffusivity (MD) voxel-
based group analysis map of the paralytic dogs; (F) Mean diffusivity (MD) voxel-based
group analysis map of the furious dogs; (G and I) FLAIR signal voxel-based group analysis
map of the paralytic dogs; (H and J) FLAIR signal voxel-based group analysis map of the
furious dogs. Macrostructural or cellular damage (represented by increased FLAIR signals
in G–J) was relatively minimal in rabies virus-infected dog brains. These areas were
mostly confined to the brain stem in dogs with paralytic rabies (G) and to the cerebral
hemispheres in dogs with furious rabies (J). Impaired neural tract integrity with microstructural damage (represented by diminished FA) was evident more frequently in the
case of paralytic rabies at the brain stem (A) in comparison to dogs with furious rabies (B)
and more frequently at cerebral hemispheres in furious rabies (J) compared to paralytic
rabies (I). Decreased MD (indicative of cytotoxic edema) was noted more frequently in
dogs with paralytic (E) than with furious (F) rabies. There was no evidence of BBB damage
(or increased MD, not shown). Increased FA, representing faster than normal diffusion of
water along the tracts, was found in the cerebral hemispheres more in dogs with furious
(D) than with paralytic (C) rabies. (See Page 11 in Color Section at the back of the book.)

ACKNOWLEDGMENTS

We thank Ramathibodi Hospital and Ramathibodi Foundation (Advanced Diagnostic Imaging and Image-Guided Minimal Invasive Therapy Center) and Chulalongkorn Hospital (Department of Medicine) and Thai Red Cross Society for support of the imaging studies and of patient and animal care. This chapter was supported from grants by Thailand Research Fund and National Science and Technology Development Agency and Thai Red Cross Society. The work on advanced MRI and whole brain DTI probabilistic tractography mapping has been supported by Thai Government Fund (Development of Brain Mapping Project).

REFERENCES

Assaf, Y., and Pasternak, O. (2008). Diffusion tensor imaging (DTI)-based white matter mapping in brain research: A review. *J. Mol. Neurosci.* **34**:51–61.

Awasthi, M., Parmar, H., Patankar, T., and Castillo, M. (2001). Imaging findings in rabies encephalitis. *AJNR Am. J. Neuroradiol.* **22**:677–680.

Barker, P. (2009). Clinical MR Spectroscopy. Cambridge University Press, New York.

Barker, P., and Lin, D. (2006). In vivo proton MR spectroscopy of the human brain. *Prog. Nucl. Magn. Reson. Spectrosc.* **49**:99–128.

Burton, E. C., Burns, D. K., Opatowsky, M. J., El-Feky, W. H., Fischbach, B., Melton, L., Sanchez, E., Randall, H., Watkins, D. L., Chang, J., and Klintmalm, G. (2005). Rabies encephalomyelitis: Clinical, neuroradiological, and pathological findings in 4 transplant recipients. *Arch. Neurol.* **62**:873–882.

Chavhan, G. B., Babyn, P. S., Thomas, B., Shroff, M. M., and Haacke, E. M. (2009). Principles, techniques, and applications of T2-based MR imaging and its special applications. *Radiographics* **29**:1433–1449.

de Backer, M. E., Nabuurs, R. J. A., van Buchem, M. A., and van der Weerd, L. (2010). MR-based molecular imaging of the brain: The next frontier. *AJNR Am. J. Neuroradiol.* **31**:1577–1583.

Desai, R. V., Jain, V., Singh, P., Singhi, S., and Radotra, B. D. (2002). Radiculomyelitic rabies: Can MR imaging help? *AJNR Am. J. Neuroradiol.* **23**:632–634.

Dirk, W., Norbert, S., Gerald, B. M., Brian, J. S., Antao, T. D., Andrew, A. M., and Michael, W. W. (2001). Short echo time multislice proton magnetic resonance spectroscopic imaging in human brain: Metabolite distributions and reliability. *Magn. Reson. Imaging* **19**:1073–1080.

Gillard, J. W. A. B. P. (2009). Clinical MR Neuroimaging. Cambridge University Press, New York.

Goldman, L. W. (2007). Principles of CT and CT technology. *J. Nucl. Med. Technol.* **35**:115–128.

Haacke, E. M., Mittal, S., Wu, Z., Neelavalli, J., and Cheng, Y.-C. N. (2009). Susceptibility-weighted imaging: Technical aspects and clinical applications. Part 1. *AJNR Am. J. Neuroradiol.* **30**:19–30.

Hagmann, P., Jonasson, L., Maeder, P., Thiran, J.-P., Wedeen, V. J., and Meuli, R. (2006). Understanding diffusion MR imaging techniques: From scalar diffusion-weighted imaging to diffusion tensor imaging and beyond. *Radiographics* **26**(Suppl. 1):S205–S223.

Hemachudha, T., and Phuapradit, P. (1997). Rabies. *Curr. Opin. Neurol.* **10**:260–267.

Hemachudha, T., and Wilde, H. (2009). Rabies. *In* Physicians' Information and Educational Resource (PIER) Online. (D. R., Goldmann, ed.), American College of Physicians, USA.

Hemachudha, T., Laothamatas, J., and Rupprecht, C. E. (2002). Human rabies: A disease of complex neuropathogenetic mechanisms and diagnostic challenges. *Lancet Neurol.* **1**:101–109.

Hemachudha, T., Sunsaneewitayakul, B., Mitrabhakdi, E., Suankratay, C., Laothamathas, J., Wacharapluesadee, S., Khawplod, P., and Wilde, H. (2003). Paralytic complications following intravenous rabies immune globulin treatment in a patient with furious rabies. *Int. J. Infect. Dis.* **7**:76–77.

Hemachudha, T., Wacharapluesadee, S., Mitrabhakdi, E., Wilde, H., Morimoto, K., and Lewis, R. (2005). Pathophysiology of human paralytic rabies. *J. Neurovirol.* **11**:93–100.

Hoehn, M., Himmelreich, U., Kruttwig, K., and Wiedermann, D. (2008). Molecular and cellular MR imaging: Potentials and challenges for neurological applications. *J. Magn. Reson. Imaging* **27**:941–954.

Jacobs, M. A., Ibrahim, T. S., and Ouwerkerk, R. (2007). MR imaging: Brief overview and emerging applications. *Radiographics* **27**:1213–1229.

Jansen, J. F. A., Backes, W. H., Nicolay, K., and Kooi, M. E. (2006). ^{1}H MR spectroscopy of the brain: Absolute quantification of metabolites. *Radiology* **240**:318–332.

Johnson, T., and Nath, A. (2009). Neurological complications of immune reconstitution in HIV-infected populations. *In* "Neurology in the Year 2010" (R. T. Johnson, ed.), Vol. 1184, pp. 106–120.

Kalita, J., Misra, U. K., Pandey, S., and Dhole, T. N. (2003). A comparison of clinical and radiological findings in adults and children with Japanese encephalitis. *Arch. Neurol.* **60**:1760–1764.

Kastrup, O., Wanke, I., and Maschke, M. (2005). Neuroimaging of infections. *NeuroRX* **2**:324–332.

Kastrup, O., Wanke, I., and Maschke, M. (2008). Neuroimaging of infections of the central nervous system. *Semin. Neurol.* **28**(511):522.

Kiroğlu, Y., Calli, C., Yunten, N., Kitis, O., Kocaman, A., Karabulut, N., Isaev, H., and Yagci, B. (2006). Diffusion-weighted MR imaging of viral encephalitis. *Neuroradiology* **48**:875–880.

Laothamatas, J., Hemachudha, T., Mitrabhakdi, E., Wannakrairot, P., and Tulayadaechanont, S. (2003). MR imaging in human rabies. *AJNR Am. J. Neuroradiol.* **24**:1102–1109.

Laothamatas, J., Wacharapluesadee, S., Lumlertdacha, B., Ampawong, S., Tepsumethanon, V., Shuangshoti, S., Phumesin, P., Asavaphatiboon, S., Worapruekjaru, L., Avihingsanon, Y., Israsena, N., Lafon, M., *et al.* (2008). Furious and paralytic rabies of canine origin: Neuroimaging with virological and cytokine studies. *J. Neurovirol.* **14**:119–129.

Lee, S.-K., Kim, D. I., Kim, J., Kim, D. J., Kim, H. D., Kim, D. S., and Mori, S. (2005). Diffusion-tensor MR imaging and fiber tractography: A new method of describing aberrant fiber connections in developmental CNS anomalies. *Radiographics* **25**:53–65.

Long, C. M., and Bulte, J. W. (2009). In vivo tracking of cellular therapeutics using magnetic resonance imaging. *Expert Opin. Biol. Ther.* **9**:293–306.

Mark, E. M. (2006). MR spectroscopy: Truly molecular imaging; past, present and future. *Neuroimaging Clin. N. Am.* **16**:605–618.

Mitrabhakdi, E., Shuangshoti, S., Wannakrairot, P., Lewis, R., Susuki, K., Laothamatas, J., and Hemachudha, T. (2005). Difference in neuropathogenetic mechanisms in human furious and paralytic rabies. *J. Neurol. Sci.* **238**:3–10.

Mittal, S., Wu, Z., Neelavalli, J., and Haacke, E. M. (2009). Susceptibility-weighted imaging: Technical aspects and clinical applications, part 2. *AJNR Am. J. Neuroradiol.* **30**:232–252.

Nucifora, P. G. P., Verma, R., Lee, S.-K., and Melhem, E. R. (2007). Diffusion-tensor MR imaging and tractography: Exploring brain microstructure and connectivity. *Radiology* **245**:367–384.

Pleasure, S. J., and Fischbein, N. J. (2000). Correlation of clinical and neuroimaging findings in a case of rabies encephalitis. *Arch. Neurol.* **57**:1765–1769.

Poustchi-Amin, M., Mirowitz, S. A., Brown, J. J., McKinstry, R. C., and Li, T. (2001). Principles and applications of echo-planar imaging: A review for the general radiologist. *Radiographics* **21:**767–779.

Prakash, M., Kumar, S., and Gupta, R. K. (2004). Diffusion-weighted MR imaging in Japanese encephalitis. *J. Comput. Assist. Tomogr.* **28:**756–761.

Rauscher, A., Sedlacik, J., Barth, M., Mentzel, H.-J., and Reichenbach, J. R. (2005). Magnetic susceptibility-weighted MR phase imaging of the human brain. *AJNR Am. J. Neuroradiol.* **26:**736–742.

Sheikh, K. A., Ramos-Alvarez, M., Jackson, A. C., Li, C. Y., Asbury, A. K., and Griffin, J. W. (2005). Overlap of pathology in paralytic rabies and axonal Guillain–Barré syndrome. *Ann. Neurol.* **57:**768–772.

Simonson, T. M., Magnotta, V. A., Ehrhardt, J. C., Crosby, D. L., Fisher, D. J., and Yuh, W. T. (1996). Echo-planar FLAIR imaging in evaluation of intracranial lesions. *Radiographics* **16:**575–584.

Thomas, L. C., Pia, C. S., and Brian, D. R. (2006). Diffusion imaging: Insight to cell status and cytoarchitecture. *Neuroimaging Clin. N. Am.* **16:**619–632.

Tong, K. A., Ashwal, S., Obenaus, A., Nickerson, J. P., Kido, D., and Haacke, E. M. (2008). Susceptibility-weighted MR imaging: A review of clinical applications in children. *AJNR Am. J. Neuroradiol.* **29:**9–17.

van Thiel, P. (2009). Fatal human rabies due to Duvenhage virus from a bat in Kenya: Failure of treatment with coma-induction, ketamine, and antiviral drugs. *PLoS Negl. Trop. Dis.* **3:**e428.

Willoughby, R. E., Roy-Burman, A., Martin, K. W., Christensen, J. C., Westenkirschner, D. F., Fleck, J. D., Glaser, C., Hyland, K., and Rupprecht, C. E. (2008). Generalised cranial artery spasm in human rabies. *Dev. Biol. (Basel)* **131:**367–375.

Yael, R., and Robert, E. L. (2007). Recent advances in magnetic resonance neurospectroscopy. *Neurotherapeutics* **4:**330–345.

CHAPTER **15**

Rabies Virus Infection and MicroRNAs

Nipan Israsena,* Aekkapol Mahavihakanont,† and **Thiravat Hemachudha†**

Abstract   Endogenous RNA-silencing mechanisms have been shown to play a role in regulating viral and host processes during the course of infection. Such interactive processes may involve host cellular and/or viral-encoded microRNAs (miRNAs). Rabies is unique not only in terms of its invariably fatal course once disease signs develop, but it also has a variable incubation period (eclipse phase). It has been recently shown that cells or tissues of different

---

* Department of Pharmacology, Faculty of Medicine, Chulalongkorn University, Bangkok, Thailand
† Department of Medicine (Neurology) and WHO Collaborating Center in Research and Training on Viral Zoonoses, Faculty of Medicine, Chulalongkorn University, Bangkok, Thailand

Advances in Virus Research, Volume 79
ISSN 0065-3527, DOI: 10.1016/B978-0-12-387040-7.00015-9

origin have their own specific miRNAs that, in theory, may impact on viral transcription and replication. This may possibly explain, in part, why rabies virus remains dormant at the inoculation site in rabies patients for long periods. Owing to the RNA interference (RNAi) technology, it has been possible to introduce exogenously designed artificial short interfering RNAs (siRNAs) and miRNAs into virus-infected cells for therapeutic purposes. Successful attempts in using RNAi for prevention and treatment of DNA and RNA virus infections both *in vitro* and *in vivo* experiments have been reported. The fact that rabies remains incurable has stimulated the development of the therapeutic RNAi strategy. We describe herein preliminary evidence that cellular miRNA may play a role in suppressing viral replication, explaining the eclipse phase, and that artificially designed multitargeting miRNA can successfully inhibit rabies virus transcription and replication *in vitro*.

I. INTRODUCTION

Short interfering RNAs (siRNAs) and microRNAs (miRNAs) are two relatively well-defined classes of small RNAs involved in RNA silencing, a mechanism for sequence-specific gene silencing regulated by RNAs of 19–30 nucleotides (nt) in length (Carthew and Sontheimer, 2009). siRNAs are usually derived from long double-stranded RNA (dsRNA) of exogenous origin. In contrast, miRNAs are endogenously encoded small RNAs generated from the dsRNA region of hairpin-shaped precursors. Evidence suggests that both classes of small RNAs play important roles in viral pathogenesis (Lu and Liston, 2009; Skalsky and Cullen, 2010). In this chapter, we discuss the potential role of noncoding RNA, especially miRNAs, in rabies pathogenesis as well as progress and roadblocks in developing a therapeutic strategy against rabies using an artificial miRNA (amiRNA) approach.

II. MICRORNAS

A. miRNA biogenesis

miRNAs are small, single-stranded RNA, 18–25 nt long encoded in the genome of diverse organisms, including plants (Jones-Rhoades *et al.*, 2006), worms (Lee *et al.*, 1993; Reinhart *et al.*, 2000), flies (Brennecke *et al.*, 2003), and humans (Bartel, 2004; Lagos-Quintana *et al.*, 2001; Lim *et al.*, 2003), that regulate gene expression by binding to the 3′-untranslated region (UTR) of specific mRNAs. These miRNAs are derived from long RNA transcripts containing single or multiple stem-loop structures called primary transcripts of the miRNA genes (pri-miRNAs). Pri-miRNA transcripts can be found as independent transcripts or within the intron of protein-encoding genes. They are generated by RNA polymerase II and contain a 5′-cap and polyA tail (Lee *et al.*, 2004). The first step of mature (18- to 25-nt) miRNA biogenesis involves the recognition and nuclear cleavage of the RNA stem-loop structure of the pri-miRNA by the cellular RNAse III enzyme Drosha and its copartner dsRNA-binding protein, DiGeorge syndrome critical region gene 8 (DGCR8) to form the 60- to 70-nt pre-miRNA (Lee *et al.*, 2003). The cleavage leaves a 2-nt overhang at the 3′-end of pre-miRNA which is recognized and transported out of the nucleus by Ran-GTP and a receptor, Exportin 5 (Lund *et al.*, 2004; Yi *et al.*, 2003). Upon reaching the cytoplasm, GTP hydrolysis results in release of the pre-miRNA, 3′ 2-nt overhang is then bound by a second cellular RNase III enzyme called Dicer. Dicer removes the terminal loop from pre-miRNA and generates miRNA duplex intermediate. Usually, only one strand of the duplex (miRNA strand) is stabilized and incorporated into a multiple protein nuclease complex, the RNA-induced silencing complex (RISC), whereas the other strand (passenger strand) is released and degraded. The miRNA acts as a guide to direct RISC to complementary targets and regulates protein expression by promoting translational repression, mRNA degradation, and mRNA cleavage (Cullen, 2004; Khvorova *et al.*, 2003; Kim, 2005; Kim *et al.*, 2009) (Fig. 1). Although it was generally believed that perfect or near perfect complementary pairing between miRNA and mRNA is required for mRNA cleavage and degradation, whereas imperfect complementary pairing leads to translation block, miRNAs can target mRNAs containing only partially complementary sequences to degradation pathway (Bagga *et al.*, 2005). New evidence suggests that mRNA degradation, not translational block, may be the main pathway used by mammalian miRNAs that leads to a reduction in target proteins level (Guo and Lu, 2010). In plants, most known targets of miRNAs are silenced by perfectly complementary miRNA. In contrast, most known miRNA targets in animals are only partially complementary to their cognate miRNAs (Sontheimer and Carthew, 2005). The pairing of nucleotide 2–8 of miRNA (seed region) is crucial for target recognition.

B. Functions

The latest version (16th) of the largest miRNA database MiRBase (http://microrna.sanger.ac.uk) contains 17,341 mature miRNAs, from 142 species, including over 700 human miRNAs. As each miRNA has the potential to target over 200 different transcripts, it is possible that miRNAs regulate up to 30% of all human protein-coding genes (Lewis *et al.*, 2005). While siRNAs function mainly as natural defenses against viruses, miRNAs are found to be involved in regulating a wide variety of important

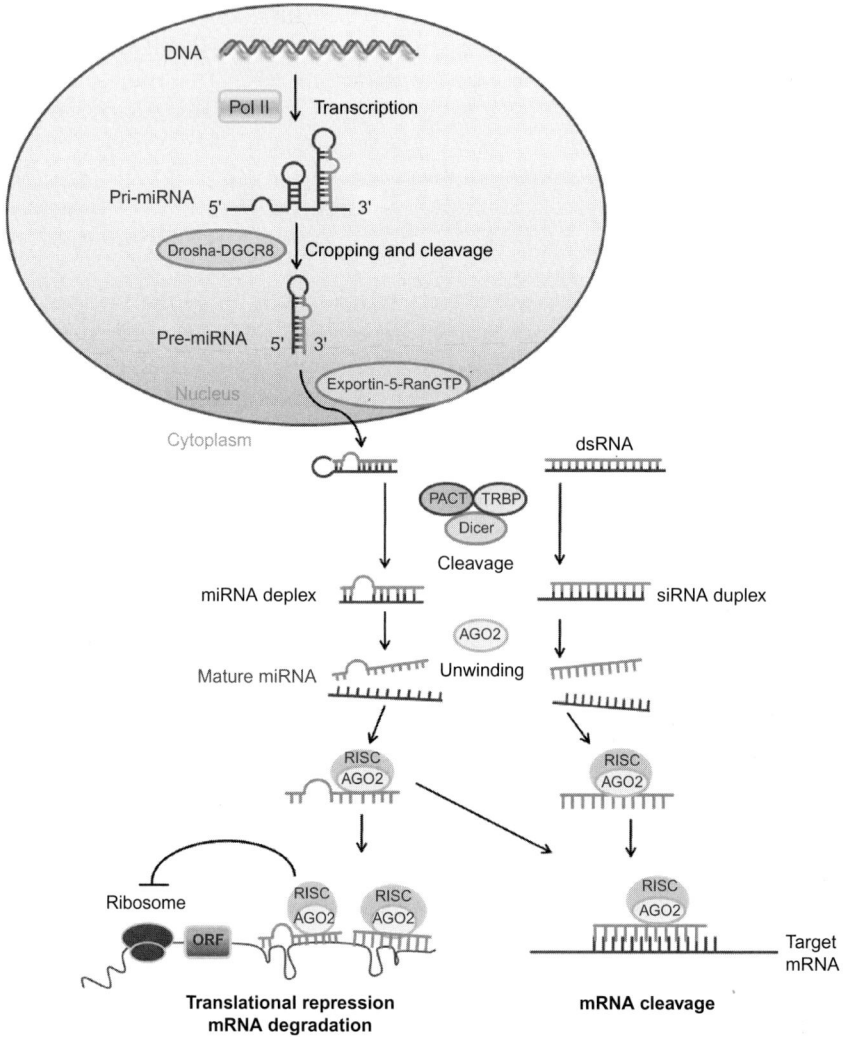

FIGURE 1   The microRNA (miRNA) biogenesis. The miRNA biogenesis pathway requires two RNase III type enzymes, Drocha and Dicer, generating pri-miRNA, pre-miRNA, and mature miRNA. Mature miRNA combines with multiple protein nuclease complexes resulting in the formation of the RISC, which is able to regulate the mRNA downstream.

cellular processes, ranging from development (Carrington and Ambros, 2003; Stefani and Slack, 2008), cellular differentiation (Kim *et al.*, 2006), proliferation (Brennecke *et al.*, 2003), and apoptosis (Jovanovic and Hengartner, 2006; Xu *et al.*, 2003) to cancer transformation (Dalmay and Edwards, 2006). Many miRNAs are ubiquitously expressed, whereas others are expressed in a cell-type-specific manner. Certain viruses can produce viral-encoded miRNAs that regulate both viral and host cell gene expression suitable for each stage of the viral life cycle (Cullen, 2009; Dykxhoorn, 2007; Schutz and Sarnow, 2006).

III. miRNAS AND VIRUSES

A. Roles of cellular and virally encoded miRNAs in viral diseases

Viral survival and replication are highly dependent on host cellular machinery. There has been growing evidence that host cellular miRNAs can moderate the viral life cycle and cell-type-specific miRNAs may contribute to the tissue tropisms of viruses (Perez et al., 2009; Umbach and Cullen, 2009). In most cases, it has been shown that endogenous miRNAs can, at least partially, reduce viral replication. For example, human miR-32 has been reported to restrict the replication of primate foamy virus type 1 (PFV-1) (Lecellier et al., 2005), whereas miR24 and miR93 interfere with the function of vesicular stomatitis virus (VSV) P and L genes (Otsuka et al., 2007). When miRNA processing is inhibited, the replication rate of viruses, such as influenza A virus (Song et al., 2010), VSV (Otsuka et al., 2007), herpes simplex virus 1 (HSV-1) (Gupta et al., 2006), and human immunodeficiency virus (HIV-1) (Triboulet et al., 2007; Yeung et al., 2005), is increased. Recent studies have showed that interferon beta can mediate antiviral effects through upregulation of endogenous miRNAs (Pedersen et al., 2007, Witwer et al., 2010). Many viruses globally repress Pol II transcription in infected cells and, therefore, repress miRNA biogenesis. In contrast, some viruses use host cellular miRNA to facilitate viral replication. It has been shown that liver-specific human miR-122 targets the 5'-UTR of hepatitis C virus (HCV) RNA and promotes HCV replication (Jopling et al., 2005). However, inhibition of mir-122 reduces the viral load in chimpanzees chronically infected with HCV (Roberts and Jopling, 2010). In Epstein–Barr virus (EBV) infection, the switch from latency stage to lytic replication involves miR200b and miR429 (Ellis-Connell et al., 2010). Specific cellular miRNAs can be induced by specific viral infections (Triboulet et al., 2007). EBV induces the expression of several cellular miRNAs, including miR155 that plays an important role in promoting transformation of B cells (Cameron et al., 2008; Linnstaedt et al., 2010).

To date, more than 200 virally encoded miRNAs have been reported. Virally encoded miRNAs have been found mainly with DNA viruses. Viruses within the Herpesviridae family, such as cytomegalovirus (CMV) (Grey et al., 2005; Pfeffer et al., 2005), EBV, and Kaposi's sarcoma-associated herpesvirus (KSHV) (Cai and Cullen, 2006), encode several miRNA

(9–23 miRNA) within the viral genome. Adenovirus (Aparicio *et al.*, 2006) and SV40 virus (Sullivan *et al.*, 2005), also nuclear DNA viruses, contain a single miRNA. As cleavage of the pri-miRNA by Drosha occurs in the nucleus, it has been speculated that cytoplasmic viruses may not be able to generate miRNA (Cullen, 2010).

Current evidence suggests that viruses use their miRNAs to manipulate the cellular environment and viral gene expression to favor their long-term survival (Skalsky and Cullen, 2010). Most known cellular targets of viral-encoded miRNAs are involved in either modulating cellular immune responses or apoptosis (Choy *et al.*, 2008; Umbach and Cullen, 2009). Regulation of viral protein production at different stages of the life cycle helps promote immune evasion. For example, SV40 miRNAs inhibit viral T-antigen RNA in the late stage of infection, thus, reducing infected cell susceptibility to killing by cytotoxic T-cells (Sullivan *et al.*, 2005). HSV-1 miRNAs, which are expressed at high level during latency, but not during productive viral replication, downregulate the immediate-early transactivators ICP0 and ICP4, both of which play a key role in the induction of lytic replication, therefore, maintaining latency stage (Umbach *et al.*, 2008).

B. Potential roles of cellular miRNAs in rabies virus infection

It would be intriguing to know whether cellular miRNAs play any role in rabies pathogenesis. Recent studies in VSV, a negative sense single-stranded RNA virus, closely related to rabies virus (RABV), showed that miR24 and miR93 could contribute to viral susceptibility by binding to viral *L* and *P* genes (Otsuka *et al.*, 2007). It was also shown that VSV infection induced expression of miR706 which inhibits apoptosis pathway and therefore may be involved in strategy for survival of VSV (Lian *et al.*, 2010). Computational predictions using a ViTa bioinformatics program (Hsu *et al.*, 2007) identify several candidate miRNAs that may bind to either RABV transcripts or RABV genome. Moreover, we found that when Drosha was knocked down, RABV can replicate at a faster rate (Israsena, unpublished data) (Fig. 2A and B).

Of a few endogenous miRNA candidates identified, we focused on miR-133, which is specifically expressed in skeletal muscle (Chen *et al.*, 2006) in which RABV may enter and remain latent for variable periods of time, from days to year(s) (Jackson, 2008). miR-133 has been predicted to bind to both N and G transcripts (Fig. 3A and B). To address whether hsa-mir-133 influenced RABV replication, we transfected Neuro-2a with an miRNA-133 mimic before challenge with attenuated RABV (HEP-Flury). On comparison between Neuro-2a cells transfected with control miRNA and muscle-specific miR133 mimic, the results showed that there was marked reduction of expression of viral protein

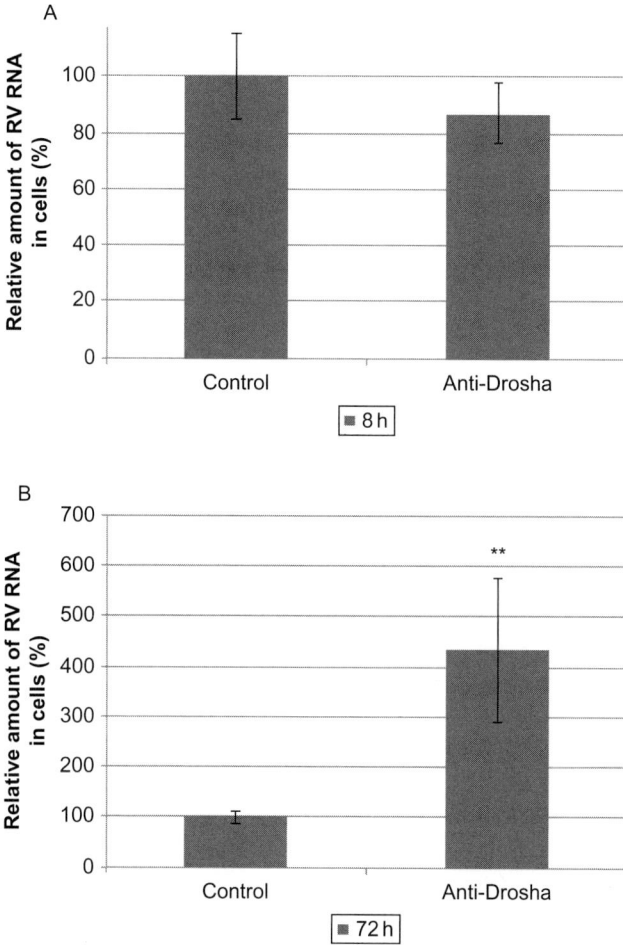

FIGURE 2   SiRNA against Drosha promotes rabies virus propagation. Neuro2A cells were transfected with anti-Drosha siRNA. Twelve hours after transfection, the cells were infected with RABV. Eight hours (A) and 72 h (B) after infection, the levels of viral genome were determined by real-time PCR. **, the results were significantly different ($P < 0.05$).

(as shown by immunofluorescence staining) only in the case of miR133 (Fig. 3C).

Wild-type RABVs may have differences in mutations, either at coding (either as nonsynonymous or synonymous pattern) or noncoding regions or both. Therefore, it is possible that miRNAs, which recognize target genes through nucleotide pairings in different host cells/tissues in the body of infected hosts, can affect the properties of RABV and even have effects on the clinical manifestations or outcomes of patients. In addition,

A

miR133a	uGUCGACCAACUUCCCCUGguu
	‖‖¦‖ ‖‖‖ ‖‖‖‖‖‖‖
Nucleoprotein	gCAGTTCTTTG-AGGGGACatg

B

miR133a	ugUCGACCAACUUCCCCUGGUU
	‖ ‖ ‖‖ ‖ ‖ ‖‖‖‖‖‖‖‖
Glycoprotein	caATCGGGCTCCA-GGGACCAA

C   Control

hsa-miR-133a mimic

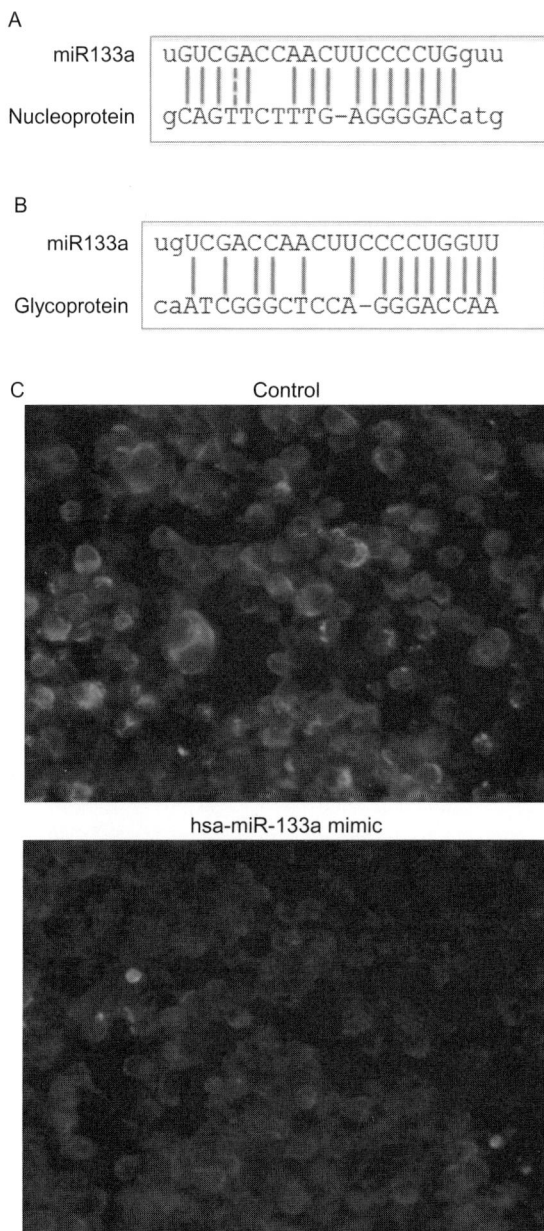

FIGURE 3   Effect of miR133 on rabies virus. (A) A schematic diagram depicting the location of the hsa-miR-133a in association with CVS N mRNA. (B) A diagram showing the location of potential binding of hsa-miR-133a to CVS G mRNA. (C) Neuro2a cells transfected with miRNA mimic hsa-miR-133 or control miRNA were challenged with RABV (HEP-Flury). Forty-eight hours after infection, cells were fixed and subjected to direct-immunofluorescent staining with FITC-conjugated anti-N antibody (C). Note the reduction in FITC staining in hsa-miR-133a treated group. (See Page 12 in Color Section at the back of the book.)

the pressure constraints by cell-type-specific miRNA suppression may promote mutations in that specific corresponding region of the RABV genome (Fig. 4).

It remains to be determined to what extent that tissue-specific endogenous miRNA(s) play roles in tissue tropism and in the variable incubation periods in patients with rabies.

C. Viral-encoded RNA: Does it exist in RABV infection?

It is still debatable whether RNA viruses can generate miRNA. This is due to the fact that most RNA viruses replicate in the cytoplasm and excision of genomically encoded miRNA in stem-loop structure, theoretically, would induce the cleavage and degradation of the RNA viral genome. Large-scale small RNA cloning studies failed to identify viral-encoded miRNAs from various viruses with RNA genomes (Pfeffer *et al.*, 2005)

Recently, it has been shown that RNA viruses can be engineered to produce functional miRNA (Rouha *et al.*, 2010; Varble *et al.*, 2010). Cytoplasmic viral miRNA can be processed by noncanonical mechanisms, which is a Dicer-dependent, DGCR8-independent pathway (Shapiro *et al.*, 2010). In RABV infection, bioinformatics analysis using the Vir-mir

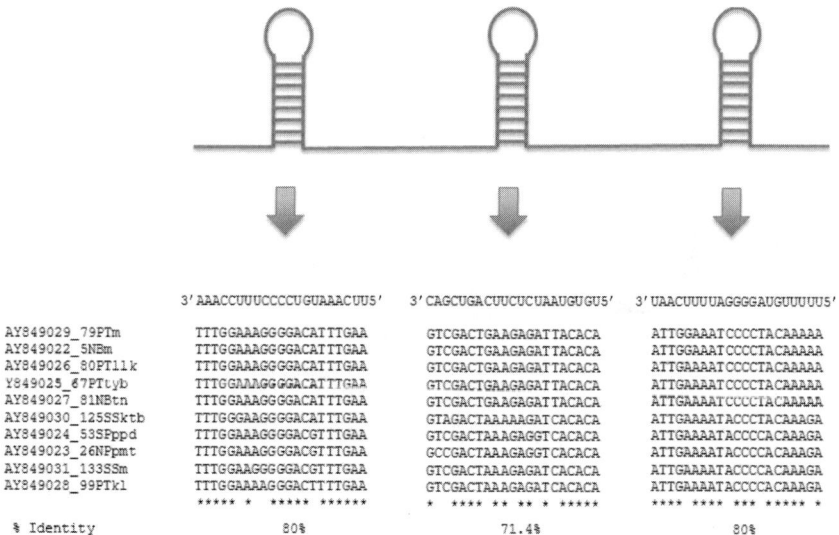

	3′ AAACCUUUCCCCUGUAAACUU5′	3′ CAGCUGACUUCUCUAAUGUGU5′	3′ UAACUUUUAGGGGAUGUUUUU5′
AY849029_79PTm	TTTGGAAAGGGGACATTTGAA	GTCGACTGAAGAGATTACACA	ATTGGAAATCCCCTACAAAAA
AY849022_5NBm	TTTGGAAAGGGGACATTTGAA	GTCGACTGAAGAGATTACACA	ATTGGAAATCCCCTACAAAAA
AY849026_80PT11k	TTTGGAAAGGGGACATTTGAA	GTCGACTGAAGAGATTACACA	ATTGAAAATCCCCTACAAAAA
Y849025_67PTtyb	TTTGGAAAGGGGACATTTGAA	GTCGACTGAAGAGATTACACA	ATTGAAAATCCCCTACAAAAA
AY849027_81NBtn	TTTGGAAAGGGGACATTTGAA	GTCGACTGAAGAGATTACACA	ATTGAAAATCCCCTACAAAAA
AY849030_125SSktb	TTTGGGAAGGGGACATTTGAA	GTAGACTAAAAAGATCACACA	ATTGAAAATACCCTACAAAGA
AY849024_53SPppd	TTTGGAAAGGGGACGTTTGAA	GTCGACTAAAGAGGTCACACA	ATTGAAAATACCCCACAAAGA
AY849023_26NPpmt	TTTGGAAAGGGGACGTTTGAA	GCCGACTAAAGAGGTCACACA	ATTGAAAATACCCCACAAAGA
AY849031_133SSm	TTTGGAAGGGGGACGTTTGAA	GTCGACTAAAGAGATCACACA	ATTGAAAATACCCCACAAAGA
AY849028_99PTk1	TTTGGAAAAGGGACTTTTGAA	GTCGACTAAAGAGATCACACA	ATTGAAAATACCCCACAAAGA
	***** * ***** ******	* **** ** ** * *****	**** **** *** ***** *
% Identity	80%	71.4%	80%

FIGURE 4   Diagram showing genetic variability of wild-type RABV in Thailand and its effect on miRNA target selection. Based on sequences of RABV N gene from 237 samples of rabies infected dogs in Thailand during 1998–2002 (Denduagboripant *et al.*, 2005), any prechosen 22-nt target sequences for amiR inhibition will have a small but significant chance for not forming a perfect base-pairing with unknown wild-type RABV NmRNA.

database (Li *et al.*, 2008) identifies two potential stem-loop structures within the *L* gene transcript and also in the intergenic region of some RABV strains. We also found that incorporation of an miRNA precursor within HEP-Flury genome can produce functional miRNA and does not interfere with viral replication (Israsena *et al.*, unpublished data). It is still unclear whether wild-type RABV can produce miRNA or a distinct form of noncoding RNA other than leader RNA and whether this may play a role in rabies pathogenesis.

IV. INHIBITION OF RABIES VIRAL REPLICATION BY siRNA/amiRNA

Rabies is a fatal human disease that remains a serious public health problem in many countries. More than 50,000 persons die of rabies each year (World Health Organization, 2005). Once the symptoms develop, there is no effective treatment (Hemachudha *et al.*, 2006). RNAi technology has rapidly evolved to become one of the promising approaches for the treatment of viral infections. RNAi can be initiated in target cells by either applying exogenous synthetic dsRNA molecules or using plasmid/viral vector constructs containing short-hairpin RNA (shRNA) or a pre-miRNA backbone that can be processed into amiRNAs. It has been demonstrated that expression of amiRNAs is more effective and less toxic than the regular shRNA vectors (Boden *et al.*, 2004; Li and Ding, 2006; McBride *et al.*, 2008; Qu *et al.*, 2007). Results from many *in vivo* studies (McCaffrey *et al.*, 2003) and a phase I clinical trial (DeVincenzo *et al.*, 2010) provide the proof-of-concept for the use of an RNAi as a therapeutic agent in humans. We will discuss the progress that has been made and roadblocks needed to overcome to develop siRNA/miRNA into new therapeutic modalities for RABV infection.

There have been many approaches to inhibit viral infections such as inhibiting viral RNA replication, silencing viral accessories, inhibiting the assembly of viral particles, and blocking virus–host interactions. The proteins of the RNP complex, nucleoprotein (N), phosphoprotein (P), and polymerase (L), are important for both viral transcription and replication. Therefore, they are considered as candidates for siRNA/miRNA inhibition. Pioneering studies in searching for genetic suppressor elements that inhibit RABV replication also identified rabies N and P as effective targets (Wunner *et al.*, 2004). It has been shown in VSV infection that siRNA against PmRNA can reduce viral replication (Barik, 2004).

In RABV infection, it has been reported that siRNA designed against NmRNA can partially protect BHK-21 cells from rabies viral infection as shown by a reduction of fluorescent intensity with the direct fluorescent antibody test (Brandao *et al.*, 2007). Further, the application of amiRNA designed against NmRNA prior to or after infection of neural cells with RABV significantly reduced rabies viral mRNA and its replication (Israsena *et al.*, 2009). These results suggest that N may be a viable target for inhibition. It is possible that siRNA/miRNA designed against P and L mRNA could also be strong inhibitors of RABV replication. Recent studies have demonstrated the important role of P protein in suppressing the IFN pathway (Ito *et al.*, 2010) and, therefore, promotion of innate immune responses to RABV may be possible by inhibiting P mRNA.

Similar to what has been previously shown in the case of other negative dsRNA viruses, such as VSV and respiratory syncytial virus (RSV), the RABV genome is protected from the RNAi pathway (Israsena *et al.*, unpublished data). Yet, it is still unclear whether targeting viral genome can alter its pathogenicity. Recombinant VSVs, which incorporate miRNA target sequences in the viral genome, showed significant reduction in neurotoxicity in the presence of amiRNA as compared to wild-type virus, and these recombinant viruses showed distinct tissue tropism (Kelly and Russell, 2009; Kelly *et al.*, 2010).

One of the major concerns in using siRNA against RNA viruses is the high rate of viral mutations that can lead to the loss of siRNA efficacy. As RNAi relies upon a nearly perfect sequence complementary between a siRNA molecule and the viral RNA target, the accumulation of mutations can render that virus to become resistant to RNAi suppression. This phenomenon has been observed in chronic HIV infection (Das *et al.*, 2004). Although cellular miRNA can inhibit mRNA translation when there is (are) mismatch(s) in base pairing outside the seeding region of the miRNA, a near perfect base pairing is still required for mRNA cleavage. Analysis of data from sequences of amiRNA against those of RABV demonstrated that amiRNA construct activity can be reduced when mismatching with target sequences occurs at critical sites (Israsena *et al.*, 2009). This issue is of particular concern if amiRNA is to be developed as a therapeutic option. In the clinical setting, the patient must receive treatment as early as possible. Data from country-wide survey of wild-type rabies sequences suggested that even within the conserved region of rabies N gene (Denduangboripant *et al.*, 2005), one-third of nucleotides studied showed significant degree of genetic variability (5–49%). Because these variable nucleotides are present in every 10–15 nt of the gene, it is not possible to predesigned amiRNA that can perfectly match the wild-type virus even within the same country. This potential limitation may be solved by using vectors containing multiple RNAi molecules such as amiRNA, long-hairpin RNAs (lhRNA), and modified hairpin RNA (mhRNAs; Haasnoot *et al.*, 2007) to enable simultaneous targeting of different sites. Efficient inhibition by lhRNAs has been reported for viruses, such as HIV-1 and HBV (Konstantinova *et al.*, 2006; Liu *et al.*, 2008; Weinberg *et al.*, 2007).

MRI studies suggest that, unlike other causes of viral encephalitis, the blood–brain barrier (BBB) remains intact until a late stage of RABV infection (Laothamatas *et al.*, 2003). Intactness of the BBB precludes entry of therapeutic agents from blood to brain. Safe and effective methods for delivery of siRNA/miRNA to the CNS remain an important unsolved issue. One possible approach for siRNA delivery is by intravenous treatment with modified RABV G incorporated with antiviral siRNA. It has been shown that this strategy can protect mice against fatal West Nile viral encephalitis (Kumar *et al.*, 2007). Another potential strategy is by using viral vectors. Recently, it has been shown that combined systemic injection of SV40 virus with mannitol, which temporarily breaks down the BBB, can effectively deliver transgenes to adult neurons in several regions of the CNS (Louboutin *et al.*, 2010). An appropriate delivery system needs to be developed and tested further in an *in vivo* model.

V. CONCLUSIONS

After decades of studies, several aspects of rabies pathogenesis, such as mechanisms explaining the variable incubation period, virulence, and diversity of clinical manifestations, are still unclear and there is no effective treatment available. Further research on the relationship between noncoding RNA and RABV infection may shed some light on these unanswered questions. Strategies using siRNA/amiRNA to inhibit RABV replication have begun to show promise in an *in vitro* study (Brandao *et al.*, 2007; Israsena *et al.*, 2009). It remains to be seen whether these strategies can be developed into viable therapeutic options. Much work is needed to be done to solve the problem of the delivery issue and long-term efficacy. Due to the limitation of cellular gene silencing machinery, it is very likely that this RNAi approach has to be applied in conjunction with other measures in the real clinical setting.

REFERENCES

Aparicio, O., Razquin, N., Zaratiegui, M., Narvaiza, I., and Fortes, P. (2006). Adenovirus virus-associated RNA is processed to functional interfering RNAs involved in virus production. *J. Virol.* **80:**1376–1384.

Bagga, S., Bracht, J., Hunter, S., Massirer, K., Holtz, J., Eachus, R., and Pasquinelli, A. E. (2005). Regulation by let-7 and lin-4 miRNAs results in target mRNA degradation. *Cell* **122:**553–563.

Barik, S. (2004). Control of nonsegmented negative-strand RNA virus replication by siRNA. *Virus Res.* **102:**27–35.

Bartel, D. P. (2004). MicroRNAs: Genomics, biogenesis, mechanism, and function. *Cell* **116:**281–297.

Boden, D., Pusch, O., Silbermann, R., Lee, F., Tucker, L., and Ramratnam, B. (2004). Enhanced gene silencing of HIV-1 specific siRNA using microRNA designed hairpins. *Nucleic Acids Res.* **32:**1154–1158.

Brandao, P. E., Castilho, J. G., Fahl, W., Carnieli, P., Jr., Oliveira Rde, N., Macedo, C. I., Carrieri, M. L., and Kotait, I. (2007). Short-interfering RNAs as antivirals against rabies. *Braz. J. Infect. Dis.* **11:**224–225.

Brennecke, J., Hipfner, D. R., Stark, A., Russell, R. B., and Cohen, S. M. (2003). Bantam encodes a developmentally regulated microRNA that controls cell proliferation and regulates the proapoptotic gene hid in Drosophila. *Cell* **113:**25–36.

Cai, X., and Cullen, B. R. (2006). Transcriptional origin of Kaposi's sarcoma-associated herpesvirus microRNAs. *J. Virol.* **80:**2234–2242.

Cameron, J. E., Fewell, C., Yin, Q., McBride, J., Wang, X., Lin, Z., and Flemington, E. K. (2008). Epstein-Barr virus growth/latency III program alters cellular microRNA expression. *Virology* **382:**257–266.

Carrington, J. C., and Ambros, V. (2003). Role of microRNAs in plant and animal development. *Science* **301:**336–338.

Carthew, R. W., and Sontheimer, E. J. (2009). Origins and mechanisms of miRNAs and siRNAs. *Cell* **136:**642–655.

Chen, J. F., Mandel, E. M., Thomson, J. M., Wu, Q., Callis, T. E., Hammond, S. M., Conlon, F. L., and Wang, D. Z. (2006). The role of microRNA-1 and microRNA-133 in skeletal muscle proliferation and differentiation. *Nat. Genet.* **38:**228–233.

Choy, E. Y., Siu, K. L., Kok, K. H., Lung, R. W., Tsang, C. M., To, K. F., Kwong, D. L., Tsao, S. W., and Jin, D. Y. (2008). An Epstein-Barr virus-encoded microRNA targets PUMA to promote host cell survival. *J. Exp. Med.* **205:**2551–2560.

Cullen, B. R. (2004). Transcription and processing of human microRNA precursors. *Mol. Cell* **16:**861–865.

Cullen, B. R. (2009). Viral and cellular messenger RNA targets of viral microRNAs. *Nature* **457:**421–425.

Cullen, B. R. (2010). Five questions about viruses and microRNAs. *PLoS Pathog.* **6:**e1000787.

Dalmay, T., and Edwards, D. R. (2006). MicroRNAs and the hallmarks of cancer. *Oncogene* **25:**6170–6175.

Das, A. T., Brummelkamp, T. R., Westerhout, E. M., Vink, M., Madiredjo, M., Bernards, R., and Berkhout, B. (2004). Human immunodeficiency virus type 1 escapes from RNA interference-mediated inhibition. *J. Virol.* **78:**2601–2605.

Denduangboripant, J., Wacharapluesadee, S., Lumlertdacha, B., Ruankaew, N., Hoonsuwan, W., Puanghat, A., and Hemachudha, T. (2005). Transmission dynamics of rabies virus in Thailand: Implications for disease control. *BMC Infect. Dis.* **5:**52.

DeVincenzo, J., Lambkin-Williams, R., Wilkinson, T., Cehelsky, J., Nochur, S., Walsh, E., Meyers, R., Gollob, J., and Vaishnaw, A. (2010). A randomized, double-blind, placebo-controlled study of an RNAi-based therapy directed against respiratory syncytial virus. *Proc. Natl. Acad. Sci. USA* **107:**8800–8805.

Dykxhoorn, D. M. (2007). MicroRNAs in viral replication and pathogenesis. *DNA Cell Biol.* **26:**239–249.

Ellis-Connell, A. L., Iempridee, T., Xu, I., and Mertz, J. E. (2010). Cellular microRNAs 200b and 429 regulate the Epstein-Barr virus switch between latency and lytic replication. *J. Virol.* **84:**10329–10343.

Grey, F., Antoniewicz, A., Allen, E., Saugstad, J., McShea, A., Carrington, J. C., and Nelson, J. (2005). Identification and characterization of human cytomegalovirus-encoded micro-RNAs. *J. Virol.* **79:**12095–12099.

Guo, L., and Lu, Z. (2010). The fate of miRNA* strand through evolutionary analysis: Implication for degradation as merely carrier strand or potential regulatory molecule? *PLoS ONE* **5:**e11387.

Gupta, A., Gartner, J. J., Sethupathy, P., Hatzigeorgiou, A. G., and Fraser, N. W. (2006). Anti-apoptotic function of a microRNA encoded by the HSV-1 latency-associated transcript. *Nature* **442**:82–85.

Haasnoot, J., Westerhout, E. M., and Berkhout, B. (2007). RNA interference against viruses: Strike and counterstrike. *Nat. Biotechnol.* **25**:1435–1443.

Hemachudha, T., Sunsaneewitayakul, B., Desudchit, T., Suankratay, C., Sittipunt, C., Wacharapluesadee, S., Khawplod, P., Wilde, H., and Jackson, A. C. (2006). Failure of therapeutic coma and ketamine for therapy of human rabies. *J. Neurovirol.* **12**:407–409.

Hsu, P. W., Lin, L. Z., Hsu, S. D., Hsu, J. B., and Huang, H. D. (2007). ViTa: Prediction of host microRNAs targets on viruses. *Nucleic Acids Res.* **35**:D381–D385.

Israsena, N., Supavonwong, P., Ratanasetyuth, N., Khawplod, P., and Hemachudha, T. (2009). Inhibition of rabies virus replication by multiple artificial microRNAs. *Antiviral Res.* **84**:76–83.

Ito, N., Moseley, G. W., Blondel, D., Shimizu, K., Rowe, C. L., Ito, Y., Masatani, T., Nakagawa, K., Jans, D. A., and Sugiyama, M. (2010). Role of interferon antagonist activity of rabies virus phosphoprotein in viral pathogenicity. *J. Virol.* **84**:6699–6710.

Jackson, A. C. (2008). Rabies. *Neurol. Clin.* **26**:717–726, ix.

Jones-Rhoades, M. W., Bartel, D. P., and Bartel, B. (2006). MicroRNAS and their regulatory roles in plants. *Annu. Rev. Plant Biol.* **57**:19–53.

Jopling, C. L., Yi, M., Lancaster, A. M., Lemon, S. M., and Sarnow, P. (2005). Modulation of hepatitis C virus RNA abundance by a liver-specific microRNA. *Science* **309**:1577–1581.

Jovanovic, M., and Hengartner, M. O. (2006). miRNAs and apoptosis: RNAs to die for. *Oncogene* **25**:6176–6187.

Kelly, E. J., and Russell, S. J. (2009). MicroRNAs and the regulation of vector tropism. *Mol. Ther.* **17**:409–416.

Kelly, E. J., Nace, R., Barber, G. N., and Russell, S. J. (2010). Attenuation of vesicular stomatitis virus encephalitis through microRNA targeting. *J. Virol.* **84**:1550–1562.

Khvorova, A., Reynolds, A., and Jayasena, S. D. (2003). Functional siRNAs and miRNAs exhibit strand bias. *Cell* **115**:209–216.

Kim, V. N. (2005). MicroRNA biogenesis: Coordinated cropping and dicing. *Nat. Rev. Mol. Cell Biol.* **6**:376–385.

Kim, H. K., Lee, Y. S., Sivaprasad, U., Malhotra, A., and Dutta, A. (2006). Muscle-specific microRNA miR-206 promotes muscle differentiation. *J. Cell Biol.* **174**:677–687.

Kim, W., Benhamed, M., Servet, C., Latrasse, D., Zhang, W., Delarue, M., and Zhou, D. X. (2009). Histone acetyltransferase GCN5 interferes with the miRNA pathway in Arabidopsis. *Cell Res.* **19**:899–909.

Konstantinova, P., de Vries, W., Haasnoot, J., ter Brake, O., de Haan, P., and Berkhout, B. (2006). Inhibition of human immunodeficiency virus type 1 by RNA interference using long-hairpin RNA. *Gene Ther.* **13**:1403–1413.

Kumar, P., Wu, H., McBride, J. L., Jung, K. E., Kim, M. H., Davidson, B. L., Lee, S. K., Shankar, P., and Manjunath, N. (2007). Transvascular delivery of small interfering RNA to the central nervous system. *Nature* **448**:39–43.

Lagos-Quintana, M., Rauhut, R., Lendeckel, W., and Tuschl, T. (2001). Identification of novel genes coding for small expressed RNAs. *Science* **294**:853–858.

Laothamatas, J., Hemachudha, T., Mitrabhakdi, E., Wannakrairot, P., and Tulayadaechanont, S. (2003). MR imaging in human rabies. *AJNR Am J. Neuroradiol.* **24**:1102–1109.

Lecellier, C. H., Dunoyer, P., Arar, K., Lehmann-Che, J., Eyquem, S., Himber, C., Saib, A., and Voinnet, O. (2005). A cellular microRNA mediates antiviral defense in human cells. *Science* **308**:557–560.

Lee, R. C., Feinbaum, R. L., and Ambros, V. (1993). The C. elegans heterochronic gene lin-4 encodes small RNAs with antisense complementarity to lin-14. *Cell* **75**:843–854.

Lee, Y., Ahn, C., Han, J., Choi, H., Kim, J., Yim, J., Lee, J., Provost, P., Radmark, O., Kim, S., and Kim, V. N. (2003). The nuclear RNase III Drosha initiates microRNA processing. *Nature* **425:**415–419.

Lee, Y., Kim, M., Han, J., Yeom, K. H., Lee, S., Baek, S. H., and Kim, V. N. (2004). MicroRNA genes are transcribed by RNA polymerase II. *EMBO J.* **23:**4051–4060.

Lewis, B. P., Burge, C. B., and Bartel, D. P. (2005). Conserved seed pairing, often flanked by adenosines, indicates that thousands of human genes are microRNA targets. *Cell* **120:**15–20.

Li, F., and Ding, S. W. (2006). Virus counterdefense: Diverse strategies for evading the RNA-silencing immunity. *Annu. Rev. Microbiol.* **60:**503–531.

Li, S. C., Shiau, C. K., and Lin, W. C. (2008). Vir-Mir db: Prediction of viral microRNA candidate hairpins. *Nucleic Acids Res.* **36:**D184–D189.

Lian, H., Liu, W., Liu, Q., Jin, H., Sun, Y., Li, J., Xia, Z., and Gao, H. (2010). A laboratory-attenuated vesicular stomatitis virus induces apoptosis and alters the cellular microRNA expression profile in BHK cells. *Arch. Virol.* **155:**1643–1653.

Lim, L. P., Glasner, M. E., Yekta, S., Burge, C. B., and Bartel, D. P. (2003). Vertebrate microRNA genes. *Science* **299:**1540.

Linnstaedt, S. D., Gottwein, E., Skalsky, R. L., Luftig, M. A., and Cullen, B. R. (2010). Virally induced cellular microRNA miR-155 plays a key role in B-cell immortalization by Epstein-Barr virus. *J. Virol.* **84:**11670–11678.

Liu, Y. P., Haasnoot, J., ter Brake, O., Berkhout, B., and Konstantinova, P. (2008). Inhibition of HIV-1 by multiple siRNAs expressed from a single microRNA polycistron. *Nucleic Acids Res.* **36:**2811–2824.

Louboutin, J. P., Chekmasova, A. A., Marusich, E., Chowdhury, J. R., and Strayer, D. S. (2010). Efficient CNS gene delivery by intravenous injection. *Nat. Methods* **7:**905–907.

Lu, L. F., and Liston, A. (2009). MicroRNA in the immune system, microRNA as an immune system. *Immunology* **127:**291–298.

Lund, E., Guttinger, S., Calado, A., Dahlberg, J. E., and Kutay, U. (2004). Nuclear export of microRNA precursors. *Science* **303:**95–98.

McBride, J. L., Boudreau, R. L., Harper, S. Q., Staber, P. D., Monteys, A. M., Martins, I., Gilmore, B. L., Burstein, H., Peluso, R. W., Polisky, B., Carter, B. J., and Davidson, B. L. (2008). Artificial miRNAs mitigate shRNA-mediated toxicity in the brain: Implications for the therapeutic development of RNAi. *Proc. Natl. Acad. Sci. USA* **105:**5868–5873.

McCaffrey, A. P., Nakai, H., Pandey, K., Huang, Z., Salazar, F. H., Xu, H., Wieland, S. F., Marion, P. L., and Kay, M. A. (2003). Inhibition of hepatitis B virus in mice by RNA interference. *Nat. Biotechnol.* **21:**639–644.

Otsuka, M., Jing, Q., Georgel, P., New, L., Chen, J., Mols, J., Kang, Y. J., Jiang, Z., Du, X., Cook, R., Das, S. C., Pattnaik, A. K., Beutler, B., and Han, J. (2007). Hypersusceptibility to vesicular stomatitis virus infection in Dicer1-deficient mice is due to impaired miR24 and miR93 expression. *Immunity* **27:**123–134.

Pedersen, I. M., Cheng, G., Wieland, S., Volinia, S., Croce, C. M., Chisari, F. V., and David, M. (2007). Interferon modulation of cellular microRNAs as an antiviral mechanism. *Nature* **449:**919–922.

Perez, J. T., Pham, A. M., Lorini, M. H., Chua, M. A., Steel, J., and tenOever, B. R. (2009). MicroRNA-mediated species-specific attenuation of influenza A virus. *Nat. Biotechnol.* **27:**572–576.

Pfeffer, S., Sewer, A., Lagos-Quintana, M., Sheridan, R., Sander, C., Grasser, F. A., van Dyk, L. F., Ho, C. K., Shuman, S., Chien, M., Russo, J. J., Ju, J., Randall, G., Lindenbach, B. D., Rice, C. M., Simon, V., Ho, D. D., Zavolan, M., and Tuschl, T. (2005). Identification of microRNAs of the herpesvirus family. *Nat. Methods* **2:**269–276.

Qu, J., Ye, J., and Fang, R. (2007). Artificial microRNA-mediated virus resistance in plants. *J. Virol.* **81:**6690–6699.

Reinhart, B. J., Slack, F. J., Basson, M., Pasquinelli, A. E., Bettinger, J. C., Rougvie, A. E., Horvitz, H. R., and Ruvkun, G. (2000). The 21-nucleotide let-7 RNA regulates developmental timing in *Caenorhabditis elegans*. *Nature* **403:**901–906.

Roberts, A. P., and Jopling, C. L. (2010). Targeting viral infection by microRNA inhibition. *Genome Biol.* **11:**201.

Rouha, H., Thurner, C., and Mandl, C. W. (2010). Functional microRNA generated from a cytoplasmic RNA virus. *Nucleic Acids Res* **38:**8328–8337.

Schutz, S., and Sarnow, P. (2006). Interaction of viruses with the mammalian RNA interference pathway. *Virology* **344:**151–157.

Shapiro, J. S., Varble, A., Pham, A. M., and Tenoever, B. R. (2010). Noncanonical cytoplasmic processing of viral microRNAs. *RNA* **16:**2068–2074.

Skalsky, R. L., and Cullen, B. R. (2010). Viruses, microRNAs, and host interactions. *Annu. Rev. Microbiol.* **64:**123–141.

Song, L., Liu, H., Gao, S., Jiang, W., and Huang, W. (2010). Cellular microRNAs inhibit replication of the H1N1 influenza A virus in infected cells. *J. Virol.* **84:**8849–8860.

Sontheimer, E. J., and Carthew, R. W. (2005). Silence from within: Endogenous siRNAs and miRNAs. *Cell* **122:**9–12.

Stefani, G., and Slack, F. J. (2008). Small non-coding RNAs in animal development. *Nat. Rev. Mol. Cell Biol.* **9:**219–230.

Sullivan, C. S., Grundhoff, A. T., Tevethia, S., Pipas, J. M., and Ganem, D. (2005). SV40-encoded microRNAs regulate viral gene expression and reduce susceptibility to cytotoxic T cells. *Nature* **435:**682–686.

Triboulet, R., Mari, B., Lin, Y. L., Chable-Bessia, C., Bennasser, Y., Lebrigand, K., Cardinaud, B., Maurin, T., Barbry, P., Baillat, V., Reynes, J., Corbeau, P., Jeang, K. T., and Benkirane, M. (2007). Suppression of microRNA-silencing pathway by HIV-1 during virus replication. *Science* **315:**1579–1582.

Umbach, J. L., and Cullen, B. R. (2009). The role of RNAi and microRNAs in animal virus replication and antiviral immunity. *Genes Dev.* **23:**1151–1164.

Umbach, J. L., Kramer, M. F., Jurak, I., Karnowski, H. W., Coen, D. M., and Cullen, B. R. (2008). MicroRNAs expressed by herpes simplex virus 1 during latent infection regulate viral mRNAs. *Nature* **454:**780–783.

Varble, A., Chua, M. A., Perez, J. T., Manicassamy, B., Garcia-Sastre, A., and tenOever, B. R. (2010). Engineered RNA viral synthesis of microRNAs. *Proc. Natl. Acad. Sci. USA* **107:**11519–11524.

Weinberg, M. S., Ely, A., Barichievy, S., Crowther, C., Mufamadi, S., Carmona, S., and Arbuthnot, P. (2007). Specific inhibition of HBV replication in vitro and in vivo with expressed long hairpin RNA. *Mol. Ther.* **15:**534–541.

Witwer, K. W., Sisk, J. M., Gama, L., and Clements, J. E. (2010). MicroRNA regulation of IFN-beta protein expression: Rapid and sensitive modulation of the innate immune response. *J. Immunol.* **184:**2369–2376.

World Health Organization(2005). WHO Expert Consultation on Rabies: First Report . World Health Organization, Geneva.

Wunner, W. H., Pallatroni, C., and Curtis, P. J. (2004). Selection of genetic inhibitors of rabies virus. *Arch. Virol.* **149:**1653–1662.

Xu, P., Vernooy, S. Y., Guo, M., and Hay, B. A. (2003). The Drosophila microRNA Mir-14 suppresses cell death and is required for normal fat metabolism. *Curr. Biol.* **13:**790–795.

Yeung, M. L., Bennasser, Y., Le, S. Y., and Jeang, K. T. (2005). siRNA, miRNA and HIV: Promises and challenges. *Cell Res.* **15:**935–946.

Yi, R., Qin, Y., Macara, I. G., and Cullen, B. R. (2003). Exportin-5 mediates the nuclear export of pre-microRNAs and short hairpin RNAs. *Genes Dev.* **17:**3011–3016.

CHAPTER 16

Design of Future Rabies Biologics and Antiviral Drugs

Todd G. Smith, Xianfu Wu, Richard Franka, and **Charles E. Rupprecht**

Contents

Abstract

In recent years, no major paradigm shifts have occurred in the utilization of new products for the prevention and control of rabies. Development of new cost-effective rabies biologics and antiviral drugs is critical in continuing to prevent and reduce disease. Current rabies vaccines are highly effective but have developed largely based on technical improvements in the vaccine industry. In the future, alternative approaches for improved vaccines, including novel avirulent rabies virus (RABV) vectors, should be pursued. Any rabies vaccine that is effective without the need for rabies immune globulin (RIG) will contribute fundamentally to disease prevention

Poxvirus and Rabies Branch, Centers for Disease Control and Prevention, Atlanta, Georgia, USA

Advances in Virus Research, Volume 79
ISSN 0065-3527, DOI: 10.1016/B978-0-12-387040-7.00016-0

by reducing the cost and complexity of postexposure prophylaxis (PEP). The lack of high quality, affordable RIG is a continuing problem. Virus-specific monoclonal antibodies (mAbs) will soon fulfill the PEP requirement for passive immunity, currently met with RIG. Several relevant strategies for mAb production, including use of transgenic mice, humanization of mouse mAbs, and generation of human immune libraries, are underway. As a result of successful PEP and pre-exposure prophylaxis in developed countries, until recently, no significant focused efforts have been devoted to RABV-specific antiviral agents. To date, combination therapy including broad spectrum antiviral agents has been successful in only one case, and reports of antiviral activity are often conflicting. Current antiviral strategies target either the nucleoprotein or phosphoprotein, but drugs targeting the viral polymerase should be considered. Considering the lag from creation of new concepts to experimental development and clinical trials, many years will likely elapse between today's ideas and tomorrow's practices.

I. INTRODUCTION

In the twenty-first century, the majority of human rabies fatalities are due to socioeconomic factors regarding the lack of applied postexposure prophylaxis (PEP) regimens, shortages of existing rabies biologics, and inadequate canine vaccination (Wunner and Briggs, 2010; Wilde, 2007). All current rabies vaccines, antibodies, and antiviral drugs were conceived and developed more than 30 years ago. Improved approaches to safety, effectiveness, and administration of rabies biologics need to remain a primary focus in modern rabies prevention and control.

II. VACCINES

A. Existing biologics

Rabies vaccine development began with live rabies viruses (RABVs) in mammalian nerve tissue vaccines (MNTV), progressed to avian tissue vaccines, and thereafter resulted in primary continuous cell-culture derived vaccines (Table I). In contrast to the intensive research into attenuated RABV from the 1880s through the 1950s, current rabies vaccines have benefited mostly from advancements in cell-culture techniques. All modern human rabies vaccines are inactivated, and no serious interest in attenuated RABV has been present for the past 50 years (Plotkin, 2000).

TABLE I   Human rabies vaccine development

Year	Name	Description	Use
	Mammalian Nerve Tissue Vaccines (MNTV)		
1885	Pasteur vaccine (PV)	Air-dried spinal cord from RABV-infected rabbits, emulsified, and injected for 10 days using less attenuated material each day[a]	
1887	Roux/Calmette	PV preserved in glycerol	
1908	Fermi vaccine	5% suspension of RABV-infected sheep brain, treated with 0.5–1.0% of phenol[b]	Still produced in Ethiopia[c]
1911	Semple vaccine	Fermi vaccine inactivated for 48–72 h at 30 °C[d]	Still used in some developing countries
1964	Fuenzalida/ Palacios vaccine	Inactivated RABV-infected neonatal (myelin-free) mouse brains, prevented vaccination-related allergic encephalomyelitis[e]	Still used in some South American countries
	Avian tissue vaccines		
1948	Flury low egg passage (LEP)	Flury RABV, 40th–50th egg-passage lyophilized from a 33% whole-embryo suspension[f]	Used for canine vaccination but retained virulence in puppies
	Flury high egg passage	Same as LEP except 180th or higher egg passage	1950s and 1960s tested in humans[g]
1956	Duck-embryo derived rabies vaccine	Pitman-Moore RABV, inactivated using β-propiolactone[h]	Used in the United States until 1980s, low antigenic responses and severe adverse reactions[i]

(continued)

TABLE I   (*continued*)

Year	Name	Description	Use
1986	Purified duck embryo vaccine	Pitman-Moore RABV, concentrated, inactivated using β-propiolactone [j]	Suggested for use in India[k]
		Cell-culture-derived vaccines	
1964	Human diploid cell vaccine (HDCV)	RABV produced in human diploid fibroblast cell line WI-38, concentrated, inactivated[l]	Not licensed in U.S. until 1980, current WHO gold-standard
1965	Purified chick embryo cell vaccine	Flury RABV produced in primary chick embryo cells, concentrated, inactivated using β-propiolactone[m]	Not licensed in U.S. until 1997
1967	Primary hamster kidney cell vaccine	RABV produced in primary hamster kidney cell, concentrated, inactivated using formalin[n]	Currently used in some countries, including Russia and China[o]
1984	Purified Vero cell rabies vaccine	Pitman-Moore RABV produced in green monkey kidney cells, concentrated, inactivated using β-propiolactone [p]	Currently in use world-wide except in U.S., comparable to HDCV

[a] Kammer and Ertl (2002); "attenuation" was achieved by using a mixture of live (active) virus and virus inactivated by desiccation at room temperature. The initial doses contained mostly inactivated virus, but each day, fresher material was used. Thus, the amount of live virus gradually increased, until the last dose using freshly prepared material which contained mostly live virus.
[b] Fermi (1908).
[c] Ayele *et al.* (2001).
[d] Semple (1911).
[e] Fuenzalida *et al.* (1964); inactivated using ultra-violet irradiation.
[f] Leach and Johnson (1940), Koprowski and Cox (1948).
[g] Ruegsegger *et al.* (1961), Sharpless *et al.* (1957).
[h] Culbertson *et al.* (1956).
[i] Vodopija and Clarke (1991).
[j] Gluck *et al.* (1984, 1986).
[k] Ashwathnarayana *et al.* (2009).
[l] Wiktor *et al.* (1964); inactivated using either treatment with phenol at 37 °C for 48 h or treatment with β-propiolactone at 4 °C for 24 h.
[m] Kondo (1965), Yoshino *et al.* (1966); Barth *et al.* (1983).
[n] Lin *et al.* (1983).
[o] Lin (1990).
[p] Fournier *et al.* (1985), Roumiantzeff *et al.* (1984), Suntharasamai *et al.* (1986).

1. Animal vaccines

All licensed animal and human rabies vaccines are derived from canine RABV variants. In the United States alone, 11 different rabies vaccines are licensed for dogs, 12 for cats, 1 for ferrets, 3 for horses, 4 for cattle, and 5 for sheep (National Association of State Public Health Veterinarians Committee, 2008). Theoretically, any one of these vaccines should protect any susceptible target species. High titer RABV vaccines generate sufficient acquired immune responses. Development of novel adjuvants for animal rabies vaccines is not necessary, and prior use has led to the development of serious adverse events, especially in cats (Hendrick *et al.*, 1994; Kass *et al.*, 1993).

A milestone in animal rabies prevention was the development of oral vaccination for wildlife. In 1978, the Evelyn–Rokitnicki–Abelseth (ERA) RABV was successfully field tested in foxes (Abelseth, 1964; Steck *et al.*, 1982). Subsequent derivatives of ERA, such as SAD-B19, SAG-1, and SAG-2, were further attenuated by clone purification and monoclonal antibody selection (Lafay *et al.*, 1994). The failure of ERA vaccines and their derivatives to induce protective immunity in some wildlife species, as well as vaccine-associated rabies cases, led to the development of a recombinant *Vaccinia* virus (V-RG) that expressed ERA glycoprotein (G protein; Wiktor *et al.*, 1984). However, neither V-RG nor ERA vaccines induced optimal immune responses in some species, such as skunks (Grosenbaugh *et al.*, 2007). Despite oral vaccination's utility for the past 30 years, the immunogenic mechanism is still largely unknown.

B. Future approaches

Even though the *Lyssavirus* genus is highly diverse, very few seed strains have been selected for vaccine development. For example, more than a century after its historical use, the Pasteur strain remains highly solicited for vaccine development. The various cell-culture vaccines are of comparable parameters, regardless of which RABV is used for production. On suitable substrates, the virus titer (yield) contributes ultimately to vaccine efficacy. Many RABV vaccines need to be concentrated by ultracentrifugation, which dramatically increases the cost. Any future approaches that improve RABV yield will improve current vaccines by making them more cost-effective. Focused research on attenuated RABV could play a role in improving virus yield. However, if such novel attenuated RABV continue to be overshadowed by historical legacies and phylogenetically restricted vaccine strains, novel vaccine development may falter.

1. DNA vaccines

DNA vaccines offer greater thermostability and lower production costs (Ertl, 2003). However, current RABV DNA vaccines are less effective than traditional vaccines (Nadin-Davis and Fehlner-Gardiner, 2008). Recently, a DNA vaccine using a modified RABV *G* gene proved more effective than the native *G* gene (Osinubi *et al.*, 2009). From a regulatory standpoint, development of a DNA vaccine is subject to additional manufacturing, immunogenicity, and safety guidelines.

2. Plant-derived vaccines

While initially promising, plant-derived vaccines have been slow to develop. Several studies have shown that RABV G protein can be produced in transgenic plants (Ashraf *et al.*, 2005; Loza-Rubio *et al.*, 2008; McGarvey *et al.*, 1995; Rojas-Anaya *et al.*, 2009), and plant-produced antigens administered orally or by injection may protect animals from lethal challenge (Ashraf *et al.*, 2005; Loza-Rubio *et al.*, 2008; Modelska *et al.*, 1998). However, these findings have not been rigorously applied to target species (e.g., dogs or wildlife). Issues related to glycosylation and antigenic load may continue to limit this approach.

3. Recombinant vaccines

In addition to poxviruses, other DNA viruses, such as human, chimpanzee and canine adenovirus, have been considered for recombinant vaccine research (Vos *et al.*, 2001; Xiang *et al.*, 2002; Yarosh *et al.*, 1996). In these studies, experimental recombinant vaccines appear more antigenic than traditional vaccines. However, several issues will require careful long-term evaluation, such as release of a replication-competent DNA virus-based vaccine as well as the high frequency of recombination in large DNA viruses.

4. Avirulent rabies virus vaccines

Residual pathogenicity is a concern with any active vaccine, especially in juvenile and immunocompromised individuals. Approaches using reverse genetics for gene rearrangement, duplication, or deletion resulted in various degrees of fitness and immunogenicity (Faber *et al.*, 2002; Ito *et al.*, 2005; Shoji *et al.*, 2004; Wu and Rupprecht, 2008). Research into attenuation for target animals would have a significant impact on vaccine development, but public perception and regulatory hurdles could thwart future developments in this area.

5. Dual rabies vaccination and immunocontraception

Population management in free-ranging animals using RABV as a vector is needed. Despite the highly attractive idea of dual rabies vaccination and immunocontraception, various scientific, regulatory, and ethical challenges face any such product. The use of RABV as a vector for immunocontraception has been reported in cell culture and preliminary studies in mice (Wu *et al.*, 2009, 2010).

III. ANTIBODIES

A. Existing biologics

The current World Health Organization (WHO) rabies PEP guide recommends that, for all category III exposures (bites, scratches, and mucosal contacts), rabies immune globulin (RIG) be infiltrated around the site. Currently, only human RIG (HRIG) and equine RIG (ERIG) are available for PEP (Table II).

HRIG is not widely available in most countries where cost is a major limiting factor. In 2004, the average per patient cost of HRIG in the United States was estimated at $761 and is now assumed to be over US$1000 (Dhankhar *et al.*, 2008; Kreindel *et al.*, 1998). Only HRIG is administered in many developed countries due to the risk of adverse events associated with ERIG.

Compared to HRIG, ERIG is more widely available and less expensive, but affordability and availability are still problems. For example, less than

TABLE II Current and future rabies virus antibodies

Status	Name	Dose	Components	Source
Currently available	Human rabies immune globulin (HRIG)	20 IU/kg	Polyclonal	Multiple
	Equine rabies immune globulin (ERIG)	40 IU/kg	Polyclonal; F(ab')$_2$ or IgG preparations	Multiple
Human clinical trials	CL184	20 IU/kg	CR57/CR4098 monoclonal cocktail	Crucell (Leiden, Netherlands)
In vivo testing	Not specified	20 IU/kg	R16F7/R14D6 monoclonal cocktail	Indian Immunologicals Ltd. (Hyderabad, India)
In vitro testing	RAB1	0.03 mg/ml	17C7 monoclonal	MassBioLogics (Jamaica Plain, MA)

18% of patients in India that required ERIG received it due to affordability (Satpathy *et al.*, 2005). Severe adverse events such as anaphylaxis and serum-sickness are often cited as problems with ERIG (Wilde and Chutivongse, 1990; Wilde *et al.*, 1989). However, several studies have found that currently available highly purified, modified ERIG only rarely caused severe adverse events (Lang *et al.*, 1998a,b; Satpathy *et al.*, 2005). In Brazil, antihistamines and corticosteroids were administered before treatment with ERIG to reduce adverse effects (Cupo *et al.*, 2001). Highly purified products can reduce adverse effects but may be cleared more rapidly reducing passive immunity before vaccine-induced antibodies are present.

Monoclonal antibodies (mAbs) that neutralize RABV have been recognized as one alternative to overcome the limitations of RIG. Theoretically, adequate supplies of mAbs could be produced in a cost-effective manner to meet the demand for PEP (Prosniak *et al.*, 2003). Using a human mAb cocktail for PEP reduces the likelihood of adverse events and is as effective as HRIG in preventing rabies in laboratory animals (Goudsmit *et al.*, 2006). Currently, one mAb cocktail is in human clinical trials (Fig. 1, Table II; reviewed in De Kruif *et al.*, 2007).

B. Future approaches

Recently, a single anti-rabies human mAb was isolated from immunized transgenic mice (Sloan *et al.*, 2007). This mAb, known as RAB1, neutralized all RABV from various sources that were tested, and two amino acid substitutions were required for neutralization escape (Table II). No RABV (out of 468 sequences) was identified with both substitutions, so theoretically, RAB1 will neutralize all these sequenced strains (Wang *et al.*, 2009). Arguments in favor of this approach include lower production costs and high conservation of the epitope in canine strains. However, if this concept is in error, then no alternate mAbs are present to neutralize the exposing virus.

Another strategy is to return to mouse hybridomas and use these to identify mAbs that have desired properties, such as high activity, binding specificity, IgG isotype, and a reliable source (Muller *et al.*, 2009). Such mouse mAbs can then be humanized to create a human mAb that has equivalent properties to the mouse mAb. Recently, Muller *et al.* (2009) followed this strategy to produce three cocktails containing two noncompeting mouse mAbs that were as effective as HRIG in animal models.

Producing mAbs from humans reduces the risks of reactions related to animal sequences. Two mAbs from immortalized B-lymphocyte lines from an immunized human were developed recently for use in India (Table II). These mAbs protected animals when given with vaccine in a PEP model either individually or in a cocktail (Nagarajan *et al.*, 2008).

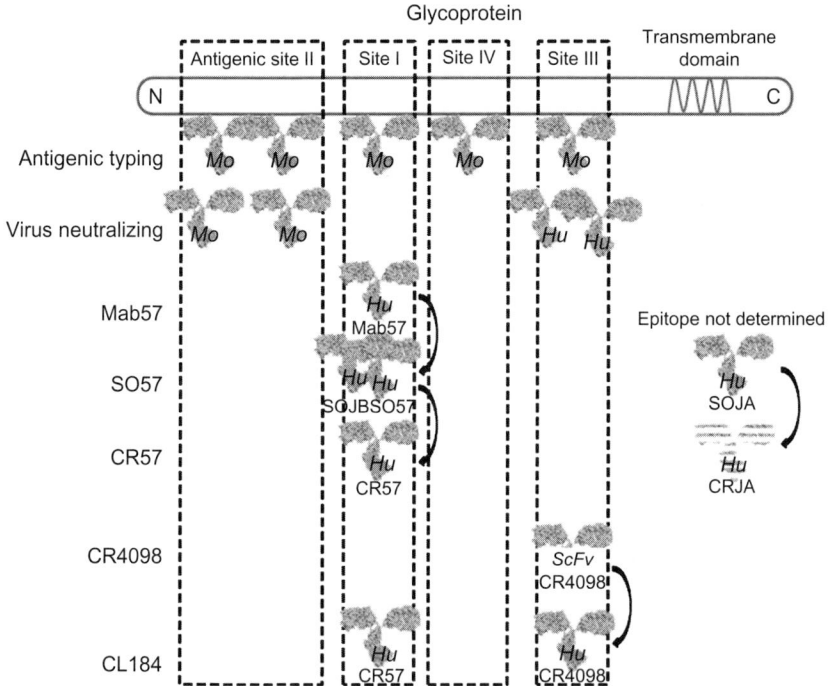

FIGURE 1 Development of RABV mAb cocktail. Panels of mouse (*Mo*) mAbs were used for *antigenic typing* and to define four major antigenic regions (Lafon *et al.*, 1983). The majority of *virus-neutralizing* antibodies (VNA) isolated from mice are specific for antigenic region II, while the majority of human mAbs isolated are specific for antigenic region III (Benmansour *et al.*, 1991). *Mab57* was isolated from vaccinated humans (*Hu*) and shown to protect laboratory animals from lethal challenge (Dietzschold *et al.*, 1990; Ueki *et al.*, 1990). SOJA and SOJB were isolated to include in a cocktail with *SO57* (Champion *et al.*, 2000; Prosniak *et al.*, 2003), but SOJB competed with SO57 binding. While SO57 was successfully reformatted as *CR57* for production in a human cell line, SOJA lost activity when reformatted (Marissen *et al.*, 2005). Single-chain variable fragments (scFv) were isolated from phage-display libraries from immunized humans (Kramer *et al.*, 2005), and *CR4098* was selected for high affinity, neutralizing activity, and compatibility with CR57 (Bakker *et al.*, 2005). In a phase I clinical trial, the CR57/CR4098 mAb cocktail, *CL184*, was found to be safe and effective (i.e., it did not cause major adverse reactions in healthy adults, and it did not interfere with induction of VNA; Bakker *et al.*, 2008).

Houimel and Dellagi (2009) selected RABV-specific antigen-binding fragments (Fabs) from immunized humans using a phage-display library. Similar to previous results (Kramer *et al.*, 2005; Sloan *et al.*, 2007), the selected Fabs were specific for G protein antigenic region III (Fig. 1) but did not compete with each other for binding in this region (Houimel and Dellagi, 2009).

Production of human mAbs in transgenic plants offers many similar benefits with the added benefit of agricultural scalability. When one mAb, SO57, was purified from transgenic plants, high levels of active protein were recovered. The plant-derived mAb had altered glycosylation, which resulted in shorter serum half-life but did not cause antigenic or allergic responses in animals. Given in a PEP animal model, this mAb protected all animals (Ko *et al.*, 2003).

C. Preliminary studies toward an anti-*Lyssavirus* mAb

The use of immunized humans for immune library construction biases libraries toward neutralization of RABV genotype 1 with lower cross-reactivity toward other *Lyssavirus* genotypes. To circumvent this limitation, mAbs can be (1) isolated from transgenic mice immunized with lyssaviruses; (2) selected from naïve immune libraries, which theoretically contain binders to any antigen; or (3) engineered from distinct heavy and light chains. With the goal of identifying and characterizing a novel anti-*Lyssavirus* mAb, we have obtained a naïve, human-heavy chain domain, phage-display library (Famm *et al.*, 2008). The library was panned using a recombinant ERA RABV expressing G proteins from Lagos and West Caucasian bat viruses following established methods (Kramer *et al.*, 2005; Lee *et al.*, 2007). After panning, potential high affinity domain antibodies (dAb) were identified by ELISA. Research is underway at our laboratory to identify virus-neutralizing dAbs and to conduct animal efficacy trials.

IV. ANTIVIRAL DRUGS

A. Existing options

Only recently has some scientific interest shifted to exploration of anti-RABV compounds, following the successful recovery of a patient with clinical rabies without use of vaccine or RIG, with treatment using an induced coma and nonspecific antiviral products (Willoughby *et al.*, 2005). The patient survived with mild neurological impairments, which partially improved after a few months (Hu *et al.*, 2007). This treatment was successful, but the mechanisms (host immune responses, effects of applied drugs, etc.) of RABV clearance remain unknown. A similar protocol has been applied in approximately 18 additional cases with less than satisfactory outcomes, and other survivors received at least partial PEP prior to development of clinical symptoms.

Previously, only a few compounds, that were successful against other viral targets, were applied to RABV (Lockhart *et al.*, 1992). The Working

Group on Management of Rabies in Humans proposed aggressive and palliative approaches for management of human rabies. For aggressive treatment, a combination therapy was recommended, including ribavirin, INF-α, and ketamine, as well as vaccine and RIG (Jackson *et al.*, 2003).

1. Ribavirin

Ribavirin is a broad spectrum antiviral drug targeting various DNA and RNA viruses by blocking RNA synthesis via inhibition of inosine 5'-monophosphate dehydrogenase (De Clercq, 2004). Activity against RABV was demonstrated in cell culture but could not be replicated in animal models (Bussereau and Ermine, 1983; Bussereau *et al.*, 1983, 1988). Ribavirin is known to skew the immune response toward a Th1-type inflammatory response (Lau *et al.*, 2002; Powers *et al.*, 1982; Tam *et al.*, 2000). Given the primacy of the humoral Th2-type response in clearance of RABV, the immunomodulatory properties of ribavirin may result in suppression or delays in antibody production (Jahrling *et al.*, 1980). Intravenous administration of ribavirin alone for treatment of rabies in humans was not successful (Kureishi *et al.*, 1992). Similarly, administration of ribavirin with IFN-α in humans did not mediate virus neutralization or clearance (Warrell *et al.*, 1989).

2. Interferon

During initiation of the innate immune response, IFN generates an intracellular environment that restricts viral replication. IFN-α interacts with cells of the innate immune system and participates in the transition to an effective adaptive immune response. In general, lyssaviruses have evolved mechanisms to counteract IFN, allowing efficient intracellular replication and propagation (Brzozka *et al.*, 2005, 2006; Lafon, 2005). In some experiments, IFN prevented replication of RABV in cell culture or protected animals when given after exposure (Atanasiu *et al.*, 1981; Baer *et al.*, 1979; Depoux, 1965; Weinmann *et al.*, 1979; Wiktor and Clark, 1972). However, in symptomatic or suspect human rabies patients, systemically or locally administered IFN showed no clinically beneficial effect. In some cases, diminished or delayed virus-neutralizing antibody titers were observed (Merigan *et al.*, 1984).

3. *N*-methyl ᴅ-aspartate (NMDA) receptor antagonists Amantadine and Ketamine

Amantadine is a noncompetitive NMDA receptor antagonist (Stoof *et al.*, 1992). Based on studies of influenza virus, amantadine prevents uncoating and release of viral RNA into the host cell (De Clercq, 2004). The potential antiviral effect against RABV was demonstrated only in limited extent in cell culture (Superti *et al.*, 1985).

Ketamine is also a noncompetitive NMDA receptor antagonist and a dissociative anesthetic. In high concentrations, it has been shown to inhibit RABV genome transcription (Lockhart *et al.*, 1992). However, such high drug concentrations most likely cannot be achieved in humans (Jackson *et al.*, 2003). Ketamine reduced the spread of RABV infection in rats (Lockhart *et al.*, 1991), but this was not confirmed in a recent more detailed study in mice and primary mouse neuronal cell cultures (Weli *et al.*, 2006). Ketamine and amantadine may have an additive effect, as they bind differently to the NMDA receptor (Bresink *et al.*, 1995; Porter and Greenamyre, 1995; Willoughby *et al.*, 2005). Amantadine specifically inhibits NMDA receptors by accelerating channel closure during channel block (Blanpied *et al.*, 2005).

B. Future approaches

The development of antiviral biologics for rabies therapy currently focuses on inhibition of virus replication, specifically targeting the phosphoprotein (P), nucleoprotein (N), or their genes. Four strong RABV inhibitory peptides were identified which affect different P protein functional domains and inhibit viral replication (Real *et al.*, 2004). Similarly, peptides derived from P protein demonstrated an inhibitory effect on virus replication in cell culture (Castel *et al.*, 2009). Wunner *et al.* (2004) used a cDNA library of short random fragments derived from the RABV genome to isolate two nucleotide fragments, from the N and P genes, that inhibited RABV replication in cell culture. Other RNA interference-based antiviral approaches using short-interfering RNAs have been developed against N mRNA (Brandao *et al.*, 2007). In all these studies, dosage and delivery present significant problems. Thus, many of these peptides are currently being used to direct the search for compounds that will have similar inhibitory properties (Tordo, 2010).

Small-molecular weight compounds, such as snake antivenom, may inhibit RABV binding, based on their binding to acetylcholine receptors, but have not shown promising results in preliminary animal studies. Screens for compounds that inhibit replication of a RABV mini-genome that expresses green fluorescent protein are being carried using high-throughput methods (Tordo, 2010). Multiple small-molecule scaffolds have been identified using cell-free protein synthesis (CFPS) that block putative steps of host-catalyzed viral capsid-related complex formation (Lingappa and Lingappa, 2005). Application of CFPS in the designing of anti-RABV products could be one key strategy in the future. Gene trap target discovery is another strategy for screening currently available, licensed drugs that inhibit nonessential human host genes that are required for viral replication (Rubin and Ruley, 2006).

Currently, no RABV-specific antiviral compounds with significant, reproducible activity in animal models have been identified. Despite significant progress in our understanding of *Lyssavirus* pathogenesis and host immune responses, clinical rabies remain almost inevitably fatal. Only limited guidance exists for confirmed human rabies cases, due to the lack of a validated animal model for experimental rabies therapeutics with critical care capacities and effective licensed antiviral agents.

V. CONCLUSIONS

Within the next decade, current cell-culture vaccines will be produced in serum-free culture media, which will reduce production costs and result in safer products. Better vaccine and alternate routes of administration may simplify the PEP regimen in the near future. The ideal "one shot" solution both for human PEP and canine PrEP is still a long-range goal and will likely require a live recombinant adenovirus or avirulent RABV vector. In the next decade, mAbs will become part of the PEP regimen and will eventually replace RIG. Significant efforts to screen compound libraries for specific RABV antiviral drugs, which can be tested in a relevant animal model, will result in better rabies therapeutics.

Use of trade names and commercial sources is for identification only and does not imply endorsement by the US Department of Health and Human Services. The findings and conclusions in this report are those of the authors and do not necessarily represent the views of the Centers for Disease Control and Prevention.

REFERENCES

Abelseth, M. K. (1964). An attenuated rabies vaccine for domestic animals produced in tissue culture. *Can. Vet. J.* **5:**279–286.

Ashraf, S., Singh, P. K., Yadav, D. K., Shahnawaz, M., Mishra, S., Sawant, S. V., and Tuli, R. (2005). High level expression of surface glycoprotein of rabies virus in tobacco leaves and its immunoprotective activity in mice. *J. Biotechnol.* **119:**1–14.

Ashwathnarayana, D. H., Madhusudana, S. N., Sampath, G., Sathpathy, D. M., Mankeshwar, R., Ravish, H. H., Ullas, P. T., Behra, T. R., Sudarshan, M. K., Gangaboraiah, M. K., and Shamanna, M. (2009). A comparative study on the safety and immunogenicity of purified duck embryo cell vaccine (PDEV, Vaxirab) with purified chick embryo cell vaccine (PCEC, Rabipur) and purified vero cell rabies vaccine (PVRV, Verorab). *Vaccine* **28:**148–151.

Atanasiu, P., Perrin, P., Segre, L., and Manganas, O. (1981). Evaluation and comparative studies of inactivated rabies vaccines obtained in the heterologous diploid and polyploid cells (HAK, BHK and VERO). *Dev. Biol. Stand.* **50:**173–182.

Ayele, W., Fekadu, M., Zewdie, B., Beyene, M., Bogale, Y., Mocha, K., and Egziabher, F. G. (2001). Immunogenicity and efficacy of Fermi-type nerve tissue rabies vaccine in mice and in humans undergoing post-exposure prophylaxis for rabies in Ethiopia. *Ethiop. Med. J.* **39:**313–321.

Baer, G. M., Moore, S. A., Shaddock, J. H., and Levy, H. B. (1979). An effective rabies treatment in exposed monkeys: A single dose of interferon inducer and vaccine. *Bull. World Health Organ.* **57:**807–813.

Bakker, A. B., Marissen, W. E., Kramer, R. A., Rice, A. B., Weldon, W. C., Niezgoda, M., Hanlon, C. A., Thijsse, S., Backus, H. H., de Kruif, J., Dietzschold, B., Rupprecht, C. E., *et al.* (2005). Novel human monoclonal antibody combination effectively neutralizing natural rabies virus variants and individual *in vitro* escape mutants. *J. Virol.* **79:**9062–9068.

Bakker, A. B., Python, C., Kissling, C. J., Pandya, P., Marissen, W. E., Brink, M. F., Lagerwerf, F., Worst, S., van Corven, E., Kostense, S., Hartmann, K., Weverling, G. J., *et al.* (2008). First administration to humans of a monoclonal antibody cocktail against rabies virus: Safety, tolerability, and neutralizing activity. *Vaccine* **26:**5922–5927.

Barth, R., Bijok, U., Grushkau, H., Smerdel, J., and Vodopija, J. (1983). Purified chicken embryo cell rabies vaccine for human use. *Lancet* **1:**700.

Benmansour, A., Leblois, H., Coulon, P., Tuffereau, C., Gaudin, Y., Flamand, A., and Lafay, F. (1991). Antigenicity of rabies virus glycoprotein. *J. Virol.* **65:**4198–4203.

Blanpied, T. A., Clarke, R. J., and Johnson, J. W. (2005). Amantadine inhibits NMDA receptors by accelerating channel closure during channel block. *J. Neurosci.* **25:**3312–3322.

Brandao, P. E., Castilho, J. G., Fahl, W., Carnieli, P., Jr., Oliveira Rde, N., Macedo, C. I., Carrieri, M. L., and Kotait, I. (2007). Short-interfering RNAs as antivirals against rabies. *Braz. J. Infect. Dis.* **11:**224–225.

Bresink, I., Danysz, W., Parsons, C. G., and Mutschler, E. (1995). Different binding affinities of NMDA receptor channel blockers in various brain regions—Indication of NMDA receptor heterogeneity. *Neuropharmacology* **34:**533–540.

Brzozka, K., Finke, S., and Conzelmann, K. K. (2005). Identification of the rabies virus alpha/beta interferon antagonist: Phosphoprotein P interferes with phosphorylation of interferon regulatory factor 3. *J. Virol.* **79:**7673–7681.

Brzozka, K., Finke, S., and Conzelmann, K. K. (2006). Inhibition of interferon signaling by rabies virus phosphoprotein P: Activation-dependent binding of STAT1 and STAT2. *J. Virol.* **80:**2675–2683.

Bussereau, F., and Ermine, A. (1983). Effects of heteropolyanions and nucleoside analogues on rabies virus: In vitro study of syntheses and viral production. *Ann. Inst. Pasteur Virol.* **134:**487–506.

Bussereau, F., Chermann, J. C., De Clercq, D., and Hannoun, C. (1983). Search for compounds which have an inhibitory effect on rhabdovirus multiplication in vitro. *Ann. Inst. Pasteur Virol.* **134:**127–134.

Bussereau, F., Picard, M., Blancou, J., and Sureau, P. (1988). Treatment of rabies in mice and foxes with antiviral compounds. *Acta Virol.* **32:**33–49.

Castel, G., Chteoui, M., Caignard, G., Prehaud, C., Mehouas, S., Real, E., Jallet, C., Jacob, Y., Ruigrok, R. W., and Tordo, N. (2009). Peptides that mimic the amino-terminal end of the rabies virus phosphoprotein have antiviral activity. *J. Virol.* **83:**10808–10820.

Champion, J. M., Kean, R. B., Rupprecht, C. E., Notkins, A. L., Koprowski, H., Dietzschold, B., and Hooper, D. C. (2000). The development of monoclonal human rabies virus-neutralizing antibodies as a substitute for pooled human immune globulin in the prophylactic treatment of rabies virus exposure. *J. Immunol. Methods* **235:**81–90.

Culbertson, C. G., Peck, F. B., Jr., and Powell, H. M. (1956). Duck-embryo rabies vaccine: Study of fixed virus vaccine grown in embryonated duck eggs and killed with beta-propiolactone (BPL). *J. Am. Med. Assoc.* **162:**1373–1376.

Cupo, P., de Azevedo-Marques, M. M., Sarti, W., and Hering, S. E. (2001). Proposal of abolition of the skin sensitivity test before equine rabies immune globulin application. *Rev. Inst. Med. Trop. São Paulo* **43:**51–53.

De Clercq, E. (2004). Antivirals and antiviral strategies. *Nat. Rev. Microbiol.* **2:**704–720.

De Kruif, J., Bakker, A. B., Marissen, W. E., Kramer, R. A., Throsby, M., Rupprecht, C. E., and Goudsmit, J. (2007). A human monoclonal antibody cocktail as a novel component of rabies postexposure prophylaxis. *Annu. Rev. Med.* **58**:359–368.

Depoux, R. (1965). Fixed rabies virus and interferon (virus rabique fixe et interféron). *C. R. Hebd. Seances Acad. Sci.* **260**:354–356.

Dhankhar, P., Vaidya, S. A., Fishbien, D. B., and Meltzer, M. I. (2008). Cost effectiveness of rabies post exposure prophylaxis in the United States. *Vaccine* **26**:4251–4255.

Dietzschold, B., Gore, M., Casali, P., Ueki, Y., Rupprecht, C. E., Notkins, A. L., and Koprowski, H. (1990). Biological characterization of human monoclonal antibodies to rabies virus. *J. Virol.* **64**:3087–3090.

Ertl, H. C. (2003). Rabies DNA vaccines for protection and therapeutic treatment. *Expert Opin. Biol. Ther.* **3**:639–644.

Faber, M., Pulmanausahakul, R., Hodawadekar, S. S., Spitsin, S., McGettigan, J. P., Schnell, M. J., and Dietzschold, B. (2002). Overexpression of the rabies virus glycoprotein results in enhancement of apoptosis and antiviral immune response. *J. Virol.* **76**:3374–3381.

Famm, K., Hansen, L., Christ, D., and Winter, G. (2008). Thermodynamically stable aggregation-resistant antibody domains through directed evolution. *J. Mol. Biol.* **376**:926–931.

Fermi, C. (1908). On immunization against rabies (über die immunisierung gegen wutkrankheit). *Med. Microbiol. Immunol.* **58**:233–276.

Fournier, P., Montagnon, B., Vincent-Falquet, J. C., Ajjan, N., Drucker, J., and Roumiantzeff, M. (1985). A new vaccine produced from rabies virus cultivated on Vero cells. *In* "Improvements in Rabies Post-exposure Treatment" (I. Vodopija, K. G. Nicholson, S. Smerdel, and U. Bijok, eds.), pp. 129–136. Zagreb Institute of Public Health, Zagreb.

Fuenzalida, E., Palacios, R., and Borgono, J. M. (1964). Antirabies antibody response in man to vaccine made from infected suckling-mouse brains. *Bull. World Health Organ.* **30**:431–436.

Gluck, R., Wegmann, A., Germanier, R., Keller, H., Hess, M. W., Kraus-Ruppert, R., and Wandeler, A. I. (1984). A new, highly immunogenic duck embryo rabies vaccine. *Lancet* **1**:844–845.

Gluck, R., Matthieu, J. M., Wegmann, A., and Mean, F. (1986). Absence of myelin basic protein in an improved purified duck embryo rabies vaccine. *Neurochem. Pathol.* **4**:69–75.

Goudsmit, J., Marissen, W. E., Weldon, W. C., Niezgoda, M., Hanlon, C. A., Rice, A. B., Kruif, J., Dietzschold, B., Bakker, A. B., and Rupprecht, C. E. (2006). Comparison of an anti-rabies human monoclonal antibody combination with human polyclonal anti-rabies immune globulin. *J. Infect. Dis.* **193**:796–801.

Grosenbaugh, D. A., Maki, J. L., Rupprecht, C. E., and Wall, D. K. (2007). Rabies challenge of captive striped skunks (Mephitis mephitis) following oral administration of a live vaccinia-vectored rabies vaccine. *J. Wildl. Dis.* **43**:124–132.

Hendrick, M. J., Shofer, F. S., Goldschmidt, M. H., Haviland, J. C., Schelling, S. H., Engler, S. J., and Gliatto, J. M. (1994). Comparison of fibrosarcomas that developed at vaccination sites and at nonvaccination sites in cats: 239 cases (1991–1992). *J. Am. Vet. Med. Assoc.* **205**:1425–1429.

Houimel, M., and Dellagi, K. (2009). Isolation and characterization of human neutralizing antibodies to rabies virus derived from a recombinant immune antibody library. *J. Virol. Methods* **161**:205–215.

Hu, W. T., Willoughby, R. E., Jr., Dhonau, H., and Mack, K. J. (2007). Long-term follow-up after treatment of rabies by induction of coma. *N. Engl. J. Med.* **357**:945–946.

Ito, N., Sugiyama, M., Yamada, K., Shimizu, K., Takayama-Ito, M., Hosokawa, J., and Minamoto, N. (2005). Characterization of M gene-deficient rabies virus with advantages of effective immunization and safety as a vaccine strain. *Microbiol. Immunol.* **49**:971–979.

Jackson, A. C., Warrell, M. J., Rupprecht, C. E., Ertl, H. C., Dietzschold, B., O'Reilly, M., Leach, R. P., Fu, Z. F., Wunner, W. H., Bleck, T. P., and Wilde, H. (2003). Management of rabies in humans. *Clin. Infect. Dis.* **36:**60–63.

Jahrling, P. B., Hesse, R. A., Eddy, G. A., Johnson, K. M., Callis, R. T., and Stephen, E. L. (1980). Lassa virus infection of rhesus monkeys: Pathogenesis and treatment with ribavirin. *J. Infect. Dis.* **141:**580–589.

Kammer, A. R., and Ertl, H. C. (2002). Rabies vaccines: From the past to the 21st century. *Hybrid. Hybridomics* **21:**123–127.

Kass, P. H., Barnes, W. G., Jr., Spangler, W. L., Chomel, B. B., and Culbertson, M. R. (1993). Epidemiologic evidence for a causal relation between vaccination and fibrosarcoma tumorigenesis in cats. *J. Am. Vet. Med. Assoc.* **203:**396–405.

Ko, K. S., Tekoah, Y., Rudd, P. M., Harvey, D. J., Dwek, R. A., Spitsin, S., Hanlon, C. A., Rupprecht, C., Dietzschold, B., Golovkin, M., and Koprowski, H. (2003). Function and glycosylation of plant-derived antiviral monoclonal antibody. *Proc. Natl. Acad. Sci. USA* **100:**8013–8018.

Kondo, A. (1965). Growth characteristics of rabies virus in primary chick embryo cells. *Virology* **27:**199–204.

Koprowski, H., and Cox, H. R. (1948). Studies on chick embryo adapted rabies virus: Culture characteristics and pathogenicity. *J. Immunol.* **60:**533–554.

Kramer, R. A., Marissen, W. E., Goudsmit, J., Visser, T. J., Clijsters-Van der Horst, M., Bakker, A. Q., de Jong, M., Jongeneelen, M., Thijsse, S., Backus, H. H., Rice, A. B., Weldon, W. C., *et al.* (2005). The human antibody repertoire specific for rabies virus glycoprotein as selected from immune libraries. *Eur. J. Immunol.* **35:**2131–2145.

Kreindel, S. M., McGuill, M., Meltzer, M., Rupprecht, C., and DeMaria, A., Jr. (1998). The cost of rabies postexposure prophylaxis: One state's experience. *Public Health Rep.* **113:**247–251.

Kureishi, A., Xu, L. Z., Wu, H., and Stiver, H. G. (1992). Rabies in China: Recommendations for control. *Bull. World Health Organ.* **70:**443–450.

Lafay, F., Benejean, J., Tuffereau, C., Flamand, A., and Coulon, P. (1994). Vaccination against rabies: Construction and characterization of SAG2, a double avirulent derivative of SADBern. *Vaccine* **12:**317–320.

Lafon, M. (2005). Modulation of the immune response in the nervous system by rabies virus. *Curr. Top. Microbiol. Immunol.* **289:**239–258.

Lafon, M., Wiktor, T. J., and Macfarlan, R. I. (1983). Antigenic sites on the CVS rabies virus glycoprotein: Analysis with monoclonal antibodies. *J. Gen. Virol.* **64:**843–851.

Lang, J., Attanath, P., Quiambao, B., Singhasivanon, V., Chanthavanich, P., Montalban, C., Lutsch, C., Pepin-Covatta, S., Le Mener, V., Miranda, M., and Sabcharoen, A. (1998a). Evaluation of the safety, immunogenicity, and pharmacokinetic profile of a new, highly purified, heat-treated equine rabies immunoglobulin, administered either alone or in association with a purified, Vero-cell rabies vaccine. *Acta Trop.* **70:**317–333.

Lang, J., Gravenstein, S., Briggs, D., Miller, B., Froeschle, J., Dukes, C., Le Mener, V., and Lutsch, C. (1998b). Evaluation of the safety and immunogenicity of a new, heat-treated human rabies immune globulin using a sham, post-exposure prophylaxis of rabies. *Biologicals* **26:**7–15.

Lau, J. Y., Tam, R. C., Liang, T. J., and Hong, Z. (2002). Mechanism of action of ribavirin in the combination treatment of chronic HCV infection. *Hepatology* **35:**1002–1009.

Leach, C. N., and Johnson, H. N. (1940). Human rabies, with special reference to virus distribution and titer. *Am. J. Trop. Med.* **s1–20:**335–340.

Lee, C. M., Iorno, N., Sierro, F., and Christ, D. (2007). Selection of human antibody fragments by phage display. *Nat. Protoc.* **2:**3001–3008.

Lin, F. T. (1990). The protective effect of the large-scale use of PHKC rabies vaccine in humans in China. *Bull. World Health Organ.* **68:**449–454.

Lin, F., Zeng, F., Lu, L., Lu, X., Zen, R., Yu, Y., and Chen, N. (1983). The primary hamster kidney cell rabies vaccine: Adaptation of viral strain, production of vaccine, and pre- and postexposure treatment. *J. Infect. Dis.* **147:**467–473.

Lingappa, V. R., and Lingappa, J. R. (2005). Recent insights into biological regulation from cell-free protein-synthesizing systems. *Mt. Sinai J. Med.* **72:**141–160.

Lockhart, B. P., Tsiang, H., Cecaldi, P. E., and Guillemer, S. (1991). Ketamine-mediated inhibition of rabies virus infection in vitro and in rat brain. *Antiviral Chem. Chemother.* **2:**9–15.

Lockhart, B. P., Tordo, N., and Tsiang, H. (1992). Inhibition of rabies virus transcription in rat cortical neurons with the dissociative anesthetic ketamine. *Antimicrob. Agents Chemother.* **36:**1750–1755.

Loza-Rubio, E., Rojas, E., Gomez, L., Olivera, M. T., and Gomez-Lim, M. A. (2008). Development of an edible rabies vaccine in maize using the Vnukovo strain. *Dev. Biol. (Basel)* **131:**477–482.

Marissen, W. E., Kramer, R. A., Rice, A., Weldon, W. C., Niezgoda, M., Faber, M., Slootstra, J. W., Meloen, R. H., Clijsters-van der Horst, M., Visser, T. J., Jongeneelen, M., Thijsse, S., et al. (2005). Novel rabies virus-neutralizing epitope recognized by human monoclonal antibody: Fine mapping and escape mutant analysis. *J. Virol.* **79:**4672–4678.

McGarvey, P. B., Hammond, J., Dienelt, M. M., Hooper, D. C., Fu, Z. F., Dietzschold, B., Koprowski, H., and Michaels, F. H. (1995). Expression of the rabies virus glycoprotein in transgenic tomatoes. *Biotechnology* **13:**1484–1487.

Merigan, T. C., Baer, G. M., Winkler, W. G., Bernard, K. W., Gibert, C. G., Chany, C., and Veronesi, R. (1984). Human leukocyte interferon administration to patients with symptomatic and suspected rabies. *Ann. Neurol.* **16:**82–87.

Modelska, A., Dietzschold, B., Sleysh, N., Fu, Z. F., Steplewski, K., Hooper, D. C., Koprowski, H., and Yusibov, V. (1998). Immunization against rabies with plant-derived antigen. *Proc. Natl. Acad. Sci. USA* **95:**2481–2485.

Muller, T., Dietzschold, B., Ertl, H., Fooks, A. R., Freuling, C., Fehlner-Gardiner, C., Kliemt, J., Meslin, F. X., Franka, R., Rupprecht, C. E., Tordo, N., Wanderler, A. I., et al. (2009). Development of a mouse monoclonal antibody cocktail for post-exposure rabies prophylaxis in humans. *PLoS Negl. Trop. Dis.* **3:**e542.

Nadin-Davis, S. A., and Fehlner-Gardiner, C. (2008). Lyssaviruses: Current trends. *Adv. Virus Res.* **71:**207–250.

Nagarajan, T., Rupprecht, C. E., Dessain, S. K., Rangarajan, P. N., Thiagarajan, D., and Srinivasan, V. A. (2008). Human monoclonal antibody and vaccine approaches to prevent human rabies. *Curr. Top. Microbiol. Immunol.* **317:**67–101.

National Association of State Public Health Veterinarians Committee(2008). Compendium of animal rabies prevention and control . *J. Am. Vet. Med. Assoc.* **232:**1478–1486.

Osinubi, M. O., Wu, X., Franka, R., Niezgoda, M., Nok, A. J., Ogunkoya, A. B., and Rupprecht, C. E. (2009). Enhancing comparative rabies DNA vaccine effectiveness through glycoprotein gene modifications. *Vaccine* **27:**7214–7218.

Plotkin, S. A. (2000). Rabies. *Clin. Infect. Dis.* **30:**4–12.

Porter, R. H., and Greenamyre, J. T. (1995). Regional variations in the pharmacology of NMDA receptor channel blockers: Implications for therapeutic potential. *J. Neurochem.* **64:**614–623.

Powers, C. N., Peavy, D. L., and Knight, V. (1982). Selective inhibition of functional lymphocyte subpopulations by ribavirin. *Antimicrob. Agents Chemother.* **22:**108–114.

Prosniak, M., Faber, M., Hanlon, C. A., Rupprecht, C. E., Hooper, D. C., and Dietzschold, B. (2003). Development of a cocktail of recombinant-expressed human rabies virus-neutralizing monoclonal antibodies for postexposure prophylaxis of rabies. *J. Infect. Dis.* **188:**53–56.

Real, E., Rain, J. C., Battaglia, V., Jallet, C., Perrin, P., Tordo, N., Chrisment, P., D'Alayer, J., Legrain, P., and Jacob, Y. (2004). Antiviral drug discovery strategy using combinatorial libraries of structurally constrained peptides. *J. Virol.* **78:**7410–7417.

Rojas-Anaya, E., Loza-Rubio, E., Olivera-Flores, M. T., and Gomez-Lim, M. (2009). Expression of rabies virus G protein in carrots (Daucus carota). *Transgenic Res.* **18:**911–919.

Roumiantzeff, M., Ajjan, N., Branche, R., Fournier, P., Montagnon, B., Trotemann, P., and Vincent-Falquet, J. C. (1984). Rabies vaccine produced in cell-culture: Production and control and clinical results. *In* "Applied Virology" (E. Kurstak, ed.), pp. 241–296. Academic Press, Orlando, FL.

Rubin, D. H., and Ruley, H. E. (2006). Cellular genetics of host susceptibility and resistance to virus infection. *Crit. Rev. Eukaryot. Gene Expr.* **16:**155–170.

Ruegsegger, J. M., Black, J., and Sharpless, G. R. (1961). Primary antirabies immunization of man with HEP flury virus vaccine. *Am. J. Public Health* **51:**706–716.

Satpathy, D. M., Sahu, T., and Behera, T. R. (2005). Equine rabies immunoglobulin: A study on its clinical safety. *J. Indian Med. Assoc.* **103**(238):241–242.

Semple, D. (1911). The preparation of a safe and efficient antirabic vaccine, Vol. 44. Sci. Mem. Med. Sanit. Dept., India.

Sharpless, G. R., Black, J., Cox, H. R., and Ruegsegger, J. M. (1957). Preliminary observations in primary antirabies immunization of man with different types of high-egg-passage Flury virus. *Bull. World Health Organ.* **17:**905–910.

Shoji, Y., Inoue, S., Nakamichi, K., Kurane, I., Sakai, T., and Morimoto, K. (2004). Generation and characterization of P gene-deficient rabies virus. *Virology* **318:**295–305.

Sloan, S. E., Hanlon, C., Weldon, W., Niezgoda, M., Blanton, J., Self, J., Rowley, K. J., Mandell, R. B., Babcock, G. J., Thomas, W. D., Jr., Rupprecht, C. E., and Ambrosino, D. M. (2007). Identification and characterization of a human monoclonal antibody that potently neutralizes a broad panel of rabies virus isolates. *Vaccine* **25:**2800–2810.

Steck, F., Wandeler, A., Bichsel, P., Capt, S., Hafliger, U., and Schneider, L. (1982). Oral immunization of foxes against rabies. Laboratory and field studies. *Comp. Immunol. Microbiol. Infect. Dis.* **5:**165–171.

Stoof, J. C., Booij, J., and Drukarch, B. (1992). Amantadine as N-methyl-D-aspartic acid receptor antagonist: New possibilities for therapeutic applications? *Clin. Neurol. Neurosurg.* **94**(Suppl.):S4–S6.

Suntharasamai, P., Chanthavanich, P., Warrell, M. J., Looareesuwan, S., Karbwang, J., Supanaranond, W., Phillips, R. E., Jansawan, W., Xueref, C., Pouradier-Duteil, X., and Warrell, D. A. (1986). Purified Vero cell rabies vaccine and human diploid cell strain vaccine: Comparison of neutralizing antibody responses to post-exposure regimens. *J. Hyg.* **96:**483–489.

Superti, F., Seganti, L., Pana, A., and Orsi, N. (1985). Effect of amantadine on rhabdovirus infection. *Drugs Exp. Clin. Res.* **11:**69–74.

Tam, R. C., Ramasamy, K., Bard, J., Pai, B., Lim, C., and Averett, D. R. (2000). The ribavirin analog ICN 17261 demonstrates reduced toxicity and antiviral effects with retention of both immunomodulatory activity and reduction of hepatitis-induced serum alanine aminotransferase levels. *Antimicrob. Agents Chemother.* **44:**1276–1283.

Tordo, N. (2010). New strategies for diagnosis and therapy of Lyssaviruses. Rabies in the Americas XXI, Guadalajara, Mexico.

Ueki, Y., Goldfarb, I. S., Harindranath, N., Gore, M., Koprowski, H., Notkins, A. L., and Casali, P. (1990). Clonal analysis of a human antibody response. Quantitation of precursors of antibody-producing cells and generation and characterization of monoclonal IgM, IgG, and IgA to rabies virus. *J. Exp. Med.* **171:**19–34.

Vodopija, I., and Clarke, H. F. (1991). Human vaccination against rabies. *In* "The Natural History of Rabies" (G. M. Baer, ed.), pp. 571–595. CRC Press, Boca Raton, FL.

Vos, A., Neubert, A., Pommerening, E., Muller, T., Dohner, L., Neubert, L., and Hughes, K. (2001). Immunogenicity of an E1-deleted recombinant human adenovirus against rabies by different routes of administration. *J. Gen. Virol.* **82**:2191–2197.

Wang, Y., Rowley, K. J., Booth, B. J., Sloan, S. E., Fehlner-Gardiner, C., Wandeler, A., Ambrosino, D. M., and Babcock, G. J. (2009). G glycoprotein amino acid residues required for RAB1 neutralization are conserved in rabies virus street isolates. Rabies in the Americas XX, Quebec City, Canada.

Warrell, M. J., White, N. J., Looareesuwan, S., Phillips, R. E., Suntharasamai, P., Chanthavanich, P., Riganti, M., Fisher-Hoch, S. P., Nicholson, K. G., Manatsathit, S., Vannaphan, S., and Warrell, D. A. (1989). Failure of interferon alfa and tribavirin in rabies encephalitis. *Br. Med. J.* **299**:830–833.

Weinmann, E., Majer, M., and Hilfenhaus, J. (1979). Intramuscular and/or intralumbar postexposure treatment of rabies virus-infected cynomolgus monkeys with human interferon. *Infect. Immun.* **24**:24–31.

Weli, S. C., Scott, C. A., Ward, C. A., and Jackson, A. C. (2006). Rabies virus infection of primary neuronal cultures and adult mice: Failure to demonstrate evidence of excitotoxicity. *J. Virol.* **80**:10270–10273.

Wiktor, T. J., and Clark, H. F. (1972). Chronic rabies virus infection of cell-cultures. *Infect. Immun.* **6**:988–995.

Wiktor, T. J., Fernandes, M. V., and Koprowski, H. (1964). Cultivation of rabies virus in human diploid cell strain Wi-38. *J. Immunol.* **93**:353–366.

Wiktor, T. J., Macfarlan, R. I., Reagan, K. J., Dietzschold, B., Curtis, P. J., Wunner, W. H., Kieny, M. P., Lathe, R., Lecocq, J. P., Mackett, M., *et al.* (1984). Protection from rabies by a vaccinia virus recombinant containing the rabies virus glycoprotein gene. *Proc. Natl. Acad. Sci. USA* **81**:7194–7198.

Wilde, H. (2007). Failures of post-exposure rabies prophylaxis. *Vaccine* **25**:7605–7609.

Wilde, H., and Chutivongse, S. (1990). Equine rabies immune globulin: A product with an undeserved poor reputation. *Am. J. Trop. Med. Hyg.* **42**:175–178.

Wilde, H., Chomchey, P., Prakongsri, S., Puyaratabandhu, P., and Chutivongse, S. (1989). Adverse effects of equine rabies immune globulin. *Vaccine* **7**:10–11.

Willoughby, R. E., Jr., Tieves, K. S., Hoffman, G. M., Ghanayem, N. S., Amlie-Lefond, C. M., Schwabe, M. J., Chusid, M. J., and Rupprecht, C. E. (2005). Survival after treatment of rabies with induction of coma. *N. Engl. J. Med.* **352**:2508–2514.

Wu, X., and Rupprecht, C. E. (2008). Glycoprotein gene relocation in rabies virus. *Virus Res.* **131**:95–99.

Wu, X., Franka, R., Svoboda, P., Pohl, J., and Rupprecht, C. E. (2009). Development of combined vaccines for rabies and immunocontraception. *Vaccine* **27**:7202–7209.

Wu, X., Franka, R., Jackson, F. R., Carson, W. C., Ellison, J. A., and Rupprecht, C. E. (2010). Two copies of GnRH fused to rabies virus glycoprotein induce efficient immunocontraception in a mouse model. Rabies in the Americas XXI, Guadalajara, Mexico.

Wunner, W. H., and Briggs, D. J. (2010). Rabies in the 21 century. *PLoS Negl. Trop. Dis.* **4**:591.

Wunner, W. H., Pallatroni, C., and Curtis, P. J. (2004). Selection of genetic inhibitors of rabies virus. *Arch. Virol.* **149**:1653–1662.

Xiang, Z., Gao, G., Reyes-Sandoval, A., Cohen, C. J., Li, Y., Bergelson, J. M., Wilson, J. M., and Ertl, H. C. (2002). Novel, chimpanzee serotype 68-based adenoviral vaccine carrier for induction of antibodies to a transgene product. *J. Virol.* **76**:2667–2675.

Yarosh, O. K., Wandeler, A. I., Graham, F. L., Campbell, J. B., and Prevec, L. (1996). Human adenovirus type 5 vectors expressing rabies glycoprotein. *Vaccine* **14**:1257–1264.

Yoshino, K., Taniguchi, S., and Arai, K. (1966). Plaque assay of rabies virus in chick embryo cells. *Arch. Virol.* **18**:370–373.

CHAPTER **17**

Therapy of Human Rabies

Alan C. Jackson*,†

Contents

Abstract

Preventive therapy for rabies, including wound cleansing and active and passive immunization after a recognized exposure, is highly efficacious. Unfortunately, there is no established therapy that is effective for patients who develop rabies encephalomyelitis. There have been several survivors from rabies and all but one received rabies vaccine prior to the onset of clinical illness. Aggressive approaches to therapy of human rabies may be appropriate in certain situations. There is no scientific rationale for the use of therapeutic coma, and there are many reports of failures using this approach. Therapeutic coma should be abandoned for the therapy of rabies. New approaches such as therapeutic hypothermia should be evaluated, in combination with other therapeutic agents. More basic research is needed on the mechanisms involved in rabies pathogenesis, which will hopefully facilitate the development of new therapeutic approaches in the future for this ancient disease.

* Department of Internal Medicine (Neurology), University of Manitoba, Winnipeg, Manitoba, Canada
† Department of Medical Microbiology, University of Manitoba, Winnipeg, Manitoba, Canada

Advances in Virus Research, Volume 79
ISSN 0065-3527, DOI: 10.1016/B978-0-12-387040-7.00017-2

I. INTRODUCTION

Worldwide, there are at least 55,000 human cases of rabies each year (World Health Organization, 2005) and perhaps as many as 75,000 or more. Rabies virus transmission almost always occurs in association with animal bites. Most human rabies cases are related to transmission where there is endemic dog rabies in resource-limited or resource-poor countries, particularly in Asia and Africa. In North America, there is rabies in wildlife, including in bats, raccoons, skunks, and foxes, and relatively few human cases occur. In the United States and Canada, most human cases are caused by bat rabies virus variants, and many of these cases are due to unrecognized bat exposures. Patients who develop rabies have a very dismal outcome. Although it is unclear why an American girl survived rabies in 2004 (Willoughby *et al.*, 2005), this favorable outcome offers hope that aggressive approaches to therapy may become more successful in the future (Jackson, 2005). Unfortunately, no effective therapy for rabies is available at this time. An improved understanding of the pathogenesis of rabies may be helpful in designing novel therapies for the future.

II. PREVENTION OF RABIES

Rabies can be very effectively prevented after a recognized exposure. It is important that current recommendations for rabies prevention (Manning *et al.*, 2008; World Health Organization, 2005), which are available in the Morbidity and Mortality Weekly Report (http://www.cdc.gov/mmwr/) and World Health Organization (http://www.who.int/en/) Web sites, are closely followed because even minor deviations can lead to failure of preventive therapy. After a human is bitten by a dog, cat, or ferret, the animal should be captured, confined, and observed for a period of at least 10 days and then examined by a veterinarian prior to its release. This approach cannot be taken with any other species, and a laboratory examination of the brain is necessary for confirmation of the presence or absence of rabies, which is also the approach if a confined animal develops signs suggestive of rabies. Effective postexposure therapy for rabies includes wound cleansing and both active and passive immunization in a previously unimmunized individual (Manning *et al.*, 2008). Active immunization is achieved with four doses of vaccine, which was recently updated from a recommendation for five doses (Rupprecht *et al.*, 2010), with the use of a modern cell-culture vaccine, including purified chick embryo cell-culture vaccine or human diploid cell vaccine (administered intramuscularly in the deltoid muscle on days 0, 3, 7, and 14). Passive immunization is performed with human rabies immune globulin at a dosage of 20 IU/kg with local infiltration into and around the wound(s); any remainder of the volume should be given intramuscularly at a site distant from the site of vaccine administration.

III. THERAPY OF RABIES

The ideal therapy for a patient with rabies is unknown. Until recently, only patients who received rabies vaccine prior to the onset of their disease had survived. A variety of approaches have proved to be unsuccessful. Therapy with human leukocyte interferon, given as high-dose intraventricular and systemic (intramuscular) administration, in three patients was not associated with a beneficial clinical effect, but this therapy was not initiated until between 8 and 14 days after the onset of symptoms (Merigan et al., 1984). Similarly, antiviral therapy with intravenous ribavirin (16 patients given doses of 16–400 mg) was unsuccessful in China (Kureishi et al., 1992). An open trial of therapy with combined intravenous and intrathecal administration of either ribavirin (one patient) or interferon-α (three patients; Warrell et al., 1989) was also unsuccessful. Anti-rabies virus hyperimmune serum of either human or equine origin has been administered intravenously and by the intrathecal routes (Basgoz and Frosch, 1998; Emmons et al., 1973; Hattwick et al., 1976; Hemachudha et al., 2003), but there was no beneficial effect.

A group of physicians with expertise in rabies and rabies researchers published an article in 2003 giving recommendations on therapies that could be considered for an aggressive approach (Jackson et al., 2003). Young and previously healthy patients with an early clinical diagnosis of rabies (prior to laboratory confirmation) and prompt initiation of therapy should offer the best opportunity for a favorable outcome (Jackson et al., 2003). Therapies for potential consideration include rabies vaccine, human rabies immune globulin, monoclonal antibodies (for the future), ribavirin, interferon-α, and ketamine. The recommendation for therapy with ketamine was based on animal studies performed at Institut Pasteur in Paris (Lockhart et al., 1991). Similar to current therapies for cancer, human immunodeficiency virus infection, and chronic hepatitis C infection, it was felt that a combination of therapies might prove effective in situations that specific therapies had failed previously.

In 2004, a patient survived rabies who had not received rabies vaccine or any other prophylactic therapy for rabies prior to the onset of clinical disease (Willoughby et al., 2005) This 15-year-old female was bitten by a bat on her left index finger. About 1 month after the bite, she developed numbness and tingling of her left hand, and over the next 3 days, she developed diplopia, bilateral partial sixth-nerve palsies, and unsteadiness. An MR imaging study of the brain was normal. On her 4th day of illness, CSF examination showed a pleocytosis (23 white blood cells/μL, predominantly lymphocytes) and mildly elevated protein. She subsequently developed fever (38.8 °C), nystagmus, left arm tremor, and hypersalivation, and the history of the bat bite was obtained at about this time. The patient was transferred to a tertiary care hospital in Milwaukee, Wisconsin 5 days after the onset of neurologic symptoms. Neutralizing anti-rabies virus antibodies were detected in sera and CSF (initially at titers of 1:102 and 1:47, respectively). Nuchal skin biopsies were negative for rabies virus antigen, rabies virus RNA was not detected in the skin biopsies or in saliva by RT-PCR, and attempts at rabies virus isolation on saliva were negative. The patient was intubated and put into a drug-induced coma, which included the noncompetitive N-methyl-D-aspartate (NMDA) antagonist ketamine, administered at 48 mg/kg/day as a continuous infusion and intravenous midazolam for 7 days. A burst-suppression pattern on her electroencephalogram was maintained and this required the use of supplemental phenobarbital. She also received antiviral therapy, including intravenous ribavirin and amantadine (200 mg/day administered enterally). The justification for amantadine was on the basis of an obscure *in vitro* study (Superti *et al.*, 1985). She improved and was discharged from hospital with neurologic deficits, and she has subsequently shown progressive neurologic improvement (Hu *et al.*, 2007).

This is the first documented survivor who had not received rabies vaccine prior to the onset of clinical rabies. As discussed in an accompanying editorial, it is unknown if therapy with one or more specific agents played an important role in the favorable outcome of this patient (Jackson, 2005). However, since that time, there have been at least 20 cases in which the main components of this approach (the "Milwaukee Protocol") have been used and fatal outcomes have resulted (Table I). There is also evidence that this protocol has been used in additional cases (Willoughby, 2009), and perhaps many others, but the details are not known and likely will never be reported. The induction of coma *per se* has not been shown to be useful in the management of infectious diseases of the nervous system, and there is no evidence supporting this approach in rabies or in other viral encephalitides. Hence, therapeutic coma should not become a routine therapy for the management of rabies. Unlike other viral infections of the nervous system, including Sindbis virus encephalomyelitis (Darman *et al.*, 2004; Nargi-Aizenman and Griffin, 2001; Nargi-Aizenman *et al.*, 2004) and human immunodeficiency virus infection (Kaul and Lipton, 2007), there is no established experimental evidence supporting excitotoxicity in rabies, and there is recent evidence in an animal model that demonstrated the lack of efficacy of ketamine therapy, which argues against this hypothesis (Weli *et al.*, 2006). Even where there is strong experimental evidence of excitotoxicity in animal models,

Case no.	Year of death	Age and sex of patient	Virus source	Country	Reference
1	2005	47 male	Kidney and pancreas transplant (dog)	Germany	Maier et al. (2010)
2	2005	46 female	Lung transplant (dog)	Germany	Maier et al. (2010)
3	2005	72 male	Kidney transplant (dog)	Germany	Maier et al. (2010)
4	2005	Unknown	Dog	India	Bagchi (2005)
5	2005	7 male	Vampire bat	Brazil	—[a]
6	2005	20–30 female	Vampire bat	Brazil	—[a]
7	2006	33 male	Dog	Thailand	Hemachudha et al. (2006)
8	2006	16 male	Bat	USA (Texas)	Houston Chronicle (2006)
9	2006	10 female	Bat	USA (Indiana)	Christenson et al. (2007)
10	2006	11 male	Dog (Philippines)	USA (California)	Christenson et al. (2007)
11	2007	73 male	Bat	Canada (Alberta)	McDermid et al. (2008)
12	2007	55 male	Dog (Morocco)	Germany	Drosten (2007)
13	2007	34 female	Bat (Kenya)	The Netherlands	van Thiel et al. (2009)
14	2008	5 male	Dog	Equatorial Guinea	Rubin et al. (2009)
15	2008	55 male	Bat	USA (Missouri)	Pue et al. (2009), Turabelidze et al. (2009)
16	2008	8 female	Cat	Colombia	Juncosa (2008)
17	2008	15 male	Vampire bat	Colombia	Badillo et al. (2009)
18	2009	37 female	Dog (South Africa)	Northern Ireland	Hunter et al. (2010)
19	2009	42 male	Dog (India)	USA (Virginia)	Troell et al. (2010)
20	2010	11 female	Cat	Romania	—[b]

[a] Personal communication from Dr. Rita Medeiros, University of Para, Belem, Brazil.
[b] Personal communication from Dr. Mihai A. Turcitu, Institute for Diagnosis and Animal Health, National Reference Laboratory for Rabies, Bucharest, Romania.

multiple clinical trials in humans have shown a lack of efficacy of neuro-protective agents in stroke (Ginsberg, 2009). Hence, a strong neuroprotec-tive effect of a therapy given to a single patient without a clear scientific rationale is not likely responsible for a favorable outcome. It is much more likely that this patient would have recovered with only supportive ther-apy and did well to tolerate the additional "insult" of therapeutic coma without having adverse effects.

The presence of neutralizing anti-rabies virus antibodies early in a patient's clinical course is likely an important factor contributing to a favorable outcome. This probably occurs in less than 20% of all patients with rabies. The presence of neutralizing anti-rabies virus antibodies is a marker of an active adaptive immune response that is essential for viral clearance (Lafon, 2007). There have been six survivors of rabies who received rabies vaccine prior to the onset of their disease (and only one who did not receive vaccine). This supports the notion that an early immune response is associated with a positive outcome. Bat rabies viruses may be less neurovirulent than canine or other variants that are responsi-ble for most human cases of rabies (Lafon, 2005), and rabies due to canine rabies virus variants may have a less favorable outcome than cases caused by bat rabies variants. A previous survivor of rabies, who received rabies vaccine prior to the onset of disease, had a good neurological recovery and was also infected with a bat rabies virus (Hattwick et al., 1972). It is unknown if the causative bat rabies virus variant in the Milwaukee case was, in some way, attenuated and different from previously isolated bat rabies virus variants because viral isolation was not successful. There is also another case with transmission of rabies from a vampire bat in Brazil, in which the patient received rabies vaccine prior to the onset of disease and was also treated with the Milwaukee protocol; this case has been reported only in preliminary form (Ministerio da Saude in Brazil, 2008). Finally, most survivors of rabies have shown neutralizing anti-rabies virus antibodies in sera and cerebrospinal fluid, but other diagnostic laboratory tests are usually negative for rabies virus antigen and RNA in fluids and tissues (brain tissues not tested). This may be because viral clearance was so effective that centrifugal spread of the infection to peripheral organ sites was reduced or rapid clearance occurred through immune-mediated mechanisms.

An aggressive approach to therapy of rabies will require the full resources of a critical care unit and has a high risk of failure. The following should all be considered a "favorable" factors for initiating an aggressive therapeutic approach: (1) therapy with dose(s) of rabies vaccine prior to the onset of illness, (2) young age, (3) healthy and immunecompetent individual, (4) rabies due to a bat rabies variant (e.g., in contrast to a canine variant), (5) early presence of neutralizing anti-rabies virus anti-bodies in serum and CSF, and (6) mild neurological disease at the time of initiation of therapy. Laboratory tests for the detection of rabies virus antigen and RNA may be persistently negative in potential rabies survivors because viral clearance has already been initiated by the individual's immune response.

IV. NEW APPROACHES

New approaches to treating human rabies need to be developed rather than repeating ineffective therapies. Finding an effective neuroprotective drug is highly unlikely with a "trial and error" approach in light of the fact that over 100 clinical trials have already shown a lack of efficacy for a single neuroprotective drug for acute stroke, whereas many of these drugs showed efficacy *in vivo* in animal models (Ginsberg, 2009). The most effective "neuroprotective" therapy for an acute brain insult is therapeutic hypothermia, in which the body temperature is reduced by a variety of cooling methods to reduce neuronal injury and improve clinical outcomes. Efficacy has been established in Australian (Bernard *et al.*, 2002) and European (The Hypothermia After Cardiac Arrest Study Group, 2002) studies for patients who remain unconscious after witnessed cardiac arrest due to ventricular fibrillation. Efficacy for hypothermia for traumatic brain injury has not yet been established (Christian *et al.*, 2008). Hypothermia decreases cerebral metabolism, production of reactive oxygen species, lipid peroxidation, and inflammatory response activity, which, at least in part, may explain its beneficial effects. There are generalized methods of inducing hypothermia and also regional methods that can be applied to the head and neck, which include use of a cooling helmet (Wang *et al.*, 2004) and intranasal cooling (Busch *et al.*, 2010; Castren *et al.*, 2010). Intranasal cooling involves spraying an inert evaporative coolant via nasal prongs that rapidly evaporates after contact with the nasopharynx, and it has the advantage that it reduces the temperature more rapidly. The regional methods are associated with less systemic adverse effects and would also be expected to have a reduced effect on a natural or rabies vaccine-induced systemic immune response, which is important for viral clearance in rabies virus infection. Rabies virus replication is generally fairly efficient at lower-than-normal body temperatures (e.g., 33 °C), particularly with infection of an epithelial cell line with a bat rabies virus variant (Morimoto *et al.*, 1996). However, there may be reduced viral spread due to inhibitory effects of hypothermia on fast axonal transport (Bisby and Jones, 1978) and *trans*-synaptic spread as well as other beneficial and neuroprotective effects. Under natural conditions, hibernation of rabies vectors likely results in "suspension" of viral replication (Sulkin *et al.*, 1960) and inhibition of viral spread by marked inhibition of axonal transport (Bisby and Jones, 1978) due to very low body temperatures (e.g., below 5–10 °C). In contrast, therapeutic mild (34 °C) or moderate (30 °C) hypothermia maintained for periods of 24–48 h would be expected to be associated with more modest but potentially beneficial effects. Entirely new approaches need to be taken for the aggressive management of human rabies, which may combine a variety of different therapeutic approaches, including, for example, hypothermia and antiviral drugs. Nevertheless, further research is also needed to gain a better understanding of basic pathogenetic mechanisms in rabies, which may open the door to novel therapeutic approaches in the future.

V. CONCLUSIONS

Although rabies can be prevented after recognized exposures, no effective therapy for human rabies is available. It remains highly doubtful that the Milwaukee Protocol will prove to be useful in the management of human rabies. Repetition of this therapy will likely impede progress in developing new effective therapies for rabies. More basic research is needed to improve our understanding of basic mechanisms underlying rabies pathogenesis in humans and animals. In the meantime, new therapeutic approaches such as hypothermia should be evaluated in combination with antiviral and other therapeutic agents to conquer this ancient disease.

REFERENCES

Badillo, R., Mantilla, J. C., and Pradilla, G. (2009). Human rabies encephalitis by a vampire bat bite in an urban area of Colombia (Spanish). *Biomédica* **29**:191–203.

Bagchi, S. (2005). Coma Therapy. The Telegraph, Calcutta. July 4, 2005.

Basgoz, N., and Frosch, M. P. (1998). Case records of the Massachusetts General Hospital: A 32-year-old woman with pharyngeal spasms and paresthesias after a dog bite. *N. Engl. J. Med.* **339**:105–112.

Bernard, S. A., Gray, T. W., Buist, M. D., Jones, B. M., Silvester, W., Gutteridge, G., and Smith, K. (2002). Treatment of comatose survivors of out-of-hospital cardiac arrest with induced hypothermia. *N. Engl. J. Med.* **346**:557–563.

Bisby, M. A., and Jones, D. L. (1978). Temperature sensitivity of axonal transport in hibernating and nonhibernating rodents. *Exp. Neurol.* **61**:74–83.

Busch, H. J., Eichwede, F., Fodisch, M., Taccone, F. S., Wobker, G., Schwab, T., Hopf, H. B., Tonner, P., Hachimi-Idrissi, S., Martens, P., Fritz, H., Bode, C., *et al.* (2010). Safety and feasibility of nasopharyngeal evaporative cooling in the emergency department setting in survivors of cardiac arrest. *Resuscitation* **81**:943–949.

Castren, M., Nordberg, P., Svensson, L., Taccone, F., Vincent, J. L., Desruelles, D., Eichwede, F., Mols, P., Schwab, T., Vergnion, M., Storm, C., Pesenti, A., *et al.* (2010). Intra-arrest transnasal evaporative cooling: A randomized, prehospital, multicenter study (PRINCE: Pre-ROSC IntraNasal Cooling Effectiveness). *Circulation* **122**:729–736.

Christenson, J. C., Holm, B. M., Lechlitner, S., Howell, J. F., Wenger, M., Roy-Burman, A., Hsieh, C. J., LaBar, L., Petru, A., Davis, S., Simons, N., Apolinario, P., et al. (2007). Human rabies—Indiana and California, 2006. MMWR Morb. Mortal. Wkly. Rep. 56:361–365.

Christian, E., Zada, G., Sung, G., and Giannotta, S. L. (2008). A review of selective hypothermia in the management of traumatic brain injury. Neurosurg. Focus 25:E9.

Darman, J., Backovic, S., Dike, S., Maragakis, N. J., Krishnan, C., Rothstein, J. D., Irani, D. N., and Kerr, D. A. (2004). Viral-induced spinal motor neuron death is non-cell-autonomous and involves glutamate excitotoxicity. J. Neurosci. 24:7566–7575.

Drosten, C. (2007). Rabies - Germany (Hamburg) ex Morocco. ProMED-mail 20070419.1287. Available at http://www.promedmail.org/Accessed December 4, 2010.

Emmons, R. W., Leonard, L. L., DeGenaro, F., Jr., Protas, E. S., Bazeley, P. L., Giammona, S. T., and Sturckow, K. (1973). A case of human rabies with prolonged survival. Intervirology 1:60–72.

Ginsberg, M. D. (2009). Current status of neuroprotection for cerebral ischemia: Synoptic overview. Stroke 40(Suppl. 3):S111–S114.

Hattwick, M. A. W., Weis, T. T., Stechschulte, C. J., Baer, G. M., and Gregg, M. B. (1972). Recovery from rabies: A case report. Ann. Intern. Med. 76:931–942.

Hattwick, M. A., Corey, L., and Creech, W. B. (1976). Clinical use of human globulin immune to rabies virus. J. Infect. Dis. 133(Suppl.):A266–A272.

Hemachudha, T., Sunsaneewitayakul, B., Mitrabhakdi, E., Suankratay, C., Laothamathas, J., Wacharapluesadee, S., Khawplod, P., and Wilde, H. (2003). Paralytic complications following intravenous rabies immune globulin treatment in a patient with furious rabies. Int. J. Infect. Dis. 7:76–77(Letter).

Hemachudha, T., Sunsaneewitayakul, B., Desudchit, T., Suankratay, C., Sittipunt, C., Wacharapluesadee, S., Khawplod, P., Wilde, H., and Jackson, A. C. (2006). Failure of therapeutic coma and ketamine for therapy of human rabies. J. Neurovirol. 12:407–409.

Houston Chronicle (2006). Rabies, human—USA (Texas) . ProMED-mail 20060513.1360. Available at http://www.promedmail.org/Accessed December 4, 2010.

Hu, W. T., Willoughby, R. E., Jr., Dhonau, H., and Mack, K. J. (2007). Long-term follow-up after treatment of rabies by induction of coma. N. Engl. J. Med. 357:945–946, (Letter).

Hunter, M., Johnson, N., Hedderwick, S., McCaughey, C., Lowry, K., McConville, J., Herron, B., McQuaid, S., Marston, D., Goddard, T., Harkess, G., Goharriz, H., et al. (2010). Immunovirological correlates in human rabies treated with therapeutic coma. J. Med. Virol. 82:1255–1265.

Jackson, A. C. (2005). Recovery from rabies. N. Engl. J. Med. 352:2549–2550, (Editorial).

Jackson, A. C., Warrell, M. J., Rupprecht, C. E., Ertl, H. C. J., Dietzschold, B., O'Reilly, M., Leach, R. P., Fu, Z. F., Wunner, W. H., Bleck, T. P., and Wilde, H. (2003). Management of rabies in humans. Clin. Infect. Dis. 36:60–63.

Juncosa, B. (2008). Hope for rabies victims: Unorthodox coma therapy shows promise. First a U.S. girl—And now two South American kids survive onset of the deadly virus. Scientific American.com. Available at, http://www.scientificamerican.com/Accessed December 4, 2010.

Kaul, M., and Lipton, S. A. (2007). Neuroinflammation and excitotoxicity in neurobiology of HIV-1 infection and AIDS: Targets for neuroprotection. In "Interaction Between Neurons and Glia in Aging and Disease" (J. O. Malva, A. C. Rego, R. A. Cunha, and C. R. Oliveira, eds.), pp. 281–308. Springer Science, New York.

Kureishi, A., Xu, L. Z., Wu, H., and Stiver, H. G. (1992). Rabies in China: Recommendations for control. Bull. World Health Organ. 70:443–450.

Lafon, M. (2005). Bat rabies—The Achilles heel of a viral killer? Lancet 366:876–877.

Lafon, M. (2007). Immunology. In "Rabies" (A. C. Jackson and W. H. Wunner, eds.), pp. 489–504. Elsevier Academic Press, London.

Lockhart, B. P., Tsiang, H., Ceccaldi, P. E., and Guillemer, S. (1991). Ketamine-mediated inhibition of rabies virus infection *in vitro* and in rat brain. *Antivir. Chem. Chemother.* **2:**9–15.

Maier, T., Schwarting, A., Mauer, D., Ross, R. S., Martens, A., Kliem, V., Wahl, J., Panning, M., Baumgarte, S., Muller, T., Pfefferle, S., Ebel, H., *et al.* (2010). Management and outcomes after multiple corneal and solid organ transplantations from a donor infected with rabies virus. *Clin. Infect. Dis.* **50:**1112–1119.

Manning, S. E., Rupprecht, C. E., Fishbein, D., Hanlon, C. A., Lumlertdacha, B., Guerra, M., Meltzer, M. I., Dhankhar, P., Vaidya, S. A., Jenkins, S. R., Sun, B., and Hull, H. F. (2008). Human rabies prevention—United States, 2008: Recommendations of the Advisory Committee on Immunization Practices. *MMWR. Morb. Mortal. Wkly. Rep.* **57(No. RR-3):**1–28.

McDermid, R. C., Saxinger, L., Lee, B., Johnstone, J., Noel Gibney, R. T., Johnson, M., and Bagshaw, S. M. (2008). Human rabies encephalitis following bat exposure: Failure of therapeutic coma. *Can. Med. Assoc. J.* **178:**557–561.

Merigan, T. C., Baer, G. M., Winkler, W. G., Bernard, K. W., Gibert, C. G., Chany, C., Veronesi, R., and Collaborative Group, R. (1984). Human leukocyte interferon administration to patients with symptomatic and suspected rabies. *Ann. Neurol.* **16:**82–87.

Ministerio da Saude in Brazil (2008). Rabies, human survival, bat—Brazil: (Pernambuco). ProMED-mail 20081114.3599. Available at http://www.promedmail.org/ Accessed December 4, 2010.

Morimoto, K., Patel, M., Corisdeo, S., Hooper, D. C., Fu, Z. F., Rupprecht, C. E., Koprowski, H., and Dietzschold, B. (1996). Characterization of a unique variant of bat rabies virus responsible for newly emerging human cases in North America. *Proc. Natl Acad. Sci. USA* **93:**5653–5658.

Nargi-Aizenman, J. L., and Griffin, D. E. (2001). Sindbis virus-induced neuronal death is both necrotic and apoptotic and is ameliorated by N-methyl-D-aspartate receptor antagonists. *J. Virol.* **75:**7114–7121.

Nargi-Aizenman, J. L., Havert, M. B., Zhang, M., Irani, D. N., Rothstein, J. D., and Griffin, D. E. (2004). Glutamate receptor antagonists protect from virus-induced neural degeneration. *Ann. Neurol.* **55:**541–549.

Pue, H. L., Turabelidze, G., Patrick, S., Grim, A., Bell, C., Reese, V., Basilan, R., Rupprecht, C., and Robertson, K. (2009). Human rabies—Missouri, 2008. *MMWR Morb. Mortal. Wkly. Rep.* **58:**1207–1209.

Rubin, J., David, D., Willoughby, R. E., Jr., Rupprecht, C. E., Garcia, C., Guarda, D. C., Zohar, Z., and Stamler, A. (2009). Applying the Milwaukee Protocol to treat canine rabies in Equatorial Guinea. *Scand. J. Infect. Dis.* **41:**372–375.

Rupprecht, C. E., Briggs, D., Brown, C. M., Franka, R., Katz, S. L., Kerr, H. D., Lett, S. M., Levin, R., Meltzer, M. I., Schaffner, W., and Cieslak, P. R. (2010). Use of a reduced (4-dose) vaccine schedule for postexposure prophylaxis to prevent human rabies: Recommendations of the advisory committee on immunization practices. *MMWR Recomm. Rep.* **59:**1–9.

Sulkin, S. E., Allen, R., Sims, R., Krutzsch, P. H., and Kim, C. (1960). Studies on the pathogenesis of rabies in bats. II. Influence of environmental temperature. *J. Exp. Med.* **112:**595–617.

Superti, F., Seganti, L., Pana, A., and Orsi, N. (1985). Effect of amantadine on rhabdovirus infection. *Drugs Exp. Clin. Res.* **11:**69–74.

The Hypothermia After Cardiac Arrest Study Group (2002). Mild therapeutic hypothermia to improve the neurologic outcome after cardiac arrest . *N. Engl. J. Med.* **346:**549–556.

Troell, P., Miller-Zuber, B., Ondrush, J., Murphy, J., Fatteh, N., Feldman, K., Mitchell, K., Willoughby, R., Glymph, C., Blanton, J., and Rupprecht, C. (2010). Human rabies—Virginia, 2009. *MMWR Morb. Mortal. Wkly. Rep.* **59:**1236–1238.

Turabelidze, G., Pue, H., Grim, A., and Patrick, S. (2009). First human rabies case in Missouri in 50 years causes death in outdoorsman. *Mo. Med.* **106:**417–419.

van Thiel, P. P., de Bie, R. M., Eftimov, F., Tepaske, R., Zaaijer, H. L., van Doornum, G. J., Schutten, M., Osterhaus, A. D., Majoie, C. B., Aronica, E., Fehlner-Gardiner, C., Wandeler, A. I., et al. (2009). Fatal human rabies due to Duvenhage virus from a bat in Kenya: Failure of treatment with coma-induction, ketamine, and antiviral drugs. *PLoS Negl. Trop. Dis.* **3**:e428.

Wang, H., Olivero, W., Lanzino, G., Elkins, W., Rose, J., Honings, D., Rodde, M., Burnham, J., and Wang, D. (2004). Rapid and selective cerebral hypothermia achieved using a cooling helmet. *J. Neurosurg.* **100**:272–277.

Warrell, M. J., White, N. J., Looareesuwan, S., Phillips, R. E., Suntharasamai, P., Chanthavanich, P., Riganti, M., Fisher-Hoch, S. P., Nicholson, K. G., Manatsathit, S., Vannaphan, S., and Warrell, D. A. (1989). Failure of interferon alfa and tribavirin in rabies encephalitis. *Br. Med. J.* **299**:830–833.

Weli, S. C., Scott, C. A., Ward, C. A., and Jackson, A. C. (2006). Rabies virus infection of primary neuronal cultures and adult mice: Failure to demonstrate evidence of excitotoxicity. *J. Virol.* **80**:10270–10273.

Willoughby, R. E., Jr. (2009). Are we getting closer to the treatment of rabies? *Future Virol.* **4**:563–570.

Willoughby, R. E., Jr., Tieves, K. S., Hoffman, G. M., Ghanayem, N. S., Amlie-Lefond, C. M., Schwabe, M. J., Chusid, M. J., and Rupprecht, C. E. (2005). Survival after treatment of rabies with induction of coma. *N. Engl. J. Med.* **352**:2508–2514.

World Health Organization (2005). WHO Expert Consultation on Rabies: First Report. World Health Organization, Geneva.

CHAPTER 18

Mathematical Models for Rabies

Vijay G. Panjeti and **Leslie A. Real**

Contents		

Abstract

Rabies virus and its associated host–pathogen population dynamics have proven a remarkable model system for developing mathematical models of infectious disease emergence and spread. Beginning with simple susceptible-infectious-removed (SIR) compartment models of fox rabies emergence and spread across Western Europe, mathematical models have now been developed to incorporate dynamics across heterogeneous landscapes, host demographic variation, and environmental stochasticity. Model structures range from systems of ordinary differential equations (ODEs) to stochastic agent-based computational simulations. We

Department of Biology and Center for Disease Ecology, Emory University, Atlanta, Georgia, USA

Advances in Virus Research, Volume 79
ISSN 0065-3527, DOI: 10.1016/B978-0-12-387040-7.00018-4

have reviewed the variety of mathematical approaches now available for analyzing dynamics in different host populations; most notably rabies virus spread in raccoon hosts.

I. INTRODUCTION

There has been a long history of mathematical models associated with the study of rabies, and in many ways the timeline of model development for rabies over the last 30 years has closely followed the development of mathematical methods within the analysis of the ecology of infectious diseases in general.

Early models of rabies dynamics were similar to early models for most other diseases and followed the basic "*SEIR*" framework where populations are subdivided into specific classes corresponding to susceptible (S), exposed (E), infectious (I), and recovered/removed (R) individuals (Anderson and May, 1979, 1981). The dynamics are encapsulated through the construction of a system of ordinary differential equations (ODEs) representing either single populations or linked metapopulations from which a variety of predictions can be drawn concerning temporal and spatial pattern.

Although these foundational models may have lacked the level of mathematical sophistication, we see in models today, there was really no need for highly complicated mathematical representations since data itself were rather limited. For instance, some recent models for describing rabies dynamics incorporate explicit spatial interactions and can account for events that are discrete in time and space. These spatially explicit models may not have provided much improvement over the earliest ODE models used 30 years ago by Anderson and May (1981), since early in the epidemic, detailed temporal history was not yet available and spatial resolution was limited to densities of individuals within large regions. At present, even though the mathematical toolkit for studying the ecological and evolutionary dynamics of a variety of infectious diseases is very robust, it is the availability of data that lags behind.

In addition to asking the question of what modeling approach works best with one's data, it is also necessary to consider what the overall goal of the modeling approach will be. With rabies systems, in general, the goals of researchers are often very different. They can range from models that are predictive, which could be used to assess the quality of different management regimes or understand spillover risks, to models that are focused on providing insights into ecological and evolutionary processes that could possibly improve parameter estimations. Although many modeling approaches can address aspects of all of these concerns, certain modeling approaches are more appropriate when properly considering the available data and the primary questions.

From a modeling perspective, rabies is particularly interesting in that the virus can infect a wide variety of mammalian hosts with different species associations in different ecological regions. In Europe, rabies has been primarily restricted to spread within the red fox (*Vulpes vulpes*), whereas in North America, rabies infects a wide range of terrestrial carnivores including raccoons (*Procyon lotor*), skunks (*Mephitis mephitis*), arctic and red foxes (*Vulpes lagopus and V. vulpes*), and coyotes (*Canis latrans*). Rabies virus also circulates among domesticated animals (especially dogs and cats) and among various bat species. Despite geographic and ecological overlap in the ranges of many of these species, the implications of multispecies host susceptibility and the community ecology of rabies has rarely been examined (Real and Childs, 2006).

Most models for rabies virus transmission have been confined to single species dynamics and, although the general framework for models across these species is similar, ecological and biological constraints between species can often make it difficult to form generalizations about dynamics. Nonetheless, there has been a distinct history associated with the structure of models applied to individual systems, which provides a general conceptual framework for understanding the biological mechanisms driving temporal and spatial pattern.

II. THE DEVELOPMENT OF THE MATHEMATICAL APPROACH TO RABIES DYNAMICS

The past decade has seen substantive developments in both mathematical and computational approaches to studying rabies virus dynamics, particularly raccoon rabies within North America. In this chapter, we will focus our discussion on these more recent developments in modeling approaches. However, in order to put contemporary analysis into an appropriate context, we will also review historical approaches.

Most of the earliest models for rabies virus transmission were developed to understand the epizootic expansion of rabies virus in red fox (*V. vulpes*) populations into Western Europe from a focus of origin in Eastern Europe following World War II. These early models utilized the basic *SEIR* compartmental framework and these models were used to derive several critical features of disease emergence and spread. Most importantly, the models were used to calculate the critical threshold for epidemic emergence and the basic reproductive number (R_0) for the virus. The value of R_0 expresses the number of secondary infections generated from a single infection in an entirely susceptible population. When R_0 is greater than 1, the infection will spread and an epidemic will result. Using R_0, it is possible to determine a threshold density of foxes (S_t) below which an epizootic cannot occur. By determining a threshold density, it could then be possible to suggest what level of population culling would be necessary in order to bring threshold density below the epizootic level.

The flowchart in Fig. 1 illustrates the basic compartmental framework similar to ones utilized for early fox rabies models.

Although the construction of the model illustrated in Fig. 1 follows the *SEIR* compartmental framework, we have omitted the inclusion of the *R* class in order to follow the convention of many of the early rabies models, since there is little or no evidence of natural recovery or the development of natural immunity where no vaccination is considered, which translates susceptibles into the removed category.

The dynamics portrayed in the flowchart can be translated into the following set of ODEs:

$$\frac{dS}{dt} = rS - \gamma SN - \beta SI \tag{1}$$

$$\frac{dE}{dt} = \beta SI - (\sigma + b + \gamma N)E \tag{2}$$

$$\frac{dI}{dt} = \sigma E - (\alpha + b + \gamma N)I \tag{3}$$

$$N = S + E + I \tag{4}$$

where S, E, and I represent densities of susceptible hosts, exposed, and infectious individuals, respectively. The intrinsic *per capita* growth is $r = a - b$, where a is the *per capita* birth rate and $1/b$ is the mean life expectancy. The rate at which individuals are exposed to rabies (E) in the

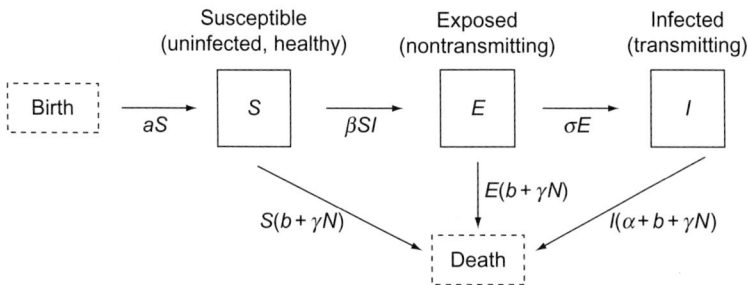

FIGURE 1 Compartment diagram of basic *SEIR* framework used in early ODE formulations for rabies. Arrows represent the directionality of each process.

population is proportional to the densities of susceptible and infectious individuals, βSI. Here β is the disease transmission parameter. The average length of time a fox remains in the exposed class before becoming infectious is $1/\sigma$. Infectious or rabid individuals have greater risk for mortality, such that $(\alpha + b)$ is the mortality rate for infectious individuals.

In order to parameterize their model for red foxes, Anderson *et al.* (1981) utilized the available estimates from then recent descriptive studies (MacDonald, 1980). The situation they considered in their models was the introduction of a few rabid foxes into a naïve population. In order to determine R_0 and the corresponding minimum density of foxes (S_t) necessary for rabies to spread, they also assumed that the host population prior to the introduction of rabies was at a stable equilibrium. From Eqs. (1) to (4), this equilibrium is simply $K = a/b$. So at the onset of the epidemic at time $t = 0$, the population size of susceptibles is then $S(t = 0) = K$. By solving Eqs. (1)–(4) simultaneously, they determined that the criteria for an epidemic ($dI/dt > 0$), for the equilibrium population size K, at the onset of the first infections is $K > S_t$, where S_t is

$$S_t = (\sigma + a)(\alpha + a)/\beta\sigma \tag{5}$$

and the relationship between K and S_t can be reformulated to define R_0:

$$R_0 = \frac{K}{S_t} = \frac{K\beta\sigma}{(\sigma + a)(\alpha + a)} \tag{6}$$

Based on the available data, Anderson *et al.* (1981) determined that the minimum threshold density of foxes was $S_t \sim 0.99$ foxes/km^2. Subsequent to their analysis, it was confirmed that almost all areas of Europe that had seen outbreaks had densities in excess of this number. Oral vaccines for rabies had not yet been developed, so the recommended control strategy was culling of fox populations in areas with densities above the threshold, S_t.

III. MODELING APPROACHES USING REACTION DIFFUSION METHODS

Concurrent to the development of the models by Anderson *et al.* (1981), fox rabies was continuing to advance southwesterly into France and Switzerland. Earlier descriptive studies had begun to investigate ecological factors that could influence the spatial propagation of virus, such as habit quality or fox densities (MacDonald, 1980; MacDonald *et al.*, 1981). Subsequent to these descriptive studies, Murray *et al.* (1986) developed a reaction-diffusion model to describe the behavior of this propagating wave. Most importantly, this model allowed predictive modeling of how a transmission barrier might be implemented at the wave front in order to halt the expansion of the epizootic. The construction of a transmission barrier or "break" was akin to that of firebreaks used to arrest the advance of major wildfires.

From the work of Anderson *et al.* (1981), a minimum density for preventing epizootics within a population had already been determined. From a practical standpoint, implementation of such large-scale culling or vaccine distribution across Europe ahead of the wave front would not be possible. However, the model developed by Murray *et al.* (1986) allowed for the estimation of movement rates for rabid foxes. It was now possible to suggest how wide and where a break could be implemented in order to halt the spatial propagation of the epidemic. The framework of the reaction diffusion formulation used by Murray *et al.* (1986) consisted of the following coupled partial differential equations (PDEs):

$$\frac{\partial S(x,t)}{\partial t} = r(1 - N/K)S - \beta SI \tag{7}$$

$$\frac{\partial E(x,t)}{\partial t} = \beta SI - (\sigma + b + rN/K)E \tag{8}$$

$$\frac{\partial I(x,t)}{\partial t} = \sigma E - (\alpha + b + rN/K)I + D\frac{\partial^2 I}{\partial x^2} \tag{9}$$

$$N = S + E + I \tag{10}$$

This one-dimensional reaction diffusion framework is almost identical to the model of Anderson *et al.* (1981); however, there are two important differences. First, Eqs. (7)–(10) implement density dependence in terms of an environmental carrying capacity K, rather than the parameter γ, which determined the strength of density dependence. However, these terms are interchangeable if we consider $\gamma = r/K$. Second, the reaction diffusion framework incorporates the diffusion term at the end of Eq. (9) that describes the movement of infectious foxes across the landscape. Here D is the diffusion coefficient that specifies the rate of movement of rabid foxes. Utilizing this type of framework, it was estimated that the rate of movement for rabid foxes was $D \sim 50$ km^2/year (Andral *et al.*, 1982; Murray *et al.*, 1986). The diffusion coefficient D tells part of the story, but in order to describe the velocity v of the traveling waves associated with the epidemic, other model parameters also have to be considered.

Similar to ODEs, the reaction diffusion formulation is composed of a system of coupled equations. In this case, the equations are PDEs. Although these equations can describe the basic properties of spatial prorogation, they make assumptions similar to that of ODEs, mainly that the population is well mixed and homogeneous and that the rates for process such as infection or birth, etc., can be considered to be constant during the course of the epidemic. An epidemic wave propagating at a velocity v in a homogenous environment will maintain the same shape as it traverses space. Mathematically this allows us to consider a solution in the form $f(x,t) = f(x - vt)$, for Eqs. (7)–(10), solving these equations simultaneously can be nontrivial; additionally, several solutions for wave velocities may be recovered, so it is necessary to evaluate all solutions. Some solutions may describe unrealistic biological scenarios, whereas others may describe the oscillations of standing waves that occur after a significant time has passed. Although the dynamics of secondary oscillations may be important, particularly for predicting recurrent epidemics, it is often possible in reaction diffusion systems to simply estimate the velocity of the initial epidemic wave by applying some assumptions that will allow us to reduce Eqs. (7)–(10) into a more tractable form. For instance, if we consider that over a small time period, Δt at the forefront of the epidemic wave, population size is relatively constant such that $a = b = 0$, it is possible to simplify Eqs. (7)–(9):

$$\frac{\partial S(x,t)}{\partial t} = -\beta SI \tag{11}$$

$$\frac{\partial E(x,t)}{\partial t} = \beta SI - \sigma E \tag{12}$$

$$\frac{\partial I(x,t)}{\partial t} = \sigma E - \alpha I + D\frac{\partial^2 I}{\partial x^2} \tag{13}$$

Additionally, since the initial epidemic process must be driven by the movement of infectious individuals into a region, we can assume that $\partial E(x,t)/\partial t \sim 0$ over Δt. This allows us to combine Eqs. (12) and (13), by setting $\beta SI = \sigma E$. Equation (13) now becomes

$$\frac{\partial I(x,t)}{\partial t} = (\beta S - \alpha)I + D\frac{\partial^2 I}{\partial x^2} \tag{14}$$

Equation (14) now has the same form as the well-known Fisher–Kolmogoroff Equation:

$$\frac{\partial u}{\partial t} = f(u) + D\frac{\partial^2 u}{\partial x^2} \tag{15}$$

which has solutions for the wave velocity $v = 2[f'(u)D]^{1/2}$; from this relation, the wave velocity from Eq. (14) is

$$v = 2[(\beta S_0 + \alpha)D]^{\frac{1}{2}} \tag{16}$$

where S_0 is the initial density of susceptibles prior to the arrival of the first rabid foxes.

The derived relation in Eq. (16) illustrates how one might investigate the roles played by host density and fox dispersal in driving the epidemic process. From a management standpoint, S_0 can suggest the level of culling or vaccination necessary to halt the epidemic wave, and D, which is related to the movement rate of infectious foxes, can suggest how wide an area in front of the epidemic should be managed. These were some of the primary relationships that Murray et al. (1986) had investigated. A more comprehensive derivation of the wave speed, including a two-dimensional formation, can be found in Murray et al. (1986). Additionally, a detailed review of early ODE and PDE frameworks in European fox rabies can also be found in Shigesada and Kawasaki (1997).

IV. METHODS FOR INCORPORATING LANDSCAPE HETEROGENEITIES

These early models by Anderson et al. (1981) and Murray et al. (1986) were important and helped illustrate the utility of basic mathematical models in analyzing disease dynamics in ecological systems. However, despite the fact that the use of these deterministic ODE and PDE frameworks in disease ecology was in many ways pioneering at that time, the methods themselves had been available for centuries, particularly in other disciplines such as physics where use of these methods was commonplace for understanding the behaviors of dynamical systems under ideal conditions. These early deterministic models yielded a number of important insights into the dynamics of the rabies virus in wildlife populations. However, due to several simplifying assumptions about the nature of the ecological interactions, several aspects of the observed dynamics remained unexplained and poorly understood. ODE and PDE approaches assume that all ecological interactions occur over a homogenous landscape and at constant rates, and that events occur continuously through time. Given that the spatial distribution of rabies often occurs over large regions, landscape heterogeneity is likely to be important. As data with finer spatial resolution became available, the importance of considering heterogeneity became evident. For instance, data describing the movement of fox rabies across Europe illustrated that the spread of the virus, particularly in areas near Switzerland and northward, was characterized by rapid movement deep into valleys and then a slower percolation of the virus into the areas neighboring those valleys (Steck et al., 1982). Similarly, in North America landscape heterogeneities drove patterns of irregular spread during the epidemic spread of the rabies virus that started in mid-1970s. These patterns became most evident in the northern United States, when the rabies virus began to enter areas of New York and Connecticut in the early 1990s. Subsequent modeling and data revealed that rivers were effective barriers to transmission, and drove close to sevenfold delays in the advance of the epidemic wave (Russell *et al.*, 2004; Smith *et al.*, 2002).

Extensions to these early models such as multidimensional reaction diffusion or optimal control have allowed the ODE and PDE frameworks to remain relevant. Extensions can be made to the traditional ODE and PDE frameworks that allow for some consideration of parameter variation, stochasticity, and even some environmental heterogeneity. Mollison and Kuulasmaa (1985) incorporated a stochastic dispersal process, which showed good agreement with estimated velocities for fox rabies. Shigesada and Kawasaki (1997) considered not only variation in rates of diffusion between classes of individuals in a reaction diffusion model but also the effect of two habitat types on those rates of diffusion.

Despite these inroads, it is difficult to fully incorporate the effects of landscape level heterogeneities or stochastic variation among all model parameters without moving to other (mostly computational) approaches, such as network models, cellular automata, interacting particle systems, or percolation-based techniques. A number of recent models have utilized these types of computational approaches to study the roles of environmental heterogeneity and stochastic effects.

Some of the earliest work to incorporate these techniques employed agent-based simulation approaches. In these models, the fate of individual hosts is tracked during the course of transmission generating overall population level dynamics over a landscape. Voigt *et al.* (1985) utilized this type of model where they considered landscape and habitat heterogeneity specific to Ontario, Canada. By using a model of the rabies virus tailored specifically to a region of interest, they were able to gain important insights into the epidemic process in Ontario and then implement specific management strategies for that region (Macinnes *et al.*, 1988; Voigt *et al.*, 1985). The effectiveness of this agent-based approach in Ontario may beg the question as to why these types of agent-based models are not more predominant. However, the effectiveness of the agent-based or individually based approach depends very much on the scale at which we are interested. This is important in terms of "scale" as applied to not only the size of the overall landscape in which one is interested but also "scale" as measure of coarseness or degree of resolution at which we need to investigate that landscape. An important work by Thulke *et al.* (1999) investigated this type of question directly by looking for differences in dynamics between models that explored rabies virus dynamics at different scales.

Smith *et al.* (2002) developed an interactive network model that incorporated local heterogeneities in an attempt to better understand the irregular spread of the rabies wave front across Connecticut in the early 1990s. Figure 2 details the algorithm they utilized in implementing their model.

The model used by Smith *et al.* (2002) considered the landscape as a network of connected townships where habitat differences among townships could be approximated as variation in local transmission rates between neighboring townships ($\lambda_{i,j}$) and global transmission among all townships (μ_{ij}). The parameters μ_i and $\lambda_{i,j}$ were fixed throughout the course of any simulation, but some degree of stochasticity was implemented since the order in which townships were chosen was based on a uniform random distribution. Smith *et al.* (2002) showed convincingly that landscape heterogeneity could help explain the irregular spread of the raccoon rabies virus across Connecticut, something which reaction diffusion frameworks had difficulty achieving. The initial application of the network approach developed for modeling spread of rabies in

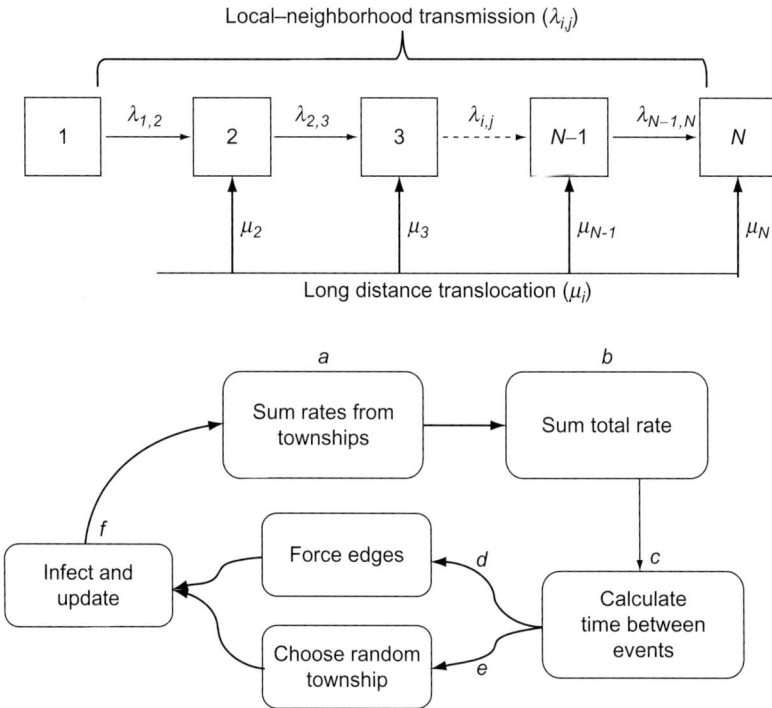

FIGURE 2 *Diagram of network model used by Smith* et al. *(2002). The landscape is subdivided into N populations. The parameters μ_i and $\lambda_{i,j}$ are rates for processes that connect populations; here μ_i describes the rate at which long distance translocation occurs in a particular population i, and $\lambda_{i,j}$ describes local movement of the virus from population i to j. The flowchart (a $\rightarrow$ f) illustrates the sequence followed for iterating and updating the model over time.*

Connecticut used the observed pattern of spread across that State to parameterize the network simulation. Russell *et al.* (2004) then used the parameterized model to predict the pattern of spread in a novel geographic region and demonstrated a remarkable correspondence between the observed and predicted spatial pattern of appearance across New York.

V. STOCHASTIC MODELS

Stochastic effects in model behavior can be explored using a variety of techniques, the simplest being the use of one or more distributions to describe a rate process (or processes) in an ODE or PDE. In these cases, the ODE or PDE is implemented algorithmically and a rate process such as *birth (a)* or *death (d)* would be sampled from an appropriate distribution. For instance, from Eq. (1) the expected number of new susceptibles in the interval dt could be implemented using a Poisson distribution with rate parameter $[rS(t)]$dt. This approach is similar to the one used by Smith *et al.* (2002) who implemented the waiting time for townships to become infected as an exponential distribution.

Unless there are pertinent ecological or computational reasons to consider the use of specific distributions for stochastic implementations, it may make more sense to implement a fully stochastic model based on the methodology developed by Gillespie (1977). In the most straightforward implementation of the Gillespie method, equations are transformed into a stochastic simulation algorithm, which allows any processes μ, in a system of equations (such as *birth, death, infection,* etc.), to occur relative to its statistical weight at a particular time τ. That is, the probability of any specific event such as *birth* or *death* occurring at a specific time τ is relative to the likelihood of all events that could occur at time τ. Gillepie's insight, which allowed the development of his well-known "direct method," stems from a reformulation of how the probability of an event occurring in an ODE or PDE system can be expressed. Earlier work by van Kampen (2001) had illustrated that in most interacting systems, a "Master Equation" could be formulated that expressed the exact probability of any process occurring at a specific time and location within the system. By evaluating the spatial component of the "Master Equation" over the entire region or area of interest, Gillespie defined a probability distribution similar to the one below.

$$P(\mu, \tau)\mathrm{d}\tau = a_\mu \exp\left(-\tau \sum^{k} |a_i|\right)\mathrm{d}\tau \qquad (17)$$

Equation (17) represents the probability that a process μ will occur at a specific time τ within the entire region being modeled by an ODE or PDE. For instance, the rate at which the process of infection, β, occurs in Eq. (8) would be dependent on the densities of S and I at time τ, so in this case, $a_{\mu=\beta} = \beta S(\tau)I(\tau)$. Following from this, the summation of a_i in Eq. (17) is over the total number of processes k, in the entire system of coupled equations. This defines the sum probability of any processes (inclusive of the processes μ being considered) occurring at the time τ. Gillespie noted that the probability distribution expressed in Eq. (17) was a joint probability distribution, such that $P(\mu,\tau) = P(\mu)P(\tau)$. If we consider this, then the probability of a specific event occurring in the time interval $d\tau$, around τ is $a_\mu(\tau)/\sum{}^k a_i(\tau)$ and the time τ, at which the event occurs is exponentially distributed.

Since the probability of an event's occurrence and the time at which the event occurs is joint, and therefore independent, Gillespie's algorithm is implemented by sampling two random numbers r_1 and r_2 from a uniform distribution. Then using the following relations, the algorithm sequentially updates the population dynamics event by event in increments of time τ.

$$\tau = (1/a_0)\ln(1/r_1) \tag{18}$$

$$\sum_{i=1}^{\mu-1} a_i < r_2 a_0 \leq \sum_{i=1}^{\mu} a_i \tag{19}$$

The relationship in Eqs. (18) and (19) describe how to implement a stochastic algorithm for almost any system of deterministic equations. Whereas in traditional deterministic equations, events and population densities are continuous, the implementation of the Gillespie method discretizes our system of ODEs, such that densities only take on and change in integer increments and all events happen at discrete times (no events occur simultaneously), which adds further realism and utility to this approach.

VI. INCORPORATING STOCHASTICITY AND SPATIAL HETEROGENEITY

Using the framework of an interacting network and the Gillespie method, it is possible to go one step further and consider that each subpopulation within a network can be described by a specific set of stochastically implemented ODEs. Here, similar to Smith et al. (2002), parameters describing local spread or long distance translocation act to couple each set of ODEs. A stochastic SEIR model formulated in this way simulates the discrete changes in the number of susceptible, exposed, infectious, and vaccinated individuals produced by births, deaths, infections, and movement within all subpopulations. This system of coupled ODEs allows the model to be easily scaled to different ecological units, promoting flexibility in employing the model for hypothesis testing using data reported at different ecological scales. In many ways, this type of approach leverages many of the best qualities of the models discussed earlier. Here we will use this framework to formulate a more sophisticated model that attempts to incorporate a high degree of biological realism based on much of the current knowledge of the rabies virus infection in raccoons in North America. The flowchart in Fig. 3 illustrates how rates and transitions between classes are specified in this type of coupled stochastic $SEIR$ model.

A spatial component is easily incorporated in this model if we consider that the index i on all classes in Fig. 3 corresponds to populations distributed across a lattice. At each location in the lattice, the local dynamics are then based upon the following set of ODE's:

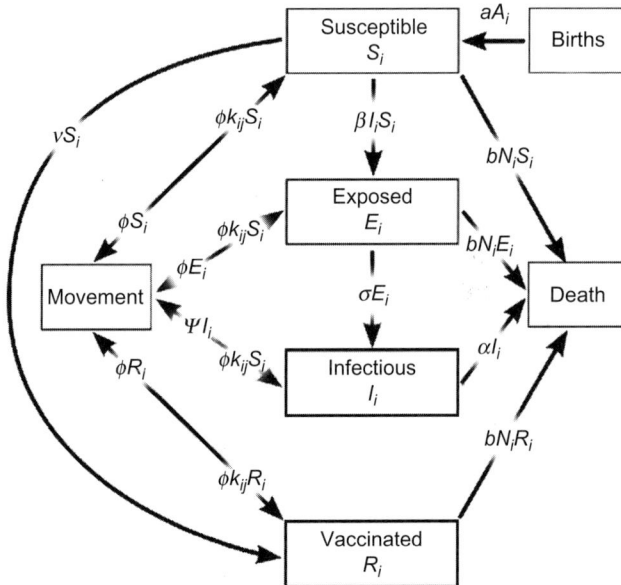

FIGURE 3 *Flowchart illustrating interactions in the model.* Here "Movement" is represented as a class, but simply indicates how the process allows for the rearrangement of individuals spatially.

$$\frac{dS}{dt} = aA_i - bN_iS_i - \beta I_iS_i - vS_i - (\phi + \phi_{\mathrm{LDT}})S_i + \sum_{j \neq i} \left(\phi k_{ij} + \phi_{\mathrm{LDT}}\hat{k}_{ij} \right) S_j$$

(20)

$$\frac{dE}{dt} = \beta I_iS_i - bN_iE_i - \sigma E_i - (\phi + \phi_{\mathrm{LDT}})E_i \sum_{j \neq i} \left(\phi k_{ij} + \phi_{\mathrm{LDT}}\hat{k}_{ij} \right) E_j \quad (21)$$

$$\frac{dI}{dt} = \sigma E_i - \alpha I_i - (\psi + \psi_{\mathrm{LDT}})I_i + \sum_{j \neq i} \left(\psi k_{ij} + \psi_{\mathrm{LDT}}\hat{k}_{ij} \right) I_j \quad (22)$$

$$\frac{dR}{dt} = vS_i - bN_iR_i - (\phi + \phi_{\mathrm{LDT}})R_i + \sum_{j \neq i} \left(\phi k_{ij} + \phi_{\mathrm{LDT}}\hat{k}_{ij} \right) R_j \quad (23)$$

$$A_i = S_i + E_i + R_i \quad (24)$$

$$N_i = S_i + E_i + I_i + R_i \quad (25)$$

Parameterization of Eqs. (20)–(25) is similar to that of earlier models presented here. In these equations, S_i, E_i, I_i, and R_i are the number of susceptible, exposed, infectious, and vaccinated individuals at location i, respectively; A_i is the total number of noninfectious individuals (Eq. (24)); and N_i is the local population size (Eq. (25)). Individuals are born into the susceptible class at a *per capita* rate, a. In the absence of rabies, the population is only subject to the density-dependent mortality rate, b, resulting in logistic population growth and a carrying capacity, $K = a/b$. In the presence of viral transmission, the rate at which susceptibles are infected is βI_iS_i, where β is the transmission rate. Infection with rabies is followed by a latency period during which the virus reproduces and infection moves toward the central nervous system and salivary glands. Latently infected individuals comprise the exposed class, E_i, and newly infected individuals enter this class at the rate of infection (βI_iS_i). Exposed individuals either die from nondisease-related, density-dependent sources (bN_iE_i) or become infectious at a rate σE_i, where $1/\sigma$ is the expected length of the latency period. The latency period ends when the virus enters the brain and salivary glands at which point an individual becomes infectious. Individuals become infectious at the rate σE_i and are removed at a rate αI_i, where $1/\alpha$ is the life expectancy once infectious.

Equations (20)–(25) also introduce several new interactions and parameters. Individuals transition into a vaccinated class, R_i, in our model at a rate, vS_i, and vaccinated individuals die from nondisease-related, density-dependent sources of mortality (bN_iR_i). Local populations are linked by local dispersal of individuals from all classes. Noninfectious individuals (S_i, E_i, R_i) emigrate from their local population at a *per capita* rate ϕ and immigrate to other locations at rate ϕk_{ij}, where i and j are location indices. The k_{ij} terms are dispersal coefficients giving the fraction of individuals migrating from location j to location i and characterize the pattern of dispersal. We include the effects of long distance translocation (LDT) by adding a separate term to Eqs. (20)–(23). The *per capita* rate of translocation is ϕ_{LDT} and ψ_{LDT} for the noninfectious (S_i, E_i, R_i) and infectious classes (I_i), respectively. LDT represents a different process and pattern of movement and we provide separate coefficients, $\hat{k}_{ij}$, quantifying the fraction of individuals that are moved from location j to location i by LDT.

Initial estimates for parameter values (Table I) are drawn from published values and USDA sources or can be estimated indirectly based on fitting our model to epidemiological patterns.

Recently, the approach described here was used to investigate the role of seasonality in dynamics of the rabies virus in raccoon hosts along the East coast in North America. Using this type of model, Duke-Sylvester *et al.* (2010) implemented a north–south latitudinal gradient in the seasonal demography of raccoon birth rates. Specifically, the implementation of the gradient allowed Duke-Sylvester *et al.* (2010) to simulate the variation in timing associated with birth pulses for raccoons in the southern United States versus further north. In their model, the larger variance around the timing of spring births associated with southern populations drove spatial synchronization of southern epidemics. However, in northern populations, where the birth pulse is often narrow, epidemics were irregular and not spatially synchronized across the landscape (Fig. 4).

These types of differences between northern and southern populations may be important, particularly in terms of surveillance strategies.

TABLE I Parameter description for the stochastic model and the associated ODEs in Eqs. (20)–(25)

Parameter	Description	Standard value
a	*Per capita* birth rate	2.67 kits/female/year
b	Natural, density-dependent death rate	2.293E−7 year^{-1}
β	Contact rate	1E−4 (animal days)$^{-1}$
v	Vaccination rate	Variable
$1/\sigma$	Latency period	50 days
$1/\alpha$	Infectious period	14 days
ϕ	Noninfectious movement rate	6E−6 day^{-1}
ϕ_{LDT}	Long distance translocation rate	6E−7 day^{-1}
ψ	Infectious movement rate	6E−6 day^{-1}
ψ_{LDT}	Long distance translocation rate	6E−7 day^{-1}
$k_{ij}, \hat{k}_{ij}$	Fraction of emigrants from j to i	Variable

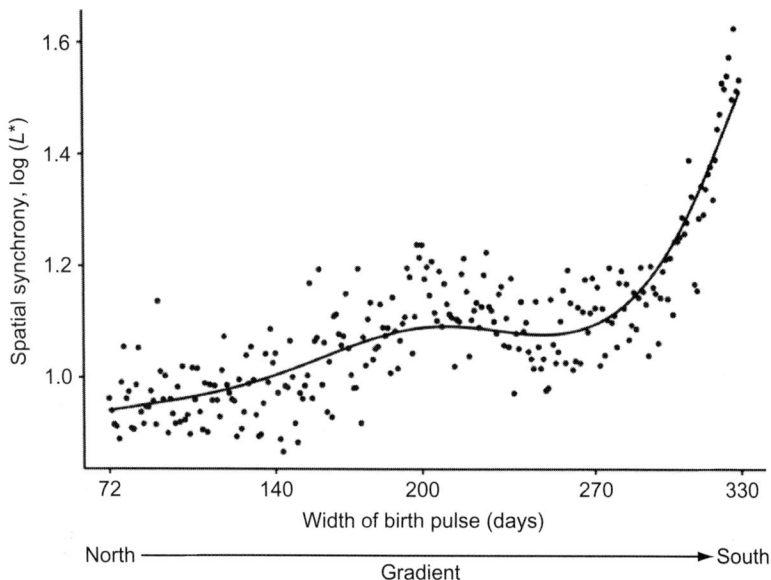

FIGURE 4   Spatial synchrony is represented as log (*L**). *L**, which is calculated by a wavelet analysis, represents the distance at which the local phase coherency is equivalent to the larger regional average correlation (Duke-Sylvester *et al.*, 2010).

Importantly, Duke-Sylvester *et al.* (2010) note that surveillance in the southern states could be reduced relative to northern locations without loss of detection ability since a single spatial location in the south is informative about neighboring spatial locations while northern locations share no common spatial information about neighbors. The potential monetary savings from a reduced surveillance effort without loss of detection is likely to be significant, and would free up more resources for other avenues, such as increased vaccination coverage.

VII. OPTIMAL CONTROL

An important detail, which separates these early ODE and PDE frameworks from contemporary approaches, is the inclusion of a vaccinated class. Once vaccines were developed and then afterward formulated into affordable easily distributed oral forms, the use of oral vaccination as a management approach for controlling rabies became more prevalent than methods associated with the culling of populations.

For diseases like rabies, where the force of infection was based on a density-dependent transmission kernel, traditional solutions for vaccination and culling strategies took the approach of determining what fraction of the population (V_f), should be vaccinated (or culled) in order to bring

$R_0 < 1$ (Coyne *et al.*, 1989). For a single population model, the solution for this vaccination fraction, V_f in terms of R_0 is trivial and is given as $V_f = 1 - 1/R_0$. If we consider that for rabies in terrestrial mammals $R_0 \sim 2$, this would suggest that around 50% of a population should be vaccinated in order to prevent an epizootic. In reality, this level of control may be relatively easy or difficult to implement depending on a number of factors, such as the density of the host population in a target area, the type of terrain or level of landscape heterogeneity in the region, and of course the amount of monetary resources available and the given cost to develop and distribute the vaccine given all these considerations.

Often a particular management strategy has a defined goal associated with the implementation of that strategy and, consequently, the full range of methods that have been developed in operations research can be employed. For example, optimal control (Lenhart and Workman, 2007) allows a reformulation of an ODE system with a vaccination class in which a specific objective is defined mathematically and the dynamics of host–pathogen transmission act as constraints on the realization of the proposed strategy. This reformulation defines an objective function that can incorporate, for instance, a cost function for vaccine delivery. A solution for the objective function, for example, can provide insight into what management strategies can both minimize costs as well as minimize the number of infected hosts. Similarly, an objective function could also be formulated to explore strategies that minimize cost and maximize the number of susceptibles. In general, the objective function can be tailored so it considers the specific goals and constraints for the management problem. Consider the system of ODEs given below.

$$\frac{dS}{dt} = -\beta SI - \varepsilon \delta S - bS \tag{26}$$

$$\frac{dI}{dt} = \beta SI - (b + \alpha)I \tag{27}$$

$$\frac{dR}{dt} = \varepsilon \delta S - bR \tag{28}$$

Here Eqs. (26)–(28) are similar to the earlier system described by Eqs. (11)–(13). However, here for the sake of simplicity, we consider a closed population and have dropped the exposed class and now incorporated a vaccinated class, R in Eq. (28). Here the parameter ε and δ represent the efficacy and rate of vaccine distribution, respectively. In order to formulate an objective function for determining optimal control, we consider that any control measure must be applied during a finite time interval $[0,T]$ and our goal is to determine the optimal control δ, from among a set of control strategies U, such that

$$U = \{\delta = (\delta_1, \ldots, \delta_n), \quad \text{where } 0 \leq \delta_i(t) \leq \delta_{\max} \quad \text{for } i = 1, 2, \ldots, n\}$$

Here δ is a normalized variable representing the density of bait distribution. In such a formulation, the upper bound $\delta_{\max}$ is usually specified to be 1, which would represent the maximum level of bait distribution that is currently possible, for rabies in North America, this is around 150 baits/ km^2 (Asano *et al.*, 2008). Now let us consider that our optimal control problem is to minimize the number of infected hosts as well as the costs of vaccination.

$$\text{Minimize} J(\delta) = \sum_{i=1}^{n} \int_0^T \left(I + \frac{\theta}{2} \delta_i^2 \right) dt \qquad (29)$$

Here θ represents a weight in the cost of the control. Additionally, we have considered that our cost function is quadratic, but in general, a cost function can be formulated in a variety of ways; combinations of linear and quadratic costs having the form $A\delta_i + B\delta_i^2$ are common. Solutions for Eq. (29) require a formulation of the Hamiltonian for our particular system. Although formulating the Hamiltonian itself is often not difficult, solutions are often nontrivial, particularly if one is dealing with a large system of ODEs and/or complicated cost functions. A detailed mathematical description of the processes can be found in Lenhart and Workman (2007), Asano *et al.* (2008), and Ding *et al.* (2007).

VIII. CONCLUSIONS

Mathematical modeling of rabies is now quite well developed embracing a large number of complexities in biological organization and interaction including the ability to incorporate environmental stochasticity and landscape heterogeneity among coupled subpopulations of hosts linked across season and ecological gradients. The power of these models has been tested against extant data sets and has proven predictive of spread in novel locations. New tools, such as optimal control, now can utilize these developed ecological models to drive management and strategic planning in conjunction with public health agencies and planners.

ACKNOWLEDGMENTS

This research was supported by the National Institutes of Health grant RO1-AI047498 to L. A. R. and by the RAPIDD Program of the Science and Technology Directorate, Department of Homeland Security and the Fogarty International Center, National Institutes of Health.

REFERENCES

Anderson, R. M., and May, R. M. (1979). Population biology of infectious diseases: Part 1. *Nature* **280:**361–367.

Anderson, R. M., and May, R. M. (1981). The population dynamics of microparasites and their invertebrate hosts. *Philos. Trans. R. Soc. Lond. B Biol. Sci.* **291:**451–524.

Anderson, R. M., Jackson, H. C., May, R. M., and Smith, A. (1981). Population dynamics of fox rabies in Europe. *Nature* **289:**765–771.

Andral, L., Artois, M., Aubert, M. F. S., and Blancou, J. (1982). Radio-tracking of rabid foxes. *Comparative Immunology, Microbiology and Infectious Diseases.* **5:**285–291.

Asano, E., Gross, L., Lenhart, S., and Real, L. A. (2008). Optimal control of vaccine distribution in a rabies metapopulation model. *Math. Biosci. Eng.* **5:**219.

Coyne, M. J., Smith, G., and McAllister, F. E. (1989). Mathematic model for the population biology of rabies in raccoons in the mid-Atlantic states. *Am. J. Vet. Res.* **50:**2148–2154.

Ding, W., Gross, L. J., Langston, K., Lenhart, S., and Real, L. A. (2007). Rabies in raccoons: Discrete time model with grid spatial component. *J. Biol. Dyn.* **1:**379–393.

Duke-Sylvester, S. M., Bolzoni, L., and Real, L. A. (2010). Strong seasonality produces spatial asynchrony in the outbreak of infectious diseases. *J. R. Soc. Interface.*

Gillespie, D. T. (1977). Exact stochastic simulation of coupled chemical-reactions. *J. Phys. Chem.* **81:**2340–2361.

Lenhart, S., and Workman, J. (2007). *Optimal Control Applied to Biological Models.* Chapman & CRC Mathematical and Computational Biology Series, Chapman & Hall, CRC Press, Boca Raton, FL.

MacDonald, D. (1980). Rabies and Wildlife: A Biologist's Perspective. Oxford University Press, Oxford.

MacDonald, D., Bunce, R., and Bacon, P. (1981). Fox populations, habitat characterization and rabies control. *J. Biogeogr.* **8:**145–151.

MacInnes, C., Tinline, R., Voigt, D., Broekhoven, L., and Rosatte, R. (1988). Planning for rabies control in Ontario. *Rev. Infect. Dis.* **10:**665–669.

Mollison, D., and Kuulasmaa, K. (1985). Spatial epidemic models: Theory and simulations. *In* "Population Dynamics of Rabies in Wildlife" (P. Bacon, ed.), pp. 291–309.

Murray, J., Stanley, E., and Brown, D. (1986). On the spatial spread of rabies among foxes. *Proc. R. Soc. Lond. B Biol. Sci.* **229:**111–150.

Real, L. A., and Childs, J. (2006). Spatial-temporal dynamics of rabies in ecological communities. *In* "Disease Ecology: Community Structure and Pathogen Dynamics" (S. K. Collinge and C. Ray, eds.), pp. 168–185. Oxford University Press, Oxford.

Russell, C., Smith, D., Waller, L., Childs, J., and Real, L. (2004). A priori prediction of disease invasion dynamics in a novel environment. *Proc. R. Soc. Lond. B Biol. Sci.* **271:**21–25.

Shigesada, N., and Kawasaki, K. (1997). Biological Invasions: Theory and Practice. Oxford University Press, Oxford.

Smith, D., Lucey, B., Waller, L., Childs, J., and Real, L. (2002). Predicting the spatial dynamics of rabies epidemics on heterogeneous landscapes. *Proc. Natl. Acad. Sci. USA* **99:**3668–3672.

Steck, F., Wandeler, A., Bicksel, P., Capt, S., Hafliger, U., and Schneider, L. (1982). Oral immunization of foxes against rabies: laboratory and field studies. *Comp. Immunol. Microbiol. Infect. Dis.* **5:**165–171.

Thulke, H. H., Grimm, V., Muller, M. S., Staubach, C., Tischendorf, L., Wissel, C., and Jeltsch, F. (1999). From pattern to practice: A scaling-down strategy for spatially explicit modelling illustrated by the spread and control of rabies. *Ecol. Modell.* **117:**179–202.

van Kampen, N. (2001). Stochastic Processes in Physics and Chemistry. Elsevier Science, Amsterdam.

Voigt, D., Tinline, R., and Broekhoven, L. (1985). A spatial simulation model for rabies control. *Popul. Dyn. Rabies Wildl.*311–349.

CHAPTER 19

Evolution of Wildlife Rabies Control Tactics

Rick Rosatte

Contents		

Abstract

The development of tactics for the control of rabies in wildlife species has evolved dramatically during the past few decades in part due to research advances. Historically, rabies control measures primarily involved the culling of target species. However, contemporary advances in the research and development of oral rabies vaccines and delivery systems for wildlife have now made it feasible to treat rabies outbreaks over thousands of square kilometers of habitat. Systems have been developed to control rabies in several of the primary wildlife vectors such as raccoon dogs, red

Ontario Ministry of Natural Resources, Wildlife Research and Development Section, Trent University, Peterborough, Ontario, Canada

Advances in Virus Research, Volume 79
ISSN 0065-3527, DOI: 10.1016/B978-0-12-387040-7.00019-6

foxes, and raccoons, and rabies has been eliminated from many jurisdictions. However, future research is needed to develop cost-effective and efficacious methods to control rabies in species such as striped skunks as well as in nonterrestrial vectors such as bats. As well, cost-effective rabies management techniques need to be adopted by developing nations so that wildlife rabies control is a realistic and achievable goal globally.

I. INTRODUCTION

Over the course of history, significant advances have been accomplished in the field of wildlife rabies control. So-called cures for rabies such as the application of boxwood or the ashes from a "mad dog's head" were suggested during historical times (Steele, 1975). However, gradually advances were made, and during much of the 1800s, rabies control was based on quarantine measures, muzzling orders, or euthanasia. Research was initiated during the mid-1800s on the development of vaccination as a method for rabies control. Significant advances were made in understanding rabies virus infections during Pasteur's experiments with rabbits. He later immunized dogs using attenuated virus from rabbits. By 1885–1886, Pasteur had vaccinated humans with vaccine derived from rabies virus-infected rabbit spinal cords (Pasteur, 1886).

The discipline of wildlife rabies control has made significant advances since the time of Pasteur. Progress has advanced to the point where globally, hundreds of thousands of square kilometers of land are being baited with millions of vaccine baits to control rabies in wildlife rabies vectors. This chapter will address the advances made with respect to rabies control tactics for wildlife.

II. HISTORICAL AND CONTEMPORARY WILDLIFE RABIES CONTROL TACTICS

Trapping and poisoning of wildlife rabies vector species such as red foxes (*Vulpes vulpes*), coyotes (*Canis latrans*), and skunks (*Mephitis mephitis*) were used as control tactics in some areas of North America during the mid-twentieth century (Ballantyne and O'Donoghue, 1954; Debbie, 1991; Rosatte *et al.*, 1986). Culling of foxes was also used historically in parts of Europe to control rabies (Matouch and Polak, 1982; Niin *et al.*, 2008). Rabies in vampire bats in Latin America was controlled by injecting anticoagulants in cattle. Bats died after feeding on the blood of cattle and this also led to the death of additional bats (Cliquet and Picard-Meyer, 2004).

Research was conducted in the United States to lower fertility of rabies vector species during the 1960s using reproductive inhibitors in an attempt to diminish rabies spread by limiting rabies vector population growth. (Storm and Sanderson, 1969a,b). However, these methods were ineffective due to a lack of target specificity (Turner and Kirkpatrick, 1996). Recently, reproductive inhibitor research has been initiated for use in dogs using a product called GonaCon™ (Bender et al., 2009). This product is also being considered for controlling raccoon populations in North America.

In the late 1960s, research focused on developing an oral rabies vaccine (ORV) delivery system for use on red foxes in North America (Baer et al., 1971; Black and Lawson, 1970, 1980; Winkler, 1992). The idea is to increase herd immunity to the point where the probability of encountering an infected animal is low (Blancou et al., 2009). Experimented with Flury LEP and HEP vaccines to orally vaccinate foxes during that period. He proved that ORV for the control of rabies in foxes was a possibility (Baer et al., 1971).

Development of an effective ORV system was slow. In view of this, some researchers focused on developing a parenteral rabies vaccination system for species of wildlife such as raccoons and striped skunks in Canada (Rosatte et al., 1990, 1992, 2001, 2009a), and foxes in Europe (Aubert et al., 1994). A tactic called trap-vaccinate-release (TVR) proved to be effective for raccoons and skunks as they could be readily captured (Rosatte et al., 1992). In addition, injectable vaccines such as Imrab® (Merial Inc., Athens, Georgia) provided protective immunity in those two species (Rosatte et al., 1990) (Fig. 1). An epizootic of raccoon rabies was eliminated in Ontario during 1999–2005 using TVR and parenteral vaccination in combination with culling and vaccinia-rabies glycoprotein (V-RG) baiting (Rosatte et al., 2001, 2009a). In fact, more than 1.2 million trap-nights were used to vaccinate about 96,000 raccoons (43–83% of the population annually) and 8000 skunks to control the disease (Rosatte et al., 2009a). TVR and culling were also used in other Canadian provinces such as New Brunswick and Quebec during the 2000s to control raccoon rabies.

The use of TVR for the control of rabies in red foxes proved not to be feasible in Canada as foxes are difficult to live-capture. However, parenteral vaccination and administration of vaccine via dart were used during the 1990s in Tanzania to protect African wild dogs (Lycaon pictus) against rabies (Gascoyne et al., 1993). Parental vaccination was also used to control rabies in endangered Ethiopian wolves where up to 70% mortality due to rabies occurred in some packs during 1991–2004 (Randall et al., 2006). In addition, TVR was used in Ohio and Massachusetts to control raccoon rabies and in Flagstaff, Arizona, to combat an outbreak of bat variant rabies in skunks (Algeo et al., 2008; Slate et al., 2009).

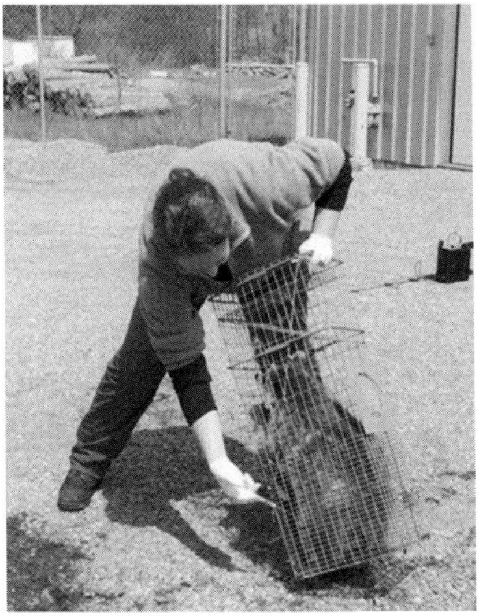

FIGURE 1 Trap-vaccinate-release was used to control raccoon rabies in Ontario during the 1980s–2000s to prevent and manage rabies incursions (photo by R. Rosatte).

Oral rabies vaccination is the most cost-effective method for rabies control in Europe and elsewhere (Muller *et al.*, 2005). Chicken-head baits containing SAD-Berne ORV were used in Switzerland during the late 1970s (this was the first time ORV was used in the field) and early 1980s to control an epizootic of rabies in red foxes (Aubert *et al.*, 1994; Steck *et al.*, 1982). During the early 1990s, baits containing SAD-B19 vaccine were used in Europe to control fox rabies (Brochier *et al.*, 2001; Pastoret *et al.*, 2004). In 2005/2006, Rabidog® SAG2 baits were used in Estonia to control rabies in red foxes and raccoon dogs. Spring and fall baiting campaigns were successful in immunizing an average of 64% of the target populations and rabies declined dramatically (Niin *et al.*, 2008).

Oral rabies vaccination of the primary terrestrial vectors [red foxes and raccoon dogs (*Nyctereutes procyonoides*)] in Europe has been extremely successful with rabies cases declining from about 21,000 in 1990 to about 5400 in 2004 (http://pasteur.fr/). In fact, many countries have attained "rabies-free" status including Switzerland, Italy, the Netherlands, Finland, France, Belgium, Luxembourg, and the Czech Republic (http://pasteur.fr/). However, the disease still persists in "hot spots" in some areas of Europe such as Poland and Lithuania and reinfections have occurred in the Czech Republic (Moutou, 2005). There was also an outbreak of rabies in urban areas of Germany during the 2000s (Muller *et al.*, 2005). In fact, "rabies-free" countries are vulnerable to the threat of illegal importation of rabies-infected animals due to the new policy of "freedom to travel" within the European Union (Bourhy *et al.*, 2005).

Recent advancements in rabies management tactics in Europe include improved vaccination protocols, a consistent vaccination strategy, increased vaccination in rabies hot-spots (at 6 week intervals), and intense rabies surveillance (8 foxes/100 km^2 area) (Muller *et al.*, 2005). In addition, research in Germany has revealed that vaccine-bait acceptance by foxes can be elevated by decreasing the distance between aircraft baiting lines (Thulke *et al.*, 2004). Success in rabies control of foxes was also attained in areas such as France (Toma, 2005) and Estonia (Niin *et al.*, 2008) by implementing vaccination campaigns during spring and summer and also by baiting around fox dens. Toma (2005) reported the use of three baiting campaigns following the last reported rabies case.

In North America, a modified live rabies virus vaccine (ERA) was used during 1989–2009 to control rabies in foxes in Ontario, Canada (MacInnes *et al.*, 2001; Rosatte *et al.*, 2007e). Control of rabies in wildlife in Ontario led to a decrease in human postexposure treatments (from 2000 per year during the 1980s to 1000 per year during the late 1990s) (Nunan *et al.*, 2002). Rabies was also eliminated in coyotes in Texas using V-RG baits and progress is also being made toward the elimination of rabies in gray foxes in Texas (Slate *et al.*, 2009). V-RG was also used in the United States and Canada in an attempt to control raccoon rabies during the 1990s and 2000s (Rosatte *et al.*, 2008; Sattler *et al.*, 2009; Slate *et al.*, 2005). In the laboratory, V-RG proved to be very effective on captive raccoons, but its performance in the field was well below expectations (Rosatte *et al.*, 2008; Sattler *et al.*, 2009). In addition, V-RG was not effective in striped skunks which also accounted for a considerable number of raccoon rabies cases in eastern North America (Hanlon *et al.*, 2002). In view of this, alternate vaccines such as ONRAB® (which is effective in raccoons and skunks) were developed for the control of raccoon rabies in North America (Rosatte *et al.*, 2009b).

III. ADVANCES IN RABIES VACCINE-BAIT DELIVERY SYSTEMS FOR WILDLIFE

In Europe, chicken-heads, fish meal, and fish oil baits containing rabies vaccine were utilized to control rabies in foxes during the 1970s and 1980s (Brochier *et al.*, 1990; Steck *et al.*, 1982). Tubingen baits containing vaccine (vaccine capsule was embedded in a mixture of fish meal and fat) were also used during the 1980s in Germany to control rabies in foxes (Muller *et al.*, 2005; Schneider and Cox, 1988). In 1985, Germany began using an automated bait manufacturing system that allowed the use of baits in other European countries (Wandeler, 1988). Vaccine baits were delivered by hand placement or via aircraft and helicopters (http://pasteur.fr/).

Significant advancements in baiting technology were made during the 1980s and 1990s, and by 1995, a 215,000 km² area of Germany was being treated for wildlife rabies control (Muller *et al.*, 2005). Recent advances include the use of a satellite navigated computer-driven aerial vaccine-bait distribution system called SURVIS (Muller *et al.*, 2005). SURVIS allows real-time calculation of bait density to determine which areas need to be targeted for additional baiting (Muller *et al.*, 2005).

During the early 1980s, experiments were initiated in Ontario, Canada, using chicken-head baits and the vaccine blister-pack that was being used in Switzerland at that time (Fig. 2) (P. Bachmann, personal communication; Steck *et al.*, 1982). However, this bait was abandoned due to potential problems with mass production. Beef tallow or fat was used as the primary ingredient in the matrix of rabies vaccine baits (ERA®) during the 1980s to the 2000s in Ontario (Bachmann *et al.*, 1990; MacInnes *et al.*, 2001; Rosatte *et al.*, 2001, 2007e, 2008). However, in view of the risk of prion diseases such as bovine spongiform encephalopathy and Creutz-feldt-Jakob disease from tainted beef products (Prusiner, 1997), Ontario conducted research to improve their bait as well as make it safer and free from the risk of prion transmission.

Ontario produced a vegetable oil-based bait containing ONRAB® (produced by Artemis Technologies Inc., Guelph, Ontario) during the late 2000s for rabies control operations (Rosatte *et al.*, 2009b) (Fig. 3). Production is about 50,000 ONRAB® baits/2 days (A. Beresford, personal communication). Ontario Ministry of Natural Resources (OMNR) aircraft are able to aerially distribute about 176,580 ONRAB® baits/day at 300 baits/km² and 0.5 km flight-line spacing (average 44,145 baits/flight at 4 flights/day) using Twin Otter aircraft and an automatic baiting machine in the aircraft (P. Bachmann, personal communication). Other types of baits used to deliver ORV to wildlife rabies vectors in

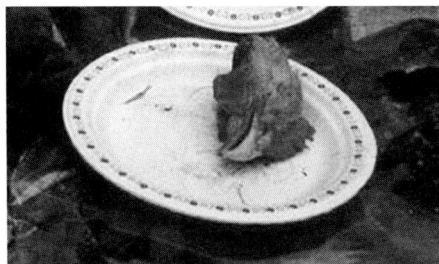

FIGURE 2 Chicken-head baits were used in Ontario during the 1970s in experiments to develop baits to deliver oral rabies vaccine to red foxes (photo by M. Pedde).

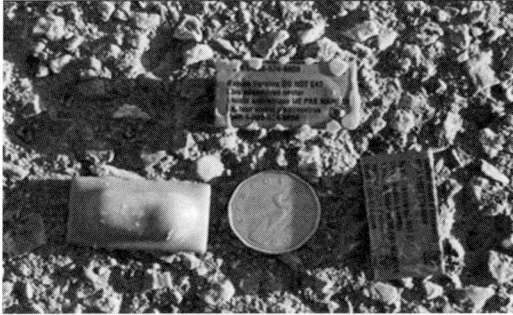

FIGURE 3 New vegetable-based ONRAB® baits are being used in Ontario, Canada, during 2010 for the control of rabies in red foxes, striped skunks, and raccoons. Baits are about 3.0 cm long (photo by R. Rosatte).

North America included Raboral V-RG®, a fish meal polymer bait manufactured by Merial Inc., Athens, Georgia. A matrix coated sachet bait containing Raboral V-RG® was also used to attempt to control raccoon rabies in North America during the 2000s (Slate *et al.*, 2005).

In North America, rabies vaccine-bait delivery systems have advanced from hand-placement of baits to distribution via small fixed winged aircraft and helicopters to large aircraft such as Twin Otter (Bachmann *et al.*, 1990). In Ontario, ERA® baits were distributed by hand during the late 1980s to control rabies in red foxes in urban landscapes such as metropolitan Toronto (Rosatte *et al.*, 2007e). During that same time-frame, progress was being made in the development of an aerial baiting system for rural Ontario landscapes. Initial experiments during the mid-1980s involved the use of baits being placed by hand down a funnel in the back of a Cessna 172 aircraft. A metronome was used to determine how many baits were exiting the aircraft to provide a rough estimate of bait density.

Significant advances were made in the 1990s in Ontario and an automated bait distribution system was developed for use in Twin Otter aircraft (Fig. 4). That system used GIS software to determine bait density and placement. By the 2000s, the system was capable of distributing in excess of 300 baits/km^2 with a flight line spacing of 0.25 km. Software has been developed in Ontario for preplanning flight lines prior to bait distribution operations. Flight lines are uploaded into the aircrafts Global Positioning System (GPS) navigational system. Progress was also made with software to provide an analytical tool for determining bait placement on the landscape, which would provide researchers with a tool to determine whether there were areas that did not receive sufficient baits as well as the accuracy of bait placement (Rosatte *et al.*, 2007c) (Fig. 5).

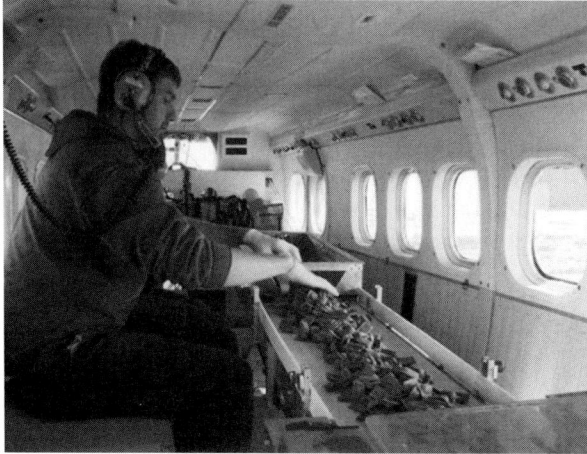

FIGURE 4   Photo of MNR staff in the back of a Twin Otter aircraft operating OES software controlled baiting machine to aerially distribute ONRAB® baits in Ontario during September 2009.

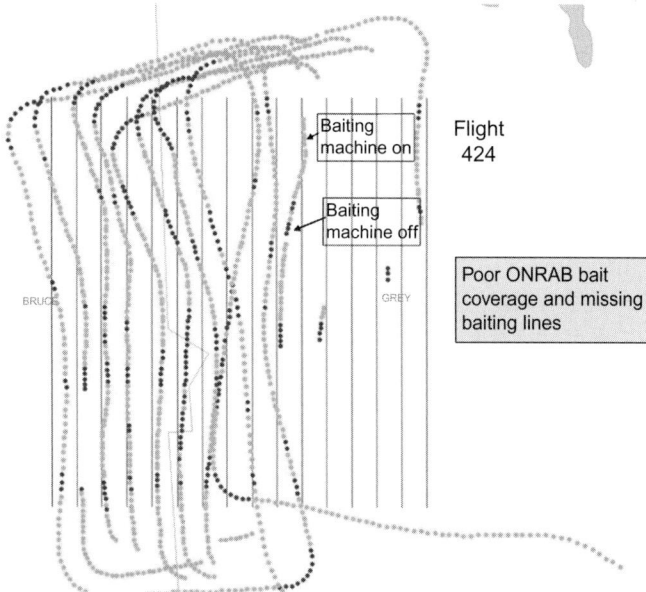

FIGURE 5   Planned flight lines with respect to actual flight line and ONRAB® bait placement in SW Ontario, Canada during September 2009 (figure by L. Brown). (See Page 13 in Color Section at the back of the book.)

Twin Otter containing automated baiting machinery capable of baiting hundreds of thousands of square kilometers of landscape can place baits at high density with GPS accuracy (Bachmann *et al.*, 1990; MacInnes *et al.*, 2001; Rosatte *et al.*, 2008, 2009b; Sidwa *et al.*, 2005). For example, in Ontario, a Twin Otter aircraft is capable of baiting a 540 km^2 area in 1 h with a bait density of 20 baits/km^2 (Johnston and Tinline, 2002). In fact, a 28,000 km^2 area was baited in 1 week in 2009 during fox rabies control operations. Even more impressive is that in the United States, a 180,000 km^2 area was baited during 2003 using 10 million rabies vaccine baits (Rosatte *et al.*, 2007c; Slate *et al.*, 2005). Ontario aircraft have distributed >60 million rabies vaccine baits in North America since 1989.

IV. ADVANCES IN WILDLIFE RABIES VACCINES

A V-RG recombinant vaccine showed great promise as an oral vaccine for wildlife in the laboratory during the 1980s when experiments were conducted on captive raccoons and foxes (Rupprecht and Kieny, 1988). V-RG worked well for the control of rabies in gray foxes and coyotes in Texas where resulting mean serum rabies antibody levels were about 61% and 63%, respectively (Slate *et al.*, 2009). However, V-RG has not proven to be effective for the control and elimination of raccoon rabies in North America where serum antibody levels in raccoons have been about 30% (Rosatte *et al.*, 2008; Slate *et al.*, 2005, 2009). The reason for the poor performance of V-RG in raccoons is unknown. Additional research is needed to improve the efficacy of V-RG in raccoons in the field.

In Europe, SAD-B19 and SAD-Berne proved to be effective in the target species such as red foxes; however, these vaccine strains were pathogenic in some rodents. In view of this, safer vaccines were developed for use in Europe during the late 1980s including V-RG, SAG1, and SAG2 (Artois *et al.*, 1997; Lambot *et al.*, 2001; Pastoret and Brochier, 1999). During the 2000s, SAG2 was used in some areas of Europe to control rabies in red foxes and raccoon dogs (Niin *et al.*, 2008).

ERA® modified live-virus rabies vaccine was first used in Ontario in the field during 1985 to orally immunize red foxes against the Arctic variant of rabies virus (MacInnes, 1988). Larger sized experiments and eventual control programs occurred in Ontario using ERA® baits during 1989–2009 (MacInnes *et al.*, 2001; Rosatte *et al.*, 2007e). However, ERA® was not effective in striped skunks or raccoons which were two other primary vectors of rabies in Ontario. In addition, ERA also was capable of causing vaccine-induced rabies in some species (foxes, raccoons, skunks, one bovine calf, and rodents) in Ontario (Black and Lawson, 1980; Fehlner-Gardiner *et al.*, 2008).

With the advancement of raccoon rabies into Ontario during 1999, an attempt was made to control the disease using V-RG baits. During 1999–2006, about 3.6 million V-RG baits were distributed in an approximate 4000–9000 km^2 area in eastern Ontario. However, vaccine efficacy in raccoons was very disappointing with seropositivity rates ranging between 7% and 28% (Rosatte et al., 2008). Therefore, a more effective vaccine, ONRAB® was developed (Rosatte et al., 2009b). ONRAB® is a human adenovirus type 5-rabies glycoprotein recombinant vaccine. Experiments in the laboratory using ONRAB® orally in a variety of species (target and nontarget) revealed low rates of recovery of the vaccine virus from the oral cavity, feces, and tissues, indicating that the vaccine would be safe for use in wildlife (Knowles et al., 2009a). A qRT-PCR (real time) technique was used to determine the quantity of vaccine present (Knowles et al., 2009b). Research advances on baits, vaccines, and delivery systems in Ontario resulted in vaccine efficacy (ONRAB®) in raccoons ranging from 79% to 90% with vaccine baiting densities of 75–400/km^2 during 2006/2007 (Rosatte et al., 2009b). During 2009, aerial and ground distribution of ONRAB® replaced TVR as a proactive tactic to prevent raccoon rabies from entering Ontario via Niagara Falls (R. Rosatte, unpublished observations). ONRAB® is also currently (2010) being used in Quebec to control raccoon rabies.

Advancements in rabies vaccine research for canine rabies control in Asia have been slow primarily due to inadequate funding, a lack of government motivation, and cultural issues (Wilde et al., 2005). In South America, outbreaks of rabies in vampire bats and transmission to humans have been attributed to the continued deforestation of the Amazon region which has resulted in the displacement of bats (Gupta, 2005). V-RG (in Vaseline) was applied to the back of vampire bats in captivity to see if their behaviors would result in the immunization of other bats in the same containment area. V-RG proved to be immunogenic and survival of bats was good (43–71%) upon challenge with rabies virus (Almeida et al., 2005, 2008a,b). In the United States, Hanlon et al. (2002) evaluated an attenuated SAG2 rabies vaccine for safety and efficacy when administered orally to skunks and raccoons. Upon challenge with rabies virus, four of five skunks and five of five raccoons survived making it a promising candidate for ORV of those species in North America (Hanlon et al., 2002). In that experiment, five of five control (unvaccinated) raccoons and four of five control skunks developed rabies upon challenge (Hanlon et al., 2002).

Research on the development of a canine adenovirus recombinant rabies vaccine (CAV2) showed promise in the laboratory for use on raccoons in North America (Slate et al., 2009). In addition, Dietzschold et al. (2004) examined the stability of several live rabies virus recombinant vaccines (called SPBNGA, SPBNGA-Cyto c, and SPBNGA-GA) for use in wildlife. Other vaccine research experiments were conducted on a lyo-philized vaccine (SAG2) for use in foxes in the Arctic regions of North America (Follmann *et al.*, 2004). A lyophilized vaccine as opposed to a liquid vaccine may be more appropriate for use in cold climates where freezing of vaccine might be a problem during baiting campaigns.

V. ADVANCES IN THE ASSESSMENT OF WILDLIFE VACCINATION SYSTEMS

During the 1970s, fluorochrome biomarkers were incorporated into test baits to determine whether oral vaccination of wildlife with baits was feasible (Wandeler *et al.*, 1982). Tetracyclines, which bind to teeth and bone and form a permanent marker have long been used as a means of determining bait acceptance by wildlife rabies vector species (Bachmann *et al.*, 1990; MacInnes *et al.*, 2001; Rosatte and Lawson, 2001). During the 1990s, Rosatte and Lawson (2001) experimented with different densities of placebo baits containing tetracycline to determine the potential for delivering ORV to raccoons in urban and rural habitats of Ontario, Canada. Advances have been made to the point where the date of bait ingestion can be determined by counting the daily growth lines in the teeth of young animals (Rosatte *et al.*, 2007c). In juvenile animals, teeth grow rapidly and daily growth lines can be detected using a microscope. Given the date the tooth was collected from the animal, the exact date the animal ingested the bait (which contained tetracycline) can be determined by the position of tetracycline in the tooth section (see Fig. 18.4 in Rosatte *et al.*, 2007c for illustrations of tooth growth lines and tetracycline deposition) (MacInnes, 1988).

The mouse neutralization test (MNT) was first used for the detection of serum rabies neutralizing antibody more than seven decades ago. It is still in use today and is an accepted reference test (Campbell and Barton, 1988). The Rapid Fluorescent Focus Inhibition Test (RFFIT) was, and still is, an accepted method to detect specific neutralizing antibodies as is the Virus Neutralization Test (Smith, 1995). Hemaglutination-based tests can also be used to measure antibody.

Since the 1970s, the enzyme-linked immunosorbent assay (ELISA) has become one of the most widely used diagnostic tests and can be utilized to measure specific immunoglobulins such as IgM (Campbell and Barton, 1988). ELISA tests may be easier and simpler to use than other tests (e.g., the MNT). However, the ELISA measures antibody binding reactions, which may not be rabies virus neutralizing antibody (Campbell and Barton, 1988). Commercial ELISA kits are available that allow quantitative detection of rabies virus antibodies in wildlife populations provided that the kits have been validated for the species in question (Shankar, 2009).

Current rabies control operations in areas such as Ontario, Canada, normally sample blood and teeth from target rabies vector populations to assess vaccine-bait uptake and vaccine efficacy and to determine the percentage of the population immunized (Rosatte *et al.*, 2009b). Rabies virus neutralizing antibody is detected in sera samples to determine the efficacy of the vaccine in stimulating an antibody response. Sampling of target populations usually occurs 5–6 weeks postbaiting to allow the target species time to find baits as well as to ensure that sufficient time has passed for the vaccine to have produced an immune response.

Also key to the assessment of the effectiveness of rabies control programs is the ability to diagnose new rabies cases as soon as possible in an area where control has been implemented, to allow for control before the disease becomes established or enters an enzootic phase. Historically, the gold standard diagnostic rabies test has been the Fluorescent Antibody Test (FAT) and it has 98–100% reliability in diagnosing rabies cases (Shankar, 2009). The use of direct Rapid Immunohistochemical Tests (dRIT) in the field for diagnosis of rabies surveillance specimens has decreased the time in which researchers can receive rabies diagnostic test results (Blanton *et al.*, 2006). This advancement allows for a faster response time for controlling new rabies outbreaks. Research advances have included the development of tests which are more sensitive than the FAT including reverse transcription-polymerase chain reaction (RT-PCR) and PCR-TaqMan tests for detecting viral RNA in samples of saliva and blood (Cliquet and Picard-Meyer, 2004; Shankar, 2009). A TaqMan real-time PCR was used to detect minute quantities of virus in brain tissues of skunks and raccoons (Szanto, 2009). In that research project, 10 of 721 samples were positive by PCR, but negative by FAT (Szanto, 2009) proving it to be a useful tool for rabies diagnosis.

VI. ADVANCES IN CONTINGENCY AND MANAGEMENT PLANNING FOR WILDLIFE RABIES CONTROL

Historically, there was very little advanced planning for wildlife rabies control programs. Initially, the premise was that the best way to get rid of the problem was to remove it—that is, population reduction or killing the vector. If a case of rabies occurred, the solution was simple—send a team out to trap and kill the species that was transmitting the disease (Rosatte *et al.*, 1986). However, significant advancements have been made in the area of contingency and management planning for rabies control. Some jurisdictions plan the course of action to follow well in advance of an outbreak. For example, RABMEDCONTROL is a European program that has the objective of eliminating rabies in North Africa. Research advances and data are forwarded to health agencies to facilitate the design of effective strategies to eliminate rabies from North Africa (http://pasteur.fr/). Research on the complex Serengeti ecosystem revealed that rabies (a southern Africa canid-associated virus infection) only occurs sporadically in wildlife (e.g., in certain jackal and mongoose species) and management plans that target dogs should reduce the risk of rabies in wildlife populations (Lembo *et al.*, 2008).

In Europe, rabies management planning calls for the vaccination of vectors for at least 2 years after the last case has been reported (Muller *et al.*, 2005). The management goal in Germany is for all foxes to have access to rabies vaccine baits (Thulke *et al.*, 2004). In addition, the European Commission subsidized wildlife rabies management programs in Europe beginning in 1989 on the condition that the programs are coordinated among countries especially along border areas (Cliquet and Picard-Meyer, 2004).

Preparation of contingency plans before epizootics occur is crucial to successful rabies control programs (Rosatte *et al.*, 1997, 2007c). Part of successful contingency planning is to have proactive research programs in place well in advance of the impending epizootic so that the most effective tactic can be employed when actual cases occur. In fact, in Ontario, proactive TVR programs were implemented in Niagara Falls as part of a research project 5 years prior to the first case of raccoon rabies being reported in that province (Rosatte *et al.*, 1997, 2009a). Incredibly, raccoon rabies has yet (July 2010) to be reported in Niagara Falls, Ontario, despite the disease being enzootic in the nearby Niagara Falls, New York area. However, the disease was reported in eastern Ontario during 1999, and the contingency plan was put into practice. Population reduction and TVR were used to contain the outbreak of raccoon rabies during 1999 and 2000 (Rosatte *et al.*, 2001). The Ontario raccoon rabies contingency plan was modified during subsequent years to adapt to the rabies situation, for example, in response to some cases only TVR was used (Rosatte *et al.*, 2009a).

A GIS-based, real-time rabies surveillance database and Internet mapping application (RabID) was developed in the United States to evaluate wildlife rabies vaccination programs and provide input for rabies management planning (Blanton *et al.*, 2006). Wildlife rabies control program success is dependent upon timely and accurate rabies surveillance data so that a response to a rabies outbreak can be immediate with no time lags. By using dRIT in the field for testing of surveillance specimens, results can be posted in real time the same day. This is a significant advancement over the old system that could take up to 4 weeks to receive, test, and post results of potentially rabid animals (Blanton *et al.*, 2006).

Significant advancements have also been made in rabies management planning. Interjurisdictional collaboration has been vital for the implementation of ORV programs in the Americas. The North American Rabies

Management Plan was signed by representatives from Canada, the United States, and Mexico at the September 2008 Rabies in the Americas conference (Slate *et al.*, 2009). The plan establishes a framework to build long-term rabies management goals among the signing countries and promotes information sharing in relation to ORV research, wildlife management, population control, and surveillance techniques (Slate *et al.*, 2009). The Canadian Rabies Committee (CRC) was established in 2007 to address prevention and management of rabies and includes members from public health, agriculture, and wildlife agencies. The CRC produced a Canadian Rabies Management Plan that was signed at the 20th Rabies in the Americas Conference in Quebec City, 2009. Both the Canadian and North American rabies management plans are significant advancements that will promote "state-of-the-art" rabies-related research and management.

VII. ADVANCES IN TECHNOLOGIES FOR STUDYING THE ECOLOGY OF THE RABIES VIRUS AND WILDLIFE RABIES VECTOR SPECIES

To design an effective wildlife rabies control tactic, information on the ecology of the target species as well as the virus is critical. In Canada, the Ontario wildlife rabies control program evolved from one of studying the ecology of rabies vector species (Johnston and Beauregard, 1969; Rosatte and Lariviere, 2003; Voigt, 1987) to development of systems to deliver vaccine to those species. The use of radio-telemetry has advanced the knowledge of rabies vector species ecology and thus the ability to design effective rabies control tactics. Telemetry was used to study the ecology of red foxes, raccoons, and striped skunks in metropolitan Toronto (Rosatte *et al.*, 1991). The data were used to develop an effective wildlife rabies management plan and the disease was eventually eliminated in terrestrial mammals from that urban complex (Rosatte *et al.*, 2007e).

Ecological studies on raccoons in Ontario using state-of-the-art GPS collars (accurate to 5 m) enabled researchers to determine intimate details on the ecology of raccoons including home range, denning and breeding periods, animal movements, and periods of high contact (Rosatte *et al.*, 2010a,b). This information was used during the 1990s and 2000s in Ontario for designing wildlife rabies control response tactics (Rosatte *et al.*, 2001, 2009a,b). Telemetry revealed that raccoons were active between March and November during any given year in Ontario (Rosatte *et al.*, 2010a). Mark-recapture studies also revealed that raccoon movement was substantial during the summer/early fall periods (Rosatte *et al.*, 2007a). Home range studies using telemetry revealed habitats that received high use by raccoons that could be targeted for baiting (Rosatte *et al.*, 2010a; Totton *et al.*, 2004). Bait acceptance studies also proved that the optimal time for baiting raccoons was August and September in Ontario (Rosatte and Lawson, 2001; Rosatte *et al.*, 2007a,b,c).

Rabies case data were used to estimate the incubation period of raccoon rabies in Ontario, Canada (Tinline *et al.*, 2002). In addition, an analysis of rabies case data in Ontario revealed critical information on the behavior, movements, and demographics of rabid raccoons that assisted with the development of an effective rabies management program in Canada (Rosatte *et al.*, 2006). Other studies revealed a correlation between the presence of porcupine quills in raccoons (indicating aberrant behavior) and a diagnosis of rabies in eastern Canada which is valuable information for rabies surveillance operations and detecting new cases in an area previously free of reported rabies (Rosatte *et al.*, 2007d). Rabies vector ecological data can be used to optimize rabies vaccine bait-distribution using GPS navigational systems in aircraft, which should lead to efficacious wildlife rabies control and eradication programs (Rosatte *et al.*, 2007c).

Mark-recapture studies have also been used to estimate rabies vector density, which will assist in determining the density of baits necessary to reach the target population (Rosatte *et al.*, 2009a). Telemetry and bait-acceptance studies have also revealed that the majority of rabies vaccine baits are consumed within 1–3 weeks of bait placement (Bachmann *et al.*, 1990; Blackwell *et al.*, 2004). Mark-recapture also provides data so that an estimation of the percentage of the population that is vaccinated or removed by TVR or PIC tactics can be calculated (Rosatte *et al.*, 2009a).

Advances in research have also been accomplished with respect to the use of genetics to study the ecology of rabies vector species. Estimates of raccoon dispersal in Ontario, Canada, were acquired using parentage and spatial genetic analysis of raccoons. Potential travel corridors for rabies-infected raccoons were identified and the data were used for disease management planning in Ontario during the 2000s (Cullingham *et al.*, 2008). Molecular research was conducted comparing rabies virus isolates from the Greenland, Arctic, North America, the former Soviet Union, and Baltic regions (Mansfield *et al.*, 2006). They concluded that there was evidence of the cross-border movement of rabies in Arctic regions. However, in another study, Kuzmin *et al.* (2004) compared isolates from Eurasia, Africa, and North America using nucleoprotein gene sequences and concluded that the molecular evidence suggested that the current fox rabies epizootic in the former Soviet Union formed independently from those in western and Central Europe.

One of the more recent advances in rabies research tools is the genetic variant analysis of rabies virus to map the spread of virus in wildlife vector species (e.g., red foxes and striped skunks). Using this technology, Nadine-Davis *et al.* (2006) identified four primary genetic variants for Ontario, Canada. Genetic differences among the viral strains were used to identify the origin of the variants. This research suggested that failure to completely eliminate rabies in SW Ontario was not due to incursions from other areas, but due to a failure to completely interrupt the cycle of rabies transmission among the wildlife vectors (Nadine-Davis *et al.*, 2006). This research reinforces the fact that rabies control activities need to occur over the long-term and that striped skunks play a major role in maintaining the Arctic variant of rabies virus in southern Ontario, Canada (Nadine-Davis *et al.*, 2006).

Rabies epizoological patterns in Mexico were also described by Velasco-Villa *et al.* (2005) through the use of genetic and antigenic analysis of isolates from Mexican wildlife during 1976–2002. They suggest that there were two origins for rabies in Mexico—one that evolved from canine rabies virus and the other from vampire bat rabies virus. They also propose that a skunk rabies focus in north central Mexico is related (shared a common ancestor) to bat rabies foci in North America.

It is also important to have knowledge of the metapopulation structure of rabies vector species to understand the dynamics of epizootics. This can be attained by using mark-recapture study data in population models which will determine which populations may be most vulnerable to a disease outbreak. Broadfoot *et al.* (2001) used population models to identify raccoon and skunk metapopulations in Toronto and targeted these for potential control operations should a rabies outbreak occur in that metropolitan complex.

The use of models for researching the dynamics of rabies vector species and disease has also advanced significantly over the past few decades. During the 1980s, deterministic models (mathematical models without the use of random variation of variables) were used to study fox rabies dynamics in Europe (Anderson *et al.*, 1981). During the late 1980s and early 1990s, stochastic models (range of values for variables used) were developed using animal behavioral data (Voigt *et al.*, 1985). Other researchers including Smith *et al.* (2002) and Russell *et al.* (2005) used models to demonstrate how the geography of the landscape can affect rabies spread. Rees *et al.* (2009) used a landscape genetic model to understand the variables affecting the spread of raccoon rabies in Ontario, Canada.

Recently, models incorporating vector ecological data have been used to optimize rabies vaccine-bait delivery systems (Rosatte *et al.*, 2007c). In Germany, Thulke *et al.* (2004) used a simulation model combining space use by foxes and aircraft baiting lines to design an effective ORV strategy to control rabies in that species. They surmised that an increase in vaccine-bait density did not necessarily translate to an increase in bait acceptance by foxes. In fact, their study indicated that 5–10% of fox groups did not have any vaccine baits in their spatial area of utilization. They also found an increase in fox bait acceptance when the spacing between flight lines was decreased. This was also shown to be true for skunks in Ontario (R. Rosatte, unpublished observations).

Eisinger and Thulke (2008) predicted (based on modeling vector population ecology data) that a lower rabies management effort (i.e., baits/km^2) could be used than what was currently being implemented in Europe. They suggested that a new approach using fewer vaccine baits for fox rabies control would create a significant economic benefit with a target of 18–20 baits/km^2 and achieving a herd immunity in foxes of >70%. However, in some areas of Europe, control of rabies was achieved with <70% immunity in foxes (Eisinger and Thulke, 2008). They suggested that by reducing vector immunity targets by 10% and by using fewer vaccine baits (14 km^{-2}) that up to one-third of the rabies management resources currently being used would be saved.

VIII. SUMMARY

Significant research advances directed toward the control, elimination, and eradication of rabies have been made during the past few decades. Research has progressed so that control of the disease does not rely solely upon culling techniques. In fact, oral rabies vaccination has proven to be a feasible and effective method to control rabies in wildlife vectors. Rabies has been eliminated in large expanses of Europe and North America. However, ORV strategies need to be adopted by developing nations, especially for the control of canine rabies and resultant spillover to wildlife (Rupprecht et al., 2006). Research should be continued to further investigate the complex relationship of canine rabies and spillover to wildlife populations in areas such as South Africa. In addition, research is needed to determine the level of herd immunity in primary rabies vector species at which rabies will disappear from the target population to increase the cost effectiveness of control programs. Research is also needed to preserve genetically unique populations (e.g., African wild dogs) from this deadly disease (Ogun et al., 2010).

Research advances in wildlife rabies control techniques have been highly effective in areas such as Ontario, Canada. For example, raccoon rabies has been eliminated, and the province is realizing a $6M–$10M annual savings in rabies-associated costs (Rosatte et al., 2008, 2009a). However, globally there is a significant amount of research that needs to be addressed including knowledge of rabies transmission among bats, bat ecology, and improved techniques to immunize insectivorous as well as hematophagous bats.

Although an effective system to orally immunize free-ranging skunks in Canada has been developed, research is needed to develop an effective vaccine bait for skunks in more southern climates (Ramey and Mills,

2008). The matrix of vaccine baits that are effective in northern climates such as Canada may not withstand the higher temperatures of southern climates. In addition, the control of raccoon rabies in the United States has been challenging and research with respect to the development of new effective vaccine baits is critical to control the disease before the enzootic expands in a westerly direction. Research is also needed to more completely understand the viral host shift that occurred during an outbreak of bat variant rabies in skunks in Arizona in 2001 and reemergence of rabies in gray foxes during 2008/2009 (Slate *et al.*, 2009).

Large-scale ORV operations employing aircraft and GPS precision are being used globally to control wildlife rabies today. However, research is still needed to determine the number of baits to distribute as well as spatial distribution patterns for baiting to maximize bait uptake by wildlife vectors and also minimize rabies management costs. The cost of vaccine baits alone approaches 85–90% of ORV program costs and research is desperately needed to develop more affordable vaccines, especially for use by developing nations. In addition, research in model development to assist with rabies management decisions is needed along with research to determine the effect that other diseases such as canine distemper may have on an animals' ability to develop an immune response following contact with ORV.

REFERENCES

Algeo, T., Chipman, R., Bjorldand, B., Chandler, M., Wang, X., Slate, D., and Rupprecht, C. (2008). Anatomy of the Cape Cod oral rabies vaccination program. *In* "23rd Vertebrate Pest Conference Proceedings", (R. Timm and M. Madon, eds.), pp. 264–269. University of California, Davis, CA.

Almeida, M., Martorelli, L., Aires, C., Sallum, P., and Massad, E. (2008a). Indirect oral immunization of captive vampires (*Desmodus rotundus*). *Virus Res.* **111**:77–82.

Almeida, M., Martorelli, L., Aires, C., Barros, K., and Massad, E. (2008b). Vaccinating the vampire bat (*Desmodus rotundus*). *Virus Res.* **137**:275–277.

Anderson, R. M., Jackson, H. C., May, R. M., and Smith, M. (1981). Population dynamics of fox rabies in Europe. *Nature* **289**:765–771.

Artois, M., Cliquet, F., Barrat, J., and Schumacher, C. (1997). Effectiveness of SAG1 oral vaccine for long-term protection of red foxes (*Vulpes vulpes*) against rabies. *Vet. Rec.* **140**:57–59.

Aubert, M., Masson, E., Artois, M., and Barrat, J. (1994). Oral wildlife rabies vaccination field trials in Europe with recent emphasis on France. *In* "Lyssaviruses", (C. Rupprecht, B. Dietzschold, and H. Koprowski, eds.), pp. 219–243. Springer-Verlag, Berlin.

Bachmann, P., Bramwell, R. N., Fraser, S. J., Gilmore, D. H., Johnston, D. H., Lawson, K. F., MacInnes, C. D., Matejka, F. O., Miles, H. E., Pedde, M. A., and Voigt, D. R. (1990). Wild carnivore acceptance of baits for delivery of liquid rabies vaccine. *J. Wildl. Dis.* **26**:486–501.

Baer, G. M., Abelseth, M. K., and Debbie, J. G. (1971). Oral vaccination of foxes against rabies. *Am. J. Epidemiol.* **93**:487–490.

Ballantyne, E., and O'Donoghue, J. (1954). Rabies control in Alberta. *J. Am. Vet. Med. Assoc.* **125**:316–326.

Bender, S., Bergman, D., Wenning, K., Miller, L., Slate, D., Jackson, F., and Rupprecht, C. (2009). No adverse effects of simultaneous vaccination with the immuno-contraceptive GonaCon™ and a commercial rabies vaccine on rabies virus neutralizing antibody production in dogs. *Vaccine* **27:**7210–7213.

Black, J. G., and Lawson, K. F. (1970). Sylvatic rabies studies in the silver fox (*Vulpes vulpes*): Susceptibility and immune response. *Can. J. Comp. Med.* **34:**309–311.

Black, J. G., and Lawson, K. F. (1980). Safety and efficacy of immunizing foxes (*Vulpes vulpes*) using baits containing attenuated rabies virus vaccine. *Can. J. Comp. Med.* **44:**169–176.

Blackwell, B., Seamans, T., White, R., Patton, Z., Bush, R., and Cepek, J. (2004). Exposure time of oral rabies vaccine baits relative to baiting density and raccoon population density. *J. Wildl. Dis.* **40:**222–229.

Blancou, J., Artois, M., Gilot-Fromont, E., Kaden, V., Rossi, S., Smith, G., Hutchings, M., Chambers, M., Houghton, S., and Delahay, R. (2009). Options for the control of disease 1: Targeting the infectious or parasitic agent. *In* "Management of Disease in Wild Mammals", (R. Delahay, G. Smith, and M. Hutchings, eds.), pp. 97–120. Springer, Japan.

Blanton, J., Manangan, A., Manangan, J., Hanlon, C., Slate, D., and Rupprecht, C. (2006). Development of a GIS based real time Internet mapping tool for rabies surveillance. *Int. J. Health Geophys.* **5:**47. doi: 10.1186/1476-072x-5-47.

Bourhy, H., Docheux, L., Strudy, C., and Mailles, A. (2005). Rabies in Europe 2005. *Eurosurveillance* **10**(11):pii = 575.

Broadfoot, J., Rosatte, R., and O'Leary, D. (2001). Raccoon and skunk population models for urban disease control planning in Ontario, Canada. *EcologicalApplications* **11:**295–303.

Brochier, B., Thomas, I., Baudin, B., Leveau, B., Pastoret, P., Languet, B., Chappuis, G., Desmettre, P., Blancou, J., and Artois, M. (1990). Use of a vaccinia-rabies recombinant virus for the oral vaccination of foxes against rabies. *Vaccine* **8:**101–104.

Brochier, B., Deschamps, P., Costy, F., Leuris, J., Villers, M., Peharpre, D., Mosselmans, F., Beier, R., Lecomte, L., Mullier, P., Roland, H., Bauduin, B., *et al.* (2001). Elimination of sylvatic rabies in Belgium by oral vaccination of the red fox (*Vulpes vulpes*). *Ann. Méd. Vét.* **145:**293–305.

Campbell, J. B., and Barton, L. (1988). Serodiagnosis of rabies: Antibody tests. *In* "Rabies", (J. B. Campbell and K. M. Charlton, eds.), pp. 223–241. Kluwer Academic Publishers, Norwell, MA.

Cliquet, F., and Picard-Meyer, E. (2004). Rabies and rabies-related viruses: A modern perspective on an ancient disease. *Rev. Sci. Tech. L'Office Int. Epizootics* **23:**625–642.

Cullingham, C., Pond, B., Kyle, K., Rosatte, R., and White, B. (2008). Combining direct and indirect genetic methods to estimate dispersal for informing wildlife disease management decisions. *Mol. Ecol.* **17:**4874–4886.

Debbie, J. (1991). Rabies control in terrestrial wildlife by population reduction. *In* "The Natural History of Rabies", (G. Baer, ed.), 2nd edn., pp. 477–484. CRC Press, Boca Raton, FL.

Dietzschold, M., Faber, M., Mattis, J., Pak, K., Schnell, M., and Dietzschold, B. (2004). *In vitro* growth and stability of recombinant rabies virus designed for vaccination of wildlife. *Vaccine* **23:**518–524.

Eisinger, D., and Thulke, H. (2008). Spatial pattern formation facilitates eradication of infectious disease. *J. Appl. Ecol.* **45:**415–423.

Fehlner-Gardiner, C., Nadine-Davis, S., Armstrong, J., Muldoon, F., Bachmann, P., and Wandeler, A. (2008). ERA vaccine-induced cases of rabies in wildlife and domestic animals in Ontario, Canada, 1989–2004. *J. Wildl. Dis.* **44:**71–85.

Follmann, E., Ritter, D., and Hartbauer, D. (2004). Oral vaccination of captive arctic foxes with lyophilized SAG2 rabies vaccine. *J. Wildl. Dis.* **40:**328–334.

Gascoyne, S., King, A., Laurenson, M., Borner, M., Schildger, B., and Barrat, J. (1993). Aspects of rabies infection and control in the conservation of the African wild dog (*Lycaon pictus*) in the Serengeti region, Tanzania. *Onderstepoort J. Vet. Res.* **60:**415–420.

Gupta, R. (2005). Recent outbreak of rabies infections in Brazil transmitted by vampire bats. *Eurosurveillance* **10**(45)**:pii** = 2831.

Hanlon, C., Niezgoda, M., Morrill, P., and Rupprecht, C. (2002). Oral efficacy of an attenuated rabies virus vaccine in skunks and raccoons. *J. Wildl. Dis.* **38:**420–427.

Johnston, D. H., and Beauregard, M. (1969). Rabies epidemiology in Ontario. *Bull. Wildl. Dis. Assoc.* **5:**357–370.

Johnston, D. H., and Tinline, R. R. (2002). Rabies control in wildlife. *In* "Rabies", (A. Jackson and W. Wunner, eds.), pp. 445–471. Academic Press, San Diego, CA.

Knowles, M. K., Nadin-Davis, S. A., Sheen, M., Rosatte, R., Mueller, R., and Beresford, A. (2009a). Safety studies on an adenovirus recombinant vaccine for rabies (AdRG1.3-ONRAB®) in target and non-target species. *Vaccine* **27:**6619–6626.

Knowles, M. K., Roberts, D., Craig, S., Sheen, M., Nadin-Davis, S., and Wandeler, A. (2009b). In vitro and in vivo genetic stability studies of a human adenovirus type 5 recombinant rabies glycoprotein vaccine (ONRAB®). *Vaccine* **27:**2662–2668.

Kuzmin, I., Botvinkin, A., McElhinney, L., Smith, J., Orciari, L., Hughes, G., Fooks, A., and Rupprecht, C. (2004). Molecular epidemiology of terrestrial rabies in the former Soviet Union. *J. Wildl. Dis.* **40:**617–631.

Lambot, M., Blasco, E., Barrat, J., Cliquet, F., Brochier, B., Renders, C., Krafft, N., Bailly, J., Munier, M., Aubert, M., and Pastoret, P. (2001). Humoral and cell-mediated immune responses of foxes (*Vulpes vulpes*) after experimental primary and secondary oral vaccination using SAG₂ and V-RG vaccines. *Vaccine* **19:**1827–1835.

Lembo, T., Hampson, K., Haydon, D., Craft, M., Dobson, A., Dushoff, J., Ernest, E., Kaare, M., Mlengeya, T., Meatzel, C., and Cleveland, S. (2008). Exploring reservoir dynamics: A case study of rabies in the Serengeti ecosystem. *J. Appl. Ecol.* **45:**1246–1257.

MacInnes, C. D. (1988). Control of wildlife rabies: The Americas. *In* "Rabies", (J. B. Campbell and K. M. Charlton, eds.), pp. 381–405. Kluwer Academic Publishers, Norwell, MA.

MacInnes, C. D., Smith, S. M., Tinline, R. R., Ayers, N. R., Bachmann, P., Ball, D. G. A., Cader, L. A., Crosgrey, S. J., Fielding, C., Hauschildt, P., Honig, J. M., Johnston, D. H., *et al.* (2001). Elimination of rabies from red foxes in eastern Ontario. *J. Wildl. Dis.* **37:**119–132.

Mansfield, K., Racloz, V., McElhimney, L., Marston, D., Johnson, N., Ronsholt, L., Christensen, L., Neuvonen, E., Botvinkin, A., Rupprecht, C., and Fooks, A. (2006). Molecular epidemiological study of Arctic rabies virus isolates from Greenland, and comparison with isolates from throughout the Arctic and Baltic regions. *Virus Res.* **116:**1–10.

Matouch, O., and Polak, L. (1982). Rabies epizootiology and control in Czechoslovakia. *Comp. Immunol. Microbiol. Infect. Dis.* **5:**303–307.

Moutou, F. (2005). Knowledge of zoology can help clarify problems in epidemiology. *Eurosurveillance* **10**(11)**:pii** = 582.

Muller, T., Selhorst, T., and Potzsch, C. (2005). Fox rabies in Germany—An update. *Eurosurveillance* **10:**581.

Nadine-Davis, S., Muldoon, F., and Wandeler, A. (2006). Persistence of genetic variants of the Arctic fox strain of rabies virus in southern Ontario. *Can. J. Vet. Res.* **70:**11–19.

Niin, E., Laine, M., Guiot, A., Demerson, J., and Cliquet, F. (2008). Rabies in Estonia before and after the first campaigns of oral vaccination of wildlife with SAG2 vaccine bait. *Vaccine* **26:**3556–3565.

Nunan, C., Tinline, R., Honig, J., Ball, D., Hauschildt, P., and LeBer, C. (2002). Post exposure treatment and animal rabies, Ontario 1958–2000. *Emerg. Infect. Dis.* **8:**214–217.

Ogun, A., Okonko, I., Udeze, A., Shittu, I., Garba, K., Fowotade, A., Adewale, O., Fajobi, E., Onoja, B., Babalola, E., and Adedeji, A. (2010). Feasibility and factors affecting global elimination and possible eradication of rabies in the world. *J. Gen. Mol. Virol.* **2**:001–0027.

Pasteur, L. (1886). Resultats de l'application de la methode pour prevenir la rage après morsure. *C. R. Acad. Sci.* **102**:459.

Pastoret, P., and Brochier, B. (1999). Epidemiology and control of fox rabies in Europe. *Vaccine* **17**:1750–1754.

Pastoret, P., Kappeler, A., and Aubert, M. (2004). European rabies control and its history. *In* "Historical Perspective of Rabies in Europe and the Mediterranean Basin", (A. King, A. Fooks, M. Aubert, and A. Wandeler, eds.), pp. 337–350. OIE. World Organization for Animal Health Publishers, Paris, France.

Prusiner, S. (1997). Prion diseases and the BSE crisis. *Science* **278**:245–251.

Ramey, C., and Mills, K. (2008). Synopsis of the Shoshone River skunk rabies epizootic in northwestern Wyoming. *Proc. Vertebrate Pest Conf.* **23**:259–263.

Randall, D., Marino, J., Haydon, D., Sillero-Zubiri, C., Knobel, D., Tallents, L., MacDonald, D., and Laurenson, M. (2006). An integrated disease management strategy for the control of rabies in Ethiopian wolves. *Biol. Conserv.* **131**:151–162.

Rees, E., Pond, B., Cullingham, C., Tinline, R., Ball, D., Kyle, C., and White, B. (2009). Landscape modeling spatial bottlenecks: Implications for raccoon rabies disease spread. *Biol. Lett.* **5**:387–390.

Rosatte, R., and Lariviere, S. (2003). Skunks. *In* "Wild Mammals of North America; Biology, Management and Conservation", (G. Feldhamer, B. Thompson, and J. Chapman, eds.), 2nd edn., pp. 692–707. Johns Hopkins University Press, Baltimore, MD.

Rosatte, R., and Lawson, K. (2001). Acceptance of baits for delivery of oral rabies vaccine to raccoons. *J. Wildl. Dis.* **37**:730–739.

Rosatte, R., Pybus, M., and Gunson, J. (1986). Population reduction as a factor in the control of skunk rabies in Alberta. *J. Wildl. Dis.* **22**:459–467.

Rosatte, R., Howard, D., Campbell, J., and MacInnes, C. (1990). Intramuscular vaccination of skunks and raccoons against rabies. *J. Wildl. Dis.* **26**:225–230.

Rosatte, R., Power, M., and MacInnes, C. (1991). Ecology of urban skunks, raccoons, and foxes in Metropolitan Toronto. *In* "Wildlife Conservation in Metropolitan Environments", (L. Adams and D. Leedy, eds.), pp. 31–38. National Institute for Urban Wildlife, Columbia, MD.

Rosatte, R. C., Power, M. J., and MacInnes, C. D. (1992). Trap-vaccinate-release and oral vaccination techniques for rabies control in urban skunks, raccoons and foxes. *J. Wildl. Dis.* **28**:562–571.

Rosatte, R., MacInnes, C., Williams, R., and Williams, O. (1997). A proactive prevention strategy for raccoon rabies in Ontario, Canada. *Wildl. Soc. Bull.* **25**:110–116.

Rosatte, R. C., Donovan, D., Allan, M., Howes, L., Silver, A., Bennett, K., MacInnes, C., Davies, C., Wandeler, A., and Radford, B. (2001). Emergency response to raccoon rabies introduction in Ontario. *J. Wildl. Dis.* **37**:265–279.

Rosatte, R., Sobey, K., Donovan, D., Bruce, L., Allan, M., Silver, A., Bennett, K., Gibson, M., Simpson, H., Davies, J. C., Wandeler, A., and Muldoon, F. (2006). Behaviour, movements, and demographics of rabid raccoons in Ontario, Canada: Management implications. *J. Wildl. Dis.* **42**:589–605.

Rosatte, R., MacDonald, E., Sobey, K., Donovan, D., Bruce, L., Allan, M., Silver, A., Bennett, K., Brown, L., MacDonald, K., Gibson, M., Buchanan, T., *et al.* (2007a). The elimination of raccoon rabies from Wolfe Island, Ontario: Animal density and movements. *J. Wildl. Dis.* **43**:242–250.

Rosatte, R., Sobey, K., Donovan, D., Allan, M., Bruce, L., Buchanan, T., and Davies, J. C. (2007b). Raccoon density and movements after population reduction to control rabies. *J. Wildl. Manage.* **71**:2373–2378.

Rosatte, R., Tinline, R., and Johnston, D. (2007c). Rabies control in wild carnivores. *In* "Rabies", (A. Jackson and W. Wunner, eds.), 2nd edn., pp. 595–634. Academic Press, San Diego, CA.

Rosatte, R., Wandeler, A., Muldoon, F., and Campbell, D. (2007d). Porcupine quills in raccoons as an indicator of rabies, distemper, or both diseases: Disease management implications. *Can. Vet. J.* **48:**299–300.

Rosatte, R. C., Power, M., Donovan, D., Davies, J. C., Allan, M., Bachmann, P., Stevenson, B., Wandeler, A., and Muldoon, F. (2007e). Elimination of arctic variant rabies in red foxes, metropolitan Toronto. *Emerg. Infect. Dis.* **13**(1):25–27.

Rosatte, R. C., Allan, M., Bachmann, P., Sobey, K., Donovan, D., Davies, J. C., Silver, A., Bennett, K., Brown, L., Stevenson, B., Buchanan, T., Bruce, L., *et al.* (2008). Prevalence of tetracycline and rabies virus antibody in raccoons, skunks, and foxes following aerial distribution of V-RG baits to control raccoon rabies in Ontario, Canada. *J. Wildl. Dis.* **45:**772–784.

Rosatte, R., Donovan, D., Davies, J. C., Allan, M., Bruce, L., Buchanan, T., Sobey, K., Stevenson, B., Gibson, M., MacDonald, T., Whalen, M., Muldoon, F., *et al.* (2009a). The control of raccoon rabies in Ontario, Canada: Proactive and reactive tactics, 1994–2007. *J. Wildl. Dis.* **45:**772–784.

Rosatte, R. C., Donovan, D., Davies, J. C., Allan, A., Bachmann, P., Stevenson, B., Sobey, K., Brown, L., Silver, A., Bennett, K., Buchanan, T., Bruce, L., *et al.* (2009b). Aerial distribution of ONRAB® baits as a tactic to control rabies in raccoons and striped skunks in Ontario, Canada. *J. Wildl. Dis.* **45:**363–374.

Rosatte, R., Ryckman, M., Ing, K., Proceviat, S., Allan, M., Bruce, L., Donovan, D., and Davies, J. C. (2010a). Density, movements, and survival of raccoons in Ontario, Canada: Implications for disease spread and management. *J. Mammal.* **91:**122 135.

Rosatte, R., Ryckman, M., Meech, S., Proceviat, S., Bruce, L., Donovan, D., and Davies, J. C. (2010b). Home range, movements and survival of rehabilitated raccoons (*Procyon lotor*) in Ontario, Canada. *J. Wildl. Rehabil.* **30:**7–12.

Rupprecht, C., and Kieny, M. (1988). Development of a vaccinia-rabies glycoprotein recombinant virus vaccine. *In* "Rabies", (J. B. Campbell and C. M. Charlton, eds.), pp. 335–364. Kluwer Academic Publishers, Norwell, MA.

Rupprecht, C., Willoughby, C., and Slate, D. (2006). Current and future trends in the prevention, treatment and control of rabies. *Expert Rev. Anti-Infect. Ther.* **4:**1021–1038.

Russell, C., Smith, D., Childs, J., and Real, L. (2005). Predictive spatial dynamics and strategic planning for raccoon rabies emergence in Ohio. *PLoS Biol.* **3:**382–388.

Sattler, A., Krogwold, R., Wittum, T., Rupprecht, C., Algeo, T., Slate, D., Smith, K., Hale, R., Nohrenberg, G., Lovell, C., Niezgoda, M., Montoney, A., *et al.* (2009). Influence of oral rabies vaccine bait density on rabies seroprevalence in wild raccoons. *Vaccine* **27:**7187–7193.

Schneider, L., and Cox, J. (1988). Eradications of rabies through oral vaccination. The German field trial. *In* "Vaccination to Control Rabies in Foxes", (P. Pastoret, B. Brochier, I. Thomas, and J. Blancou, eds.), pp. 22–38. Commission of the European Communities, Luxembourg.

Shankar, B. (2009). Advances in diagnosis of rabies. *Vet. World* **2:**74–78.

Sidwa, T., Wilson, P., Moore, G., Oertli, E., Hicks, B., Rohde, R., and Johnston, D. (2005). Evaluation of oral rabies vaccination programs for control of rabies epizootics in coyotes and gray foxes: 1995–2003. *J. Am. Vet. Med. Assoc.* **227:**785–792.

Slate, D., Rupprecht, C., Rooney, J., Donovan, D., Lein, D., and Chipman, R. (2005). Status of oral rabies vaccination in wild carnivores in the United States. *Virus Res.* **111:**68–76.

Slate, D., Algeo, T., Nelson, K., Chipman, R., Donovan, D., Blanton, J., Niezgoda, M., and Rupprecht, C. (2009). Oral rabies vaccination in North America: Opportunities complexities and challenges. *PLOS Negl. Trop. Dis.* **3**(12):e549. doi: 10.1371/journalpntd.0000549.

Smith, J. S. (1995). Rabies virus. *In* "Manual of Clinical Microbiology", (P. Murray, E. Baron, M. Pfaller, F. Tenover, and R. Yolken, eds.), pp. 997–1003. American Society for Microbiology, Washington, DC.

Smith, D. L., Brendan, L., Waller, L., Childs, J., and Real, L. (2002). Predicting the spatial dynamics of rabies epidemics on heterogeneous landscapes. *Proc. Natl. Acad. Sci. USA* **99**:3668–3672.

Steck, F., Wandeler, A., Bichsel, P., Capt, S., and Schneider, L. (1982). Oral immunisation of foxes against rabies. A field study. *Zentralbl Veterinärmed.* **29**:372–396.

Steele, J. (1975). History of rabies. *In* "The Natural History of Rabies", (G. M. Baer, ed.), Vol. 1, pp. 1–29. Academic Press, New York, NY.

Storm, G., and Sanderson, G. (1969a). Effect of medroxyprogesterone acetate (Provera) on productivity in captive foxes. *J. Mammal.* **50**:147–149.

Storm, G., and Sanderson, G. (1969b). Results of a field test to control striped skunks with diethylstilbestrol. *Trans. Ill. State Acad. Sci.* **62**:193–197.

Szanto, A. (2009). Molecular Genetics of the Raccoon Rabies Virus. Trent University, Peterborough, Ontario, Canada, PhD Dissertation, 132 pp.

Thulke, T., Selhorst, T., Muller, T., Wyszomirski, T., Muller, U., and Breitenmoser, U. (2004). Assessing anti-rabies baiting-what happens on the ground. *Biomedical Central, Infectious Diseases* **4**:. doi: 10.1186/1471-2334-4-9.

Tinline, R., Rosatte, R., and MacInnes, C. (2002). Estimating the incubation period of raccoon rabies: A time–space clustering approach. *Prev. Vet. Med.* **56**:89–103.

Toma, B. (2005). Fox rabies in France. *Eurosurveillance* **10**(11):pii = 577.

Totton, S., Rosatte, R., Tinline, R., and Bigler, L. (2004). Seasonal home ranges of raccoons, *Procyon lotor*, using a common feeding site in rural eastern Ontario: Rabies management implications. *Can. Field Nat.* **118**:65–71.

Turner, J., Jr., and Kirkpatrick, J. (1996). New methods for selective contraception in wildlife. *In* "Contraception in Wildlife", (P. Cohn, E. Plotka, and U. Seal, eds.), pp. 191–208. The Edwin Mellen Press, Lewiston, NY.

Velasco-Villa, A., Orciari, L., Souza, V., Juarez-Islas, V., Gomez-Sierra, M., Castillo, A., and Rupprecht, C. (2005). Molecular epizootiology of rabies associated with terrestrial carnivores in Mexico. *Virus Res.* **111**:13–27.

Voigt, D. (1987). Red fox. *In* "Wild Furbearer Management and Conservation in North America", (M. Novak, J. Baker, M. Obbard, and B. Malloch, eds.), pp. 379–393. Ontario Trappers Association Publishers, North Bay, ON.

Voigt, D. R., Tinline, R. R., and Broekhoven, L. H. (1985). Spatial simulation model for rabies control. *In* "Population Dynamics of Rabies in Wildlife", (P. J. Bacon, ed.), pp. 311–349. Academic Press, London.

Wandeler, A. (1988). Control of Wildlife rabies: Europe. *In* "Rabies", (J. B. Campbell and K. M. Charlton, eds.), pp. 365–380. Kluwer Academic Publishers, Norwell, MA.

Wandeler, A., Bauder, W., Prochaska, S., and Steck, F. (1982). Small mammal studies in a SAD baiting area. *Comp. Immunol. Microbiol. Infect. Dis.* **5**:173–176.

Wilde, H., Khawplod, P., Khamoltham, T., Hemachadha, T., Tepsumethanon, V., Lumlerdacha, B., Mitmoonpitak, C., and Sitprija, V. (2005). Rabies control in south and southeast Asia. *Vaccine* **23**:2284–2289.

Winkler, W. G. (1992). A review of the development of the oral vaccination technique for immunizing wildlife against rabies. *In* "Wildlife Rabies Control", (K. Bögel, F. Meslin, and M. Kaplan, eds.), pp. 82–96. Wells Medical, Kent, England.

CHAPTER 20

Understanding Effects of Barriers on the Spread and Control of Rabies

Erin E. Rees,* Bruce A. Pond,† Rowland R. Tinline,‡,1 and Denise Bélanger*

Contents

Abstract

This chapter reviews the evidence for the impact of natural and anthropogenic barriers on the spread of rabies using evidence mainly drawn from the epidemics of fox and raccoon variant rabies virus over the past 60 years in North America. Those barriers have both directed and inhibited the spread of rabies and, at a regional scale,

* Faculté de médecine vétérinaire, Département de pathologie et microbiologie, GREZOSP Université de Montréal, Saint-Hyacinthe, Quebec, Canada
† Wildlife Research and Development Section, Ontario Ministry of Natural Resources, Peterborough, Ontario, Canada
‡ Department of Geography, Queen's University, Kingston, Ontario, Canada
1 Corresponding author: rowland.tinline@sympatico.ca

Advances in Virus Research, Volume 79
ISSN 0065-3527, DOI: 10.1016/B978-0-12-387040-7.00020-2

have been integrated with rabies control efforts in North America. Few studies have been done, however, to examine how the texture (grain) and configuration of the habitat at finer scales affect rabies control, particularly the massive oral vaccination campaigns in operation along the Atlantic coast and southeastern Canada (Ontario, Québec, New Brunswick). To explore these questions, the authors used stochastic simulation. The model of choice was the Ontario Rabies Model (ORM) adapted for use on the high performance computing resources network in Québec (RQCHP—Réseau québécois de calcul de haute performance; http://rqchp.qc.ca). The combination of the ORM and RQCHP allowed us to run many thousands of experiments to explore interactions between nine landscape grain/configuration combinations and vaccination barriers with varying widths and immunity levels. Our results show that breaches of vaccine barriers increase as the grain size of the landscape increases and as the landscape becomes more structured. We caution that mid levels of vaccination can be counterproductive resulting in rabies persistence rather than control. We also note that our model/computing system has the flexibility and capacity to explore a wide range of questions pertinent to improving the efficacy of rabies control.

I. THE CONCEPT AND MECHANISMS OF BARRIERS

In the spread and persistence of rabies, barriers manifest themselves at various scales from the cell wall to the landform boundary. In this chapter, our focus is on barriers at landscape scale (tens to thousands of kilometers in extent), scales at which barriers affect the transmission of rabies between animals and affect the spread within a landscape. By affecting transmission, barriers also affect the persistence of rabies within an area. Our approach is threefold: (1) to explore the concept and mechanisms of barriers; (2) to review recent research investigations that describe and attempt to quantify the impact of barriers on rabies spread and persistence; and (3) through the application of a spatially explicit simulation model, to explore the effectiveness of various vaccination barriers under different patterns of host species habitat.

Landscape-scale barriers reduce rabies spread and persistence through two epidemiologically important causal pathways by (1) shortening the reach of the vector species, that is, the distance which any single vector or host organism moves in the course of passing on the rabies virus, and (2) reducing the rate at which one infected host successfully passes on infection to other hosts. These are not mutually exclusive or independent mechanisms. One can imagine a barrier region through which travel by the vector is impeded or blocked; this would have the effect of reducing the average distance that vectors would travel prior to becoming infectious. In addition, the habitat of such a region could also be of poor quality with low densities of susceptible host species, which reduces the likelihood of successful disease transmission.

The distinction is useful in understanding the characteristics of barriers, which are critical to assessing their effect on rabies spread and persistence. Barriers can be characterized as having (1) a degree of permeability, that is, the likelihood that a vector will be capable of passing through the barrier, and (2) a level of susceptible host species density, which directly influences the probability that an infective host will successfully pass on the infection before losing the ability to infect other hosts. It is obvious that the other side of the barrier coin is connectivity and that higher permeability and higher host density imply connectivity with respect to rabies spread.

Both of these characteristics must be considered in the context of particular spatial scales. Two aspects that are often conflated in common usage of the term "scale" are extent and grain (Dungan *et al.*, 2002). Extent is the size of a region of interest and grain is a measure of size of the smallest spatial unit which is spatially homogeneous with respect to a phenomenon of interest, for example, host density, land use, or habitat type. Alternatively, grain can be considered the smallest size at which objects, such as forest patches, can be identified with the techniques at hand. Extent and grain together are necessary to enable consideration of landscape heterogeneity in terms of habitat or susceptible host density at a particular grain size, relative to the extent of a study area. Not only does susceptible host density have an effect on the transmission of rabies virus through a region, but the pattern of variability in the density also has an effect. There has been considerable attention focused in epidemiological modeling on the effects of landscape heterogeneity on disease spread and persistence (e.g., Ferrari and Lookingbill, 2009; Keeling, 1999; McCallum and Dobson, 2002; Real and Biek, 2007).

The fields of conservation biology and landscape ecology, in the analysis of habitat fragmentation, have recognized the correlated but separate effects of habitat amount and habitat configuration, or habitat fragmentation *per se* on species persistence in a landscape (Andren, 1994; Fahrig, 2003). The separation of concepts, amount from configuration, is important in assessing the barrier effects of habitat and concomitant host density patterns on disease spread and persistence. In the case of rabies, amount refers to the density of susceptible hosts and configuration is the pattern of host density variation, for example, the average size and separation of high density patches. The effect of habitat on fragmentation, while holding the amount of habitat constant, is to reduce wildlife populations' likelihood of persistence. Given the same amount of habitat, less fragmented landscapes with larger patches of suitable habitat are generally more likely to support self-sustaining wildlife populations than landscapes with smaller more fragmented patches (Fahrig, 2003). However, Fahrig (2003) proposed that more research on the independent effects of habitat loss and habitat fragmentation is necessary to identify factors which influence the positive versus negative effects of fragmentation *per se*. When habitat available for a species becomes scarce and fragmented, the species may be able to sustain itself in a region as a metapopulation through a continual process of recolonization of patches where local extinctions have occurred (Hanski, 1999; Levins, 1970).

There is an analogue with infectious diseases, in which diseases function as metapopulations, where the disease habitat is the population of host organisms (Nee, 2007), and the disease moves among patches where the susceptible host density and infection interactions are sufficient for the disease to establish itself and persist for a time. The likelihood of persistence is a function of the size of the host's activity space and the number, spacing, and size of patches with sufficient susceptible host density. Landscapes with levels and patterns of host density in which disease will not persist are barriers to the disease. Water bodies such as rivers and lakes may influence the spread of rabies by preventing the passage of host vectors or by reducing the distance or altering the direction that they are able to carry rabies. A number of studies have attempted to detect and estimate the magnitude of these effects on rabies spread (e.g., Rees *et al.*, 2008b; Smith *et al.*, 2002). Topography also influences rabies spread. In particular, mountainous areas may physically impede movement of vector species, and characteristically have lower densities of host species, which lowers disease transmission rates. There is evidence of topographic barriers to rabies spread, in North America in both fox and raccoon rabies incidence data (Biek *et al.*, 2007; Tinline and MacInnes, 2004) and in Europe in fox rabies incidence (Wandeler *et al.*, 1988). Therefore, average host density across a region is only one dimension in understanding disease spread; the pattern or configuration of variation in that density may be equally important.

The design of barriers to combat disease, through lowering susceptible host densities by broad scale vaccination, culling, or fertility controls, should take into account the potential for landscape pattern to interact with control efforts and influence their effectiveness. Distribution of oral vaccines is the most cost effective of the aforementioned methods for large-scale rabies control. For example, vaccination of host species in strategically defined areas has been used successfully to practically eliminate fox rabies (MacInnes *et al.*, 2001) and prevent the spread and persistence of raccoon rabies in Ontario (Rosatte *et al.*, 2009) and Québec, Canada (Bélanger *et al.*, 2010), and in various regions of the eastern United States (Russell *et al.*, 2005; Sterner *et al.*, 2009). Vaccination zones in which herd immunity is achieved serve as barriers to protect uninfected areas from rabies spread and reduce the chance of disease persistence in infected areas by lowering susceptible host species densities. Since controlled replication of landscapes for empirically assessing effects of landscape configuration on rabies spread is impossible, in the final section we use a spatially explicit simulation model to examine the effect of two elements of landscape pattern on the spread of rabies and its interaction with vaccination barriers of various extents and levels of achieved immunity.

II. ASSESSING BARRIER EFFECTS

A variety of analytical tools have been brought to bear on the problem of estimating the effect of physical barriers on the spread of rabies. The simplest approach is mapping and statistical analysis of temporal and spatial patterns in reported rabies cases over time with respect to a number of landscape features which, as described above, are hypothesized to affect rabies spread. A second approach is simulation modeling, wherein a model is built based on knowledge and hypotheses about host and disease behaviors and then is used to project disease scenarios under conditions for which there have not been opportunities to observe system behavior, to identify characteristics or parameters to which model outcomes are sensitive. Both epizootic patterns as well as genetic evidence from both host and disease have been used to validate these models.

A. Rivers

Sayers *et al.* (1985) mapped rabies cases in Baden-Württemburg, Germany between 1963 and 1971. They temporally pooled cases over 3-month periods and applied a Gaussian spatial filter; from the resulting surface map, they identified local maxima or foci of rabies occurrence. The foci were mapped over successive time periods to construct trajectories of disease intensity. The resulting trajectory map clearly showed the influence of the Danube River blocking two of the trajectories and it identified where on the river there were breakthroughs to the south. Using incidence records, Wandeler *et al.* (1988) also identified the role of rivers as natural barriers and bridges as connections for the spread of fox rabies in Europe.

Two approaches to estimating the magnitude of the effect of river barriers on the spread of the raccoon rabies strain through Connecticut, USA, have been taken by Lucey *et al.* (2002) and Smith *et al.* (2002). In Connecticut, rabies entered in the southwest corner of the state and spread northeastward, crossing the state and infecting all townships but one in a span of 49 months. There are three large rivers which cross the state aligned approximately perpendicularly to the direction of the rabies spread. The two analyses used township-level rabies case data to determine the date of first incidence for each of 169 townships in the state. Lucey *et al.* (2002), modifying a method originally developed and applied by Ball (1985), estimated trend surfaces, linear to quartic, for the date of first incidence in townships to assess the regional spatial temporal trend in rabies passage through Connecticut. The higher order trend surfaces captured some local variation in the predicted surface of date of first incidence. The variation in the trend surface indicated an overall reduction in rate of spread due to rivers of 22%.

Smith *et al.* (2002) developed a stochastic simulation model of the passage of the disease into a township from adjacent townships as a function of the infection state of the adjacent townships and a number of habitat and river barrier variables. Parameters for five configurations of the model were estimated and compared using the incidence data to identify the best fitting model and to assess the effect of the rivers on the rate of spread of rabies across the state. The best fitting model was one with a river barrier effect, and that model indicated that the rivers caused a sevenfold decrease in the local rate of transmission between adjacent townships and a 30% overall reduction in spread. They attributed the difference of their estimate with the 22% estimate of Lucey *et al.* (2002) to the greater regional influence incorporated in the trend surface estimation methodology. Smith *et al.* (2002) went on to use the model to estimate that without the river barriers rabies would have crossed the state between 11 and 16 months sooner than observed.

Cullingham *et al.* (2009) demonstrated, through genetic structure analysis of nuclear DNA markers in raccoons, the differential permeability of the St. Lawrence and the Niagara Rivers, which form part of the border between New York State and Ontario. From the lack of genetic structure coincident with the St. Lawrence River, they inferred a freer interchange of raccoon genetic material here than in Niagara. The St. Lawrence region was the location of the only observed incursion of raccoon rabies into Ontario. They also recognized that the differential structuring of raccoon genetics by the two rivers might be also be due to the more constricted interface between New York and Ontario at Niagara, compared to the longer St. Lawrence River frontier between the two jurisdictions. Both these interfaces are separated by Lake Ontario, a barrier completely impermeable to raccoons and the disease. Rees *et al.* (2009) used genetic simulation modeling to explore this spatial bottleneck effect created by the location of the large impermeable Lakes Ontario and Erie and the relatively narrow (50 km) terrestrial interface between them afforded by the Niagara Peninsula. They found that the genetic differentiation in nuclear DNA in the raccoon host species observed in field data could have arisen simply because of the landscape constriction. They argue that this factor, in conjunction with the barrier effect of the Niagara River and a raccoon vaccination program, has provided a successful barrier to raccoon spread into Ontario. At a coarser grain and larger extent, Biek *et al.* (2007), through examination of RNA sequences in the rabies virus, also note the role of the Great Lakes and the Atlantic Ocean as physical barriers in bringing rabies incidence to a demographic plateau.

Rees *et al.* (2008b) used landscape genetics analysis of neutral mitochondrial genetic markers and the Ontario Rabies Model (ORM; Tinline *et al.*, 2011), a spatially explicit, individual-based simulation model of raccoon populations to estimate the degree of permeability of the Niagara River to raccoons and by inference to rabies. The ORM has the capability of tagging individual raccoons with neutral genetic markers and passing these genetic characteristics to their offspring. By simulating 250 years of colonization by raccoons from New York across the Niagara River, into Ontario with variable levels of permeability assigned to the river barrier in the model, it was possible to match the emergent spatial genetic structure in the model with that assessed from contemporary field samples of raccoon DNA. The comparison indicated that the river permeability to raccoon movement was approximately 50%.

There are several other examples of the use of rivers in conjunction with vaccination in particular to create a *cordon sanitaire* to isolate areas from invasion by rabies. Ontario has used the combination of oral vaccination, trap–vaccinate–release, and localized depopulation along the Niagara and St. Lawrence rivers to reinforce the barrier effect (Rosatte *et al.*, 2010). The Texas Department of Health used oral vaccination to successfully contain the invasion of canine rabies in coyotes from Mexico across the Rio Grande and subsequently pushed the disease back to the Rio Grande (USDA, 2007). The United states began a National Rabies Management Program in 1997 with a major focus on preventing the spread of raccoon-variant rabies from the eastern seaboard into central United States. A 48–118 km wide oral vaccination zone was placed from Ohio south to Alabama along the Appalachian Ridge to complement natural barriers such as rivers, lakes, and poor habitat along mountain ridges. There have been breaches of this combined barrier, but they have been contained with additional vaccination measures (Sterner *et al.*, 2009).

B. Topography

We have noted previously that topography, through the combined effects of elevation, terrain ruggedness, and associated vegetation types and land use differences, has an effect on the spread of infectious disease by influencing the likelihood of successful disease transmission. Certain types of topography, for example, those of high elevation, steep slopes, and rugged terrain, may constrain movement and shorten the reach of vectors. Additionally, poor raccoon habitat and low raccoon densities, often associated with these topographic types, lower the likelihood of successful disease transmission. The north–south extent of raccoon rabies in its spread in eastern North America from a 1977 focus in West Virginia indicates a strong barrier effect of the Appalachian and Allegheny Mountains spatially constraining rabies to the eastern seaboard (Biek *et al.*, 2007). At a smaller extent, this elevation effect is evident at the current northern limit of raccoon rabies range. It is clear from data on the time of first incidence at the township level in Vermont and New York that the Adirondack Mountains have acted as a barrier, directing, in a sense the incidence of rabies around the high ground (Russell *et al.* 2003). Figures 1 and 2 illustrate this effect. Figure 1 shows the total number of rabies cases by township during over the initial invasion period (1990–2003) of New York State (Owen, 2004). Figure 2 presents a 4th order trend surface of the first date of rabies incidence by township in Vermont (Laura Bigler, personal communication, November 2010, unpublished data) and

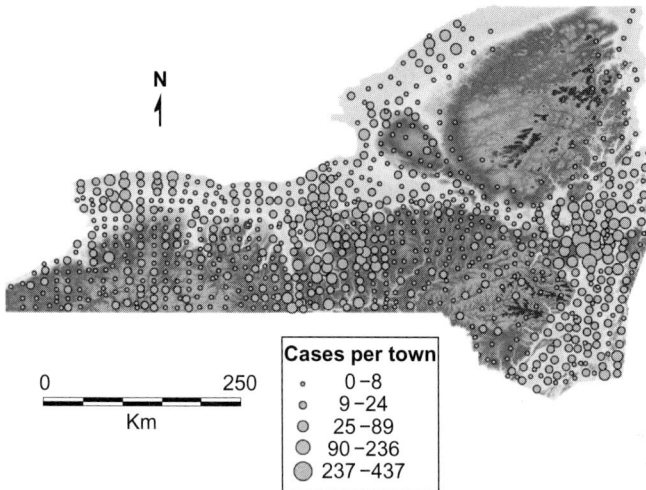

FIGURE 1   Rabies cases per town in New York during the initial invasion of the raccoon rabies variant, 1990–2003 (Owen, 2004). (See Page 13 in Color Section at the back of the book.)

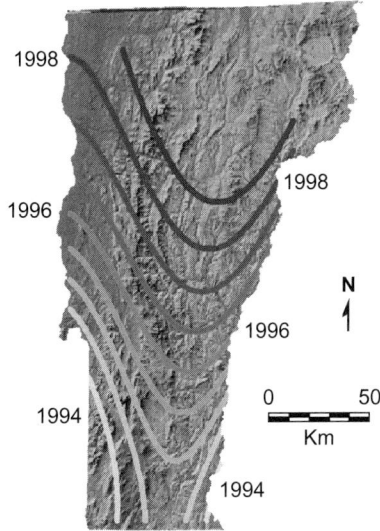

FIGURE 2   Fourth order trend surface of the date of first rabies case by township in Vermont (Laura Bigler, personal communication, 2010). (See Page 14 in Color Section at the back of the book.)

shows how the centrally located Green Mountains impeded the progress through central Vermont while the elevation corridors provided by the Champlain Valley the west and the Connecticut River valley on the east facilitated the northward spread of rabies.

Slate *et al.* (2005) argue that higher elevations in the Appalachian and Adirondack Mountains are generally characterized by short growing seasons, infertile soils and contiguous forest habitats more typical of northern latitudes, such as mixed conifers and northern hardwoods, or a boreal mix of spruce, fir, and aspen. As such, these habitats do not generally support robust raccoon populations often found in habitats at lower elevations. Population density index information collected by United States Department of Agriculture (USDA), Animal and Plant Health Inspection Service (APHIS), and Wildlife Services are in general agreement with these density-habitat relationships at higher elevations. Earlier work in New England also supports this conclusion (Godin, 1977).

Raccoon densities at a local level are difficult to estimate precisely. A number of studies, however, demonstrate the effect of habitat on rabies spread and persistence which are presumed to be an effect of host density on disease transmission rates. Smith *et al.* (2005) used modeling to investigate long distance rabies transmissions in Connecticut, similar to their earlier study (Smith *et al.*, 2002). They showed that increased forested habitats within a township slowed the overland spread of rabies by a factor of 3. They also found an interaction of forest cover and rivers slowed rabies spread to the point that, in heavily forested townships, the model predicted rabies would never cross rivers, whereas in lightly forest townships, the river effect slowed rabies spread by a factor of 2. This effect is most likely due to variability in raccoon density, where agricultural and settled areas typically support much higher raccoon densities, with accompanying higher disease transmission rates.

Genetic evidence of the rabies virus supports this hypothesis that areas of low host density act as disease barriers. Real *et al.* (2005) showed that two variants of arctic fox rabies virus, entering southern Ontario, one on the east through Québec and one on the west from Northern Ontario have retained this genetic differentiation. Each was separated from the other by the higher elevation, and generally forested Frontenac Axis of the Canadian Shield.

Tinline and MacInnes (2004) examined rabies incidence and landscape in southern Ontario in a different way. Using time series correlations of rabies incidence between adjacent townships, they were able to identify 12 clusters of townships which they termed "rabies units." Each unit had a distinctive period that was out of phase with adjacent units so that as rabies peaked in one unit it was waxing or waning in adjacent units. Further, units had similar host species composition, and unit boundaries followed the predominant physiographic features in southern Ontario. They argued that the out-of-phase relationships between units appeared to be an important mechanism for the persistence of rabies in southern Ontario. They also noted that there was a strong correlation between the spatial pattern of rabies units and the geographical localization of *N* gene variation of rabies viruses circulating in Ontario (Nadin-Davis *et al.*, 1999). Ontario used these geographic units to initiate its successful oral vaccination campaign against fox rabies. The campaign began by using vaccination along the physical barriers between units in southeastern and south central Ontario to further isolate those units. Subsequent control efforts concentrated on vaccinating within units when incidence was waning.

C. Fine-grained habitat heterogeneity

To this point, our examples have dealt with analyses and control measures over relatively large areas such as townships or counties. This is partly the result of the spatial unit at which jurisdictions collect rabies data and partly due to the lack of detailed information about host behavior at finer scales. As a result, much rabies research and control planning have made the limiting assumption of homogeneous habitat and/or host population density over wide areas. Recently, however, there is a growing recognition that local, fine-grained habitat configuration, characterized by attributes such as connectivity, interior habitat patch size, isolation, may have a critical influence on disease spread and persistence and, more importantly, on the efficacy of disease control efforts (Gilligan and van den Bosch, 2008). For example, McCallum and Dobson (2002) use meta-population models to identify the advantages of corridors and other connections for species conservation in fragmented landscapes as opposed to the disadvantages due to disease spread that metapopulation connectivity might enhance. From the point of view of species conservation, they concluded that the benefits of connectivity that allow the host species to move through a landscape more than offset the costs that enhanced disease transmission might impose on the species of conservation concern.

Su *et al.* (2009) have also examined the effects of habitat arrangement, specifically spatial clustering of habitat patches, on predator-prey dynamics through simulation of a predator–prey–disease system. Of particular interest, they explored the response of a disease in the prey population to landscape structure, both the amount of habitat and the degree of clustering of the extant habitat. As expected, they demonstrated a sharp decline in prey numbers and incidence of disease in prey, as the total amount of habitat is reduced. However, they also showed that clustering of habitat units into larger patches of good habitat mitigated some of the effects of habitat loss on the prey species abundance, as well as on the prevalence of disease. The disease is more likely to persist in a landscape where there are larger clumps of habitat units. From a rabies management perspective, these findings raise some interesting questions about how various landscape types would influence the effectiveness of a vaccination barrier in halting the spread and, ultimately, the persistence of rabies in a region. Given the general paucity of data on microscale host/disease behavior, we believe the most efficient way to explore these questions is through simulation modeling. Our initial efforts are described in the next section.

III. ASSESSING INTERACTION OF VACCINATION BARRIERS AND HABITAT PATTERNS

Our work was motivated by the raccoon rabies dynamics in Vermont and Québec. Raccoon rabies has been detected in Vermont since 1994 (USDA, 2007). In 2000, the Government of Québec put in place an enhanced surveillance program along the border of Québec and Vermont (Messier, 2001). Raccoon rabies was finally detected in May 2006, initiating a control program to eradicate the disease from Québec. Disease surveillance efforts were increased and maintained for succeeding years. The last two rabies cases in Québec's epidemic were detected in the spring of 2009. After 2 years of no rabies cases, despite constant surveillance effort, Québec can be declared disease-free, according to the definition of the World Health Organization (WHO, 2005). Under these circumstances, the Government of Québec has shifted the focus of disease control toward preventing another outbreak caused by a rabies invasion from Vermont. Since rabies control programs are economically and logistically expensive (Sterner *et al.*, 2009), our challenge was to examine how habitat structure impacts the effectiveness of oral vaccination strategies with the long-term goal of designing better and less expensive vaccination programs.

The landscape in Québec along the Vermont border ranges from large-scale farming operations to a mosaic of smaller agricultural plots and woodlots, to more contiguous forest and mountainous terrain. To begin our analysis, we felt that this landscape (and most others) could be represented by three general patterns of alternating good and poor habitat: patches, corridors, and bars where corridors are parallel to the direction of spread and bars are perpendicular to the direction of spread. Further, those patterns would be exhibited at different levels of aggregation, which we termed fine, medium, and coarse grain. To examine the interaction between vaccine barriers and these patterns, we chose different barrier widths and different levels of immunity within those barriers. Finally, we decided that stochastic simulation modeling was the only feasible means of assessing the contribution of all these factors to the effectiveness of a given vaccination program.

A. Methods

1. The simulation modeling environment

Our choice for simulation modeling was the ORM. There were four reasons for this choice. First, as Tinline *et al.* (2011) discuss, the ORM is an object-oriented stochastic spatial model of animal population dynamics that deals with individual animals and tracks the spread of infectious disease over landscapes configured as hexagonal cells where the carrying capacity of each cell (defined as K in subsequent paragraphs) is user-defined. Hence, carrying capacity becomes a surrogate for habitat quality. The ORM permits these cells to be any size, but in this study, we have accepted the default size for each cell of just over 10 km^2 per cell, the scale typical of the spatial resolution in field studies used to parameterize the model. Second, the ORM has an ArcGIS (Environmental Systems Research Institute, Inc., Redlands, California) interface that makes it easier to graphically define landscapes. ArcGIS is a widely used GIS software package in North America. Third, the ORM has been adapted to run under Linux and, therefore, we were able to use the high performance computing resources from a consortium of universities in Québec (RQCHP). Using such a resource allowed us to design multi-factorial experiments with enough trials per experiment to adequately assess the output variance was created by stochasticity in the model. Finally, the biology and parameter estimation in the ORM were derived from detailed field studies of raccoon behavior in southern Ontario and calibrated with other work in southern Québec and northern New York. Thus, for these areas of the world, we are confident that the ORM parameterization is a reasonable representation of reality.

2. Vaccination strategies

Our concern was the ability of various vaccination strategies to prevent a rabies invasion from an endemic area (in the south) into an adjacent disease-free area in the north (Fig. 3). The endemic zone has no spatial heterogeneity, as its sole purpose is to serve as a continuous source of rabid raccoons threatening to infect the disease-free area. An oral vaccination barrier was placed along the northern side of the border between these areas. The vaccination barriers tested were 20, 30, and 50 km wide and had achieved population immunities of 0%, 20%, 40%, 60%, and 80%. Achieved immunity means that the specified proportion of the population is immune to challenges from the rabies virus for 52 weeks, with the barrier being renewed annually to maintain the designated level of immunity through-out the simulation. In total, we applied 13 unique vaccination strategies as defined by a full-factorial design of barrier levels and population immunity levels $\geq$ 20%, and a strategy with 0% population immunity (i.e., no disease control) to act as a control for assessing the effect of vaccination.

3. Landscapes

We created 10 unique landscapes (Fig. 3). Each landscape is a rectangle of 40×70 hexagonal cells and represents 28,953 km^2. Every cell has a defined target population of raccoons, K, to act as a direct indicator of habitat quality (Rees et al., 2008a; Tinline et al., 2011). Cells with higher values of K can support greater densities of raccoons, as is assumed to occur in better-quality habitats. K does not influence movement beha-viors; rather, there is a feedback with mortality rate to bias the cell population toward K. Therefore, K acts to enhance or reduce disease transmission, given the cell population size. Our intent is to mimic field conditions that influence rabies spread and persistence. For example, in forested mountainous areas, raccoon densities are low because this is not a preferred habitat (Godin, 1977), and thus, the incidence of rabies is lower in these areas. In our experiments, we used extreme, but ecologi-cally realistic, values for raccoon density. Habitat in the model landscapes are differentiated from each other through the spatial arrangement of 800 low-quality habitat cells ($K = 20$; $\sim$2 raccoons/km^2) and 1600 high-quality habitat cells ($K = 120$; $\sim$12 raccoons/km^2; Rees et al., 2008b). In the 10 most southerly rows (400 cells) of all landscapes is the endemic zone. This zone is spatially homogeneous with respect to habitat (K), by assigning cells a

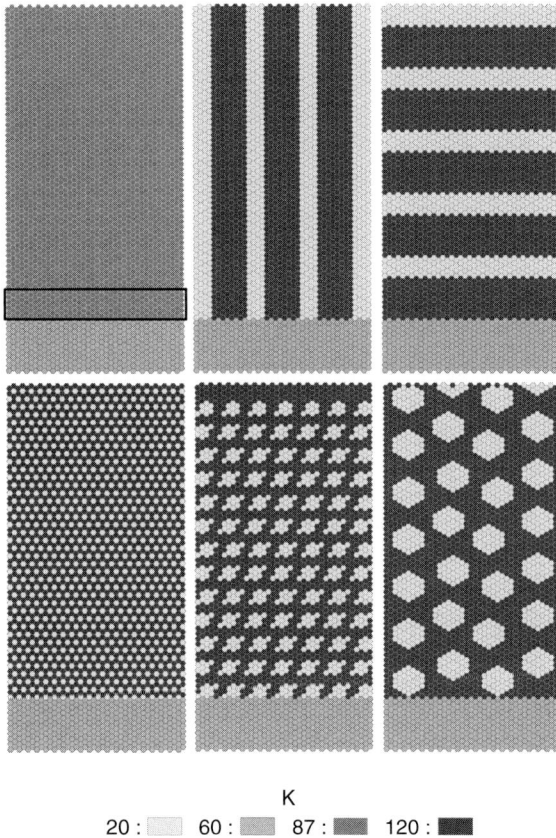

FIGURE 3 *Six of the ten landscape configurations in our experiments.* The southern tier of 10 rows in all landscapes is the endemic area with $K = 20$. The northern tier of 60 rows shows varying arrangements of high-quality habitat ($K = 60$, dark colored cells) and low-quality habitat ($K = 87$, light colored cells). The bottom left, center, and right landscapes illustrate arrangements with fine, medium, and coarse patches (1, 9, and 30 cells, respectively) of low-quality habitat. The upper center and upper right landscapes illustrate a corridor and a bar landscape 8 cells wide. The upper left landscape is our reference landscape. The upper tier of cells is isotropic with $K = 120$, the mean value of high and low densities in all other arrangements. In addition, the rectangle on the isotropic arrangement shows the placement of an example vaccination barrier 20 km wide between the endemic area and the northern tier of cells. (See Page 15 in Color Section at the back of the book.)

value of $K = 60$ to represent average-quality raccoon habitat found at mid-latitudes (~ 6 raccoons/km^2; Rees *et al.*, 2008b).

These spatial arrangements had two organizing principles. We created three fundamental configurations of landscape heterogeneity through the arrangement of the low- and high-quality cells, as structured into patches, bars, or corridors (Fig. 3). For each configuration, there were three textural grains for clustering the low-quality cells into fine, medium, and coarse aggregations as exemplified by decreasing edge to area ratios. Our intent was to represent variation in raccoon habitat that occurs at different configurations and grains. For instance, the low-quality cells forming bars and corridors at the coarsest scale are analogous to forested mountain ranges in New England that are found to be poor habitat for raccoons (Godin, 1977; Pedlar *et al.*, 1997). In our simulations, rabies flows south to north, therefore, east–west oriented bars are expected to impede disease spread and north–south oriented corridors are expected to facilitate disease spread. Contrary to bar and corridor linear features, patches mimic variation in habitat quality that occurs in clumps, for example, poor-quality habitat of isolated mountains surrounded by good-quality habitat in the agricultural valleys, as found in Vermont. The medium and fine grains of these landscape configurations enabled us to test for the interaction between grain size and the effectiveness of the vaccination scenarios. For example, one vaccination strategy may be more appropriate to combat rabies in a large-scale patchy mountain-valley landscape like Vermont, while an alternate vaccination strategy may be more appropriate for a finer grain patchy landscape of woodlots and agricultural fields in southwestern Québec. Likewise, the three different landscape configurations enabled us to test for the interaction between the arrangement of available habitat and the effectiveness of vaccination scenarios. We also created a landscape that is entirely homogeneous to act as a reference to the influence of spatial heterogeneity. This isotropic landscape also has an endemic rabies zone in the most southerly 10 rows, but all cells to the north have $K = 87$, which is the average K for the heterogeneous landscapes. Therefore, average habitat quality (i.e., overall landscape density) was equal among the 10 landscapes, meaning that total landscape density did not confound the influence of spatial heterogeneity on disease dynamics and vaccination effectiveness.

4. Simulation specifications

For each of our 10 landscapes, a raccoon population was grown from one breeding pair into a stable population that inhabits the entire landscape. This is necessary to create a starting population for our rabies simulations where raccoon densities reflect the spatial heterogeneity in habitat quality. This process takes 140 model years. For each simulation trial, we run the model another 10 years before introducing rabies. This ensures that the population dynamic processes in ORM sufficiently randomize the populations such that there is a unique starting population for each landscape and for each trial. Thus, the entire simulation lasts 20 years, the first 10 years randomize the populations and the last 10 years are used for experimentation. Hence, in all subsequent paragraphs, we only refer to the last 10 years as progressing from year 1 to 10. This 10-year window is sufficient to show an adequate response to vaccination and to evaluate its effects. For this investigation, a larger window would only increase running time without contributing further insight on the effect of vaccination.

In years 1 and 5, we seeded rabies along the southernmost extent of the landscapes at week 20 to correspond to the spring peak in raccoon rabies cases (Jenkins *et al.*, 1988). Initial experiments demonstrated that this is sufficient to ensure that rabies is continually present in the southern tier of 400 cells. Vaccination strategies are also initiated in year 1, north of the endemic area, occurring yearly at week 32 (mid-August) as is typical timing for delivery of oral vaccines at mid-latitudes in northeastern North America (Rosatte *et al.*, 2001).

Overall, we applied 13 vaccination strategies to each of the 10 landscapes and ran these combinations for 100 trials each to capture the variation in the system. All experiments were run on high-performance computing facilities (i.e., RQCHP). These systems enabled us to run approximately 1000 of the 13,000 trials in parallel. Since each trial lasts up to 30 min on a standard computing node, we were able to reduce the running time of 13,000 trials in serial at 6500 h (270 days) to approximately 4 h. Within the Linux environment of RQCHP we used a Perl script to process the model output for calculating the response variables.

5. Analysis of model response

We used multivariate regression analyses to test for the effects of population immunity, vaccination barrier width, and landscape configuration and texture on characteristics of the simulated disease dynamics. Response variables were calculated from the perspective of a resource manager wanting to evaluate the efficacy of vaccination strategies in the light of differing landscape heterogeneities. Hence, we tested the influence of the aforementioned effects on the total number of rabies cases over 10 years within the vaccination barrier and the probability of breaching a vaccination barrier. We used mixed effects multiple regression (gamm4 package in R; www.r-project.org) with a random effect to control for a lack of independence among the 100 trials run for each model specification. Previous experimentation indicated that the success of rabies to propagate within a vaccination barrier depended on the local arrangement of low- and high-quality cells where the disease enters the vaccination zone. Since the local arrangement within a vaccination zone may be slightly different from the mean habitat quality for the study area, we controlled for this effect by including a covariate defining the average quality of habitat cells within the vaccination zone, avgK. We also included the width of the vaccination barrier, VacWd, since it controls the size of the area for calculating the response variables. We used Akaike information criterion (AIC) to identify the top *a priori* models (Burnham and Anderson, 2002). A lower AIC value indicates greater support for the model given the data. Support for the top models is effectively equal when their difference in AIC from the top model is less than or equal to two (i.e., ΔAIC $\leq$ 2.0.) The beta coefficients are reported in reference to the isotropic landscape (no texture) and no vaccination (0% population immunity).

B. Results

1. Number of rabies cases within a vaccination barrier

There is effectively equal support in favor of the top two models explaining the number of rabies cases within a vaccination barrier based on population immunity, landscape grain and configuration (ΔAIC $\leq$ 2.0; Table I). There are a higher number of rabies cases at intermediary levels of population immunity, with higher vaccination levels becoming less effective in coarser grained landscapes (Fig. 4). Further, at lower levels of population immunity, vaccination is most effective in the patch and corridor landscapes; however, at higher levels of population immunity, vaccination is most effective in the isotropic landscape (Fig. 5).

The predominant trends in our results indicate that vaccination effectiveness (1) decreases with increasing coarseness of landscape grain and (2) decreases with landscape configuration from isotropic to patch to corridor to bar. For example, the mean number of rabies cases over 10 years of

TABLE I AIC model rankings of factors affecting the number of rabies cases within a vaccination barrier based on five levels of population immunity (PopImmC: 0%, 20%, 40%, 60%, and 80%), four landscape configurations (LandCfig: isotropic, patch, bar, corridor), and four textural grains (LandText: none, fine, medium, coarse). In this table Control = factors controlling for the average habitat quality (avgK) and the width of the vaccination barrier (VacWd).

Model	Np	AIC	ΔAIC
Control + PopImmC + LandText + PopImmC*LandText	6	263,401	0.0
Control + PopImmC + LandCfig + PopImmC*LandCfig	6	263,403	2.0
Control + PopImmC + LandText	5	263,598	197.0
Control + PopImmC + LandCfig	5	263,599	198.0
Control + PopImmC	4	263,651	250.0
Control + LandText	4	263,890	489.0
Control + LandCfig	4	263,891	490.0
Control	3	263,939	538.0

Np is the number of parameters, AIC is Akaike's Information Criterion, ΔAIC is relative to the most parsimonious model.

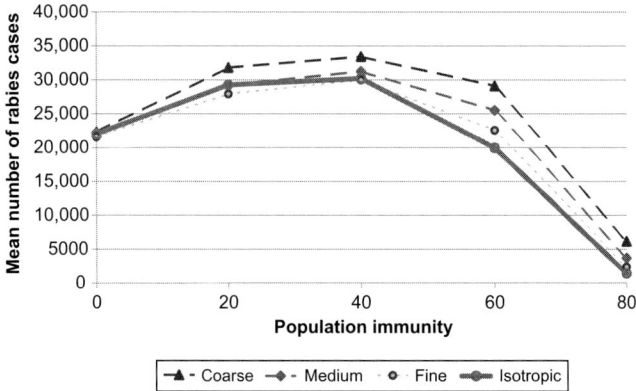

FIGURE 4 Mean number of rabies cases within all vaccination barriers for landscape grains: isotropic (none), fine, medium, and coarse, relative to levels of population immunity (0%, 20%, 40%, 60%, and 80%).

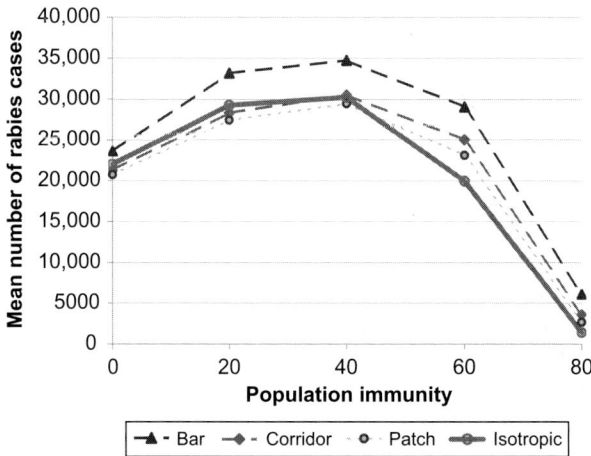

FIGURE 5 Mean number of rabies cases within all vaccination barriers for the landscape configurations: isotropic, patch, corridor, and bar, relative to levels of population immunity (0%, 20%, 40%, 60%, and 80%).

simulation in a 50-km vaccination barrier using 60% population immunity is highest at the coarsest grain and for the bar landscape (Fig. 6).

2. Probability of breaching a vaccination barrier

The probability of rabies breaching a vaccination barrier is influenced by population immunity and landscape texture and configuration (Table II). In the top model, increasing levels population immunity and vaccination

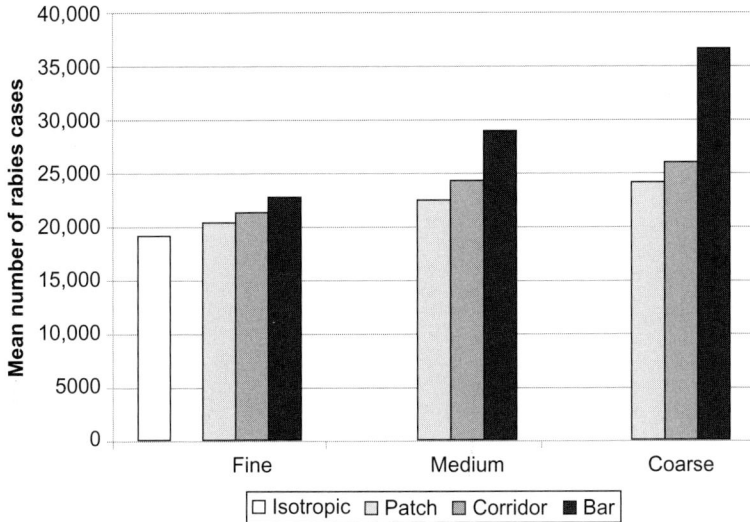

FIGURE 6   Mean number of rabies cases over 10 years of simulation within a 50-km vaccination barrier of 60% population immunity.

TABLE II   AIC model rankings of factors affecting the probability of rabies breaching a vaccination barrier based on five levels of population immunity (PopImmC: 0%, 20%, 40%, 60%, 80%), four landscape configurations (LandCfig: isotropic, patch, bar, corridor), and four textural grains (LandText: none, fine, medium, coarse). In this table Control = factors controlling for the average habitat quality (avgK) and the width of the vaccination barrier (VacWd).

Model	Np	AIC	ΔAIC
Control + PopImmC	4	2386	0.0
Control + PopImmC + LandText	5	2387	1.0
Control + PopImmC + LandCfig + PopImmC*LandCfig	6	2387	1.0
Control + PopImmC + VacWd*PopImmC	5	2393	7.0
Control + LandText	4	2554	168.0
Control	3	2556	170.0
Control + LandCfig	4	2559	173.0

Np is the number of parameters, AIC is Akaike's Information Criterion, ΔAIC is relative to the most parsimonious model.

barrier width decreases the probability of rabies breaching a barrier (Table III). The results for all levels of vaccination width, population, immunity, landscape configuration and texture (Table IV) indicate that the combined effects of high population immunity and barrier widths are necessary to minimize the risk of disease invasions. Rabies breaches are less likely in the bar and coarser grained landscapes at lower levels of

TABLE III Parameter estimates and standard errors for the top model of factors affecting the probability of rabies breaching a vaccination barrier

Variable	β	SE
Intercept	16.10	4.12
avgK	0.02	0.04
VacWd	-0.21	0.03
PopImm 20%	0.75	1.95
PopImm 40%	0.01	1.63
PopImm 60%	-0.39	1.54
PopImm 80%	-11.33	1.28

TABLE IV Percentage of rabies breaches that occur relative to vaccination barrier width (km) and level of population immunity (PI), given landscape texture: none (isotropic), fine, medium, and coarse, and landscape configuration: isotropic, patch, corridor, and bar

		Vaccination barrier width					Vaccination barrier width		
	PI	20	30	50		PI	20	30	50
Isotropic	0	100.0	100.0	100.0	Isotropic	0	100.0	100.0	100.0
	20	100.0	100.0	100.0		20	100.0	100.0	100.0
	40	100.0	100.0	100.0		40	100.0	100.0	100.0
	60	100.0	100.0	100.0		60	100.0	100.0	100.0
	80	66.0	15.0	0.0		80	66.0	15.0	0.0
Fine	0	100.0	100.0	100.0	Patch	0	100.0	100.0	100.0
	20	100.0	100.0	100.0		20	100.0	100.0	100.0
	40	100.0	100.0	100.0		40	100.0	100.0	100.0
	60	100.0	100.0	100.0		60	100.0	100.0	100.0
	80	77.7	28.1	0.7		80	81.0	36.8	3.3
Medium	0	100.0	100.0	100.0	Corridor	0	100.0	100.0	100.0
	20	100.0	100.0	100.0		20	100.0	100.0	100.0
	40	100.0	100.0	100.0		40	100.0	100.0	100.0
	60	100.0	100.0	100.0		60	100.0	100.0	100.0
	80	93.0	47.0	3.1		80	93.7	54.2	8.3
Coarse	0	100.0	100.0	99.0	Bar	0	100.0	100.0	99.0
	20	100.0	100.0	99.7		20	100.0	100.0	99.7
	40	100.0	100.0	99.0		40	100.0	100.0	99.0
	60	100.0	100.0	97.3		60	100.0	100.0	97.3
	80	98.0	71.7	12.7		80	94.0	55.7	4.8

vaccination; however, at 80% population immunity, this trend is reversed and more breaches occur for coarser grained landscapes and the bar and corridor configurations (Figs. 7 and 8). With regard to vaccination barrier width, rabies breaches are more likely in coarser grained landscapes. This effect decreases with increasing barrier width, but to a lesser degree than the finer grained landscapes. Further, rabies breaches are more likely in

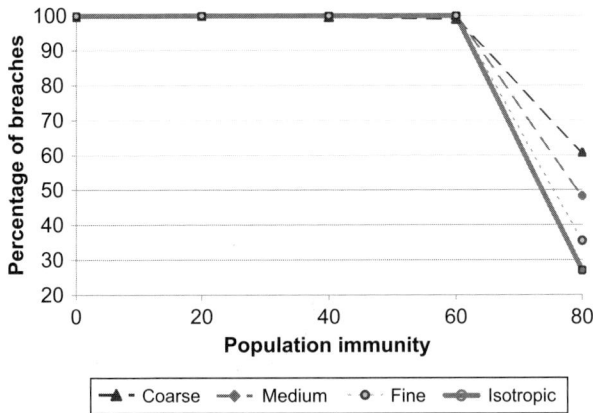

FIGURE 7 Percentage of rabies cases breaching the vaccination barrier for landscape textures: isotropic (none), fine, medium, and coarse relative to levels of population immunity (0%, 20%, 40%, 60%, and 80%) within all vaccination barriers.

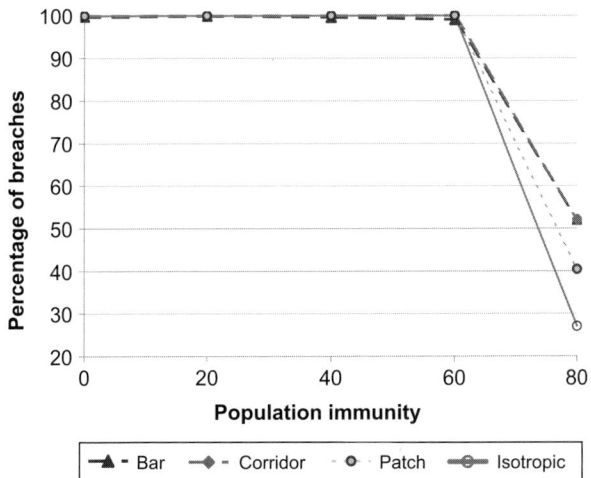

FIGURE 8 Percentage of rabies cases breaching the vaccination barrier for the four landscape configurations (isotropic, patch, bar, corridor) relative to levels of population immunity (0%, 20%, 40%, 60%, and 80%) within all vaccination barriers.

the bar landscape followed by the corridor, patch, and isotropic land-scapes. Increasing barrier width decreases the likelihood of breaches at a slower rate in the bar landscape followed by the corridor, patch, and isotropic landscapes.

3. Interpretation

It is not surprising that our results show that high levels of population immunity coupled with increasing barrier width reduce the number of rabies cases in the vaccination zone and the probability of breaches of the zone. It might be considered surprising, however, that mid-levels of immu-nity, coarse texture, and bar/corridor-like landscape configurations increase the number of rabies cases in the vaccination zone and increase the probability of breaches. In our opinion, the disease dynamics observed in our experiments are analogous to metapopulation dynamics observed in animal populations. A metapopulation consists of subpopulations of ani-mals that are separated in space and time but are connected through either immigration or emigration or both (Hanski and Gaggiotti, 2004). Persis-tence of animal populations is more likely when their size is small enough to not exhaust habitat resources, but large enough to avoid extinction through environmental stochastic events. Therefore, persistent popula-tions have a successful balance in their rates of births, deaths, immigration, and emigration to maintain sufficient numbers for population survival, given the size and quality of their habitat. Hence, we interpret our results as a metapopulation effect of rabies acting as separated subpopulations of animals that live in a spatiotemporal distribution of available habitat existing as the raccoon hosts. In coarser textured landscapes there are large patches of available good-quality, high-density habitat. Within these patches, there is higher probability of disease transmission. As a consequence, rabies can infect high numbers of raccoons over a short period of time and then exhaust the supply of susceptible individuals. However, before the disease wanes in that patch, it is likely that infected animals transferred rabies to neighboring high-density patches, enabling rabies to easily spread across the landscape. We observed this effect in our experiments in that rabies was more likely to breach the vaccination barrier in coarser grained landscapes and/or strongly configured land-scapes (bars and corridors) at the highest population immunity (80%). The highest level of population immunity prevented an exhaustion of susceptible in the high-quality habitat, such that there remained a suffi-cient number of infected individuals that heighten the probability of breaching the barrier. At finer textures, vaccination was more effective because the average density of susceptible raccoons is lower within the activity space of a rabid animal. The lessons for resource managers are that the selection of the location of vaccine barriers can affect success and that expectations about success must be tempered with an understanding of landscape texture and configuration.

Intermediate levels of population immunity of 20%, 40%, and sometimes 60% also seem to create a similar effect as we observed more rabies cases within the vaccination zone (Figs. 4 and 5) than at 0% or 80% levels of immunity. Thus, another important message to managers is that insufficient vaccination can result in more rabies cases than if no control is applied. This result can be understood when considering the number of rabies cases over the 10 years of simulation such as our isotropic landscape (Fig. 9). When no vaccination was used, a massive rabies outbreak occurred at years 4 and 5 within the vaccination zone, exhausting the stock of susceptible hosts. However, at mid-levels of population immunity, there was a smaller initial peak. This meant that a source of susceptible raccoons was conserved via vaccination and this reservoir then reproduced to a sufficient level within 4 years to spark a secondary outbreak. As a consequence, the two peaks at intermediary vaccination levels resulted in an overall higher number of rabies cases, given the temporal window of 10 simulation years. This trend was also observed in the other landscapes. Therefore, in situations where disease control managers are unable to achieve high levels of immunity, it may be advantageous to delay vaccination until the cycling of rabies incidence is at a minimum. At the trough of the cycle, the host population will be smaller and fewer animals will need to be vaccinated to protect the population. We noted previously that this strategy was used to combat

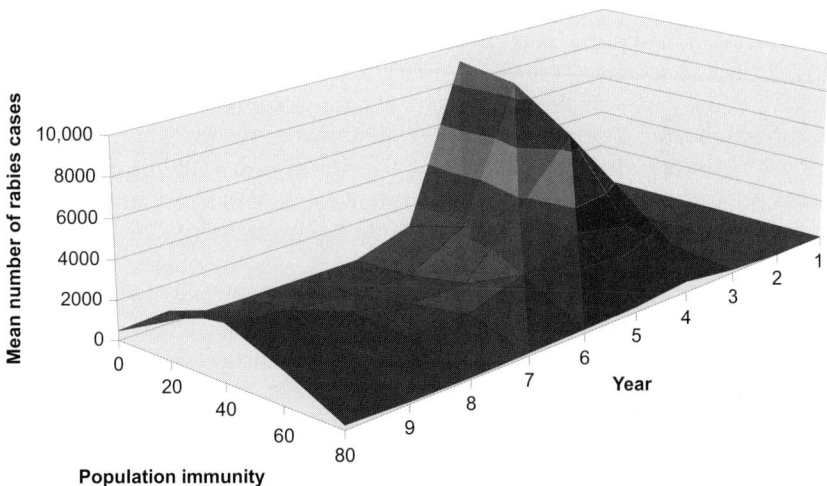

FIGURE 9 Number of rabies cases per year in a 50-km vaccination zone for all levels of population immunity in the isotropic landscape. (See Page 16 in Color Section at the back of the book.)

fox rabies in Ontario (Tinline and MacInnes, 2004). Vaccination was focused along the extents of the infected zone to prevent further disease spread and to let the disease reduce the number of susceptible foxes in the core of the infected area. When overall disease incidence and population were low, vaccines were distributed over the entire infected area and herd immunity was more easily achieved. The concern for using a delayed vaccination approach is the risk to humans in areas where the disease is not controlled. More rabies cases increase the risk of rabid animal-to-human interactions, and this may be unacceptable since the goal of public health programs is to reduce this risk to human welfare whenever possible.

IV. DISCUSSION

This chapter has reviewed the field evidence for barrier effects on the spread and persistence of rabies and noted that the effects at the township and county scales are clear and, in some instances, can be quantified. We noted, too, that there was a paucity of studies at finer scales, no doubt a reflection of the scale of data collection and detailed knowledge of animal behaviors. We argued that the efficiency of vaccination control strategies could be enhanced with further insight into the effects of landscape configuration and texture on vaccination strategies. While an increasing number of studies have reported using simulation to examine the impact of habitat on the dynamics of the spread of infection within a population, there are still few studies published on how vaccination and the spatial structure of a host population interact (Gilligan and van den Bosch, 2008). To this end, we adapted the ORM, an individual and cell based simulation model, to use the high performance computing resources of a consortium of universities in Québec (RQCHP). The ORM permitted us to examine habitat heterogeneity and epidemic behavior at fine scales and by using the high performance RQCHP facility we were able to run a large enough number of experiments to gain insight into the underlying variation in the scenarios we examined.

While our findings are preliminary, we are confident they illustrate that landscape texture and configuration do affect the success of vaccination control strategies. It is important to note that insights from our model outcomes provide understanding of factor effects relative to each other. Further work must be done to establish the link between our simulation values and an actual landscape. However, we have developed a useful tool to experiment with vaccination strategies in a controlled environment. From a management perspective, we see future work in five general areas: (1) developing further understanding about when and how to adapt vaccination strategies for a given landscape to maximize effectiveness and minimize cost; (2) categorizing landscapes and associating those categories with appropriate vaccination strategies; (3) exploring the joint impact of culling and fertility control (both are options in the ORM) with vaccination on rabies spread and persistence; (4) operationalizing measures that could prove useful to resources managers such as the rate of disease spread within a vaccination zone and the nature of breaches of the vaccination zone; and (5) understanding the sensitivity of the dynamics of an epidemic to changes in animal behavior such as the distribution of dispersal distances, as done by Cross *et al.* (2005), and which appear to vary with latitude in North America (Rees *et al.*, 2008b).

ACKNOWLEDGMENTS

Many people contributed to making this chapter possible. In particular, we are indebted to Jacques Richer at the University of Montréal and David Ball at Queen's University, Kingston, Ontario for their insight and extensive work in adapting the ORM to work under Linux on the high performance computing resources (RQCHP—Réseau québécois de calcul de haute performance; http://rqchp.qc.ca). These gave us the ability to run thousands of multifactor experiments. Jacques Richer and Daniel Stubbs were also very helpful in designing the scripts to compute selected response variables from the massive output generated by those experiments. The option of making and dealing with thousands of simulations opens a new era for experimentation with the ORM. We are also thankful to Antoinette Ludwig and her colleagues from GREZOSP for their validation experiments on the ORM using the resources of RQCHP. Those experiments played a significant role in debugging the ORM and assuring us that the ORM was operating as designed. We thank the Rabies Research Unit of the Ontario Ministry of Natural Resources for permission to use and modify the ORM. Finally, we are grateful to the Government of Québec for funding this project to support the design of effective rabies control programs.

REFERENCES

Andren, H. (1994). Effects of habitat fragmentation on birds and mammals in landscapes with different proportions of suitable habitat: A review. *Oikos* **71**:355–366.

Ball, F. G. (1985). Front-wave velocity and fox habitat heterogeneity. *In* "Population Dynamics of Rabies in Wildlife" (P. J. Bacon, ed.), Chapter 11, pp. 255–289. Academic Press Inc., London.

Bélanger, D., Canac-Marquis, P., Chamberland, G., Courtois, R., Lelièvre, F., and Mainguy, J. (2010). *Bilan des activités réalisées en 2009 dans le cadre gouvernemental de lutte contre la rage du raton laveur.* Ministère des Ressources naturelles et de la Faune-Direction de l'expertise sur la faune et ses habitats, service de la biodiversité et des maladies de la faune, Québec.

Biek, R., Henderson, J. C., Waller, L., Rupprecht, C. E., and Real, L. A. (2007). A high-resolution genetic signature of demographic and spatial expansion in epizootic rabies virus. *Proc. Natl. Acad. Sci. USA* **104**:7993–7998.

Burnham, K. P., and Anderson, D. R. (2002). Model Selection and Multimodel Inference: A Practical Information-Theoretic Approach. Springer-Verlag Inc., New York.

Cross, P. C., Lloyd-Smith, J. O., Johnson, P. L. F., and Getz, W. M. (2005). Dueling timescales of host movement and disease recovery determine invasion of disease in structured populations. *Ecol. Lett.* **8**:587–595.

Cullingham, C. I., Kyle, C. J., Pond, B. A., Rees, E. E., and White, B. N. (2009). Differential permeability of rivers to raccoon gene flow corresponds to rabies incidence in Ontario, Canada. *Mol. Ecol.* **18**:43–53.

Dungan, J. L., Perry, J. N., Dale, M. R. T., Legendre, P., Citron-Pousty, S., Fortin, M. J., Jakomulska, A., Miriti, M., and Rosenberg, M. S. (2002). A balanced view of scale in spatial statistical analysis. *Ecography* **25**:626–640.

Fahrig, L. (2003). Effects of habitat fragmentation on biodiversity. *Annu. Rev. Ecol. Evol. Syst.* **34**:487–515.

Ferrari, J. R., and Lookingbill, T. R. (2009). Initial conditions and their effect on invasion velocity across heterogeneous landscapes. *Biol. Invasions* **11**:1247–1258.

Gilligan, C. A., and van den Bosch, F. (2008). Epidemiological models for invasion and persistence of pathogens. *Annu. Rev. Phytopathol.* **46**:385–418.

Godin, A. J. (1977). Wild mammals of New England. Johns Hopkins University Press, Baltimore.

Hanski, I. (1999). Metapopulation Ecology. Oxford University Press, Oxford.

Hanski, I., and Gaggiotti, O. E. (2004). Ecology, Genetics, and Evolution of Metapopulations. Elsevier Academic Press, Burlington, MA.

Jenkins, S. R., Perry, B. D., and Winkler, W. G. (1988). Ecology and epidemiology of raccoon rabies. *Rev. Infect. Dis.* **10**:S620–S625.

Keeling, M. J. (1999). The effects of local spatial structure on epidemiological invasions. *Proc. R. Soc. Lond. B* **266**:859–867.

Levins, R. (1970). Extinction. *In* "Some Mathematical Problems in Biology", (M. Gesternhaber, ed.), pp. 77–107. American Mathematical Society, Providence, RI.

Lucey, B. T., Russell, C. A., Smith, D., Wilson, M. L., Long, A., Waller, L. A., Childs, J. E., and Real, L. A. (2002). Spatiotemporal analysis of epizootic raccoon rabies propagation in Connecticut, 1991–1995. *Vector Borne Zoonotic Dis.* **2**:77–86.

MacInnes, C. D., Smith, S. M., Tinline, R. R., Ayers, N. R., Bachmann, P., Ball, D. G. A., Calder, L. A., Crosgrey, S. J., Fielding, C., Hauschildt, P., Honig, J. M., Johnston, D. H., *et al.* (2001). Elimination of rabies from red foxes in Eastern Ontario. *J. Wildl. Dis.* **37**:119–132.

McCallum, H., and Dobson, A. (2002). Disease, habitat fragmentation and conservation. *Proc. R. Soc. Lond. B* **269**:2041–2049.

Messier, A. (2001). La problématique de l'épizootie de rage du raton laveur appréhendée au Québec. 4th rapport annuel. Gouvernement du Québec, Québec.

Nadin-Davis, S. A., Sampath, M. I., Casey, G. A., Tinline, R. R., and Wandeler, A. I. (1999). Phylogeographic patterns exhibited by Ontario rabies virus variants. *Epidemiol. Infect.* **123**:325–336.

Nee, A. (2007). Metapopulations and their spatial dynamics. *In* "Theoretical Ecology", (R. May and A. McLean, eds.), Chapter 4, pp. 35–45. Oxford University Press, Oxford.

Owen, M. (2004). Analysis of the Spread and Distribution of Raccoon Rabies in New York State, 1990–2003. Queen's University. (GIMS senior paper).

Pedlar, J. H., Fahrig, L., and Merriam, G. H. (1997). Raccoon habitat use at 2 spatial scales. *J. Wildl. Dis.* **61**:102–112.

Real, L., and Biek, R. (2007). Spatial dynamics and genetics of infectious disease on heterogeneous landscapes. *J.R. Soc. Interface* **4**:935–948.

Real, L. A., Henderson, J. C., Biek, R., Snaman, J., Jack, T. L., Childs, J. E., Stahl, E., Waller, L., Tinline, R., and Nadin-David, S. (2005). Unifying the spatial population dynamics and molecular evolution of epidemic rabies virus. *Proc. Natl. Acad. Sci. USA* **102**:12107–12111.

Rees, E. E., Pond, B. A., Phillips, J. R., and Murray, D. L. (2008a). Raccoon ecology database: A resource for population dynamics modelling and meta-analysis. *Ecol. Inform.* **3**:87–96.

Rees, E. E., Pond, B. A., Cullingham, C. I., Tinline, R. R., Ball, D., Kyle, C. J., and White, B. N. (2008b). Assessing a landscape barrier using genetic simulation modelling: Implications for raccoon rabies management. *Prev. Vet. Med.* **86**:107–123.

Rees, E. E., Pond, B. A., Cullingham, C. I., Tinline, R. R., Ball, D., Kyle, C. J., and White, B. N. (2009). Landscape modeling spatial bottlenecks: Implications for raccoon rabies disease spread. *Biol. Lett.* **5:**387–390.

Rosatte, R. C., Donovan, D., Allan, M., Howes, L. A., Silver, A., Bennett, K., MacInnes, D., Davies, C., Wandeler, A. I., and Radford, B. (2001). Emergency response to raccoon rabies introduction into Ontario. *J. Wildl. Dis.* **37:**265–279.

Rosatte, R. C., Donovan, D., Allan, M., Bruce, L., Buchannan, T., Sobey, K., Stevenson, B., Gibson, M., Macdonald, T., Whalen, M., Davies, J. C., Muldoon, F., *et al.* (2009). The control of raccoon rabies in Ontario Canada: Proactive and reactive tactics, 1994–2007. *J. Wildl. Dis.* **45:**772–784.

Rosatte, R. C., Ryckman, M., Ing, K., Proceviat, S., Allan, M., Bruce, L., Donovan, D., and Davies, C. J. (2010). Density, movements, and survival of raccoons in Ontario, Canada: Implications for disease spread and management. *J. Mammal.* **91:**122–135.

Russell, C. A., Smith, D., Waller, L. A., Childs, J. E., and Real, L. A. (2003). *A priori* prediction of disease invasion dynamics in a novel environment. *Proc. R. Soc. Lond. B* **271:**21–25.

Russell, C. A., Smith, D., Childs, J. E., and Real, L. A. (2005). Predictive spatial dynamics and strategic planning for raccoon rabies emergence in Ohio. *PLoS Biol.* **3:**382–388.

Sayers, B. M., Ross, A. J., Saengcharoenrat, P., and Mansourian, B. G. (1985). Pattern analysis of the case occurrences of fox rabies in Europe. *In* "Population Dynamics of Rabies in Wildlife", (P. J. Bacon, ed.), Chapter 10, pp. 235–254. Academic Press Inc., London.

Slate, D., Rupprecht, C. E., Rooney, J. A., Donovan, D., Lein, D. H., and Chipman, R. B. (2005). Status of oral rabies vaccination in wild carnivores in the United States. *Virus Res.* **111:**68–76.

Smith, D., Lucey, B. T., Waller, L. A., Childs, J. E., and Real, L. A. (2002). Predicting the spatial dynamics of rabies epidemics on heterogeneous landscapes. *Proc. Natl. Acad. Sci. USA* **99:**3668–3672.

Smith, D., Waller, L. A., Russell, C. A., Childs, J. E., and Real, L. A. (2005). Assessing the role of long-distance translocation and spatial heterogeneity in the raccoon rabies epidemic in Connecticut. *Prev. Vet. Med.* **71:**225–240.

Sterner, R. T., Meltzer, M. I., Shwiff, S. A., and Slate, D. (2009). Tactics and economics of wildlife oral rabies vaccination Canada and the United States. *Emerg. Infect. Dis.* **15:**1176–1184.

Su, M., Hui, C., Zhang, Y., and Li, Z. (2009). How does the spatial structure of habitat loss affect the eco-epidemic dynamics? *Ecol. Modell.* **220:**51–59.

Tinline, R. R., and MacInnes, C. D. (2004). Ecogeographic patterns of rabies in southern Ontario based on time series analysis. *J. Wildl. Dis.* **40:**212–221.

Tinline, R. R., Ball, D., and Broadfoot, J. D. (2011). The Ontario Rabies Model. Wildlife Research and Development Section, Ontario Ministry of Natural Resources, Peterborough, Canada.

USDA, (2007). Cooperative Rabies Management Plan Management Program National Report. United States Department of Agriculture, Washington.

Wandeler, A. I., Capt, S., Gerber, H., Kappeler, A., and Kipfer, R. (1988). Rabies epidemiology, natural barriers and fox vaccination. *Parassitologia* **30:**53–57.

WHO, (2005). WHO Expert Consultation Rabies . World Health Organization, Geneva.

CHAPTER 21

Rabies Research in Resource–Poor Countries

Henry Wilde* and **Boonlert Lumlertdacha**[†]

Abstract

Many cost-benefit/effective rabies research projects need to be carried out in less-developed canine-endemic regions. Among these are educational approaches directed at the public and governments. They would address effective primary wound care, availability, and proper use of vaccines and immunoglobulins, better reporting of rabies, final elimination of dangerous nerve tissue-derived vaccines, and the recognition that rabies is still expanding its geographic range. Such efforts could also reduce deaths in victims who had received no or less than adequate postexposure prophylaxis. There is a need for new technology in canine population control and sustainable vaccination. We have virtually no workable plans on how to control bat rabies, particularly that from hematophagous bats. Preexposure vaccination of villagers in vampire rabies-endemic regions may be one temporary solution. Current efforts to reduce further the time required and vaccine dose required for effective postexposure vaccination need to be encouraged. We still have incomplete understanding of the transport channels from inoculation site to rabies virus antibody generating cells. The minimum antigen dose required to achieve a consistently protective and lasting immune response has been established for intramuscular vaccine administration, but is only estimated for intradermal use. Greater knowledge may have clinical benefits, particularly in the application of intradermal reduced dose vaccination methods. Curing human rabies is still an unattained goal that challenges new innovative researchers.

* WHO-CC for Research and Training on Viral Zoonoses, Faculty of Medicine, Chulalongkorn University, Bangkok, Thailand
† Queen Saovabha Memorial Institute, Thai Red Cross Society, Bangkok, Thailand

Advances in Virus Research, Volume 79
ISSN 0065-3527, DOI: 10.1016/B978-0-12-387040-7.00021-4

Human rabies cases occurring in Western countries are rare and usually receive much media attention. However, human rabies is not uncommon in many developing canine-endemic countries. Over 55,000 humans die of rabies worldwide every year (WHO, 2010). Most diagnoses are based on clinical findings alone and the disease is widely underreported. Most of the cases come from Asia and Africa, but rabies is expanding its range (Clifton, 2010; Windiyaningsih et al., 2004). A recent WHO report (WHO and Bill Gates Consultation, 2009) lists that almost 50% of rabies cases are in children under 15 years. Almost all have had no postexposure prophylaxis (PEP) or it was inadequate. If they received PEP, they often were not treated with rabies immunoglobulin or it was not injected into bite wounds as recommended in current guidelines. Diagnosis is usually based on clinical findings, which are not always classical (furious or paralytic). Misdiagnoses are not uncommon (Bronnert et al., 2007; Srinivasan et al., 2005; Windiyaningsih et al., 2004). Government statistics are often not supported by reliable clinical or laboratory evidence. An example would be the rabies outbreak on Flores Island, Indonesia in 1999 where there were over 100 reported human rabies deaths. Only one patient, based on chart reviews by a WHO consultant, was reported to have the paralytic form of rabies resembling Guillain–Barré syndrome (Windiyaningsih et al., 2004). This suggests that there may have been at least another 20–30 misdiagnosed and not identified victims with the paralytic form, because paralytic rabies, worldwide, represents 20–30% of actual cases. Rabies is not a reportable disease in several countries that have a large canine reservoir of the virus. India has an estimated 25 million dogs with 80% of these categorized as not or only partially restricted in movements. This occurs in a human population of 1.15 billion where there are 20,000 estimated annual human rabies deaths per year (Knobel et al., 2005; Sudarshan et al., 2008). The rabies situation is similar in Pakistan where only one facility in Islamabad will, on special demand, carry out a dog necropsy and use the fluorescent antibody test. There has not yet been an attempt in Pakistan to start surveillance of canine rabies, which is the first step toward control. This is in spite of vigorous efforts by the Pakistani Infectious Diseases Society to persuade the government to develop a viable rabies control plan (Parviz et al., 2004). There is a need for more and better epidemiologic studies of rabies.

The situation is not much better in several other Asian countries such as Bangladesh, Cambodia, and Nepal as well as in parts of the Russian Federation and in most of the former, now independent, Soviet Republics (Kuzmin et al., 2004). How does this dismal picture reflect on the management of human cases and on potential research that might help to alter it? Human animal bites are often treated by traditional healers. Curry paste applied to wounds is one popular treatment in much of Pakistan and India, and is, the usual first aid applied not only in villages but also in large cities (Parviz *et al.*, 2004). Victims often do not consult a health care provider until relatively late and then mostly for wound infection (Parviz *et al.*, 2004). The primary doctor or nurse, who first sees an animal bite patient, usually does not wash and disinfect wounds and may not even have a facility to do so. We noted this while visiting several large government animal bite clinics in India and Pakistan where over 100 bites are treated daily, and where we did not see a facility to cleanse wounds. There was not even a water faucet where victims could wash their own injuries. All Asian countries, except for Pakistan, have either abolished or are in the final process of abolishing the use of nerve tissue-derived rabies vaccines. However, the WHO-approved products, that should replace Semple or suckling mouse vaccines, are expensive and not widely available. Human and equine immunoglobulins are unavailable to the majority of victims in most of south and southeast Asia. Few public facilities in the region are able to provide WHO-level PEP free of charge and the majority of animal bite victims come from the very poorest segments of society. These great problems deserve study by health economists and others for ways to reduce costs and make vaccines and biologicals more readily available to the poor.

Nevertheless, these rabies-endemic, less-developed regions are the natural location for selected cost-effective clinical and laboratory-bench research projects. They are also places where there are many needs for better clinical facilities and a dearth of funding sources. What is the future for research in such an environment? Grant providers and senior government officials are well aware of the fact that we know all that is needed to know in order to provide effective PEP and eventually eradicate canine rabies. They are more likely to sponsor research that produces early visible results in terms of reduction of human deaths and the canine rabies prevalence. More complex and basic research is difficult to carry out in most of these countries. However, a small group of devoted rabies researchers have succeeded to establish islands of productive clinical and even basic science research. Some of this work actually has allowed us to better understand the pathophysiology and immunology of rabies in humans and dogs and to devise more cost-effective immunization schedules. Much of it was done on minimum budgets, often using funding derived from clinical service fees or donations.

Working in a canine rabies-endemic country as clinicians, what would we name on a "wish list" for studies that are likely to provide early clinical benefits? Rapid inexpensive and simple diagnostic technology for measuring neutralizing rabies antibody might be able to replace the difficult, labor-intensive, and costly rabies fluorescent focus inhibition test (RFFIT). We know from studies in Tunisia, Thailand, and Finland that one shot rabies vaccination does not result in lasting protective immunity in dogs that are often severely mauled around the face resulting in large viral inocula. Improved canine vaccines might reduce or eliminate the reported 3–6% rabies occurrence among vaccinated dogs in Thailand and Tunisia (Haddad *et al.*, 1987; Sage *et al.*, 1993; Sihvonen *et al.*, 1995; Tepsumethanon *et al.*, 1991).

The Centers for Disease Control and Prevention in the United States has reduced the so-called Gold Standard Essen PEP schedule from five to four injections and allowed it to be completed in 14 days (Rupprecht *et al.*, 2010). Further shortening of intramuscular and intradermal WHO-approved PEP regimens can be anticipated as we develop greater confidence in the potency of the currently WHO-recognized rabies vaccines. This would reduce the often significant travel costs for impoverished rural patients as well as the number of dropouts from the lengthy and costly old PEP regimens which, with the now abolished eight-site intradermal schedule, could go on for 3 months and deter patients from starting any PEP (Shantavasinkul, 2010; WHO, 2010).

Reduced dose intradermal rabies vaccine was first introduced for public PEP in Thailand (Chutivongse *et al.*, 1990; Phanuphak *et al.*, 1987; Warrell *et al.*, 1984). Other Asian countries (Philippines, Sri Lanka, India, and Pakistan) have subsequently adopted it as well. Intradermal inoculation at reduced dose is now increasingly applied for vaccinating against other viral diseases such as hepatitis B, influenza, Japanese encephalitis, polio, and others (Mohammed *et al.*, 2010; Nicolas and Guy, 2008).

Tissue and avian culture rabies vaccines have been used for decades. WHO has established criteria for recognizing such vaccines on the basis of published immunogenicity studies. It then lists them in guidelines when found potent and safe. Many local regulatory authorities require such recognition by WHO before licensing any new rabies vaccine products. Some such government regulatory agencies demand additional costly and lengthy immunogenicity and safety studies carried out in their countries before approval. Better criteria for evidence-based reliable international approval of these biologicals, including the soon to arrive monoclonal rabies antibody cocktails, need to be developed and effectively implemented. WHO approval of such products now requires at least one independent published immunogenicity and safety study that meets Good Clinical Practice criteria before being recognized (WHO, 2010). Much of this work will have to be carried out in canine-endemic regions of the world.

Interesting new research suggests that the mechanism of recognition of antigen and its transport differs if antigens are deposited into muscle or fat rather than skin. The antigen transporters are more efficient and rapid in bringing rabies virus RNA from skin to immune receptor cells at regional lymph nodes than when first deposited in muscle or fat (Saraya *et al.*, 2010).

We need to know more about the dynamics of the transport of rabies virus from the inoculation site to nearby nerve tissue when introduced by a bite, and how cellular and humoral defense systems handle dormant virus in skin and muscle. These mechanisms are not yet well understood and an improved understanding may have clinical significance. This offers great opportunities for further basic research. Clarification of these mechanisms may also help to better publicize and introduce the economical and effective intradermal vaccination schedules which still meet resistance from health-care providers and some local regulatory authorities.

The rabies vaccine antigen content at the level where antibody levels reach a virtual plateau after immunization is known. The lowest WHO acceptable antigen content for tissue or avian culture vaccines has been listed as 2.5 IU/mL. This level was agreed on some 30 years ago for use with the intramuscular "full dose" schedules. Current lyophilized tissue culture rabies vaccines are dispensed with either 0.5 or 1.0 mL diluent. It is still controversial whether the lowest intradermal dose should remain the same for vaccines supplied with 0.5 or 1.0 mL diluent. An effective antigen content per 0.1 mL WHO-recommended intradermal dose is >0.5 IU with 0.5 mL diluent or 0.25 IU with 1.0 mL diluent (WHO, 2010; WHO and Bill Gates Consultation, 2009).

The lowest effective and WHO acceptable vaccine antigen content per reduced intradermal dose of 0.1 mL has not yet been established by adequate published immunogenicity trials. This has led to some controversy and uncertainties that damage the wider introduction of the less expensive vaccine-saving intradermal PEP schedules. A well-designed immunogenicity study could easily settle this troubling issue and needs to be encouraged.

Curing rabies in humans has received much media attention in recent years due to the survival of a teenage girl in Milwaukee, USA, who was put into deep brain wave burst suppression anesthesia and who received a cocktail of drugs never previously documented to have antirabies virus activity (Willoughby *et al.*, 2005). She, as well a previous survivor, developed early rabies antibody in serum and spinal fluid and no viable virus could ever be isolated during stormy hospital courses. It is likely that both subjects experienced a vigorous autogenous immune response to the infection which was responsible for their near complete neurological recovery. We currently know of no effective pharmaceuticals which, either alone or in combination, will eliminate the virus from the CNS. Laboratory and animal studies to identify new and effective drugs need to be encouraged. Nevertheless, human experimentation is better deferred until there is solid evidence of laboratory benefit. However, intensive life support efforts in patients with early disease and evidence of an active immune response should be attempted, particularly in hospitals that have experienced staff, tertiary care capabilities, and funding for such costly and resource-demanding management.

A method of male and female dog sterilization, which can be carried out in mass programs by trained lay personnel, is also on the "wish list" of many Asian public health officials and animal welfare workers. Additional research into the dynamics of rabies transmission and the immune response in bitches and their puppies may allow us to better understand how we can prevent the high prevalence of rabies in very young dogs and when to better immunize them. Above all, public health scientists need to be encouraged to find more effective and culturally acceptable methods to educate the public and governments to use existing knowledge to control and perhaps even eliminate rabies among canine vectors.

REFERENCES

Bronnert, J., Wilde, H., Tepsumethanon, V., Lumlertdacha, B., and Hemachudha, T. (2007). Organ transplantations and rabies transmission. *J. Travel Med.* **14**(3):177–180.

Chutivongse, S., Wilde, H., Supich, C., Baer, G. M., and Fishbein, D. B. (1990). Postexposure prophylaxis for rabies with antiserum and intradermal vaccination. *Lancet* **335** (8694):896–898.

Clifton, M. (2010). How not to fight a rabies epidemic: A history in Bali. *Asian Biomed.* **4**:663–670.

Haddad, N., Blacou, J., Grilli, A., and Ben Osman, F. (1987). Etude de la reponse immunitaire des chiens Tunisians a la vaccination antirabique. *Maghreb Vet.* **3**:61–64.

Knobel, D. L., Cleaveland, S., Coleman, P. G., Fèvre, E. M., Meltzer, M. I., Miranda, M. E., Shaw, A., Zinsstag, J., and Meslin, F. X. (2005). Re-evaluating the burden of rabies in Africa and Asia. *Bull. World Health Organ.* **83**(5):360–368.

Kuzmin, I. V., Botvinkin, A. D., McElhinney, L. M., Smith, J. S., Orciari, L. A., Hughes, G. J., Fooks, A. R., and Rupprecht, C. E. (2004). Molecular epidemiology of terrestrial rabies in the former Soviet Union. *J. Wildl. Dis.* **40**(4):617–631.

Mohammed, A. J., Al Awaiddy, S., Bawikar, S., Kurup, P. J., Elamir, E., Shaban, M. M. A., Sharif, S. M., Van der Avoort, H. G. A. M., Pallansch, M. A., Malankar, P., Burton, A., Sreevatsava, M., *et al.* (2010). Fractional doses of inactivated poliovirus vaccine in Oman. *New Engl. J. Med.* **362**(25):2351–2359.

Nicolas, J. F., and Guy, B. (2008). Intradermal, epidermal and transcutaneous vaccination: From immunology to clinical practice. *Expert Rev. Vaccines* **7**:1201–1214.

Parviz, S., Chotani, R., McCormick, J., Fisher-Hoch, S., and Luby, S. (2004). Rabies deaths in Pakistan: Results of ineffective post-exposure treatment. *Int. J. Infect. Dis.* **8**(6):346–352.

Phanuphak, P., Khawplod, P., Srivichayakul, S., Siriprasarub, W., Ubol, S., and Thaweepathomwat, M. (1987). Humoral and cell-mediated immune responses to various economical regimens of purified vero cell rabies vaccine. *Asian Pac. J. Allergy Immunol.* **5**:33–37.

Rupprecht, C. E., Briggs, D., Brown, C. M., Franka, R., Katz, S. L., Kerr, H. D., Lett, S. M., Levis, R., Meltzer, M. I., Schaffner, W., and Cieslak, P. R. (2010). Use of a reduced (4-dose) vaccine schedule for postexposure prophylaxis to prevent human rabies: Recommendations of the advisory committee on immunization practices. *MMWR Recomm. Rep.* **59** (RR-2):1–9.

Sage, G., Khawplod, P., Wilde, H., Lobaugh, C., Hemachudha, T., Tepsumethanon, W., and Lumlertdaecha, B. (1993). Immune response to rabies vaccine in Alaskan dogs: Failure to achieve a consistently protective antibody response. *Trans. R. Soc. Trop. Med. Hyg.* **87** (5):593–595.

Saraya, A., Wacharapluesadee, S., Khawplod, P., Tepsumethanon, S., Briggs, D., Asawavichienjinda, T., and Hemachudha, T. (2010). A preliminary study of chemo- and cytokine responses in rabies vaccine recipients of intradermal and intramuscular regimens. *Vaccine* **28**(29):4553–4557.

Shantavasinkul, P. (2010). The one week four-site postexposure prophylaxis regimen. WHO. Human and dog rabies prevention and control. Report WHO/Gates Foundation Consultation Abbecy, France October 2009. WHO/HTM/NDT/2010.1.

Sihvonen, L., Kulonen, K., Neuvonen, E., and Pekkonen, K. (1995). Rabies antibodies in vaccinated dogs. *Acta Vet. Scand.* **36**:87–91.

Srinivasan, A., Burton, E. C., Kuehnert, M. J., Rupprecht, C., Sutker, W. L., Ksiazek, T. G., Paddock, C. D., Guarner, J., Shieh, W. J., Goldsmith, C., Hanlon, C. A., Zoretic, J., *et al.* (2005). Transmission of rabies virus from organ donor to four transplant recipients. *N. Engl. J. Med.* **352**:1103–1111.

Sudarshan, M. K., Bhardwaj, S., Mahendra, B. J., Sharma, H., Sanjay, T. V., Ashwathnarayana, D. H., and Bilagumba, G. (2008). An immunogenicity, safety and post-marketing surveillance of a novel adsorbed human diploid cell rabies vaccine (Rabivax®) in Indian subjects. *Hum. Vaccin.* **4**(4):275–279.

Tepsumethanon, W., Polsuwan, C., Lumlertdacha, B., Khawplod, P., Hemachudha, T., Chutivongse, S., Wilde, H., Chiewbamrungkiat, M., and Phanuphak, P. (1991). Immune response to rabies vaccine in Thai dogs: A preliminary report. *Vaccine* **9**(9):627–630.

Warrell, M. J., Suntharasamai, P., Nicholson, K. G., Warrell, D. A., Chanthavanich, P., Viravan, C., Sinhaseni, A., Phanfung, R., Xueref, C., and Vincent-Falquet, J. C. (1984). Multi-site intradermal and multi-site subcutaneous rabies vaccination: Improved economical regimens. *Lancet* **1**(8382):874–876.

WHO (2010). Rabies vaccines position paper . *WHO Wkly. Epidemiol. Rec.* **32**(85):309–320.

WHO, Bill Gates Consultation (2009). Human and dog rabies prevention and control . Annecy, France. WHO/HTM/NTD/NZD/2010.1 Geneva.

Willoughby, R. E., Jr., Tieves, K. S., Hoffman, G. M., Ghanayem, N. S., Amlie-Lefond, C. M., Schwabe, M. J., Chusid, M. J., and Rupprecht, C. E. (2005). Survival after treatment of rabies with induction of coma. *N. Engl. J. Med.* **352**(24):2508–2514.

Windiyaningsih, C., Wilde, H., Meslin, F. X., Suroso, T., and Widarso, H. S. (2004). The rabies epidemic on Flores Island, Indonesia (1998-2000). *Med. Assoc. Thai.* **87**:1530–1538.

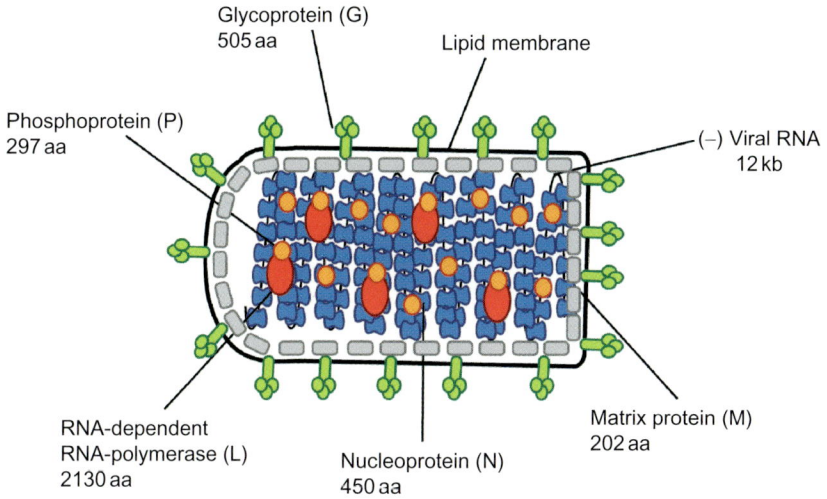

Figure 1, Aurélie A. V. Albertini *et al.*   (See Page 3 of this Volume)

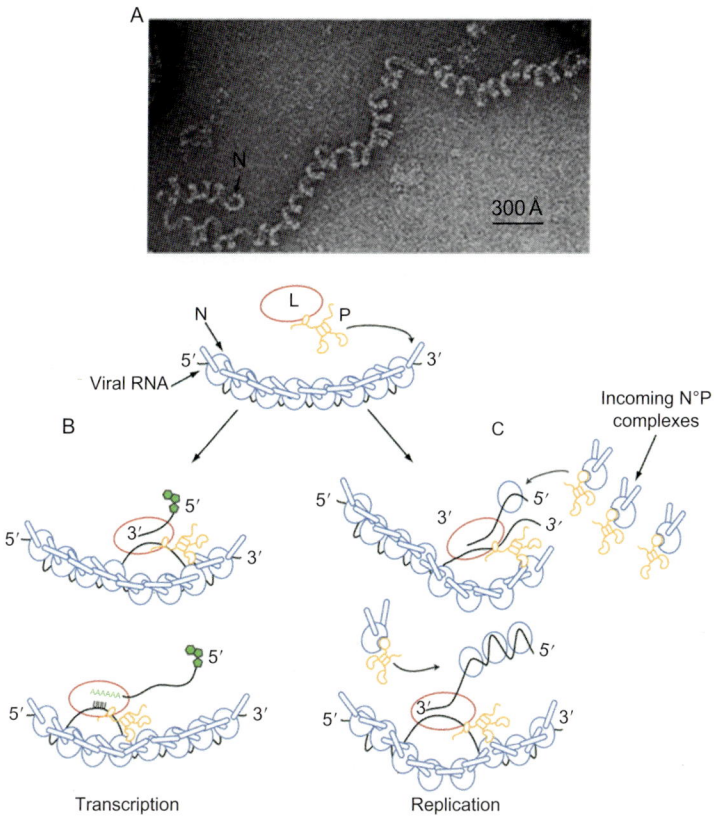

Figure 4, Aurélie A. V. Albertini *et al.*   (See Page 7 of this Volume)

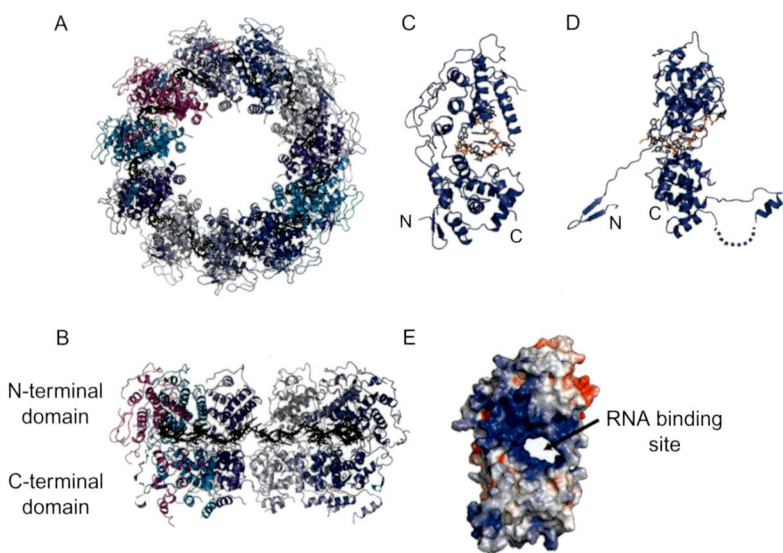

A

B
N-terminal
domain

C-terminal
domain

C

N   C

D

N   C

E

RNA binding
site

Figure 5, Aurélie A. V. Albertini *et al.* (See Page 11 of this Volume)

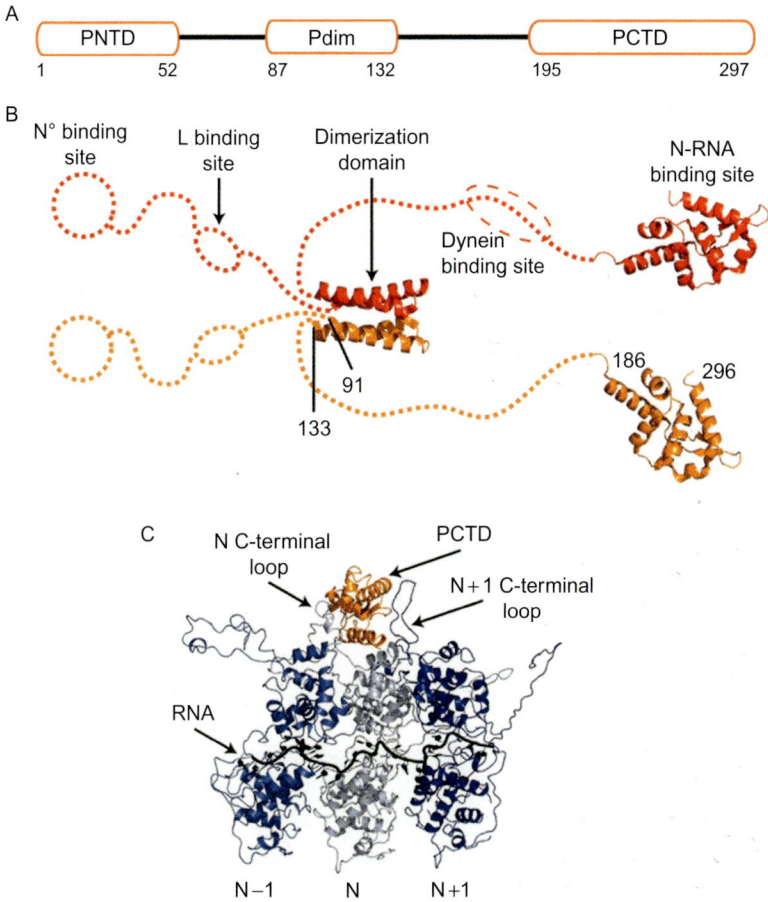

A

PNTD   Pdim   PCTD

1   52   87   132   195   297

B

N° binding site   L binding site   Dimerization domain   N-RNA binding site

Dynein binding site

91

133

186   296

C

N C-terminal loop   PCTD   N+1 C-terminal loop

RNA

N−1   N   N+1

Figure 6, Aurélie A. V. Albertini *et al.* (See Page 12 of this Volume)

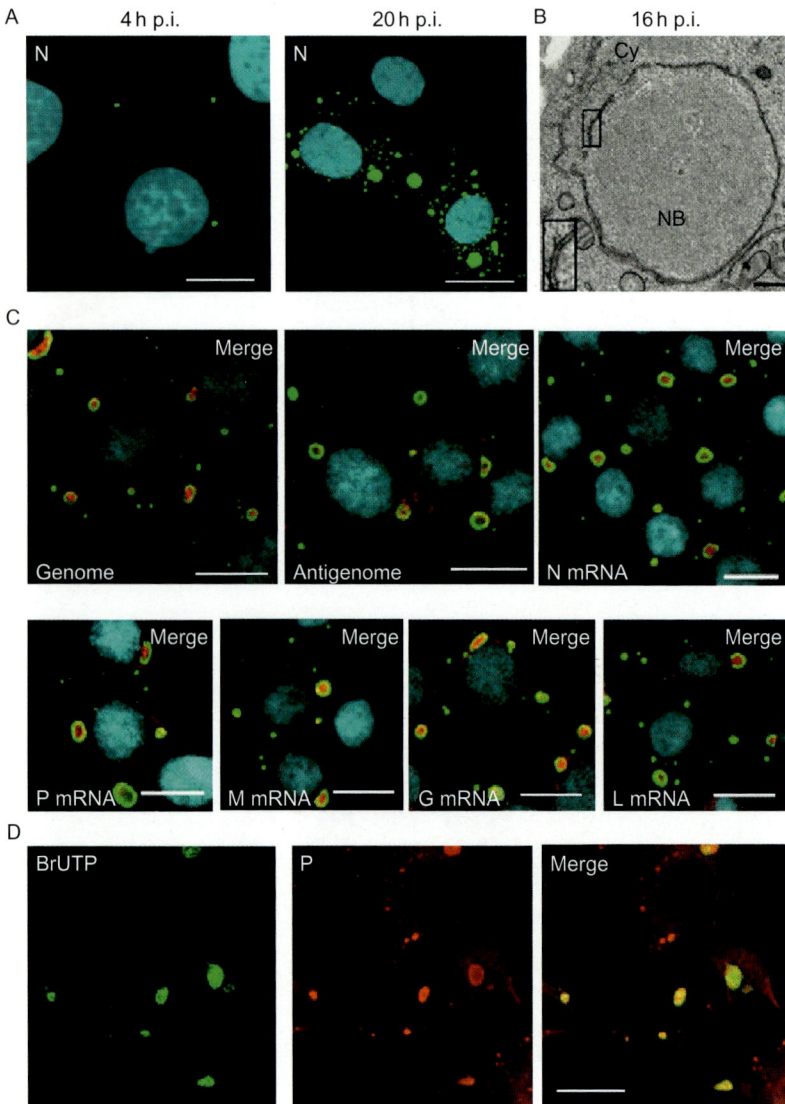

A   4 h p.i.   20 h p.i.   B   16 h p.i.

C

D

Figure 8, Aurélie A. V. Albertini *et al.* (See Page 17 of this Volume)

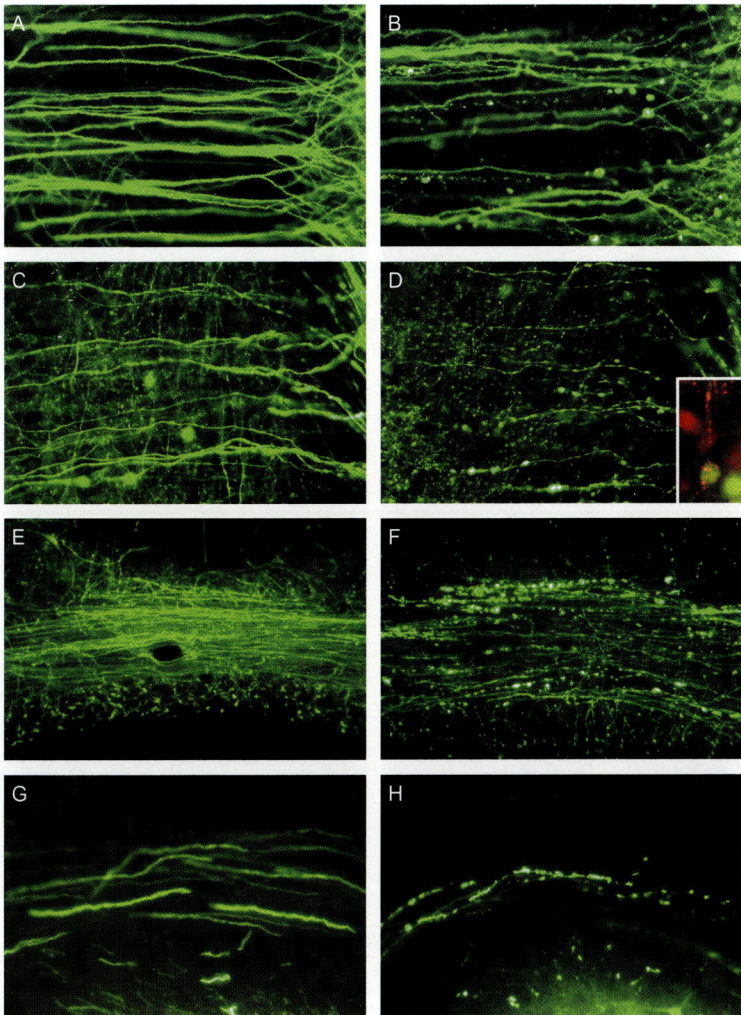

Figure 1, Alan C. Jackson *et al.* (See Page 130 of this Volume)

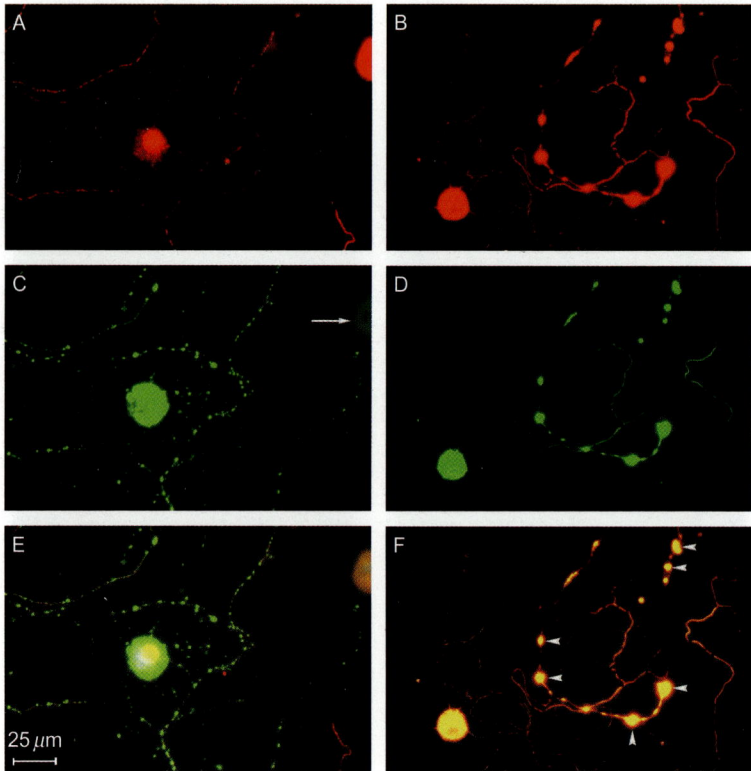

Figure 2, Alan C. Jackson *et al.* (See Page 132 of this Volume)

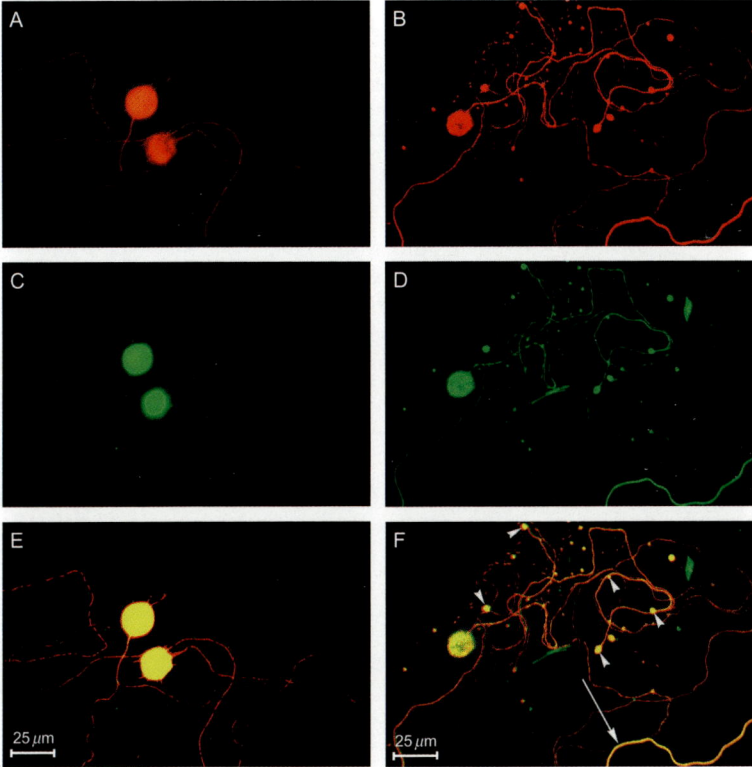

Figure 3, Alan C. Jackson *et al.* (See Page 134 of this Volume)

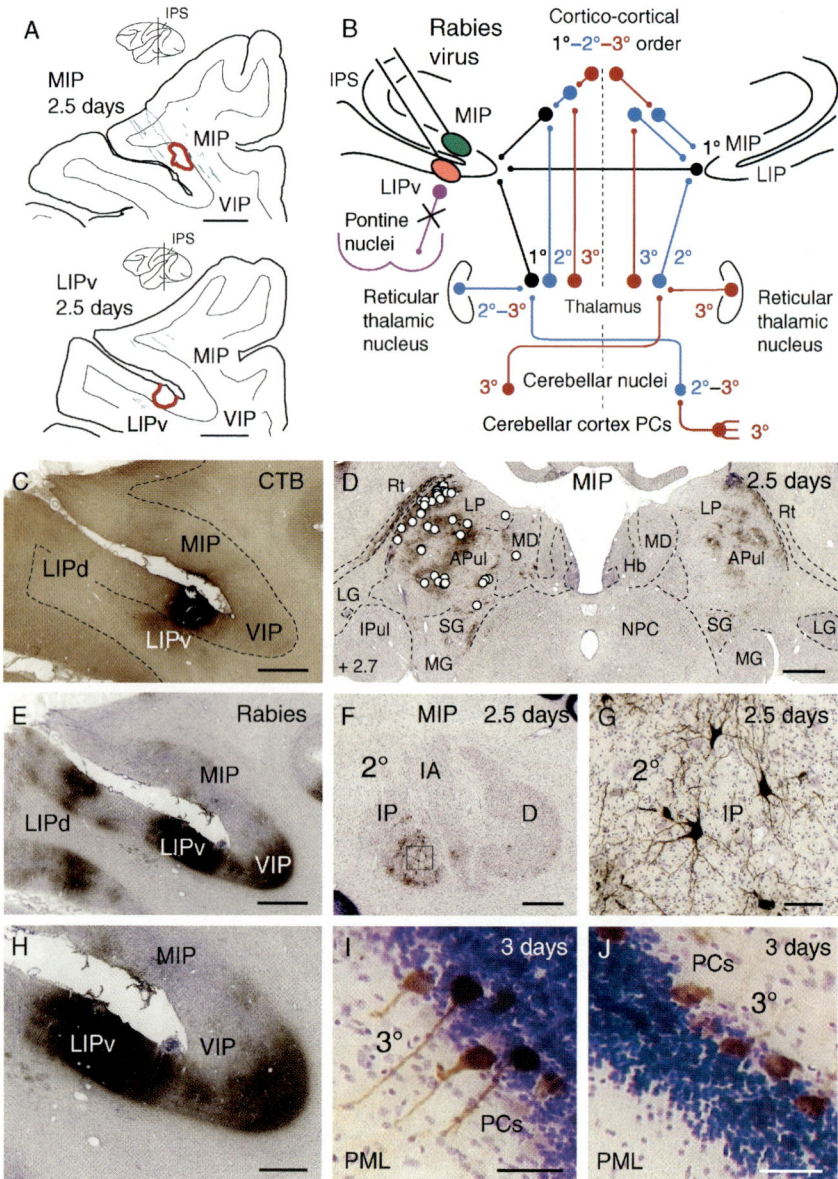

Figure 6, Gabriella Ugolini   (See Page 178 of this Volume)

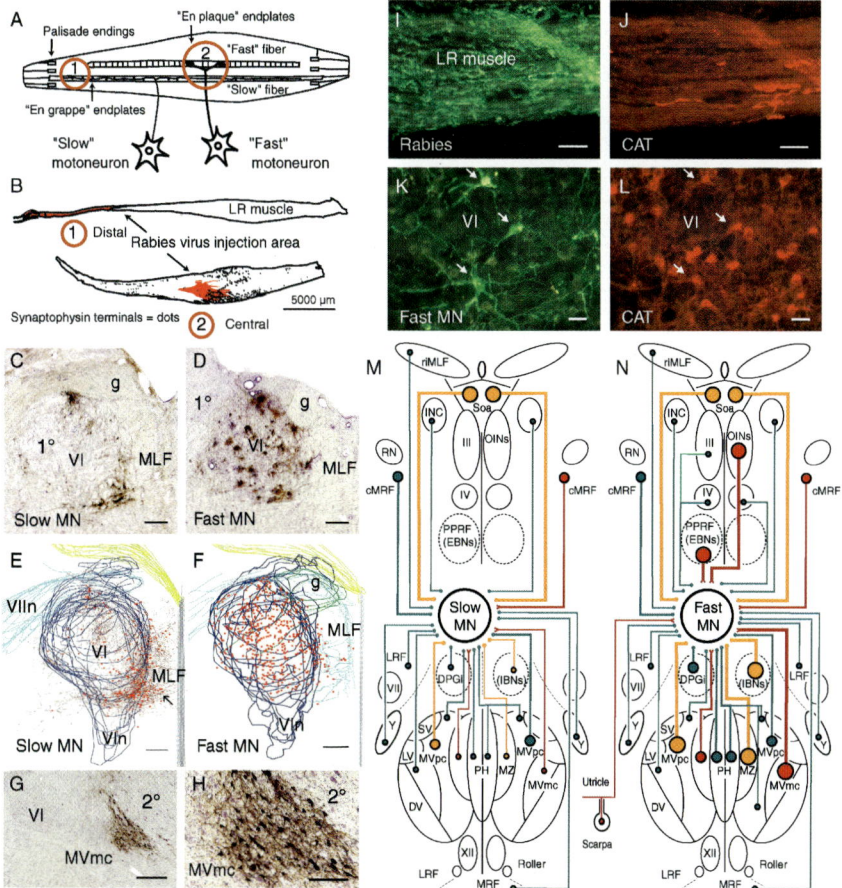

Figure 7, Gabriella Ugolini (See Page 181 of this Volume)

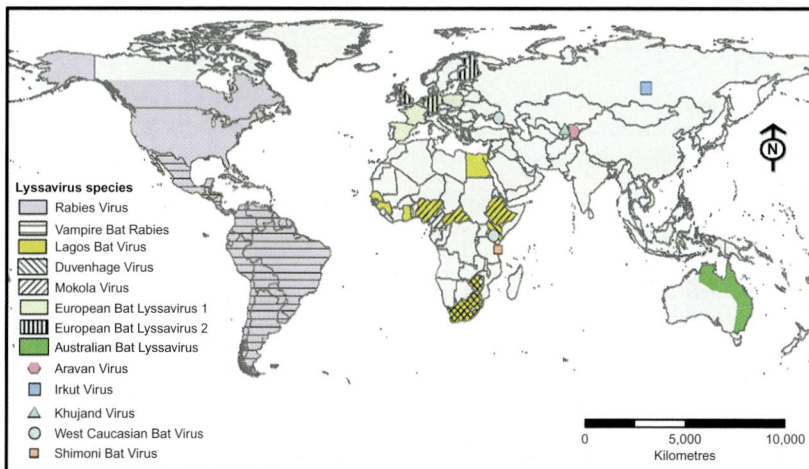

Figure 1, Ashley C. Banyard et al. (See Page 242 of this Volume)

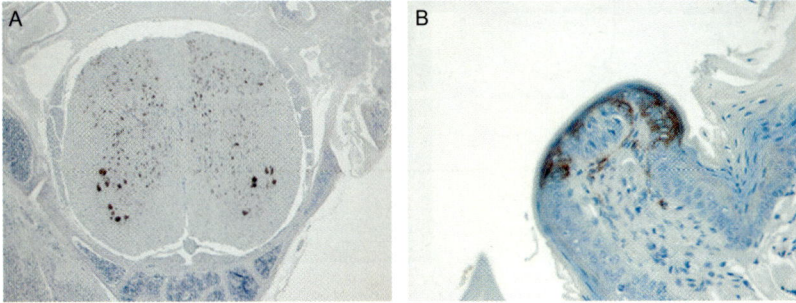

Figure 3, Ashley C. Banyard et al. (See Page 246 of this Volume)

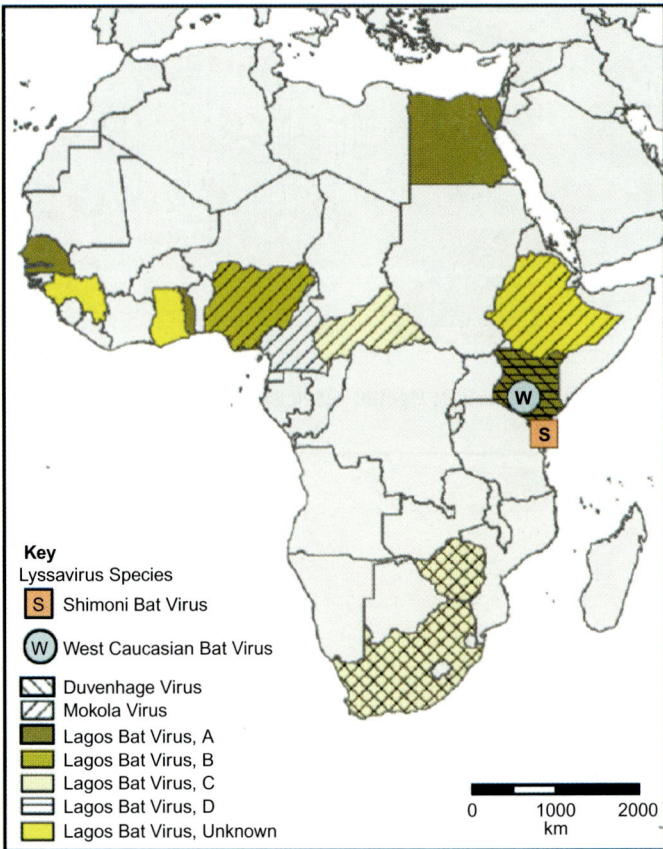

Key

Lyssavirus Species

| S | Shimoni Bat Virus |

| W | West Caucasian Bat Virus |

	Duvenhage Virus
	Mokola Virus
	Lagos Bat Virus, A
	Lagos Bat Virus, B
	Lagos Bat Virus, C
	Lagos Bat Virus, D
	Lagos Bat Virus, Unknown

0   1000   2000
km

Figure 5, Ashley C. Banyard et al. (See Page 255 of this Volume)

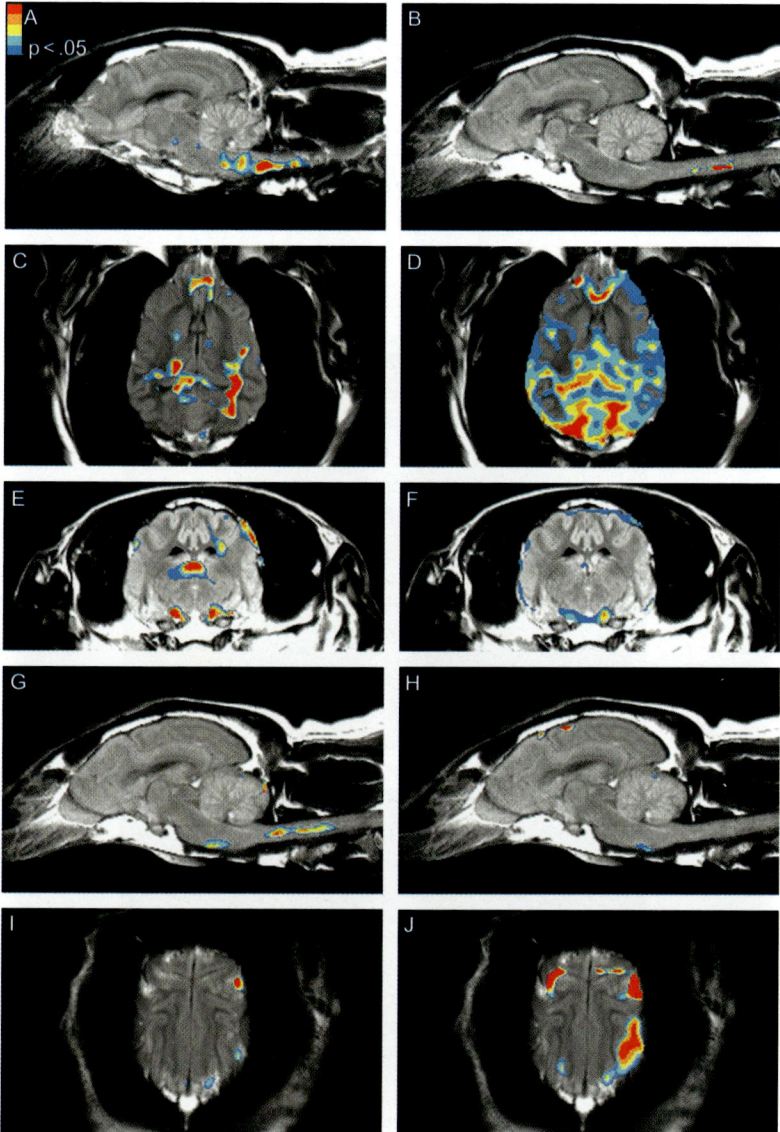

Figure 9, Jiraporn Laothamatas et al. (See Page 323 of this Volume)

A

miR133a | uGUCGACCAACUUCCCCUGguu
||||¦| ||| ||||||||
Nucleoprotein | gCAGTTCTTTG-AGGGGACatg

B

miR133a | ugUCGACCAACUUCCCCUGGUU
|||||| | |||||||||
Glycoprotein | caATCGGGCTCCA-GGGACCAA

C   Control

hsa-miR-133a mimic

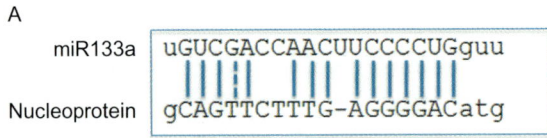

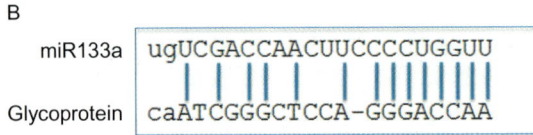

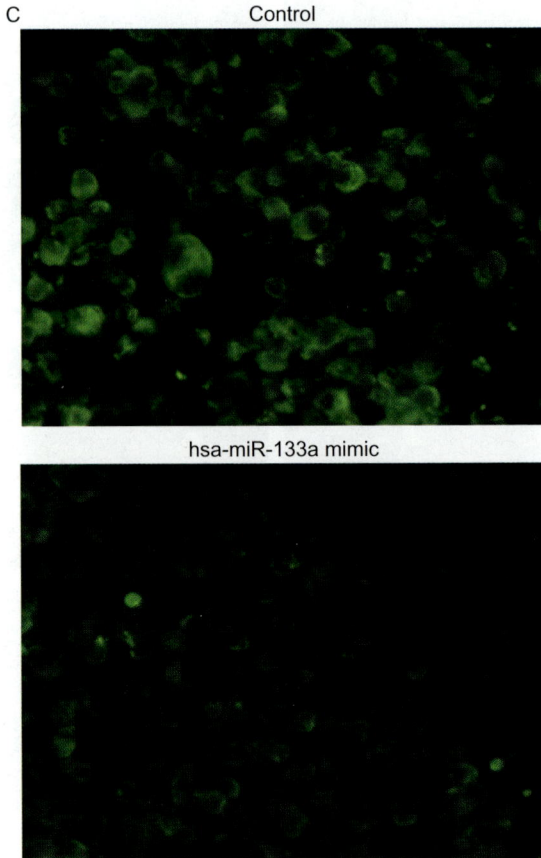

Figure 3, Nipan Israsena *et al.* (See Page 336 of this Volume)

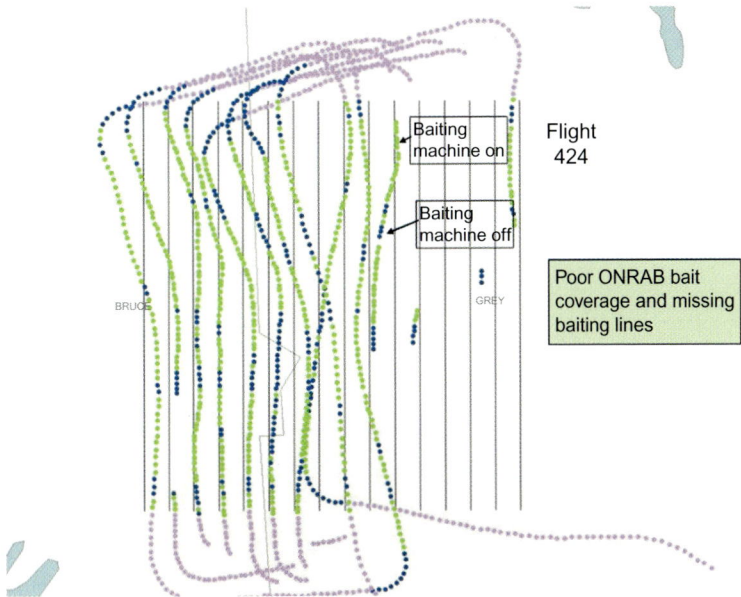

Figure 5, Rick Rosatte (See Page 404 of this Volume)

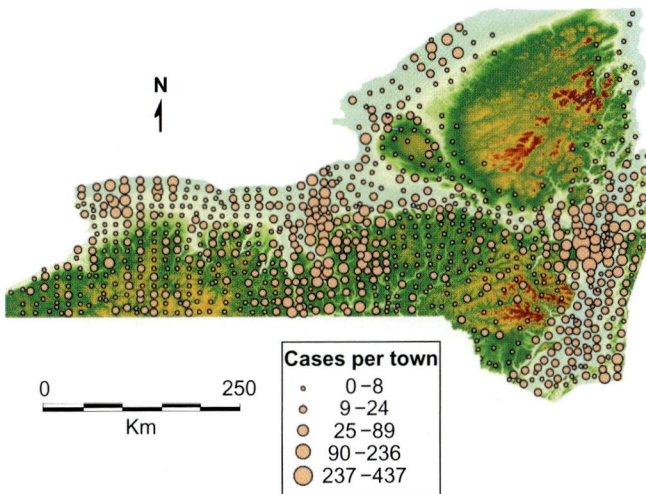

Figure 1, Erin E. Rees *et al.* (See Page 428 of this Volume)

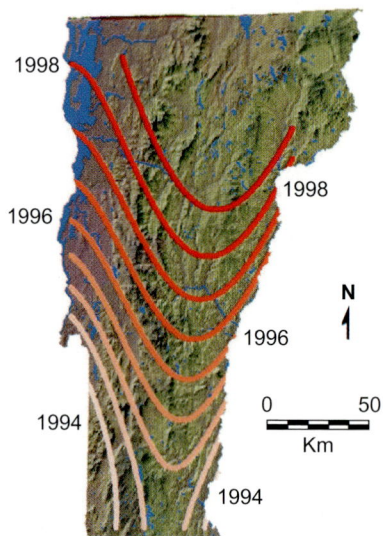

Figure 2, Erin E. Rees *et al.* (See Page 429 of this Volume)

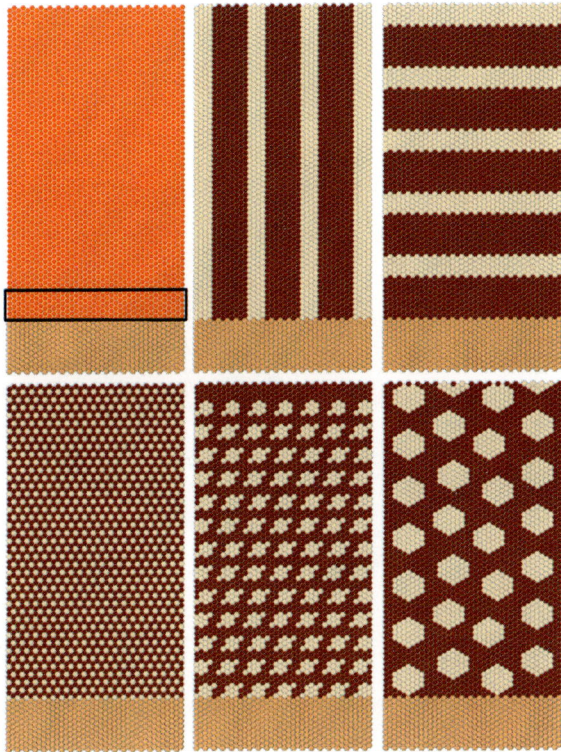

K

20 : ▨ 60 : ▨ 87 : ▨ 120 : ▨

Figure 3, Erin E. Rees *et al.*   (See Page 434 of this Volume)

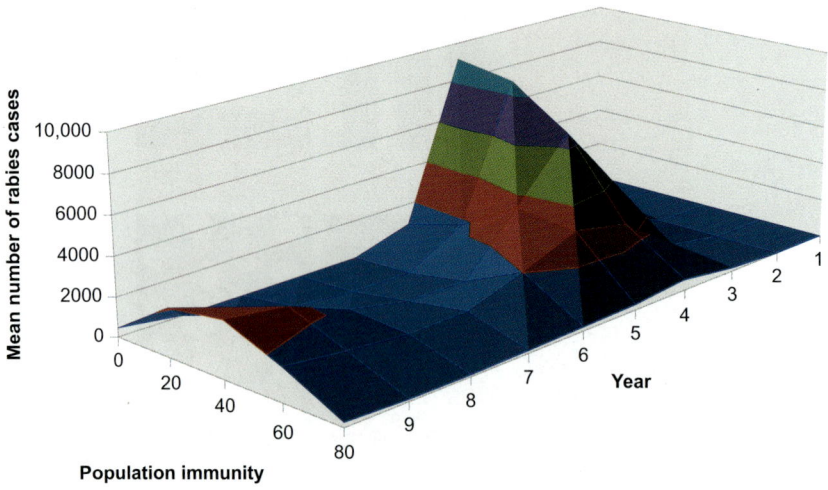

Figure 9, Erin E. Rees *et al.* (See Page 443 of this Volume)

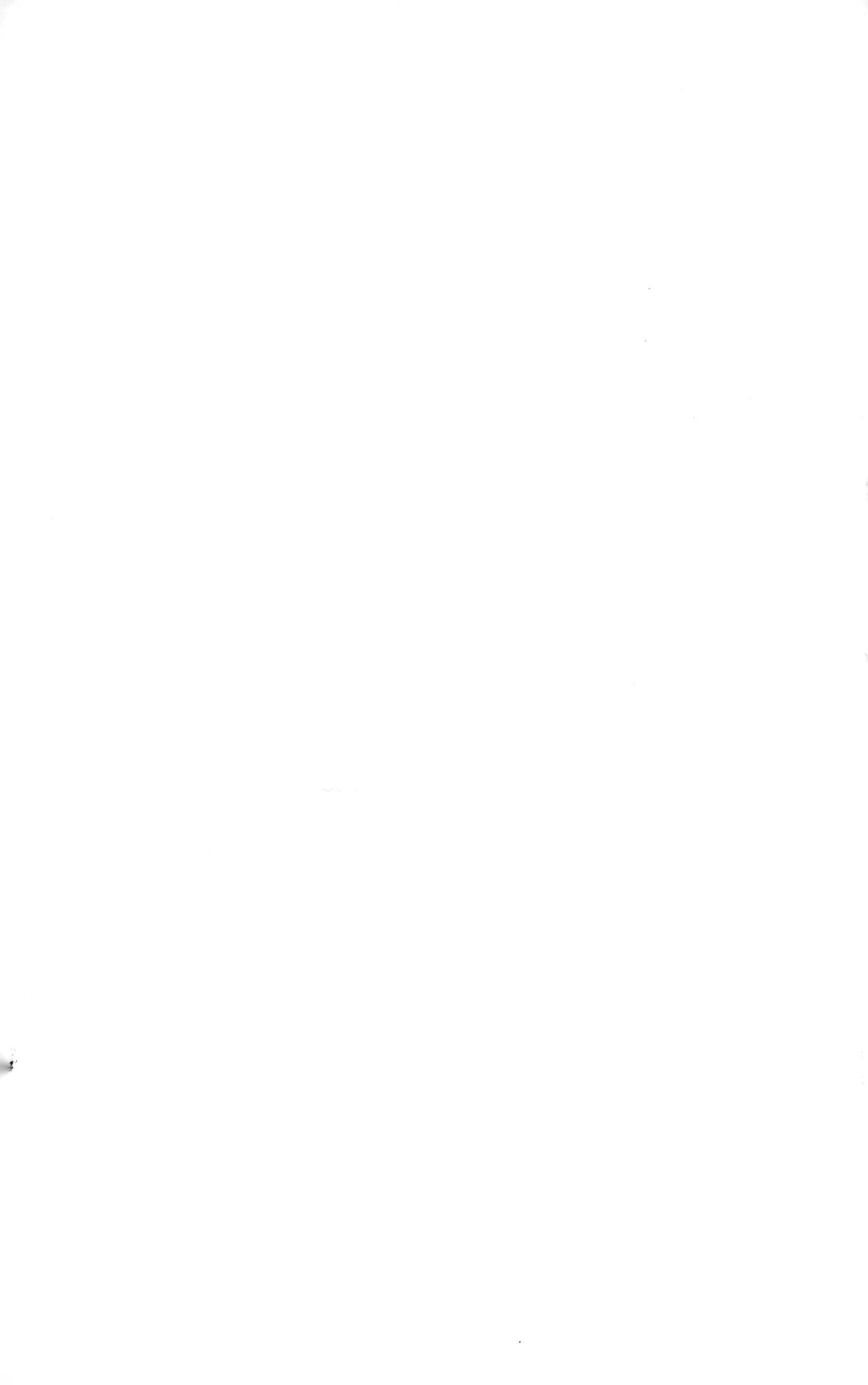